Textbook of Cardiac Critical Care

Editor-in-Chief:

Poonam Malhotra Kapoor, MD, DNB, MNAMS, FIACTA, FTEE, FISCU
Professor
Department of Cardiac Anaesthesia and Critical Care
Cardiac Thoracic Center
All India Institute of Medical Sciences (AIIMS)
New Delhi, India;
President
Indian Association of Cardiovascular and Thoracic Anaesthesiologists (IACTA);
The Society of Cardiac Anaesthesia
Delhi and National Capital Region;
Southwest Asia and Africa Chapter
Extracorporeal Life Support Organization (SWAAC ELSO)

Co-Editors:

H. K. Chopra, MD
Chief Consultant
Department of Cardiology
Moolchand Hospital
New Delhi, India

K. K. Kapur, MD, DM
Senior Cardiologist
Department of Cardiology
Apollo Hospitals
Sarita Vihar, New Delhi, India

Muralidhar Kanchi, MD
Director (Academic), Senior Consultant, and Professor
Department of Anaesthesia and Intensive Care
Narayana Hrudayalaya Hospitals
Bangalore, Karnataka, India;
Professor
Department of International Health
University of Minnesota
Minnesota, USA

Naman Shastri, MD, FASE, FEACVI, FIACTA
Chief Consultant
Cardiac Anaesthesiologist and Intensivist
Epic Hospital
Ahmedabad, Gujarat, India

Thieme
Delhi • Stuttgart • New York • Rio de Janeiro

Publishing Director: Ritu Sharma
Senior Development Editor: Dr. Gurvinder Kaur
Director-Editorial Services: Rachna Sinha
Project Manager: Madhumita Dey
Managing Director & CEO: Ajit Kohli

Thieme Medical and Scientific Publishers Private Limited.
A - 12, Second Floor, Sector - 2, Noida - 201 301,
Uttar Pradesh, India, +911204556600
Email: customerservice@thieme.in
www.thieme.in

Cover design: © Thieme
Cover image source: © peterschreiber.media/stock.adobe.com
Typesetting by RECTO Graphics, India

Printed in India

5 4 3 2 1

ISBN: 978-93-92819-10-0
Also available as an e-book:
eISBN (PDF): 978-93-95390-18-7
eISBN (epub): 978-93-95390-19-4

Important note: Medicine is an ever-changing science undergoing continual development. Research and clinical experience are continually expanding our knowledge, in particular, our knowledge of proper treatment and drug therapy. Insofar as this book mentions any dosage or application, readers may rest assured that the authors, editors, and publishers have made every effort to ensure that such references are in accordance with **the state of knowledge at the time of production of the book**.

Nevertheless, this does not involve, imply, or express any guarantee or responsibility on the part of the publishers in respect to any dosage instructions and forms of applications stated in the book. **Every user is requested to examine carefully** the manufacturers' leaflets accompanying each drug and to check, if necessary, in consultation with a physician or specialist, whether the dosage schedules mentioned therein or the contraindications stated by the manufacturers differ from the statements made in the present book. Such examination is particularly important with drugs that are either rarely used or have been newly released in the market. Every dosage schedule or every form of application used is entirely at the user's own risk and responsibility. The authors and publishers request every user to report to the publishers any discrepancies or inaccuracies noticed. If errors in this work are found after publication, errata will be posted at www.thieme.com on the product description page.

Some of the product names, patents, and registered designs referred to in this book are in fact registered trademarks or proprietary names even though specific reference to this fact is not always made in the text. Therefore, the appearance of a name without designation as proprietary is not to be construed as a representation by the publisher that it is in the public domain.

Thieme addresses people of all gender identities equally. We encourage our authors to use gender-neutral or gender-equal expressions wherever the context allows.

In fond memory of my loving father

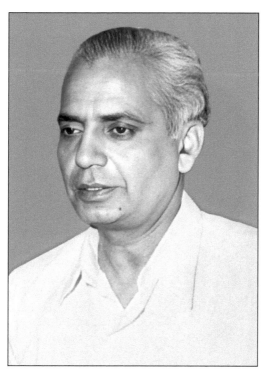

Dr K. K. Malhotra
(4.7.1929–4.1.2011)

My mentor, guide, who even after 12 years of his demise continues to inspire and encourage me, each moment.
An extraordinary physician and human being with boundless affection, witty, hardworking, and godly qualities.

Dedicated to

IACTA
(Indian Association of Cardiovascular Thoracic Anaesthesiologists),
whom I served and gained from for the last consecutive 25 years, without a break.

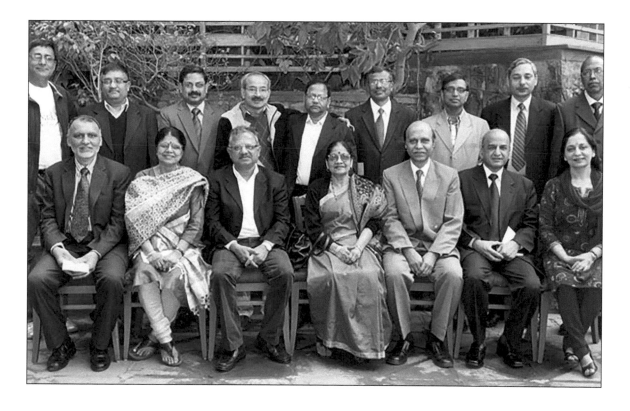

Contents

Section 1: Cardiac Critical Care

Contents

Contents

Foreword

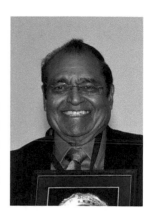

Cardiac critical care medicine is a rapidly expanding field. Recent progress in medical science and technology has led to a significant increase in the number of patients with life-threatening conditions who can benefit from increasingly wide-ranging monitoring and care, especially in the cardiac critical care intensive care unit (ICU). Significant resources are currently invested in the complex effort to discover and develop new approaches dedicated to improving the progress of these patients and to ensure a fast clinical and functional recovery.

The emerging technology overlaps in different fields such as echocardiography, use of extracorporeal membrane devices, ventricular assist devices, hemodynamic monitoring, and pain and sepsis management in the ICU. The merger of so many diverse disciplines has required a vision of forward thinking and innovation, thus replacing the conventional way of management of critical care patients to achieve new dimensions in the field. Cardiac critical care is thus a convergence of different specialties brought together by overlapping emerging technologies, imaging and diagnostics being the chief common point.

Textbook of Cardiac Critical Care is written primarily for cardiology, cardiac anesthesia, cardiac surgery, and all cardiac critical care students, junior faculties, and MBBS students. It is the aim of all contributors that the readers enjoy the text and have a take-home message from it. This book has accomplished the same in totality.

I wish the editors and authors of the book all success in their enriching endeavor.

Navin C. Nanda, MD, DSc (Med) (Hon), DSc (Hon), FACC, FAHA, FISCU(D)
Distinguished Professor
Department of Medicine and Cardiovascular Disease
University of Alabama
Birmingham, Alabama, USA

Foreword

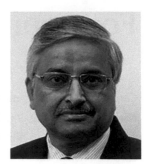

Textbook of Cardiac Critical Care has been passionately written by authors who despite being busy clinicians carry the enthusiasm of being dedicated academicians as well. The motivation behind this book is to disseminate quality clinical information for budding aspirants and young talents in the specialization of critical care, anesthesia, cardiology, and pulmonology.

I must congratulate Dr Poonam Malhotra Kapoor for being at the forefront of this project. Her drive and enthusiasm have been an inspiration not only for her co-authors but also for several other practising clinicians who aspire to be as good in research and academics. This book coming from a prestigious department of All India Institute of Medical Sciences (AIIMS), New Delhi adds another feather in the cap of the institute's academic division and goes to length to emphasize that AIIMS New Delhi has and will always lead the way in bringing out the best clinical and academic information for students, researchers, and clinicians. The institute's student, Dr. Sunny Duttagupta, being involved in developing the project with Thieme Publishers, adds more to the fact that AIIMS, New Delhi contributes toward the growth and development of science, medical research, and clinical publishing in a multidimensional way and brings out professionals who enthusiastically contributes toward dissemination of quality clinical information, taking care of emerging technologies and best practices.

I congratulate Thieme Medical Publishers, India, for collaborating with the authors for bringing out this book which shall set an unprecedented example in education and enlightenment of postgraduate students, researchers, and clinicians in management of critical care patients with a holistic approach.

Randeep Guleria, MD, DM
Former Director and Professor
All India Institute of Medical Sciences
New Delhi, India;
Chairman
Institute of Internal Medicine and Respiratory and Sleep Medicine;
Director
Medanta Medical School
Medanta—The Medicity
Gurgaon, Haryana, India

Foreword

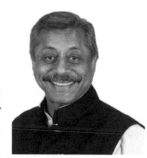

This meticulously written book, *Textbook of Cardiac Critical Care*, puts forward an urgent concept where different clinical specialties need to come together to bring out innovative modalities of clinical practices for positive outcome in treating critical patients. The book centrally addresses how to manage patients under various challenging situations, which makes it an engaging text to read along. The book is bound to engage clinicians and researchers from the field of critical care management as well as from other specialties. This textbook will serve as a stepping stone towards a structured training course in this field, which till date is lacking and needs development. Going forward, a book like this will and should be used as a reference material for academicians and organizers to teach their students and fellows. I congratulate Dr Poonam Malhotra Kapoor and her co-authors along with the entire publishing team of Thieme India for publishing this book of esteem importance in the current and future context of critical care of patients and associated academic training.

The content shows excellent scientific rigor which both the authors and the publisher have executed in developing the book. The language and presentation have a continuous flow, and the book is easy to understand even for young clinicians, trainees, research fellows in cardiology, cardiac surgery and intensive care, anesthesia etc. who are aspiring to develop a career in this field.

Naresh Trehan, Diplomate (The American Board of Surgery, USA),
Diplomate (The American Board of Cardiothoracic Surgery, USA)
Chairman and Managing Director
Medanta—The Medicity;
Chairman
Medanta Heart Institute
Gurgaon, Haryana, India

Foreword

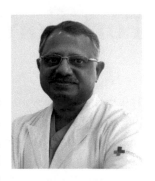

This textbook deals with extracorporeal membrane oxygenation (ECMO), which is a very important critical care subject in the 2023, besides other important topics on COVID-19, echocardiography, and pediatric intensive care. ECMO involves a huge infrastructure in the ICU and operation room, and it is difficult to know whether the institute doing ECMO has garnered all the necessary facts and reached the right standard of patients monitoring during ECMO. That is precisely where this book comes in, written by experienced ECMO physicians, who have toiled their way performing ECMO on patients in the ICU. This textbook will give the reader an opportunity to know the depth and breadth of ECMO in different case scenarios.

It is with extreme pleasure, I wish to congratulate Dr (Prof.) Poonam Malhotra Kapoor and her set of co-authors for bringing out an engaging content addressing critical care management of patients with cardiovascular anomalies, pulmonary complications etc. in both pre- and postoperative scenarios.

This textbook is, therefore, highly recommended for aspiring young clinicians who aim to contribute and serve critical care management of high-risk patients and also for clinicians who would like to get acquainted with emerging technologies and best practices in this arena.

Dr Poonam Malhotra Kapoor, as an experienced cardiac anesthesiologist in one of India's premier medical institutions, is well suited to take this onerous task of editing and writing this *Textbook of Cardiac Critical Care*, and she has done this most admirably. I highly recommend this book and I am confident that it will achieve the success it deserves.

I must congratulate Thieme India for partnering with her and her fellow co-authors for developing and publishing this engaging book for a huge target clinical audience.

Yatin Mehta, MD, MNAMS, FRCA, FAMS, FIACTA, FICCM, FTEE
Chairman
Institute of Critical Care and Anesthesiology
Medanta—The Medicity
Gurgaon, Haryana, India

Preface

Cardiac care has changed significantly over the last two decades and great progress has been made in the management of cardiac diseases. Integration of technology with clinical wisdom has led to better management of cardiac disease in hospital setting and this has resulted in overall better clinical outcomes for the patients in the long term.

In the present scenario, a lot of literature is available in the field of cardiology. However, we felt the lack of consolidated literature for management of cardiac conditions in acute critical care setting. Therefore, our goal was to create an academic resource to address the issues of critical care cardiology and accumulate the views and ideas from experts in this field. The problems we encounter in India are at times unique and offer specific challenges. Cost optimization remains a priority. Hence, this book focuses on specific issues faced by Indian physicians who manage Indian patients. We hope that you will appreciate our maiden effort in this ever-growing field of cardiac critical care and be gracious to forgive any oversight on our part. We would look forward to your comments and suggestions to improve this resource in future.

When written in Chinese, the word "crisis" is composed of two characters, one represents danger and the other opportunity. That defines the practice of critical care cardiology where a high-risk disease represents the danger. On the other hand, a good long-term outcome with minimal morbidity in most patients who tide over the acute crisis represents the opportunity.

This focused textbook is an amalgamation of ideas and views from key opinion leaders in the field of intensive care for cardiac patients. It covers many unique chapters in cardiac critical care. It mainly focuses on specific issues faced by Indian physicians who have to manage Indian patients and their unique problems.

I would like to acknowledge Dr Pranav Kapoor and Dr Rohan Kapur for their contribution in providing images throughout the book.

This book is dedicated to each and every member of IACTA—the silent, brave soldiers who form the backbone of cardiac critical care, who are unseen by the patients and administrators and yet they march forward in smaller numbers than the surgeons and cardiologists for safe patient outcomes.

I would like to express my sincere thanks to Mr Vij for granting me permission to use images from my book, *Manual Of Extracorporeal Membrane Oxygenation (ECMO) In The ICU*, published under Jaypee Publications in 2014. In case if there is a miss in crediting any figure, I would be happy to duly acknowledge the same in the subsequent editions.

Poonam Malhotra Kapoor, MD, DNB, MNAMS, FIACTA, FTEE, FISCU

About the Editors

Editor-in-Chief

Poonam Malhotra Kapoor, MD, DNB, MNAMS, FIACTA, FTEE, FISCU, is currently working as a Professor, Department of Cardiac Anaesthesia and Critical Care, Cardiac Thoracic Center, All India Institute of Medical Sciences (AIIMS), New Delhi, India. She is the President of the Indian Association of Cardiovascular and Thoracic Anaesthesiologists (IACTA) and The Society of Cardiac Anaesthesia—Delhi and National Capital Region (NCR). Dr Kapoor is the President (2022–2023) of the Southwest Asia and Africa Chapter of the Extracorporeal Life Support Organization (SWAAC ELSO). She is the Past President of ECMO Society of India and the Chairman of Academics and Founder Secretary of The Simulation Society. She is the co-founder of the IACTA Education and Research Cell and Indian College of Cardiac Anaesthesia. She is also the Editor-in-Chief of *Journal of Cardiac Critical Care* and Former Chief Editor of *Annals of Cardiac Anaesthesia*. She is also the examiner for various courses and universities such as DM, IGNOU, DNB Cardiac Anaesthesia, and Delhi University. She is an author of the bestseller books on *Manual of Extracorporeal Membrane Oxygenation (ECMO) in the ICU, Transesophageal Echocardiography of the Tricuspid and Pulmonary Valves, Transesophageal Echocardiography of Congenital Heart Diseases,* and *Review of Cardiac Anesthesia and Cardiac Critical Care with 2100 MCQs* (two editions). She has more than 310 publications in indexed journals worldwide.

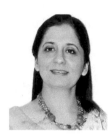

Co-Editors

H. K. Chopra, MD, is currently working as Chief Consultant, Department of Cardiology, Moolchand Hospital, New Delhi, India. He was the Chairman of National CSI Affairs from 2016 to 2018. He is the Editor-in-Chief of *ACCI-El-2018*; Hon. Editor of *Cardio Diabetes Update 2017*; Hon. Editor of *Atrial Fibrillation Update 2016*; Hon. Editor of *STEMI Update 2015*; Hon. Editor of *CSI Cardiology Update 2014*; Hon. Editor of *Heart Protection Book 2013*; Hon. Editor of *Textbook of Cardiology 2012*; and Formerly Editor of *Indian Heart Journal* and *JIAE*. He is the Chairman of CME/COP Committee; Member of Moolchand Medcity; Member of Editorial Board of *EHJ* and *ARJ*; and Co-Chairman of Health Committee, ASSOCHAM and SCOPE.

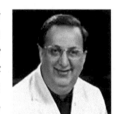

K. K. Kapur, MD, DM, is currently working as Senior Cardiologist at Apollo Hospitals, Sarita Vihar, New Delhi, India. He has several publications on echocardiography at international level. He is a member of the editorial board of many reputed journals and member of many societies in the field of cardiology. He is also recipient of innumerable awards and rewards and is a great orator of many quest lectures at national and international levels. Dr Kapur has in his merit many fellowships and achievements. He introduced fetal echocardiography and renal Doppler in 1990 for the first time in India.

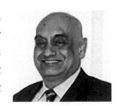

Muralidhar Kanchi, MD, is currently Director (Academic), Senior Consultant, and Professor of Anaesthesia and Intensive Care, Narayana Hrudayalaya Hospitals, Bangalore, Karnataka, India. He is also Professor of International Health at University of Minnesota, Minnesota, USA. He is member of the editorial board of many journals and member of several societies. He is the recipient of many prestigious awards for his lectures at national and international levels.

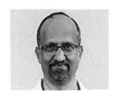

Naman Shastri, MD, FASE, FEACVI, FIACTA is currently Chief Consultant, Cardiac Anaesthesiologist and Intensivist at Epic Hospital, Ahmedabad, Gujarat, India. He is the Director of National 3D Echocardiography workshop. He is fellow of American Society of Echocardiography and European Association of Cardiovascular Imaging. He is faculty academics at U. N. Mehta Institute of Cardiology, Ahmedabad, Gujarat, India. He is among the board of reviewers of *Annals of Cardiac Anaesthesia, Indian Academy of Echocardiography, Indian Journal of Pharmacology,* and *Journal of Cardiac Critical Care.*

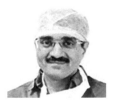

Contributors

Ajay Gandhi
Associate Director
Clinical Affairs
Werfen
Gurugram, Haryana, India

Ajmer Singh
Director
Cardiac Anaesthesia
Institute of Critical Care and Anesthesiology
Medanta—The Medicity
Gurgaon, Haryana, India

Ameya Karanjkar
Senior Resident
Department of Cardiac Anaesthesiology and Critical Care
Cardiac Thoracic Centre
All India Institute of Medical Sciences
New Delhi, India

Amita Sharma
Senior Resident
Department of Cardiac Anaesthesiology and Critical Care
Cardiac Thoracic Centre
All India Institute of Medical Sciences
New Delhi, India

Anju Grewal
Professor and Head
Department of Anaesthesiology
Dayanand Medical College and Hospital
Ludhiana, Punjab, India

Anshu Joshi
Consultant
Department of Paediatrics
Joshi Pediatrics Clinic
Chittorgarh, Rajasthan, India

Archana Malhotra Jain
Consultant (Hony)
Emergency Medicine
Health and Wellness Clinic
Pune, Maharashtra, India

Arindham Choudhary
Additional Professor
Department of Cardiac Anaesthesiology and Critical Care
Cardiac Thoracic Centre
All India Institute of Medical Sciences
New Delhi, India

Bahsa J. Khan
Senior Consultant Pulmonologist;
Lead pulmonologist—CTEPH
Narayana Institute of Cardiac Sciences
Bangalore, Karnataka, India

Chirojit Mukherjee
Head
Department of Anaesthesiology and Intensive Care
Leipzig Heart Center;
The Helios Park Clinic
Leipzig, Germany

Deepak Padmanabhan
Assistant Professor
Department of Cardiology
Sri Jayadeva Institute of Cardiovascular Sciences and Research
Bangalore, Karnataka, India

Lieutenant Colonel Devarakonda Bhargava Venkata
Associate Professor
Department of Cardiothoracic Anaesthesiology
Armed Forces Medical College
Pune, Maharashtra, India

Devi Prasad Shetty
Chairman;
Senior Consultant Cardiothoracic Surgeon;
Surgical Lead—CTEPH
Narayana Institute of Cardiac Sciences
Bangalore, Karnataka, India

Devishree Das
Senior Resident
Department of Cardiac Anaesthesiology and Critical Care
Cardiac Thoracic Centre
All India Institute of Medical Sciences
New Delhi, India

G. Srinivas
Scientist 'G' and Acting Head
Department of Biochemistry
Sree Chitra Tirunal Institute for Medical Sciences and Technology
Thiruvananthapuram, Kerala, India

Gaurav Kochhar
Medanta Institute of Anaesthesiology and Critical Care
Medanta—The Medicity
Gurgaon, Haryana, India

Gunjan Chanchlani
Fellow of Indian College of Critical Care Medicine;
Associate Editor
Critical Care Communication (ISCCM Newsletter);
AHA–BLS and ACLS Instructor;
International BASIC Course Instructor (CUHK);
Consultant, Critical Care
Mumbai, Maharashtra, India

Gurpreet Singh Wander
Professor and Head;
Chief Cardiologist;
Vice Principal;
Dayanand Medical College and Hospital
Ludhiana, Punjab, India

H. K. Chopra, MD
Chief Consultant
Department of Cardiology
Moolchand Hospital
New Delhi, India

Hema C. Nair
Locum Consultant
Department of Anaesthesia and Critical Care
Royal Papworth Hospital
Cambridge, UK

Iti Shri
Associate Professor
Department of Cardiac Anaesthesia
Atal Bihari Vajpayee Institute of Medical Sciences (ABVIMS);
Dr. Ram Manohar Lohia Hospital
New Delhi, India

Jess Jose
Resident
Department of Anaesthesiology
Atal Bihari Vajpayee Institute of Medical Sciences (ABVIMS);
Dr. Ram Manohar Lohia Hospital
New Delhi, India

Joerg Ender
Director
Department for Anesthesiology and Intensive Care Medicine
Leipzig Heart Center
Leipzig, Germany

Julius Punnen
Senior Consultant Cardiothoracic Surgeon;
Surgical Lead—Heart and Lung Transplantation and Mechanical
    Circulatory Support
Narayana Institute of Cardiac Sciences
Bangalore, Karnataka, India

Jumana Yusuf Haji
Consultant
Cardiac Critical care
Sir H. N. Reliance Foundation Hospital
Mumbai, Maharashtra, India

K. K. Kapur
Senior Cardiologist
Department of Cardiology
Apollo Hospitals
Sarita Vihar, New Delhi, India

Kanwal Kapur
Senior Consultant
Department of Cardiologist
Apollo Hospitals
New Delhi, India

Kanwal Preet Sodhi
Director and Head
Department of Critical Care
Deep Hospital
Ludhiana, Punjab, India

Kathirvel Subramaniam
Professor and Chief
Cardiothoracic Anesthesiology Division;
Director of Perioperative Echocardiography
Department of Anesthesiology and Perioperative Medicine
University of Pittsburgh
Pittsburgh, USA

Keshava Murthy
Consultant
Department of Anaesthesiologist
Narayana Hrudayalaya Hospitals
Bengaluru, Karnataka, India

Klaus Gorlinger
Senior Consultant
Department of Anaesthesiology and Intensive Care Medicine
University Hospital Essen
University Duisburg-Essen
Essen, Germany

Komal Purabiya
Senior Therapy Development Specialist—TAVI, ECMO Specialist,
    Perfusionist
India Medtronic Private Limited
Mumbai, Maharashtra, India

Kul Aggarwal
Professor of Clinical Medicine
Division of Cardiology
University of Missouri
Columbia, Missouri, USA

Manjula Sarkar
Professor
In-charge Cardiac Anaesthesia
Dr. DY Patil Medical College
Navi Mumbai, Maharashtra, India

Manoj Sahu
Professor
Department of Cardio Thoracic and Vascular Surgery
All India Institute of Medical Sciences
New Delhi, India

Minati Choudhury
Professor
Department of Cardiac Anaesthesiology and Critical Care
Cardiac Thoracic Centre
All India Institute of Medical Sciences
New Delhi, India

Mohit Prakash
Senior Resident
Department of Cardiac Anaesthesiology and Critical Care
Cardiac Thoracic Centre
All India Institute of Medical Sciences
New Delhi, India

Muralidhar Kanchi
Director (Academic), Senior Consultant, and Professor
Department of Anaesthesia and Intensive Care
Narayana Hrudayalaya Hospitals
Bangalore, Karnataka, India;
Professor
Department of International Health
University of Minnesota
Minnesota, USA

Naman Shastri
Chief Consultant
Cardiac Anaesthesiologist and Intensivist
EPIC Hospital
Ahmedabad, Gujarat, India

Naveen Garg
Senior Officer and In-charge
Non-invasive Cardiac Lab
B. K. Hospital
Faridabad, Haryana, India

Navin C. Nanda
Distinguished Professor
Department of Medicine and Cardiovascular Disease
University of Alabama
Birmingham, USA

Neeti Makhija
Professor
Department of Cardiac Anaesthesiology and Critical Care
Cardiac Thoracic Centre
All India Institute of Medical Sciences
New Delhi, India

Nisha Shetty
Clinical Application and Product Specialist
Getinge Medical India Pvt Ltd
Chennai, Tamil Nadu, India

Omer Mohammed Mujahid
Senior Resident
Department of Cardiac Anaesthesiology
Cardiac Thoracic Centre
All India Institute of Medical Sciences
New Delhi, India

P. Praveen
Senior Resident
Department of Cardiac Anaesthesiology and Critical Care
Cardiac Thoracic Centre
All India Institute of Medical Sciences
New Delhi, India

Parag Ghardhe
Professor
Department of Cardiac Anaesthesiology and Critical Care
Cardiac Thoracic Centre
All India Institute of Medical Sciences
New Delhi, India

Poonam Malhotra Kapoor
Professor
Department of Cardiac Anaesthesia and Critical Care
Cardiac Thoracic Center
All India Institute of Medical Sciences (AIIMS)
New Delhi, India;
President
Indian Association of Cardiovascular and Thoracic
    Anaesthesiologists (IACTA);
The Society of Cardiac Anaesthesia
Delhi and National Capital Region;
Southwest Asia and Africa Chapter
Extracorporeal Life Support Organization (SWAAC ELSO)

Prachee Sathe
Director
Department of Critical Care Medicine
Ruby Hall Clinic
Pune, Maharashtra, India

Pradeep Narayan
Senior Consultant
Department of Cardiac Surgery
NH Rabindranath Tagore International Institute of Cardiac Sciences
Kolkata, West Bengal, India

Prajakta Davne
Perfusionist and ECMO Specialist
Getinge Medical India Pvt Ltd
Chennai, Tamil Nadu, India

Pranav Kapoor
Junior Resident
MS Orthopaedics
Sharda University
Noida, Uttar Pradesh, India

Pranay Oza
Chief Cardiac Intensivist and ECMO Specialist
Riddhi Vinayak Critical Care and Cardiac Centre Hospital
Mumbai, Maharashtra, India

Prashant Sakhwalkar
Junior Consultant
Department of Critical Care Medicine
Ruby Hall Clinic
Pune, Maharashtra, India

Pravin Saxena
Director
Cardiac Anaesthesia
Institute of Anaesthesiology and Critical Care
Medanta—The Medicity
Gurgaon, Haryana, India

Priya Menon
Senior Consultant
Department of Critical care
Amrita Institute of Medical Science
Kochi, Kerala, India

Raghu B.
Consultant Anaesthesiologist
Narayana Hrudayalaya Health City
Narayana Hrudayalaya Hospitals
Bangalore, Karnataka, India

Rajiv Gupta
Senior Perfusionist
Department of Cardiothoracic and Vascular Surgery (CTVS)
Cardiac Thoracic Centre
All India Institute of Medical Sciences
New Delhi, India

S. Rajmohan
Senior Resident
Department of Cardiac Anaesthesiology and Critical Care
Cardiac Thoracic Centre
All India Institute of Medical Sciences
New Delhi, India

Ramesh Chand Kashav
Professor and Head
Department of Cardiac Anaesthesiology
Atal Bihari Vajpayee Institute of Medical Sciences (ABVIMS);
Dr. Ram Manohar Lohia Hospital
New Delhi, India

Randeep Guleria
Former Director and Professor
All India Institute of Medical Sciences
New Delhi, India;
Chairman
Institute of Internal Medicine and Respiratory and Sleep Medicine;
Director
Medanta Medical School
Medanta—The Medicity
Gurgaon, Haryana, India

Rashmi Singh
Senior Resident
Department of Cardiac Anaesthesiology and Critical Care
Cardiac Thoracic Centre
All India Institute of Medical Sciences
New Delhi, India

Ritu Airan
Senior Perfusionist
Department of Cardiothoracic and Vascular Surgery CTVS
Cardiac Thoracic Centre
All India Institute of Medical Sciences
New Delhi, India

Rohan Kapur
Junior Resident
Department of Critical Medicine
All India Institute of Medical Sciences
New Delhi, India

Rohan Magoon
Assistant Professor
Department of Cardiac Anaesthesiology
Atal Bihari Vajpayee Institute of Medical Sciences (ABVIMS);
Dr. Ram Manohar Lohia Hospital
New Delhi, India

Rupa Sreedhar
Professor and Head
Department of Anaesthesia
Sree Chitra Tirunal Institute for Medical Sciences and Technology
Thiruvananthapuram, Kerala, India

Russell D'Souza
Director Of Education
International Program UNESCO Chair
Bioethics University Of Haifa
Dandenong, Victoria, Australia

Sambhunath Das
Professor
Department of Cardiac Anaesthesiology and Critical Care
Cardiac Thoracic Centre
All India Institute of Medical Sciences
New Delhi, India

Sanchita Garg
Senior Resident
Department of Cardiac Anaesthesiology and Critical Care
Cardiac Thoracic Centre
All India Institute of Medical Sciences
New Delhi, India

Sandeep Chauhan
Professor and Head
Department of Cardiac Anaesthesiology and Critical Care
Cardiac Thoracic Centre
All India Institute of Medical Sciences
New Delhi, India

Sandeep Sharan
Senior Resident
Department of Cardiac Anaesthesiology and Critical Care
Cardiac Thoracic Centre
All India Institute of Medical Sciences
New Delhi, India

Sarvesh Pal Singh
Additional Professor
Department of Cardio Thoracic and Vascular Surgery
All India Institute of Medical Sciences
New Delhi, India

Saurabh Mittal
Assistant Professor
Department of Pulmonary Medicine and Sleep Disorders
All India institute of Medical Sciences
New Delhi, India

Shashank Viswanathan
Consultant
Department of Cardiac Anaesthesia
Narayana Institute of Cardiac Sciences
Bengaluru, Karnataka, India

Shivani Aggarwal
Senior Resident
Department of Cardiac Anaesthesiology and Critical Care
Cardiac Thoracic Centre
All India Institute of Medical Sciences
New Delhi, India

Sindhuja Ramarathinam
Product Manager—CA and CP
Getinge Medical India Pvt Ltd
Chennai, Tamil Nadu, India

Sonali Kore
Assistant Professor
Department of Anaesthesia
Dr. DY Patil Medical College
Navi Mumbai, Maharashtra, India

Souvik Dey
Senior Resident
Department of Cardiac Anaesthesia
Atal Bihari Vajpayee Institute of Medical Sciences (ABVIMS);
Dr. Ram Manohar Lohia Hospital
New Delhi, India

Contributors

Sukesan Subin
Associate Professor
Department of Anesthesiology
Sree Chitra Tirunal Institute for Medical Sciences and Technology
Trivandrum, Kerala India

Sumit Aggarwal
Senior Resident
Department of Cardiac Anaesthesiology and Critical Care
Cardiac Thoracic Centre
All India Institute of Medical Sciences
New Delhi, India

Suruchi Hasija
Additional Professor
Department of Cardiac Anaesthesiology and Critical Care
Cardiac Thoracic Centre
All India Institute of Medical Sciences
New Delhi, India

Tanveer Singh Kundra
Assistant Professor
Department of Anaesthesiology and Intensive Care
Government Medical College
Patiala, Punjab, India

Tarun Kumar Patra
Senior Resident
Department of Cardiac Anaesthesiology and Critical Care
Cardiac Thoracic Centre
All India Institute of Medical Sciences
New Delhi, India

Tejas Suri
Assistant Professor
Department of Pulmonary Medicine and Sleep Disorders
All India institute of Medical Sciences
New Delhi, India

Vandana Bhardwaj
Senior Resident
Department of Cardiac Anaesthesiology and Critical Care
Cardiac Thoracic Centre
All India Institute of Medical Sciences
New Delhi, India

Varun Shetty
Consultant Cardiothoracic Surgeon
Narayana Institute of Cardiac Sciences
Bangalore, Karnataka, India

Venkat Goyal
Consultant
Department of Cardiology
Riddhi Vinayak Critical Care and Cardiac Centre Hospital
Mumbai, Maharashtra, India

Vijay Hadda
Professor
Department of Pulmonary Medicine and Sleep Disorders
All India institute of Medical Sciences
New Delhi, India

Vishwas Malik
Professor
Department of Cardiac Anaesthesiology and Critical Care
Cardiac Thoracic Centre
All India Institute of Medical Sciences
New Delhi, India

Vivek Gupta
Consultant
Cardiac Anaesthesia and Critical Care
Dayanand Medical College and Hospital
Ludhiana, Punjab, India

Yatin Mehta
Chairman
Institute of Critical Care and Anesthesiology
Medanta—The Medicity
Gurgaon, Haryana, India

1

Surgical Anatomy of the Heart

Poonam Malhotra Kapoor, Neeti Makhija, Minati Choudhury,
Sandeep Chauhan, and Suruchi Hasija

Introduction

A sound knowledge of normal human heart is the basis for a proper interpretation of an echocardiographic examination. This holds good from an anatomical and physiological perspective. An in-depth knowledge of cardiac anatomy is absolutely essential for an echocardiographer to image a three-dimensional (3D) form of the cardiac structure from two-dimensional (2D) echocardiographic images and thus identify any abnormal anatomical finding. Even though 3D echocardiography has made this 3D reconstruction quite easy, the old adage that "The eyes see only what the mind knows" holds true.

Human heart is normally situated in the middle of the mediastinum as if hung inside the pericardial sac. Pericardial sac is not a single free hanging sac but in fact is made up of two different sacs adherent with each other. The outer fibrous pericardium is attached, and at many sites is continuous with the fascia surrounding the adjacent structures. It is continuous with the adventitia of great vessels superiorly. It is attached to the parietal pleura laterally, with the fascia covering the esophagus, lower part of trachea and bronchi, and the descending aorta posteriorly, completely fused to the central tendon of diaphragm inferiorly and loosely attached to the pleura, sternum, adjacent parts of ribs, and intercostal spaces anteriorly. This superior and inferior attachment of fibrous pericardium stabilizes the heart in the middle of the thoracic cavity, between the lungs.

Inner serous pericardium closely lines the fibrous pericardium but reflects onto the intrapericardial portions of the great arteries and veins to become continuous with the pericardium of the heart. The serous pericardium thus incorporates both the outer parietal layer and the inner visceral layer. The latter covers both the heart and the pericardial. These reflections onto the arteries (aorta and pulmonary artery—the arterial mesocardium) and veins (superior and inferior vena cava [SVC and IVC], and pulmonary veins—the venous mesocardium) appear as two different tubes, and this results in the formation of the two sinuses within the serous pericardial sac. The transverse sinus is between the arterial mesocardium anteriorly and the venous mesocardium posteriorly. The oblique sinus is in fact a cul-de-sac between the inverted U-shaped limbs of the venous mesocardium and lies posterior to the body of left atrium (LA) between the left and right pulmonary veins (**Fig. 1.1**). The space between the parietal and visceral portions of the serous pericardium is a potential space and has very minimal fluid between them which lubricates the continuously moving heart. Excessive amount of fluid can result in pericardial effusion and might even impair the filling of heart chambers, especially the right-sided chambers, resulting in pericardial tamponade.

Right Atrium

One of the structurally complex chambers of the heart, the right atrium (RA) lies anterior and to the right of the LA and forms the right border of the cardiac silhouette. It receives the venous blood from systemic circulation through the SVC, IVC, and the coronary sinus (CS) and empties into the right ventricle (RV) through the tricuspid valve (TV). RA is distinctly made of two parts. The smooth posterior part is the sinus venarum, which is developed from the right horn of sinus venosus. The SVC and IVC drain into this region which is continuous from the SVC inlet superiorly to the IVC inlet inferiorly. The trabeculated anterior part is the atrial appendage which is developed from the primitive atrium. This appendage encircles and overlaps the aortic root in a variable fashion. RA appendage is smooth, blunt, and has a broad base of attachment to the rest of RA unlike the LA appendage which has a hooked appearance with sharp fronds and a narrow base of attachment to the rest of LA (**Fig. 1.2**).

Externally, a variably conspicuous groove, the sulcus terminalis, runs from the SVC toward the IVC separating the sinus venarum from the atrial appendage (**Fig. 1.2**) and it corresponds to a more prominent distinctive inner ridge, the cristae terminalis. The crista terminal as shown in **Fig. 1.3** is a thick muscle ridge, which arises from the septal portion of the RA. It runs along the anterior edge of the base of the appendage and runs upward to skirt the anterior margin of

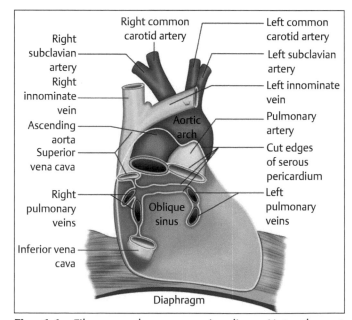

Fig. 1.1 Fibrous and serous pericardium. Note the cut edges of reflections of the serous pericardium.

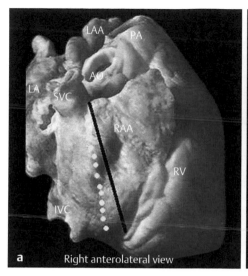

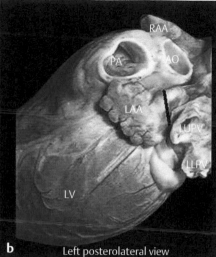

Fig. 1.2 (a, b) Morphological differences of right atrial (RA) and left atrial (LA) appendages. *Black lines* show the width of attachment of the two appendages. *Yellow dotted line* is along the sulcus terminalis. Abbreviations: AO, aorta; IVC, inferior vena cava; LA, left atrium; LAA, left atrial appendage; LLPV, left lower pulmonary vein; LUPV, left upper pulmonary vein; LV, left ventricle; PA, pulmonary artery; RAA, right atrial appendage; RV, right ventricle; SVC, superior vena cava.

the junction of SVC with RA then turns vertically down to the right margin of the IVC orifice from where it turns inwards.

The crista terminalis runs beneath the opening of CS onto the posterior annulus of the TV along the attachment of the posterior and septal leaflets. During early fetal life, this crista gives attachment to an extensive sheet of membranous valve (valve of the right sinus venosus). Cephalic portion of this membrane gets resorbed completely during fetal life itself. Caudal portions of the valve form the Eustachian valve.[1]

The IVC orifice and the Thebesian valve guard the CS orifice (**Fig. 1.3**). Incomplete resorption of this valve of right sinus venosus would result in a network of membranous and filamentous strands within the cavity of RA and is referred to as Chiari Network (**Fig. 1.4a**). Pectinate muscles originate from the cristae terminalis at right angles and extend into the appendage and are responsible for the trabeculated appearance of the inner wall of right atrial appendage (**Fig. 1.3**).

RA can be considered as a chamber with three walls, a floor, and a roof. The posterior wall is formed by the smooth portion of sinus venarum. Externally, Waterston's groove separates the posterior wall of RA from the right pulmonary veins. The septal wall runs obliquely from a right posterior to a left anterior direction. This separates the RA chamber from the LA chamber. These posteroseptal walls have many distinct anatomical landmarks. Toward the posterior-inferior part of the septum is the thinnest area of the septum—fossa ovalis (**Figs. 1.3** and **1.4b**). This is the position of the foramen ovale in fetal life. A thin flap valve almost completely seals this fossa ovalis but in 25% of adults a probe patent opening may persist at the superior extent of the valve (**Fig. 1.3**). The margins of the fossa ovalis are thickened and the degree of their thickness depends upon the amount of fat in the interatrial groove. These margins are referred to as limbus. The superior margin known as *superior limbus* is usually more prominent than the rest and it separates the

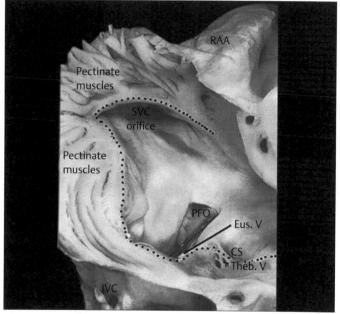

Fig. 1.3 Right atrial cavity showing the course of cristae terminalis (*black dotted line*). Note a probe exposing a patent foramen ovale (PFO). Abbreviations: CS, coronary sinus; Eus. V, eustachian valve; IVC, inferior vena cava; RAA, right atrial appendage; SVC, superior vena cava; Theb. V, Thebesian valve.

SVC from the right pulmonary veins. This corresponds to the septum secundum of fetal life. Anterior limbus corresponds to interatrial groove which runs behind the aorta.

The anterior wall of RA is formed by the trabeculated atrial appendage. Externally, the appendage appears to be blunt extension and is seen surrounding the root of aorta. Its broad base smoothly merges with the rest of RA and in fact extends down to the IVC. Internally, the appendage is trabeculated with almost parallelly arranged pectinate muscles arising at right angles from the cristae terminalis. Anterior

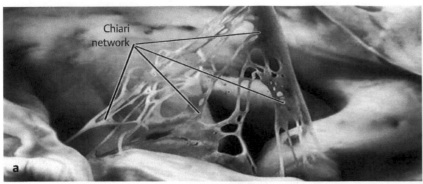

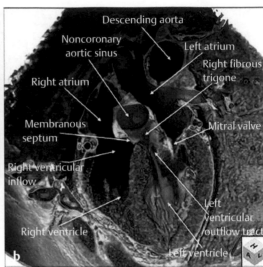

Fig. 1.4 **(a)** Specimen showing right atrial cavity and Chiari network. **(b)** The image shows the views of the heart taken from the right anterior oblique direction that produce the Valentine position, along with rotation so as to place the apex downward. The upper panel is the endocast image, while the lower panel is the virtual dissection including the walls.

and inferior to the IVC orifice this part of anterior wall where it meets the appendage shows a pouch which is called the sub-Eustachian sinus. The roof has the SVC opening into it and it curves posteriorly behind the aorta to meet the septal wall. Toward the roof, one of this pectinate muscle bands is usually more prominent and is called the septum spurium. The floor of RA has the TV opening and to the junction of the floor with the posterior wall opens the IVC.

Right Ventricle

Right ventricle (RV) propels the venous blood across the pulmonary valve which it receives from the RA through the TV. Anatomically, in a closed thorax, the RV is normally the most anterior cardiac chamber and lies directly beneath the sternum. RV lies partially inferior, anterior, and medial to RA. It lies anterior and to the right of the left ventricle (LV).

The RV is, in normal human beings, the most anterior chamber, and it lies just beneath the sternum. The RV lies anterior and to the right of the LV. The LV in a transverse section of the heart appears like an ellipsoid structure with 8- to 15-mm thick muscular walls. The RV, on the other hand, is crescent shaped with its walls thinner and measuring around 4 to 5 mm in thickness. Normally, the RV free wall curves over the interventricular septum (IVS) as if, from exterior view, piggybacking on the LV. In normal conditions the IVS bulges into the RV cavity. The IVS has more contributors to the LV than the RV, despite the fact that the IVS forms a medial border to both RV and LV. Hence, IVS appears to be predominantly belonging to LV, both anatomically and functionally. The anterior and inferior walls of the apical and central portions of RV cavity have numerous muscle bundles called trabeculae carneae which often form ridges along the inner surface of the walls or cross from one wall to the other. The moderator band is a prominent and constant

| Box 1.1 | Composition of inner LV and RV wall anatomy |

- Inlet
- Inflow AV valve
- Valve apparatus
- Trabecular body
- Outflow tract
- Outflow valve

Abbreviations: AV, atrioventricular; LV, left ventricle; RV, right ventricle.

muscle bundle which crosses the RV cavity from the lower part of IVS to the anterior wall of RV, where it joins the anterior papillary muscle. The right bundle branch traverses through the moderator band from the IVS to the RV free wall, especially the base of anterior papillary muscle of the TV.

The RV and LV have basically the same pattern of composition, as listed in **Box 1.1**.

The RV can be described functionally and anatomically as having an inflow tract, an outflow tract, and an apically situated trabecular body. The inflow tract consists of the TV as well as trabecular of the anterior and inferior walls of the RV outflow tract. As shown in **Figs. 1.5** and **1.6**, it is important to note that the RV inflow and the RV long-axis outflow both lie at an angle of 60 degrees to each other.

RV is smooth-walled and often referred to as the infundibulum or conus arteriosus. It forms the superior portion of the RV and is separated from the inflow tract by a distinct muscular ridge known as the *crista supraventricularis*. The outflow tract of the RV is also called the *conus arteriosus or the infundibulum*. It is smooth walled and it is separated from the RV inflow by a muscle ridge called the *crista supraventricularis*. This ridge moves over the anterior leaflet of the TV and attaches to the septal wall over its medial aspect and then as shown in **Fig. 1.7** it joins the anterior limb of the septal band (**Fig. 1.7**). Posteriorly, the septal band continues to join with the moderator band. This distinct septal band thus has three parts: the anterior limb, a body, and the posterior limb. These three parts with the moderator band are together called the septomarginal trabeculae (**Box 1.2**).

The septomarginal band along with crista supraventricular lar forms the rough constrictor bands of the muscle that form the outflow tract of the RV.

The atrioventricular (AV) valve between the RA and the RV is called the TV. It has the largest surface area among the four valves within the human heart. In a normal adult

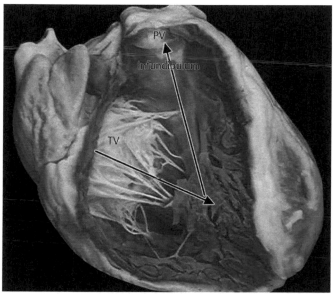

Fig. 1.5 The figure shows a front open structure of the right ventricle (RV); it also shows how the RV inflow is oriented into its outflow with the *arrows*. Abbreviations: PV, pulmonic valve; TV, tricuspid valve.

man, it has an area of 4–6 cm². The valve has a nearly vertical orientation and is aligned approximately 45 degrees to the sagittal plane so that the margins of the valve are anterosuperior, inferior, and septal, and the three cusps of TV take their name from these attachment sites. The anterosuperior and inferior leaflets are also often referred to as anterior and posterior leaflets, respectively. From a functional descriptive aspect, TV is mentioned as the TV complex, and it consists of three leaflets (anterior, posterior, and septal), the chordae tendineae, the attached papillary muscles and adjacent RV myocardium, the fibrous tricuspid annulus, and the surrounding right atrial myocardium (**Fig. 1.8**). Successful valve function depends on the integrity and coordination of these components.

The tricuspid annulus has a complex 3D structure, which differs from the more symmetric "saddle-shaped" mitral annulus. In healthy subjects TV has a nonplanar, ellipticalshaped annulus, with the posteroseptal portion being "lowest" (toward the RV apex) and the anteroseptal portion the "highest" (**Fig. 1.9**).

Septal aspect of the tricuspid annulus is interposed between the right and left trigones and because of this intertrigonal position this part of the TV annulus is relatively spared from the annular dilation. The anterior or anterosuperior leaflet (also referred to as *infundibular*) is the largest and is interposed between the AV orifice and the RV infundibulum. The posterior or inferior leaflet is the next largest cusp and is relatively more posterior in position. This posterior leaflet shows the presence of multiple scallops. The septal or medial leaflet is the smallest and is attached to the right and left fibrous trigones and the atrial and ventricular septa. These fibrous attachments make the septal leaflet and that part of the annulus relatively immobile; therefore, most

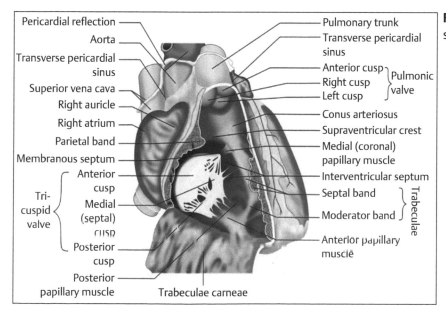

Fig. 1.6 Various structures within and surrounding the right ventricle (RV) cavity.

Pericardial reflection
Aorta
Transverse pericardial sinus
Superior vena cava
Right auricle
Right atrium
Parietal band
Membranous septum
Tricuspid valve — Anterior cusp / Medial (septal) cusp / Posterior cusp
Posterior papillary muscle
Trabeculae carneae

Pulmonary trunk
Transverse pericardial sinus
Anterior cusp / Right cusp / Left cusp — Pulmonic valve
Conus arteriosus
Supraventricular crest
Medial (coronal) papillary muscle
Interventricular septum
Septal band
Moderator band — Trabeculae
Anterior papillary muscle

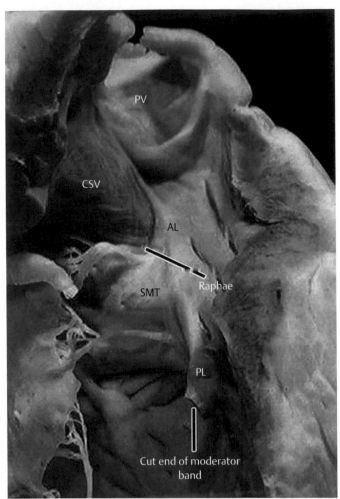

Fig. 1.7 Dissection of the right ventricle (RV) outflow tract showing the crista supraventricularis (CSV) and the septomarginal trabeculae (SMT). Note the distinct raphe between the two structures. Abbreviations: AL, anterior limb of septomarginal trabeculae; PL, posterior limb of septomarginal trabeculae; PV, pulmonary valve.

Box 1.2 Components of the septomarginal trabeculae of the right ventricle (RV) outflow tract

- The moderator band
- Septal band
  ➢ Anterior limb
  ➢ Body
  ➢ Posterior limb
- Parietal band

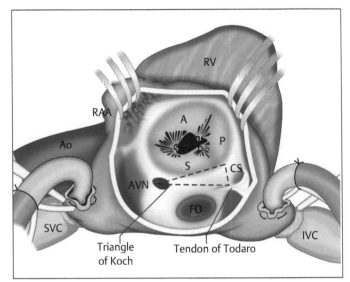

Fig. 1.8 The surgical view of the tricuspid valve (TV) from the right atrial (RA) side. Three leaflets of TV are observed: the anterior (A), posterior (P), and septal (S). Also observed, are two papillary muscle and the third rudimentary septal papillary muscle. The three main structures seen around the tricuspid valve are the AV node, the coronary sinus ostia and the todaro tendon. Abbreviations: Ao, aorta; AVN, atrioventricular node; CS, coronary sinus; FO, foramen ovale; IVC, inferior vena cava; RAA, right atrial appendage; RV, right ventricle; SVC, superior vena cava.

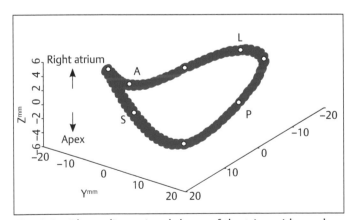

Fig. 1.9 Three-dimensional shape of the tricuspid annulus.

of the tricuspid annular descent takes place along the margins of the anterior and posterior leaflets.

The TV subvalvular apparatus consists of anterior, posterior (medial), and septal papillary muscles and their true chordae tendineae (**Fig. 1.10**). False chordae may be seen and usually connect either two papillary muscles or a papillary muscle to the ventricular wall. True chordae typically originate from the apical third of the papillary muscle but in case of the smaller septal leaflet they are seen to originate from the septal ventricular wall as well.

The anterior papillary muscle is the largest, the posterior is often bifid, trifid, or multiple, and the septal is the smallest or even at times nonexistent. The anterior papillary muscle provides chordae to the anterior leaflet only or the anterior

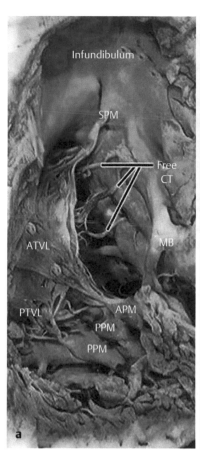

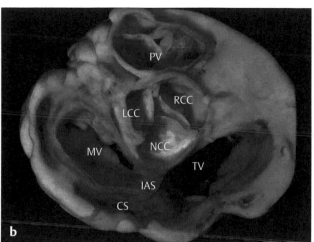

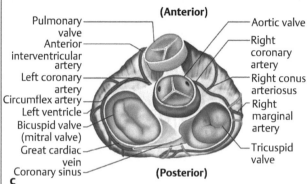

Fig. 1.10 **(a)** Dissection of right ventricle (RV) showing the tricuspid valve and subvalvular apparatus. **(b)** Cross-section through the base of a cadaveric heart showing orientation of valves and their relation. **(c)** Labeled drawing showing the orientation of heart valves and their relation to each other at the base of the heart. Abbreviations: APM, anterior papillary muscle; ATVL, anterior tricuspid valve leaflet; CS, coronary sinus; Free CT, free chordae tendineae; IAS, interatrial septum; LCC, left coronary cusp; MB, moderator band veins on the right side; MV, mitral valve; NCC, noncoronary cusp; PPM, posterior papillary muscle; PTVL, posterior tricuspid valve leaflet; PV, pulmonary valve; RCC, right coronary cusp; SPM, septal papillary muscle; TV, tricuspid valve.

and posterior leaflets. The posterior papillary muscle provides chordae to the posterior and septal leaflets; and the septal papillary provides chordae to the septal and anterior leaflets. Characteristically, the septal leaflet is also supported by chordae that arise from the ventricular septum. In addition, there may be accessory chordal attachments to the RV free wall and to the moderator band.

Pulmonic Valve

Pulmonic valve (PV) is a semilunar valve with three cusps, and it is located anterior, superior, and slightly to the left of the aortic valve. In the normal anatomical position of heart it is the most anteriorly situated valve. It is unique, in that this valve has no attachment to the fibrous skeleton of the heart which supports other three valves of a normal heart. PV is suspended at the top of the RV infundibulum and is surrounded by the infundibular muscles, separating the tunnel-shaped RV infundibulum from the pulmonary artery (**Figs. 1.5** and **1.6**). In a normal adult man it has an area of 2 to 3 cm².

Gross anatomy of the PV almost resembles the aortic valve (refer to the section on aortic valve) except that it is structurally less strong because it lies in a low pressure system. The PV has an annulus and root, similar to that of the aortic valve, from which the three cusps are suspended. Each cusp has a fibrous node of Aranti at the midpoint of the free edge as well as lunulae. The cusps or leaflets of the PV are named by their relationship to the aortic valve and are designated as the anterior or nonseptal, right and left cusps. The main difference between the PV and the aortic valve is that the cusps of the PV are supported by freestanding musculature with no direct relationship with the muscular septum, and the cusps are much thinner. None of these cusps have a fibrous continuity with the anterior leaflet of the TV unlike the aortomitral continuity. Even though the PV annulus appears to remain separate from the fibrous skeleton of the heart, it has an indirect connection with the aortic valve annulus through the tendon of infundibulum which is a part of the fibrous skeleton of the heart. This tendon runs subendocardially from the region intermediate to the right and left pulmonary valve leaflets to the region of the aortic annulus supporting the anterior aortic valve leaflet, thus providing a connection and support between the pulmonary and aortic valves.

Left Atrium

Left atrium (LA) is the most posterior chamber of the heart in normal anatomic orientation within the thorax. The LA is separated from the esophagus only by the fibrous pericardial; hence, if one gets a disease, then the other is also affected. It serves as a reservoir for oxygenated blood which drains into it from the lungs through the four pulmonary veins. It empties into the LV through the mitral valve (MV).[2]

The left atrial body has a venous component which receives the pulmonary veins, a vestibule which surrounds the mitral orifice, a blind-end appendage, and a medial wall, the interatrial septum, which it shares with the RA. The venous component and the vestibule are without obvious demarcations, but the appendage has an opening from the atrial body and this opening is called the Os (**Fig. 1.11**). As shown in **Fig. 1.11a, b** all the pulmonary veins enter the LA, posteriorly. The opening of the left-sided PVs is located more superior to those on the right side.

The transition between LA and pulmonary veins is usually smooth. Pulmonary venous drainage anatomy with four distinct ostia in the LA is present only in approximately 20 to 60% of subjects. Other common findings are the presence of a short or long common left pulmonary venous trunk in up to 75 to 80% of subjects and supernumerary pulmonary vessels.

The right and the left upper pulmonary veins project forward and upward from the hilum of the lungs to join the LA, while the right and left lower pulmonary veins project backward and downward. The right upper pulmonary vein lies just behind the SVC or RA and the left pulmonary veins are positioned between the LA appendage and descending aorta. The LA appendage Os lies in close proximity to the ostium of the left upper pulmonary vein and is separated from it by a ridge, which is in fact a fold in the atrial wall,

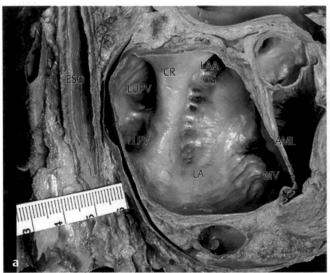

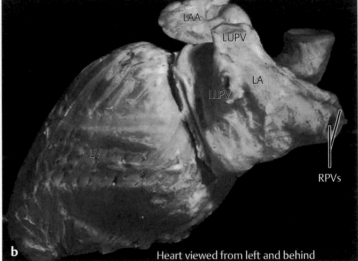

Heart viewed from left and behind

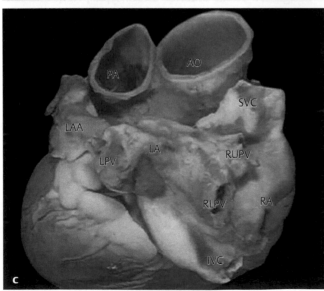

Fig. 1.11 **(a)** Sagittal section through the left atrium of a cadaver shows the proximity of the esophagus (ESO) to the posterior wall of the left atrium (LA). **(b, c)** Left atrium as viewed from the left and posterior aspect. Note the relatively superiorly placed left pulmonary veins in comparison to the right pulmonary veins (RPVs). Abbreviations: AO, aorta; AML, anterior mitral leaflet; CR, coumarin ridge; IVC, inferior vena cava; LAA OS, Os of left atrial appendage; LLPV, left lower pulmonary vein; LUPV, left upper pulmonary vein; LA, left atrium; LAA, left atrial appendage; LUPV, left upper pulmonary vein; LV, left ventricle; LPV, left pulmonary vein; MV, mitral valve; PA, pulmonary artery; RA, right atrium; RLPV, right lower pulmonary vein; RUPV, right upper pulmonary vein; SVC, superior vena cava.

and is recognized as Q-tip sign on echocardiographic imaging (**Fig. 1.11**). This ridge is often termed as *Coumadin or Warfarin ridge.* The latter is often misjudged as atrial mass or a thrombus.

Endocardial surface of the body of LA appears relatively smooth. The cavity of atrial appendage appears trabeculated by the presence of pectinate muscles and when viewed from outside it has sharp fronts and hook-shaped appearance (**Fig. 1.12**). LA wall appears uniform but shows minimal regional variations in thickness. The thickest part of the LA is superior wall, also called the LV dome. The thinnest part of the LA is the anterior wall of LA, around the aorta. It is usually the thinnest part of LA wall. The walls of the LA can be likened to a six-sided box and are described as superior wall or roof, posterior wall, posteroinferior or floor, left lateral wall, septal or medial wall, and anterior wall (**Fig. 1.11c**). The roof is formed by the tissue between the openings of the upper two pulmonary veins, and this wall continues over into the posterior surface where the lower two pulmonary veins open into LA cavity. The anterior wall lies behind the aortic root; it gets separated from each other by the transverse pericardial sinus, which lies beneath the two. MV occupies the floor. The septal surface is usually small and separates LA from RA and has the fossa ovalis in it. The left atrial surface of fossa ovalis is devoid of a rim unlike the right atrial surface (**Fig. 1.12b**).

The flap valve of foramen ovale is usually plastered down onto the anterior wall of LA and that region is characterized by a rough area on the left atrial aspect of the atrial septum and is termed *rugose septum*. When the septum is transilluminated from the RA, the fossa ovalis will be visible posterior to the rugose area (**Fig. 1.12c**).

The left atrium is wrapped by its own muscular coat, a muscular continuity between the sinus wall and the left atrial wall is common. A four-chamber echocardiography view shows that the dimensions of normal left atrial end-systolic dimensions range from 4.1 to 6.1 cm in length to 2.8 to 4.3 cm in width.

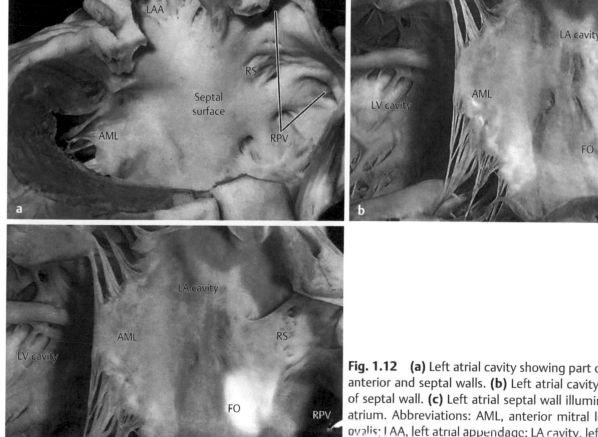

Fig. 1.12 **(a)** Left atrial cavity showing part of the roof, floor, anterior and septal walls. **(b)** Left atrial cavity showing details of septal wall. **(c)** Left atrial septal wall illuminated from right atrium. Abbreviations: AML, anterior mitral leaflet; FO, fossa ovalis; LAA, left atrial appendage; LA cavity, left atrial cavity; LV cavity, left ventricular cavity; RPV, right pulmonary veins; RS, rugose septum.

Left Ventricle

The left ventricle (LV) is a conical muscular structure with a central cavity and has a broad base and a narrow rounded apex pointing downward, anteriorly, and to the left. The LV lies anterior and superior to the RV. The LV also lies inferior, anterior, and to the left of the LA. The bulk of the diaphragmatic part of the heart is formed by the LV.

In longitudinal section, the LV chamber has an ellipsoid shape. In any transverse cross-section from the base to the apex the LV chamber appears circular. The LV chamber is surrounded by thick muscular walls measuring 8 to 15 mm in thickness. The muscles are thickest at the base of the ventricle and at the tip of the LV apex are often thin, sometimes measuring only 1 to 2 mm in thickness. The LV muscles are thickest at its base and get thinned out at the apex. Coronary arteries course along the epicardial connective tissue at varying depths. The middle part of the LV as shown in **Table 1.1** has different fiber types at the different levels of LV from subendocardium to subepicardial LV.

Unlike the RV, the left ventricle (LV) comprises three parts, namely an inlet portion, a midcavity with trabeculations and an outlet portion with an angle to each other (**Box 1.3** and **Fig. 1.13**), which has a curve gently between the inlet and outlet portion. In the LV, the inlet and outlet portions extend into the trabecular cavity portion and is separated by the anterior mitral leaflet (AML) of the MV. The septal surface of the LV is smooth as well.[1,3]

The IVS forms part of the anterior and medial wall of LV which it shares with the RV (**Fig. 1.14**). In the long axis the IVS appears triangular pointing toward the LV apex and base toward the aorta. Longitudinally, the IVS appears roughly triangular in shape with the base at the level of the aortic cusps and the pointed apex close to the LV apex (**Fig. 1.15**). IVS is muscular except for a small portion situated superiorly, just below the right coronary and the noncoronary cusps of the aortic valve, called the membranous septum. Superior portion of the membranous septum is in direct continuity with the right wall of the aortic root. The upper one-third of the septal endocardium is smooth but the remaining two-thirds are finely ridged, unlike the coarse trabeculations of RV, by the muscles of trabeculae cornea. The rest of ventricular wall is often referred to as the free wall of the LV. There are two papillary muscles forming an important part of the MV apparatus. They are the anterolateral and posteromedial papillary muscles. Their described orientation is better appreciated in the transverse short-axis cross-section of the LV (**Fig. 1.14**). The anterolateral papillary muscle (ALPM) often has a single body whereas posteromedial papillary muscle arrangement is variable. Chordae tendineae are attached to the tip and upper third of these papillary muscles. The chordate may very rarely, get muscularized and attach to the inferior aspect of the MV leaflets. The papillary muscle body may vary from long short, single, multiple to mobile or sessile. The papillary muscles generally attach to the upper third of the LV wall, with some variants in different individuals. The basal part of the papillary muscle, on imaging, shows that the base of papillary muscles generally attaches to the trabeculations of LV, rather than the LV myocardium.

Table 1.1 Muscle fibers in left ventricular (LV) wall

LV walls	Muscle fibers
Subepicardial LV wall	Oblique muscle
Middle LV wall	Circumferential LV wall
Subendocardial LV wall	Longitudinal LV wall

Box 1.3 Component structures of left ventricle (LV)

- Inlet: Mitral valve and its apparatus
- LV cavity apical trabecular zone: Comprising fine trabeculations
- Outlet zone: Support the aortic valve, which is incomplete posteriorly, and this is a part of fibrous aorta mitral continuous with the mitral valve

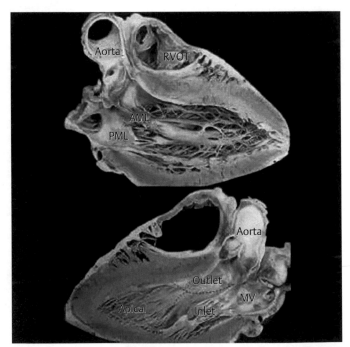

Fig. 1.13 A longitudinal cross-section of left ventricle (LV) showing the inlet and outlet and apical portions of LV. Note the absence of an infundibulum in LV and the presence of aortomitral continuity. Abbreviations: AML, anterior mitral leaflet; MV, mitral valve; PML, posterior mitral leaflet; RVOT, right ventricular outflow tract.

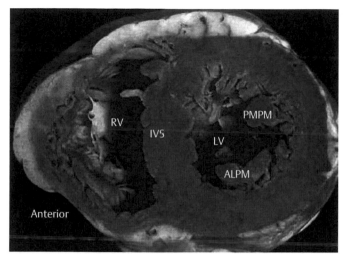

Fig. 1.14 Transverse section of the RV at the same level of the LV papillary muscles. Abbreviations: ALPM, anterolateral papillary muscle of LV; IVS, interventricular septum; LV, left ventricle; PMPM, posteromedial papillary muscle of LV; RV, right ventricle.

Mitral Valve

Mitral valve (MV) is a bicuspid valve separating the left atria (LA) from LV. If it is competent, it will only allow blood to flow from the LA to LV. It is seated completely in the fibromuscular skeleton of the heart. Grossly, MV has a valvular part and a subvalvular part. The components of the valvular part are the annulus and two leaflets. The subvalvular part consists of chordae tendineae, two papillary muscles, and part of the LV wall to which the papillary muscles are attached.[4]

Mitral Annulus

In the fibrous skeleton of the heart, there is an annulus fibrosus, which is the point where the two mitral leaflets are attached at the base of the fibrous ring. Major components of the annulus fibrosus are the two fibrous trigones (**Fig. 1.16**) which are situated close to the hinge point of the mitral leaflets—the commissures. Right fibrous trigone or the central fibrous body is situated between the tricuspid, mitral, and aortic valves. Left fibrous trigone is situated between the mitral and aortic valve toward the periphery of the fibrous skeleton, (i.e., it lies close to the left atrial appendage). This aortomitral fibrous continuity is attached near to annulus the AML of the MV, very near to the trigone. This attachment provides a rigid support to the AML. The entire AML is attached to this part of the annulus, thus occupying 40% of the total annular perimeter. This arrangement allows

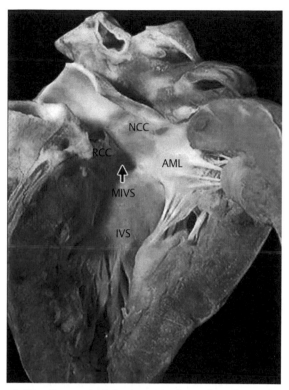

Fig. 1.15 Opened left ventricular chamber showing interventricular septum (arrow). Abbreviations: AML, anterior leaflet of mitral valve; IVS, interventricular septum (muscular); MIVS, membranous portion of interventricular septum; NCC, noncoronary cusp; RCC, right coronary cusp.

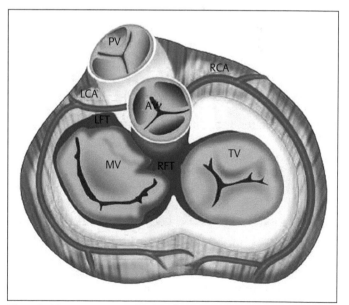

Fig. 1.16 Drawing of the base of the heart showing the fibrous skeleton of the heart. Abbreviations: AV, atrioventricular; LCA, left circumflex artery; MV, mitral valve; PV, pulmonary valve; RCA, right coronary artery; RFT, right fibrous trigone; TV, tricuspid valve.

commissural attachments to be very close to the trigones and provide rigid support to the anterior leaflet. The posterior annulus projects laterally and posteriorly from the trigones, surrounding the posterior leaflet to form the remainder of the annulus. The posterior annulus arises posterior and lateral from the trigone. It surrounds the posterior mitral leaflet (PML), thus forming remainder of the mitral annulus. The posterior annulus is weaker and thinner than the anterior annulus of the mitral leaflet. The height to width of the normal mitral annulus is 3:4. The posterior annulus is weaker around its central scallop, which gives stretch ability to the annulus.

Mitral Leaflets, Commissures and Nomenclature

The MV has two leaflets: the AMLs and PMLs. AML is also called the septal leaflet and is attached to the strongest part of the mitral annulus. It is triangular and the body of AML separates the LV inflow and LV outflow. The width (base) to free edge (length) of the AML is one-third to that of the PML. The PML is known as the mural or inferolateral leaflet. It occupies 50% of the mitral annulus; thus, its occupancy of the annulus is longer than that of AML. It has two clefts which divide the PML into lateral, middle (central), and medial scallops. The central or middle PML scallop is the largest in its surface area. The AML and the PML of the mitral valve meet at the lateral free edge, near the annulus, to form two hinge points also called commissures. There are two commissures which lie in close proximity to the fibrous trigones. Shortest distance between the commissures is anteriorly situated between the aortic valve and the MV which is occupied by the attachment of the base of the anterior leaflet and is almost a straight line. The longest distance between the commissures extends laterally and posteriorly which gives attachment to the base of the posterior leaflet and has a "C" shape. Anterolateral commissure is where the lateral scallop of the posterior leaflet joins.

The anterior leaflet lies close to the left fibrous trigone, (i.e., close to the left atrial appendage). Posteromedial commissure is where the medial scallop of the posterior leaflet joins the anterior leaflet and it lies close to the right fibrous trigone or central trigone (i.e., close to the TV).

Nomenclatures of MV: Classic anatomic nomenclature describes the three scallops of the posterior leaflet as anterolateral (lateral), middle (central), and posteromedial (medial) according to the anatomic location (**Fig. 1.17**). No division or description is made on the anterior leaflet.

Carpentier nomenclature: This is the most commonly used nomenclature and is adopted by the ASE, SCA Task force. This describes the scallops in the posterior leaflet as P1, P2, and P3, from lateral to medial, respectively; that is,

P1 corresponds to the anterolateral scallop and is close to the left atrial appendage, P2 corresponds to middle scallop, and P3 corresponds to the posteromedial scallop (**Fig. 1.18**). Here the anterior leaflet is also described as A1, A2, and A3, even though there is no anatomically discernible scalloping in the anterior leaflet. The description is in such a way that the part of anterior leaflet opposite to P1 is termed as A1 and so on.

Duran nomenclature: Here the leaflets are described according to the attachment to the papillary muscles. Parts of the MV attached to the anterior papillary muscle receives a number "1" following the description alphabet while the parts of the MV attached to the posterior papillary muscle receives a number "2" following the description alphabet. Thus, the scallops of the posterior leaflet are divided into P1, PM, and P2. P1 is closest to the left atrial appendage. PM is the middle scallop which is again arbitrarily classified as PM1 and PM2 depending upon the part of PM that is attached to the anterior or posterior papillary muscles, respectively. P2 corresponds to the medial scallop of classic anatomical nomenclature (**Fig. 1.18a**). Anterior leaflet is described as A1 and A2, the former being the part of anterior leaflet receiving chordae from the anterior papillary muscle and the latter receiving chordae from the posterior papillary muscles. The commissures are also described as C1, which is the anterolateral commissure that receives chordae from the anterior papillary muscle, and C2, which is the posteromedial commissure that receives the chordae from the posterior papillary muscle.

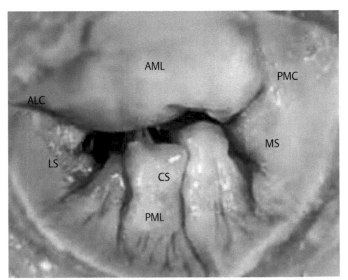

Fig. 1.17 Classic anatomical nomenclature for mitral valve leaflets in a cadaveric specimen in the surgeon's operating view. Abbreviations: ALC, anterolateral commissure; AML, anterior leaflet of mitral valve; CS, central scallop; LS, lateral scallop; MS, medial scallop; PMC, posteromedial commissure; PML, posterior leaflet of mitral valve.

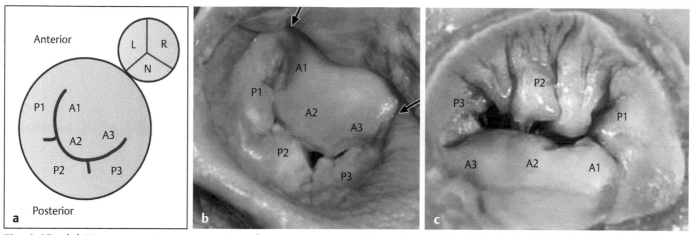

Fig. 1.18 **(a)** Diagrammatic representation of Carpentier nomenclature for mitral valve leaflets. **(b)** Carpentier nomenclature of a cadaveric mitral valve specimen in anatomical position (arrows). **(c)** Carpentier nomenclature of cadaveric mitral valve as seen from the transgastric basal short-axis view with transesophageal echocardiography (TEE).

Box 1.4 briefly outlines chordate of LV and MV as shown in **Fig. 1.19**.

Papillary Muscles

The papillary muscles originate as muscular projections from the ventricular myocardium, between the apical and middle portion of the ventricular chamber. The exact positioning of both papillary muscles may vary considerably. The anterior papillary muscle usually arises from the lateral border of the anterior wall, and the posterior papillary muscle usually originates from the medial aspect of the posterior wall where it abuts the ventricular septum. There is usually only one anterior papillary muscle with often two or three posterior papillary muscles. The volume or mass of the anterior and posterior muscle groups are usually equal. When a papillary muscle group is present, the individual muscles wrap around each other in a concave-convex fashion, allowing the whole group to act as a single unit during contraction. The base and body of the papillary muscles are anchored to the ventricular free wall by muscular or tendinous chordae known as false chords, which are believed also to serve as channels for Purkinje fibers. The tip or head of the papillary muscles taper into tendinous projections called the chordae tendineae (**Box 1.5**).

Each papillary muscle group gives off chordae tendineae in a symmetrical fashion to their respective halves of both the anterior and posterior leaflets. The blood supply to the papillary muscles is highly variable. The anterior papillary muscle is supplied by the second septal branch of the left anterior descending (LAD) artery and by a branch of the circumflex artery. The posterior papillary muscle is usually supplied from septal branches of the posterior descending

Box 1.4	Chordae arrangement in the mitral valve of LV cavity	
Chordae position	**Chordae muscle arrangement**	**Interpretation**
Chordae to AML of MV	Oblique direction (**Fig. 1.22a**) to the LV	Aids in opening and closing of the AML
Primary chordae	Attach to AML at the leaflet margin	Gives a clue of disrupted to a mitral valve prolapse
Secondary chordae	Attach to AML at the free edge (**Fig. 1.22f**): Paramedial Central strut Paracommissural chordae	Can cause mitral valve bellowing if disrupted

Each papillary muscle gives rise to single commissural chordate, which then fans out distally into five smaller chordate each, inserting at the five edges of the commissural tissue (**Fig. 1.22d**)

The posteromedial commissural chordate are usually more widely spaced and are thicker (**Fig. 1.22c**)

artery (PDA), in addition to a small branch of the circumflex artery. When the blood supply is left-dominant, the posterior papillary muscle is especially prone to ischemia. In addition to blood supply, the papillary muscles are also perfused by the diffusion of oxygen from blood in the ventricular cavity.[5]

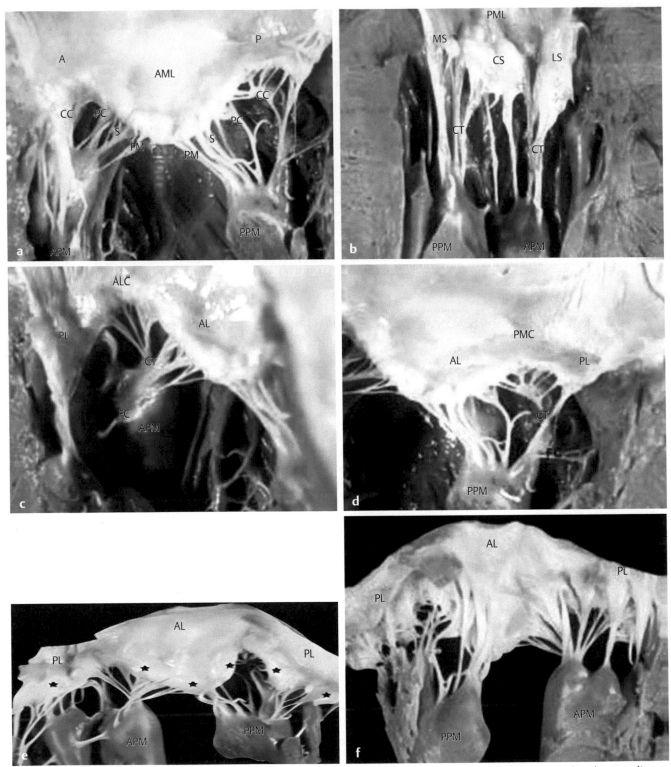

Fig. 1.19 Labeled cadaveric mitral valve specimen showing the arrangement and attachment of chordae tendineae to the leaflets. **(a)** View of the atrial surface of anterior leaflet; **(b)** atrial surface of posterior leaflet; **(c)** atrial surface of anterolateral commissure; **(d)** atrial surface of posteromedial commissure; **(e)** atrial surface view of both leaflets; **(f)** ventricular surface of both leaflets. Abbreviations: AL, anterior leaflet; ALC, anterolateral commissure; AML, anterior mitral leaflet; APM, anterior papillary muscle; CC, commissural chordae; CS, central scallop; CT, chordae tendineae; FC, false chordae; LS, lateral scallop; MS, medial scallop; PC, paracommissural chordae; PL, posterior leaflet; PM, paramedial chordae, PMC, posteromedial commissure; PML, posterior mitral leaflet; PPM, posterior papillary muscle; S, strut chordae.

Box 1.5	The papillary muscles

- Muscular projections from ventricular muscle, in between the apex and middle part of ventricle, with different origins
- Generally, one papillary muscle is anterior and two to three papillary muscles are posterior
- Both anterior and posterior papillary muscles are equal in weight and volume
- The tips of the papillary muscles taper into thinner projections known as chordate tendinae
- The whole group of papillary muscles contract together in a group
- The papillary muscle individual group gives out chordate tendinae in a symmetrical method
- Papillary muscle blood supply

Anterior papillary muscle is supplied blood by the second septal branch of the LAD and also by smaller branch of left circumflex artery	Posterior papillary muscle is supplied by septal branches of posterior descending artery and also the circumflex artery
Both papillary muscles are oxygenated in the ventricle as well	
In left dominant blood supply patients ⟷	The posterior papillary is especially prone to ischemia

Aortic Valve

Aortic valve is a semilunar valve with three symmetrical leaflets which are similar but seldom of equal size. Laterally, each leaflet is attached to the aortic root along a U-shaped line so that the upper margins remain free within the lumen of the aorta and forms a cup when it is filled with blood (**Fig. 1.20**). Three such cups when filled with blood would prevent blood from flowing from the aorta into the ventricle but would allow flow from ventricle to aorta. The lateral "U-shaped" attachment of the leaflets is in such a way that the upper parts of the three "Us" are close to each other along the circumference of the aorta at the level of sinotubular junction and the lower portions of the three "Us" are separated but forms the complete circumference of the lower end of aortic root with three triangular-shaped interleaflet areas, which in fact is a part of the left ventricular outflow tract (LVOT) (**Fig. 1.21**). The sinus of Valsalva is the dilation of the aortic root in the lateral wall of each cusp of the aortic valve. They meet each other in the lumen of aorta (i.e., the medial part of the three aortic cusps).

Diastole almost in the center of the aortic root along a line close to their free edges and when viewed from the ascending aorta will have a three-spoke star appearance which looks exactly like the Mercedes Benz sign. Three cusps of the aortic valve are named according to the coronary artery they are proximal to—right coronary cusp (RCC): close to RCA; left coronary cusp (LCC): close to LCA; and noncoronary

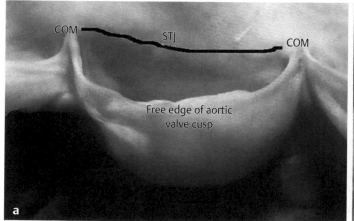

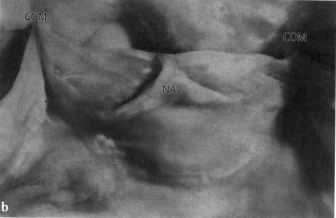

Fig. 1.20 **(a)** Anatomy of an aortic valve cusp; **(b)** aortic valve cusp in an elderly patient showing prominent nodulus arantius (NA). Abbreviations: COM, commissure; STJ, sinotubular junction.

cusp (NCC): close to interatrial septum. "Noncoronary cusp" (NCC) is not related to any coronary artery but is in close proximity to the interatrial septum and lies to the right and posterior of the three cusps. The LCC and NCC are continuous with the base of the AML. The IVS septum, near the AV valve, is next to right half of the NCC and the membranous IVS is next to the posterior part of RCC. The muscular IVS is in contact with the anterior part of RCC and LCC. The AV part of the membranous portion of IVS is adjacent to the right half of the NCC, and the interventricular part of the membranous portion of IVS is adjacent to the posterior part of the RCC. The sinotubular junction is the point where the aortic root with its valves, the ascending aorta, and all three leaflets meet each other. The region where the aortic root with its valve joins ascending aorta, which corresponds to the superior edge of the sinuses of Valsalva and also the point where upper ends of the limbs of the "U-shaped" attachment of all the leaflets meet each other is called the "sinotubular junction" (**Figs. 1.20** and **1.21**).

Anatomy of the aortic root is quite complex. Complexity arises from the semilunar pattern of the lateral attachment of the valvar leaflets. If we consider this line of attachment as the annulus then the aortic valve annulus has a crown shape (**Fig. 1.21a, b**). But most surgeons and the echocardiographers consider and measure the virtual basal ring, an imaginary ring constructed by joining together the most proximal

parts of each leaflet, as the annulus (**Fig. 1.22**). Anatomical boundary (tissue-wise) between the LV and the ascending aorta lies above this virtual basal ring and is referred to as the anatomical ventriculoaortic junction (**Fig. 1.21a, b**). The lower extent of the hemodynamic boundary between the LV and ascending aorta is at the level of the virtual basal ring where the lower ends of the "U-shaped" aortic valve leaflets are attached to the LVOT. Thus, the LVOT has a part of the aorta at the apex of the triangular interdigitations between the attachments of the leaflets, and the aortic sinuses of Valsalva have a muscular crescent of LV in their lowermost portions (**Fig. 1.21a, b** and **Fig. 1.23**).[6]

Blood Supply of the Heart

Anatomy of Coronary Artery

Human heart receives its arterial blood supply directly from the ascending aorta. The right and left coronary arteries are the only branches of the ascending aorta and arise from the right and left sinuses of Valsalva, respectively. Main arterial vessels course along the atrioventricular and interventricular grooves resembling a crown (coronary) and form a network which lies on the epicardium of the heart and thus are referred to as epicardial coronary arteries (**Fig. 1.22**).

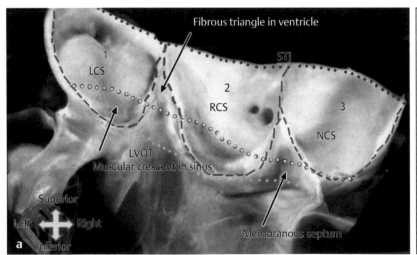
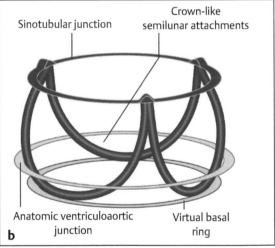

Fig. 1.21 **(a)** Cadaveric specimen of aortic root cut open through the commissure between the left and noncoronary cusps. Cusps are removed along their lateral line of attachment to the aortic wall and LVOT (*red interrupted line*). *Yellow dotted line* corresponds to the anatomic ventriculoaortic junction, *green dotted line* corresponds to the virtual basal ring, and the *blue dotted line* corresponds to the sinotubular junction (STJ). **(b)** Diagrammatic representation of aortic root. The lateral attachments of the leaflets along the annulus (*red crown shaped line*) extend from the sinotubular junction (*blue ring*) to the virtual basal ring (*green ring*). Attachments of the leaflets cross the anatomic ventriculoaortic junction (*yellow ring*). Abbreviations: LCS, left coronary sinus; LVOT, left ventricular outflow tract; NCS, noncoronary sinus; RCS, right coronary sinus.

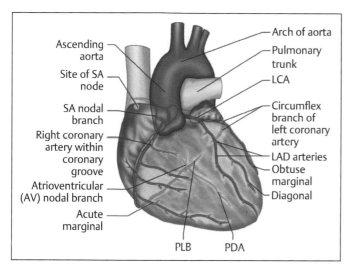

Fig. 1.22 Coronary arteries—branches and distribution. Abbreviations: LAD artery, left anterior descending artery; LCA, left coronary artery; PDA, posterior descending artery; PLB, posterolateral branch; SA, sinoatrial.

These arteries further divide into arterioles and capillaries which lie in close relation to the cardiac myocytes. Capillaries converge to form venules and epicardial veins which, in turn, drain through the CS into the RA.

Right Coronary Artery

The right coronary artery (RCA) details are given in **Box 1.6**.

The RCA courses through the anterior AV groove and travels downward toward the posterior IVS and gives off branches to supply the RV myocardium, and these branches are called "acute marginals." They supply the RV anterior wall. After it gives off the acute marginals, the RCA continues through the anterior AV groove and courses toward the diaphragmatic aspect of the heart. In a right dominant coronary circulation, which is seen in 80 to 85% cases, the RCA continues as the PDA along the posterior interventricular groove and gives off the posterolateral branch (PLB). The coronary dominance is determined, anatomically, by the coronary system which gives off the PDA and PLB branches. In a left dominant system, which is seen in 15 to 20% cases, the left circumflex artery (LCA) gives off the PLB and then continues as the PDA along the posterior interventricular groove. A left and right codominant system is a situation where the LCX gives off the PLB and the RCA continues as the PDA. The PDA has a vertical course just distal to the RCA. The AV nodal branch in patients with left dominance may also look like the PDA.

Left Coronary Artery

The LCA usually originates from the left sinus of Valsalva as the left main coronary artery (LMCA). The LMCA is normally

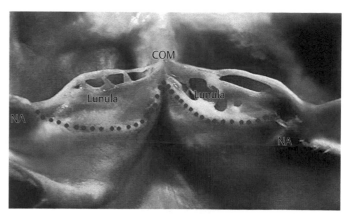

Fig. 1.23 Aortic valve cusps showing perforated lunulae. *Red dotted line* is the line of coaptation. Abbreviations: COM, commissure; NA, nodulus arantius.

Box 1.6 Anatomical features of right coronary artery (RCA)
• Arises from right sinus of Valsalva near the inferior end of the origin of LCA • Courses to right side, near pulmonary artery • Under RA passes into right AV groove • Conal artery is the first branch of RCA • Conus branch supplies RVOT and lies anteriorly • The sinoatrial artery is the other branch of RCA which supplies the SVC inflow area

Abbreviations: AV, atrioventricular; LCA, left circumflex artery; RA, right atrium; RVOT, right ventricular outflow tract; SVC, superior vena cava.

short and measures around 5 to 10 mm in length. The LMCA divides into the LAD and LCX on the left side near the pulmonary trunk. It may sometimes give a third ranch, the ramus intermedius. The LAD artery runs in the anterior interventricular sulcus, along the IVS, and gives rise to septal perforator branches which supply the anterior IVS and diagonal branches that course over the anterior wall of the LV supplying that region of the LV wall. D1, D2, D3, etc., are the diagonal branches, which arise from the proximal to distal end. The septal perforators are also likewise numbered S1, S2, S3, etc., and these are also numbered sequentially. The LCX artery runs in the left or posterior AV groove and takes a course similar to the RCA on the opposite side. The LCX artery gives off obtuse marginal (OM) branches which supply the lateral wall of the LV. These OMs are numbered sequentially from proximal to distal as OM1, OM2, OM3, etc. Further course of the LCX depends on the type of coronary dominance and has been discussed earlier. Ramus intermedius is the second branch of LMCA, after the LAD, if LMCA trifurcates. This is not an uncommon variation of LCA anatomy and here the LMCA trifurcates into LAD artery, ramus intermedius artery, and the LCX artery. Part of the LV wall supplied by this branch could be either a first diagonal territory or the first OM territory.

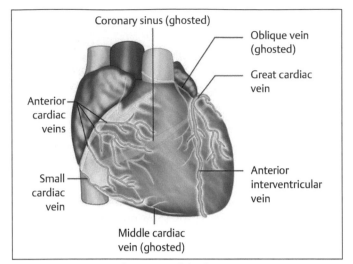

Fig. 1.24 Venous drainage of the heart—anterior view.

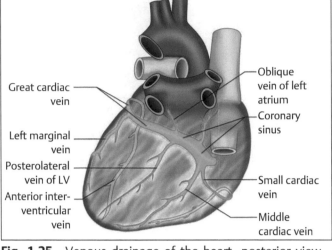

Fig. 1.25 Venous drainage of the heart—posterior view. Abbreviation: LV, left ventricle.

Venous Drainage of the Heart

The myocardium is drained by two groups of veins: the greater cardiac vein and its tributaries and the smaller cardiac veins and its tributaries or Thebesian veins. Great cardiac vein and its branches drain the anterior wall of LV and the anterior IVS. Anterior interventricular vein follows the same course as that of LAD artery in the anterior interventricular groove (**Fig. 1.24**). Closer to the base of the ventricle this vein turns left to enter the left AV groove and continues as the great cardiac vein. Other major tributaries of the great cardiac veins are the left posterior vein and the left marginal vein. This great cardiac vein joins the posterolateral vein of LV and continues as the CS (**Fig. 1.25**). Other smaller lateral veins draining the lateral walls of LV are the straight lateral vein. The most prominent vein of the greater cardiac venous system is the CS. **Box 1.7** shows the veins draining into CS. It lies in the posterior aspect of the left AV groove and receives blood from most of the myocardium and opens into the RA close to the opening of the inferior vena. The length of the CS varies from 3 to 5.5 cm and is dependent on the site of the drainage of the posterolateral vein. The valve of Vieussens is situated at this junction of the great cardiac vein and the posterolateral vein. The middle cardiac vein, also known as the posterior interventricular vein, is usually the last major tributary to join the CS close to its opening into the RA. Middle cardiac vein drains the posterior aspect of LV, inferior aspects of both ventricles, and the posterior IVS. It follows the PDA in the posterior interventricular groove and drains directly into the CS. Inferior or posterior ventricular vein drains the inferior aspect of LV and opens into the CS between the posterolateral vein and the middle cardiac vein, and it is usually mistaken for the middle cardiac vein. The CS is usually mistaken for the middle cardiac vein, because of its proximity to where the CS the drainage from the LA

myocardium is done by vein of Marshall and multiple atrial veins.[6–8]

It is the Marshal vein that is the largest trial vein which opens into the CS and courses between the left pulmonary vein and the posterior surface of the left atrial appendage. The has a embryological geneses to the left superior cava vein. When this branch remains patent after birth, it is known as the left SVC. When this vein of Marshall is completely occluded beyond the atrial level, it is known as the oblique vein of Marshall. Small cardiac veins drain the RA and portions of the posterior and posterolateral RV wall into the CS close to its opening into the RA. At its entry into the atrium the orifice of CS is guarded most often by the Thebesian valve.

Anterior aspect of the RV is drained by multiple small venous channels, the anterior cardiac veins, which drain into the RA chamber directly rather than joining the CS (**Fig. 1.24**).

The smaller cardiac venous system also known as the Thebesian venous system drains the subendocardium directly into the cavity of the cardiac chambers. The Thebesian veins are present in all four chambers of the heart, but these veins are most prominent in the right side of the heart. They help in RA drainage of the appendage and septum.

This description of the surgical anatomy of the heart is not comprehensive enough for a surgeon but it can give a fair idea to the echocardiographer regarding the normal cardiac anatomy. Slight variations in anatomy are expected in many subjects but a good understanding of the commonly encountered cardiac anatomy will help the echocardiographer to distinguish between a normal and an abnormal anatomical finding by echocardiography. In-depth knowledge of the surgical cardiac anatomy by the echocardiographer will help in better communication with the surgical team which, in turn, might translate to a better patient outcome.[9]

Conclusion

The 3D datasets of virtual dissection on patient now tells us detailed, structural anatomy of the heart, at par with a cadaveric or autopsied heart dissection. The live datasets taken in an anatomical position are attitudinally appropriate as well. This is detailed in most textbooks covering cardiac anatomy.[10-12] There are surgical normal considerations with side effects seen in ICU when anatomy is not cardiac valves can become fibrosed and calcific with age or disease, producing clinically significant stenosis requiring surgical or trans-catheter replacement. Similarly, valves may become incompetent, allowing backward flow called regurgitation, also necessitating replacement or repair.[13] Coronary arteries can become clogged with thrombus or atherosclerotic plaque, causing reduced blood supplies to cardiac muscle. This may result in angina or myocardial infarction and often requires revascularization.[14]

References

1. Ho SY. Anatomy and myoarchitecture of the left ventricular wall in normal and in disease. Eur J Echocardiogr 2009;10(8):iii3–iii7

2. Ho SY, McCarthy KP, Faletra FF. Anatomy of the left atrium for interventional echocardiography. Eur J Echocardiogr 2011;12(10):i11–i15

3. Anatomy of the heart. http://www.rjmatthewsmd.com/Definitions/anatomy_ofthe_heart.htm

4. McCarthy KP, Ring L, Rana BS. Anatomy of the mitral valve: understanding the mitral valve complex in mitral regurgitation. Eur J Echocardiogr 2010;11(10):i3–i9

5. Natale A, Raviele A. Atrial fibrillation ablation: the state of the art based on the Venice Chart International Consensus Document; Chapter 1. Anatomy of the left atrium and pulmonary veins; Hugh Calkins, Siew Y. Ho, Jose Angel Cabrera, Paolo Della Bella, Jeronimo Farre´, Josep Kautzner, Patrick Tchou

6. Habib A, Lachman N, Christensen KN, Asirvatham SJ. The anatomy of the coronary sinus venous system for the cardiac electrophysiologist. Europace 2009;11(Suppl 5):v15–v21

7. Berdajs D, Turina, M, eds. Surgical anatomy of the tricuspid valve; operative anatomy of the heart, Chapter 8.2. Springer; http://www.springer.com/medicine/surgery/book/978-3-540-69227-0

8. Kini S, Bis KG, Weaver L. Normal and variant coronary arterial and venous anatomy on high-resolution CT angiography. AJR Am J Roentgenol 2007;188(6):1665–1674

9. Mori S, Tretter JT, Spicer DE, Bolender DL, Anderson RH. What is the real cardiac anatomy? Clin Anat 2019;32(3):288–309

10. Rehman I, Rehman A. Anatomy, Thorax, Heart. In: StatPearls. Treasure Island, FL: StatPearls Publishing; January 2022

11. Spicer DE, Chowdhury UK, Anderson RH, et al. The surgical anatomy of hearts with isomeric atrial appendages—implications for surgical management. Eur J Cardiothorac Surg 2022;62(1):ezac139

12. Mill MR, Anderson RH, Cohn LH. Surgical anatomy of the heart. In: Cohn LH, Adams DH, eds. Cardiac Surgery in the Adult. 5th ed. McGraw Hill; 2017:1–30

13. Mori S, Tretter JT, Spicer DE, Bolender DL, Anderson RH. What is the real cardiac anatomy? Clin Anat. 2019;32(3):288–309

14. Rehman I, Rehman A. Anatomy, Thorax, Heart. [Updated 2022 Oct 19]. In: StatPearls [Internet]. Treasure Island (FL): StatPearls Publishing; 2022

2

Ventilator Modes in Cardiac ICU

Poonam Malhotra Kapoor, Pranay Oza, and Tarun Kumar Patra

- Introduction
- Historical Aspect
- The Cardiovascular Effects of Positive Pressure Ventilation (PPV)
- Alternative Modes to Prevent Ventilator-Induced Injury
- PRVC Mode in ARDS Prevents Barotrauma
- The Protective Lung Strategy
- When Do We Need to Start Invasive Ventilation in Cardiac ICU
- Hemodynamic Effects of Positive Pressure Ventilation (PPV) and Positive End-Expiratory Pressure (PEEP)
- Noninvasive Ventilation in Cardiac Issue
- Recruitment Maneuvers in Mechanical Ventilation

- High-Frequency Oscillatory Ventilation
- Limitations of Tidal Volume and Plateau Pressure
  - Positive End-Expiratory Pressure (PEEP)
  - Mode of Mechanical Ventilation (MV)
- Airway Pressure Release Ventilation (APRV) and a New and Important Mode of Ventilation in the Cardiac Patient
- Lung Protective Ventilation Patients with Intra-abdominal Hypertension
- Prone Ventilation
- Extracorporeal Membrane Oxygenation
- Mechanical Ventilation Settings During ECMO
- Weaning from Mechanical Ventilation
- Conclusion

Introduction

Recently, with an enormous increase in cardiac surgeries and Cath lab procedures, there has been a convolution of cardiac critical care procedures. With the ever-growing vendors producing new ventilator modes, there is also a perplexity in the mindset of the intensivist. The most commonly employed right choice is using the same breath or sequences of breath and its feedback. The cardiac interventions range from traditional revascularization and valve procedures, aortic repair to percutaneous valve insertion, ventricular assist device implantation, extracorporeal approaches, transplants, minimally invasive and robotic surgeries, the enhanced external counter pulsation (EECP). It has become quite challenging to manage an overall sicker patient population with advanced medical and surgical cardiac conditions ranging from myocardial infarction (MI), advanced heart failure, cardiogenic shock, and transplantation. These patients frequently require noninvasive or invasive mechanical ventilator support due to increased work of breathing, acute hypoxemic respiratory failure, hemodynamic instability and need for noninvasive percutaneous procedures in the Cath lab.[1-3]

Historical Aspect

Moving from Schimmelbusch masks and Yankauer masks to the Boyles machine in the early 20th century, the ventilator modes in the modern integrated anesthesia workstation have undergone revolutionary changes with many advancements from electronic flow meters to the carbon dioxide absorbers in the modern-day anesthesia machine (**Flowchart 2.1** and **Fig. 2.1a, b**), delivering low flows and low tidal volumes. The ventilator modes have advanced from "pneumatically driven" bag in bottle systems to "Piston" and turbine ventilators, which are electrically driven in most advanced intensive care units (ICUs) in the present era. The newer machines such as Draeger Zeus uses the turbine technology with a major advantage of unlimited inspiratory gas flow which is most (small) essential in a spontaneously breathing patient. Other modes in different machines like that of GE healthcare allow spontaneous ventilation, when

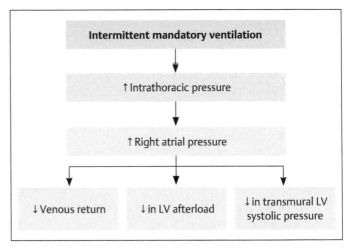

Flowchart 2.1 Hemodynamic interactions between heart and lungs. Abbreviation: LV, left ventricular.

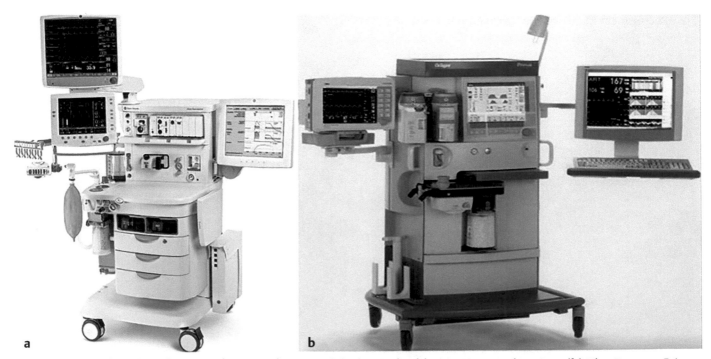

Fig. 2.1 Examples of modern anesthesia workstation. **(a)** The GE healthcare Aisys workstation. **(b)** The Draeger Primus workstation.

a laryngeal mask airway (LMA) is placed, and the synchronized intermittent mandatory ventilation is initiated.[4–7]

The Cardiovascular Effects of Positive Pressure Ventilation (PPV)

With elaborate self-testing to prevent a leak in the circuit to compliance compensation, all modern anesthesia machine ventilators ensure accuracy of delivered tidal volume. The machines today do not deliver higher tidal volumes as the decoupling valve (DV) prevents excessive fresh gas flow (FGF) beyond the limit that is set. Some newer machines like GE healthcare have electronic compensation set. Addition of both mechanical and electronic knobs actually move many mechanical parts of the machine once they are "Pressed." But the major disadvantage of the modern ventilation systems is its heavy dependence on "electricity" (**Box 2.1**).

Alternative Modes to Prevent Ventilator-Induced Injury

To prevent ventilator-induced injury to the lungs (VILI) alternative modes of ventilation were added to most modern-day ventilators, over and above the conventional ones (**Box 2.1**): conventional, biphasic pressure mode and dual control mode (closed-loop ventilation). The initial ventilator settings will depend on the type and severity of the

---

Box 2.1 Deleterious effects due to mismatch ventilation

- Patients with unstable hemodynamic status
- Acute hypoxemic failure in these patients is secondary to pulmonary edema
- Cardiogenic shock, acute respiratory distress syndrome (ARDS)
- Postoperative hypoxemia
- Pleural effusion
- Post–cardiac surgery atelectasis in ARDS
- Transfusion mismatch drug toxicity
- Barotrauma
- Transfusion-related acute lung injury (TRALI)
- Drug toxicity
- Trauma during ventilation on extracorporeal

Box 2.2 Open-lung strategy settings

- Tidal volume: 6–8 mL/kg PBW
- Plateau pressure (PPL) <30 cm H_2O
- Mode: volume control
- Respiratory rate: 10–30, to achieve pH 7.3–7.45
- I/E: 1:1–2:1
- PEEP: 10–20 cm H_2O (according to lower inflection point)

Abbreviations: IE, inspiratory expiratory ratio; PBW, predicted body weight; PEEP, positive end-expiratory pressure.

---

disease. Pressure-regulated volume control (PRVC) mode of ventilation is an advocated mode today for acute lung injury (ALI) and acute respiratory distress syndrome (ARDS). In these conditions conventional methods of ventilation will lead to overdistension of the alveoli and higher peaks inspiratory pressures would have to be set, thus delaying patient recovery. In ARDS, high ventilation pressure is to be avoided. Using the PRVC mode, the peak inspiratory pressures are kept low (**Box 2.2**).

Transition to high-frequency oscillatory ventilation (HFOV) in such a situation usually results in improvement in oxygenation and ventilation at lower airway pressures. Therefore, there is less compromise of cardiac output. HFOV has been safely used in pediatric cardiac patients with shorter ventilation times and intensive care stays. It has also been safely applied in adult patients after coronary and valvular surgeries. It may be a useful tool in balancing the ventilator and hemodynamic requirements in patient pulmonary edema and cardiac dysfunction.[8–12]

When starting invasive mechanical ventilation (MV), it is imperative to optimize the tidal volume, the inspiratory expiratory (IE) ratio, the mode of ventilation, the plateau pressure, the positive end-expiratory pressure (PEEP), and the requirement process for all types of ventilators. **Box 2.2** provides the open-lung strategy utilized for the same as depicted in **Fig. 2.2**.

PRVC Mode in ARDS Prevents Barotrauma

The PRVC mode in ARDS guarantees a "tidal volume" with minimal risk barotrauma and decelerating flow pattern, such that both ventilation and perfusion are optimal. This PRVC is a new dual-mode ventilation that offers both target volume ventilation and pressure control, but the current status on it being helpful in weaning is not known. ARDS net strategy has revolutionized the ventilator technique in patients with ARDS and has also been found to be useful in patients with pulmonary edema, and postpartum depression (PPD). In addition to this open-lung approach (OLA), other ventilator strategies such as prone ventilation, high-frequency oscillatory ventilation, noninvasive ventilation (NIV), and extracorporeal membrane oxygenation (ECMO) are also frequently applied in these patients. The nuances of these techniques pertaining to cardiac patients will be discussed herewith.

The Protective Lung Strategy

This protective lung strategy termed as lung protective ventilation (LPV) is defined as the combination of adding low-volume tidal ventilation (6–8 mL/kg predicted body weight [PBW]) to optimal PEEP levels (5–12 cm H_2O) and

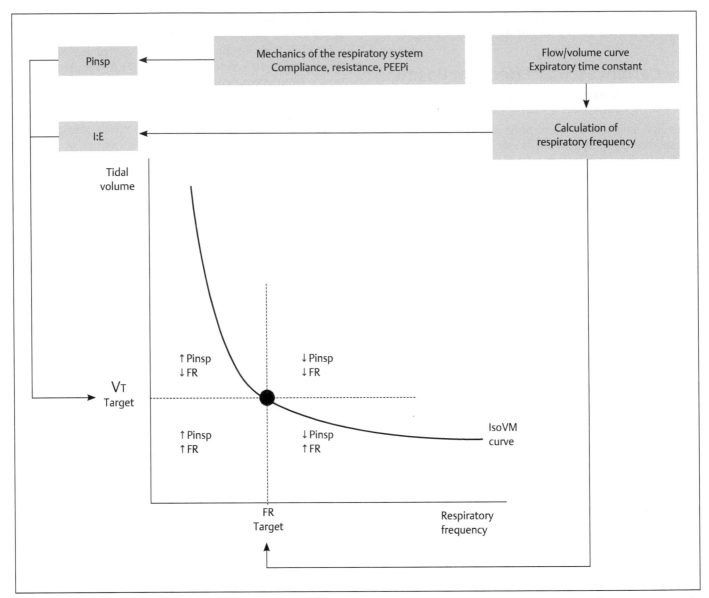

Fig. 2.2 Ventilator setting in open-lung strategy setting as in cardiac surgery. Tidal volume (Vt) against flow rate targets in open lung strategy used in mechanical of cardiac surgical patients. Abbreviations: FR, flow rate; IsoVM, minute-isovolumetric curve; Pmax, maximum inspiratory pressure limit; PEEP, positive end-expiratory pressure.

permitting permissive hypercapnia. LPV is designed to facilitate smooth operation of lung opening and closing and avoid elastase. It is achieved by simultaneously applying optimal PEEP and recruitment measures (RM), along with permissive hypercapnia. LPV is so designed such that shear forces generated by repetitive opening and closing of atelectasis lung areas can be avoided. It should be achieved with concomitant application of RM and sufficient PEEP so as to counterbalance the elastic recoil forces and to ventilate with minimum pressure amplitude to avoid pulmonary overdistension. This approach decreases the stress to the alveolocapillary membrane by preventing collapse at end expiration, thereby limiting the surfactant squeeze out and

loss of proteins. Therefore, this strategy has found place in the intraoperative period as well. Cardiac patients, however, have a sensitive hemodynamic profile due to which application of PEEP and RMs in them may prove to be detrimental, and thus require extra vigilance. Similarly, allowing permissive hypercapnia with resultant respiratory acidosis-related arrhythmia in these patients is not straightforward, and may prove to be deleterious. Thus, cardiac patients are in a special category as high PEEP, permissive hypercapnia with low tidal volume, and RMs may not be tolerated due to low compliance of the left ventricle, and exaggerated effects of vasodilatation and arrhythmias due to increased pulmonary capillary oncotic pressure (PCOP).

When Do We Need to Start Invasive Ventilation in Cardiac ICU

After cardiac surgery, most patients, even today, are shifted to the cardiac surgical ICU. Intubated weaning is fast tracked in the successive 3 to 4 hours. Generally, MV is continued in post–cardiac surgical patients, or in some others it is started or restarted, when the parameters listed in **Box 2.3** are found. FiO$_2$ is the fraction inspired oxygen when the patient is attached to the ventilation. Initially the FiO$_2$ is set at an oxygen flow of 100% (FiO$_2$ = 1). Once the patient settles on the ventilation, the flow is brought down to 0.6 or low (FiO$_2$ = 0.6) to prevent oxygen toxicity in the patient.

Hemodynamic Effects of Positive Pressure Ventilation (PPV) and Positive End-Expiratory Pressure (PEEP)

Both PEEP and PPV have deleterious as well as beneficial effects on the cardiac surgical patients. The advantages of PPV and PEEP are well enumerated in **Box 2.4**. Application of both reduces the afterload and left ventricular (LV) preload, thus reducing the pulmonary vasoconstriction and enhancing the oxygenation, but it also has some detrimental hemodynamic consequences as described in **Flowchart 2.2** which

may lead to an increase in the right ventricular (RV) afterload and reduced work of breathing.

1. Decreased venous return due to increased intrathoracic pressure and reduced caliber of inferior vena cava due to external pressure.
2. Decreased left ventricular filling due to constrictive effects of PEEP.
3. Increased RV dilatation with septal shift due to increase in RV afterload.

However, a lot of caution needs to be exercised before increasing PEEP. These are laid out as PEEP delivers continuous positive pressure which continues even at the end of expiration. PEEP has a good effect in the NIV. If continuous positive airway pressure (CPAP) only occurs on initializing it is not PEEP, but pressure support ventilation (PSV). PSV is a weaning mode of ventilation which the patient generates when he starts breathing spontaneously; thus, the effects of PEEP would vary in different patients depending on whether they are preload dependent or afterload dependent.

Noninvasive Ventilation in Cardiac Issue

NIV is used in most patients who develop acute respiratory failure (ARF) in the cardiac ICU. It has been demonstrated to effectively avoid invasive ventilation in patients with acute exacerbation of chronic obstructive pulmonary disease

---

Box 2.3   Clinical parameters necessitating invasive mechanical ventilation

- Respiratory rate (RR) >30 breaths per min (Normal 10–20)
- Tidal volume (Vt) <5 mL/kg (Normal 5–7)
- Vital capacity <15 mL/kg (Normal 65–75)
- Partial pressure of carbon dioxide (PaCO$_2$) >60 mmHg
- RR/Vt >100
- Dead space (VD)/Vt ratio >0.6 (Normal <0.3)
- Paradoxical breathing
- Partial pressure of oxygen
- Partial pressure of oxygen (PaO$_2$) <60 mmHg
- Fraction-inspired oxygen

Box 2.4   Advantages of PPV and PEEP

- Reduced LV afterload
- Reduced LV preload
- Reduced work of breath
- Relief in hypoxia-related pulmonary vasoconstriction
- Improved oxygenation to the myocardial tissue
- Keeps the alveoli recruited; this increases the FRC
- PEEP needs to be individualized as some cardiac patients are preload dependent and some afterload dependent
- Protects against VILI

Abbreviations: FRC, functional residual capacity; LV, left ventricular; PEEP, positive end-expiratory pressure; VILI, ventilator induced lung injury.

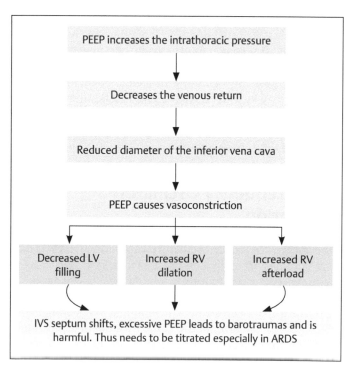

Flowchart 2.2   Deleterious effects of PEEP. Abbreviations: ARDS, acute respiratory distress syndrome; IVS, interventricular septum; LV, left ventricular; PEEP, positive end-expiratory pressure; RV, right ventricular.

(COPD), acute pulmonary edema, and immunodeficiency. It has also been found to decrease the reintubation rates in both medical and surgical patients.[13,14] Literature review suggests a beneficial role of NIV in most cardiac patients, who may be suffering from acute decompensatory heart failure or postoperative pneumonia, to prevent lung damage or pulmonary edema. There may also be associated previous lung disease, postoperative pneumonia, or cardiogenic pulmonary edema. NIV reestablishes the lung volumes and lowers the work of breaths. NIV has been found to improve lung function tests and arterial oxygenation by preventing atelectasis when applied prophylactically in cardiac surgical patients. It has been found equally effective in enabling successful weaning when applied in early postextubating period. NIV is also helpful in percutaneous procedures performed in a catheterization lab, such as transcatheter aortic valve replacement (TAVR) and endovascular aneurysm repair (EVAR).[15]

All of the above hold true for RM application as well. A common method for RM is to apply 30 cm H_2O PEEP for 30 seconds or 40 cm H_2O PEEP for 40 seconds causing sustained inflation.

Recruitment Maneuvers in Mechanical Ventilation

In both anesthesia and ARDS patient's RMs are adopted as alternatives to invasive MV. These RMs re-expand the collapsed alveoli and thus the lungs. One such method to perform it is to give a sustained PEEP of 30 to 40 cm of H_2O for up to 40 to 50 seconds. Alternatively, one may deliver high PEEP 40 and low PEEP 20, for 2 minutes in 1:1 ratio. Both RM techniques are equally efficacious. Such high airway pressures may be difficult to tolerate in a hemodynamically unstable cardiac patient. Therefore, this population subset requires extra care while incorporating protective lung strategy in their management.[8]

High-Frequency Oscillatory Ventilation

During high-frequency oscillatory ventilation (HFOV) small tidal volumes are delivered at frequencies of 3 to 15 Hz to maintain adequate minute's ventilation. Oxygenation is achieved by manipulating mean airway pressure quite similar to the use of PEEP during conventional MV. Ventilation is achieved by changing tidal volume by adjusting the amplitude and frequency. Carbon dioxide elimination increases by increasing the amplitude or by decreasing the frequency. Two recent randomized trials—the OSCILLATE (Oscillation

for ARDS treated early trial) and the OSCAR (High-frequency oscillation in ARDS trial)—did not show any reduction in hospital mortality with HFOV as compared to ARDS net strategy. However, these trials had their own set of limitations, and HFOV has been found to have theoretical as well as practical justification in cardiac patients. Continuous positive intrathoracic pressure during conventional MV impedes venous return, thereby limiting cardiac output.[9,10]

Limitations of Tidal Volume and Plateau Pressure

It is recommended by International Society of Heart Lung Transplant (ISHLT) to follow ultraprotective lung ventilation with a tidal volume less than 4 mL/kg body weight and a plateau pressure between 25 and 30 cm H_2O, with recruitment maneuvers like PEEP to prevent alveoli collapse.[16-18]

Positive End-Expiratory Pressure (PEEP)

In order to ensure adequate lung recruitment, Extracorporeal Life Support Organization (ELSO) guidelines recommend a modest PEEP of 10 cm H_2O. High PEEP during ECMO which may cause alveolar overdistension, increased alveolar strain, and hemodynamic instability by inhibiting venous return and exacerbating RV dysfunction thereby delaying heart recovery. The respiratory rates in cardiac patients may vary from 4 to 30 cycles/min but both RR and FiO_2 should be adjusted to maintain arterial oxygen saturation around 85% and above at all times. Pulmonary oxygen toxicity must be avoided at all times by reducing the FiO_2.

Mode of Mechanical Ventilation

The pressure control (PC) mode is advocated more in cases in the initial phase of postoperative period, by following a low tidal volume and a plateau pressure less than 30 cm providing the ventilation according to the target setting as previously discussed. At bedside, PC mode allows assessment of clinical improvement by daily monitoring of the increase in tidal volume. The PC mode allows minute-to-minute assessment of the tidal volume. Over a period of time, research and clinical trials have recommended starting spontaneous ventilation as early as possible, such that there is a good diaphragmatic contraction. A good mode of ventilation at this stage is airway pressure release ventilation (APRV) mode, where both muscle atrophy and prolonged ventilation due to lung rest and controlled ventilation is avoided (**Boxes 2.5–2.10** and **Fig. 2.3**). APRV is an alternative to conventional PC MV in ARDS patients in the ICU.[19]

Box 2.5   Airway pressure release ventilation

- Described as two levels of CPAP that are applied for a set period of time (high CPAP and a low CPAP)
- Inspiration occurs during high CPAP followed by a short expiration during low CPAP
- Equivalent to PCIRV for mandatory breaths

Abbreviations: CPAP, continuous positive airway pressure; PCIRV, pressure controlled inverse ratio ventilation.

Box 2.6   Indications of airway pressure release ventilation

- Protective ventilation strategy in ALI/ARDS: an oxygenation/recruitment mode
- Adequate spontaneous ventilation necessary to augment CO_2 removal and increase in venous return

Abbreviations: ALI, acute lung injury; ARDS, acute respiratory distress syndrome.

Box 2.7   Mandatory breaths and spontaneous breaths for airway pressure release ventilation

Mandatory breaths:
- Pressure controlled
- Trigger time
- Cycle time
- Limit pressure

Spontaneous breaths:
- Pressure controlled
- Trigger pressure
- Cycle pressure
- Limit pressure

Box 2.8   Settings of airway pressure release ventilation

- Inspiratory pressure set between 20 and 30 cm H_2O
- Patient should look comfortable breathing spontaneously at this pressure and be moving volumes spontaneously between 100 and 300 mL
- Expiratory pressure set between 0 and 2 to 3 cm H_2O
- Inspiratory time set between 3 and 5 seconds
- Expiratory time set between 0.5 and 1 second; longer times lead to loss of recruitment
- I:E ratio between 4:1 and 10:1
- Set rate never exceeds 20 bpm
- May take several hours before oxygenation shows improvement

Box 2.9   Noninvasive ventilation setting

Continuous positive airway pressure:
- Start with 5 cm H_2O
- Increase in increments of 2 cm H_2O, as tolerated and indicated

Bi-level positive airway pressure:
- Initial inspiratory pressure of 8–10 cm H_2O
- Initial expiratory pressure of 2–4 cm H_2O
- Increase in increments of 2–4 cm H_2O
- Maximum inspiratory pressure is 24 cm H_2O and expiratory pressure is 20 cm H_2O

Noninvasive pressure support ventilation:
- Pressure support of 8–10 cm H_2O and positive end-expiratory pressure of 2–4 cm H_2O
- Adjust as per bi-level positive airway pressure

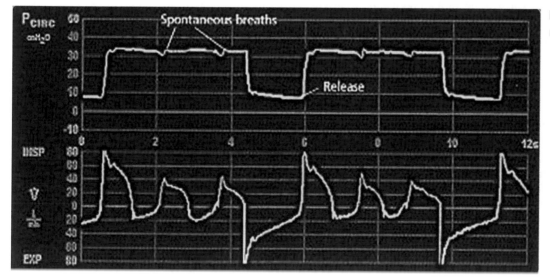

Fig. 2.3   Airway pressure release ventilation.

Box 2.10 Absolute contraindications for noninvasive ventilation (NIV)

- Cardiac or respiratory arrest
- Uncontrollable vomiting
- Hemodynamic instability or major arrhythmias
- Abnormal facial anatomy
- Upper airway obstruction
- Seizures or inability to protect the airway
- Inability to manage secretions
- Esophageal lesions or recent gastroesophageal surgery
- Inability to tolerate the mask

Box 2.11 Airway pressure release ventilation settings

Newly intubated:
- P_{high}: Set at desired plateau pressure (typically 20–35 cm H_2O)
- P_{low}: 0 cm H_2O
- T_{high}: 4–6 s
- T_{low}: 0.2–0.8 s (RLD), 0.8–1.5 s (OLD)

Transition from conventional ventilation:
- P_{high}: Plateau pressure in volume cycle mode
- P_{low}: 0 cm H_2O
- T_{high}: 4–6 s
- T_{low}: 0.2–0.8 s (RLD), 0.8–1.5 s (OLD)

Transition from HFOV: use noncompliant circuit
- P_{high}: mPaw on HFOV plus 2–4 cm H_2O
- P_{low}: 0 cm H_2O
- T_{high}: 4–6 s
- T_{low}: 0.2–0.8 s (RLD), 0.8–1.5 s (OLD)

Airway Pressure Release Ventilation (APRV) and a New and Important Mode of Ventilation in the Cardiac Patient

During APRV, the patient is given a CPAP with a shorter expiratory time. This is like an open-lung ventilation technique. A high pressure is maintained for 80 to 90% of the cycle time in which the patient undergoes spontaneous breathing (**Box 2.11**). A low-pressure setting allows ventilation and carbon dioxide clearance without alveolar collapse. Thus, it shares some similar features with other nonconventional modes of ventilation like inverse ratio ventilation (IRV) and HFOV. It also has a lung protective benefit, provided judicious selection of setting is done to ensure ventilation on the advantages portion of the pressure volume curve. APRV has also been associated with better cardiac performance in ARDS patients.[20] It has been used safely and effectively in postoperative cardiac surgical patients and acute pulmonary edema. APRV can also be applied noninvasively pre- or postintubation. It has been found to be associated with less likelihood of auto cycling from leaks common to conventional noninvasive ventilation.[21,22]

Lung Protective Ventilation Patients with Intra-abdominal Hypertension

In a review by Regli et al it has been suggested that LPV is most helpful as ventilation for portal hypertension syndrome (PHS) with raised abdominal pressure (intra-abdominal hypertension [IAH]). Although considerable progress has been made over the past decades, some important questions remain relating to the optimal ventilation management in patients with IAH. When looking after patients with IAH and ARDS requiring MV, an important first step is to measure intra-abdominal pressure (IAP)[12] and aim to reduce IAP in order to reduce airway pressures keeping in mind that small reductions in intra-abdominal volume can significantly reduce IAP and airway pressures.[23] Although challenging, the measurement of esophageal pressure as surrogate for intrathoracic pressure can provide transpulmonary pressures that can help guide ventilation. Also, note that IAH can lead to the polycompartment syndrome with the associated interactions between different compartmental pressures.[24] With respect to this, one should avoid head of bed elevation above 45 degrees in patients with high body mass index as this is associated with increase in IAP.

Prone Ventilation

Prone ventilation has been used successfully in the last 40 years in patients with ARDS. It significantly improves the patient ventilation perfusion mismatch, thus improving the oxygenation.[25,26] Prone positioning in ARDS according to recent literature reduces mortality significantly, when used in conjunction with LPV and remaining prone for a longer duration of time.[10] Proning is skilled labor and teamwork. The position itself is physiological, with a lot of deleterious effects such as kinking and dislodgement of the endotracheal tube intravenous lines (I/V) lines, chest drains and nasogastric tubes. There have also been reports about occurrence of hemodynamic instability, cardiac arrhythmias, and worsened gas exchange during prone positioning. However, protocols and nursing care guidelines might overcome these challenges. There have been multiple studies showing the feasibility, safety, and efficacy of prone ventilation in cardiac patients in the postoperative group.[26-28] There are, however, some contraindications to prone positioning as enlisted in **Box 2.12**.

Box 2.12 Prone positioning: contraindications

- Untrained staff
- Increased intracranial pressure
- Increased abdominal pressure
- Open abdominal and chest wounds
- Cervical spine precautions
- Extreme obesity

Extracorporeal Membrane Oxygenation

ECMO is partial cardiopulmonary bypass applied to a failing heart or failing lungs or used today as a bridge to recovery or while awaiting a heart lung transplant. It improves the patient's oxygenation and use of optimal lung rest ventilation settings. Venovenous (VV) ECMO can be considered for cardiac patients with isolated severe respiratory failure without hemodynamic compromise. Venoarterial (VA) ECMO is required for patients needing hemodynamic support as well. ECMO also complements cardiac surgical and cardiology procedures, heart and lung transplantation, implantation of mechanical cardiac assist devices, and extracorporeal cardiopulmonary resuscitation (i.e., CPR). Mechanical circulatory support (MCS) with VA ECMO employed in a conventional central/peripheral fashion may be used to stabilize the patient with decompensated cardiac failure having evidence of end-organ dysfunction. Patient may be transitioned to VV ECMO upon myocardial recovery to avoid upper body hypoxia.

As per the recently published International Society for Heart and Lung, for stable hemodynamic, it is essential to prevent instability with high vasopressor. ECMO is useful. The transplantation guidelines for MCS strongly recommends consideration of use of transient cardiac and lung support devices like ECMO which would stabilize the neurological and hemodynamic condition of the patient and allow these patients to be on "ECMO rest" before contemplating transplant ventricular assist devices (VAD).

Mechanical Ventilation Settings During ECMO

Cardiogenic pulmonary edema, reduced thoracic compliance, and postoperative lung damage predispose patients to develop ARDS after cardiac surgery. Factors exist which predispose after cardiac surgery, some periods to develop an ARDS like picture in the postoperative period as enumerated in **Box 2.13**. Recently published recommendations from International Society of Heart and Lung Transplantation guidelines suggest the use of a temporary mechanical support device like ECMO to tide over this period.[3]

Box 2.13 Factors predisposing to postoperative ARDS post-cardiac surgery

- Reduced thoracic compliance
- Cardiogenic pulmonary edema
- Postoperative lung damage

Box 2.14 The goal of the patient on ECMO is to minimize the ventilator-associated complications and give rest to lungs. This can be achieved by providing rest settings of the ventilator which includes:

1. Mode: PCV
2. Respiratory rate of 6–8/min
3. Peak inspiratory pressure of 30
4. PEEP: 12–15 mmHg
5. I:E ratio of 1:1
6. FiO$_2$ of 40–60%

Abbreviations: ECMO, extracorporeal membrane oxygenator; FiO2, fraction of inspired oxygen; PEEP, positive end-expiratory pressur; PCV, pressure-controlled ventilation.

Box 2.15 Lung protective ventilation in the ICU: the Berlin definition

Severity PaO$_2$/ FiO$_2$ ratio (Oxygen flow)	Mild: 200–300 mmHg with PEEP or CPAP ≥ 5 cm H$_2$O
	Moderate: 100–200 mmHg with PEEP ≥ 5 cm H$_2$O
	Severe: ≥100 mmHg with PEEP ≥ 5 cm H$_2$O
Timing	Within 1 wk of clinical insult or new or worsening respiratory symptoms
Chest imaging	Bilateral opacities
Site of origin of edema	Not fully explained by heart failure or fluid overload

Abbreviations: CPAP, continuous positive airway pressure; FiO2, fraction of inspired oxygen; PaO2, partial pressure of oxygen; PEEP, positive end-expiratory pressure.

The setting of the ECMO ventilation follows the rest LPV strategy **(Boxes 2.14–2.20)**.[29,30]

Patient with a heart etiology is more pertinent. LPV in ECMO is facilitated by direct carbon dioxide removal from the patient blood.

Weaning from Mechanical Ventilation

Weaning from MV is known to induce strong hemodynamic changes leading to weaning-induced cardiac failure and even cardiac ischemia. Cardiac patients are more predisposed to this complication. Early detection of weaning-induced pulmonary edema during spontaneous breathing trial is possible with pulmonary artery catheter (PAC), increased LV filling

Box 2.16 Ultraprotective ventilation during ECMO

- Calculate predicted body weight (PBW) using the following formula:
  - ➤ Males = 50 + 2.3 (height [in.] – 60)
  - ➤ Females = 42.5 + 2.3 (height [in.] – 60)
- Select any ventilator mode
- Set ventilator settings to achieve initial tidal volume (Vt) = 8 mL/kg PBW
- Reduce Vt by 1 mL/kg at intervals <2 h until Vt = 6 mL/kg PBW
- Set initial rate to approximately baseline minute ventilation (not >35 bpm)
- Adjust Vt and respiratory rate (RR) to achieve pH and plateau pressure goals

Abbreviations: ECMO, extracorporeal membrane oxygenator.

Box 2.17 Lower PEEP/Higher FiO_2

FiO_2	0.3	0.4	0.4	0.5	0.5	0.6	0.7	0.7	0.7	0.8	0.9	0.9	0.9	1.0
PEEP	5	5	8	8	10	10	10	12	14	14	14	16	18	18–24
Higher PEEP/Higher FiO_2														
FiO_2	0.3	0.3	0.3	0.3	0.3	0.4	0.4	0.5	0.5	0.5–0.8	0.8	0.9	1.0	1.0
PEEP	5	8	10	12	14	14	16	16	18	20	22	22	22	24

Abbreviations: FiO_2, fraction of inspired oxygen; PEEP, positive end expiratory pressure.

Box 2.18 Pulmonary hemorrhage

During pulmonary hemorrhage, we might require higher PEEP and prolonged inspiration time to achieve hemostasis. This can be done by:

- Mode: APRV
- P_{high}: around 25–30
- P_{low}: around 10–12
- T_{high}: around 4–5 s
- T_{low}: around 0.6–0.8 s
- Respiratory rate: around 10–12/min

Abbreviations: APRV, airway pressure release ventilation; PEEP, positive end-expiratory pressure.

Box 2.19 Coronary hypoxia: to be avoided in ECMO

- Coronary arteries usually gets blood from native circulation (i.e., from LV)
- With compromised LV and lungs and rest setting, coronary gets relatively hypoxic blood
- This can lead to myocardial hypoxia and cardiac stun
- In this scenario following things can be tried
  - ➤ Accept higher ventilator settings like increase FiO_2 to 60–70% and respiratory rate (RR) of –20
  - ➤ Consider HFO
  - ➤ V-AVECMO: give one return line to RA so that blood reaching native lungs and then to LV has better saturation
- Use right axillary artery for arterial cannulation instead of femoral or put an additional cannula in axillary artery

Abbreviations: ECMO, extracorporeal membrane oxygenator; FiO2, fraction of inspired oxygen; HFO, heart-forming organoids; LV, left ventricle.

Box 2.20 Plateau pressure goal: <30 cm H_2O

- Check P Plat (0.5-s inspiratory pause), at least q4h after each change in PEEP or Vt
- If P Plat >30 cm H_2O decrease initial tidal volume (Vt) by 1 mL/kg steps (minimum) 4 mL/kg
- If P Plat <25 cm H_2O and Vt < 6 mL/kg increase Vt by 1 mL/kg until P Plat >25 or Vt = 6 mL/kg
- If P Plat <30 cm and breath stacking or synchrony occurs: may increase Vt in 1 mL/kg increments to 7 or 8 mL/kg if P Plat remains <30 cm H_2O

Abbreviations: PEEP, positive end-expiratory pressure; Vt, tidal volume.

pressure with echocardiography, rise in B-type natriuretic peptide, and increase in extravascular lung water measured by transpulmonary thermodilution.[26-28] The problem of pulmonary edema can be addressed in these patients by further optimization of hemodynamics, creating more negative fluid balance and by early institution of NIV after extubation. There have also been recent reports of successful and rapid weaning after fast-track cardiac valvular surgery. ASV is a closed-loop mode of ventilation where the ventilator adjusts the inspiratory pressure in order to achieve the tidal volume associated with minimum work of breathing. In addition, there is a facility for ventilator to switch between control and support breaths depending on the absence or presence of spontaneous breathing efforts. ASV has also been found to have faster or equivalent weaning time after fast-track coronary artery bypass surgery as compared to protocolized weaning with synchronized intermittent mandatory ventilation (SIMV) with pressure support or pressure-regulated volume control with automode.[31-34]

Conclusion

Applying PPV becomes imperative in a cardiac surgery patient postoperatively. There is an increase in both RV and LV pressure after application of PEEP. To overcome this, choice of a ventilation mode should be made with the right ventilator setting, drugs,[7] and individual cardiovascular status of the patient.[8] To conclude, ventilator strategy is an important issue in cardiac intensive care. These patients, both surgical and medical, have limited reserve in tolerating conventional ARDS net ventilator strategy.[23,34] This needs modification in order to avoid permissive hypercapnia high PEEP, and recruitment. Alternative ventilator strategies such as HFOV, prone positioning, and ECMO are quite safe and useful in these patients. NIV has both a preventive and curative role in ARF in cardiac patients. Clinicians should be mindful of the specific clinical scenario and implement various ventilator strategies accordingly to enhance clinical outcome. Cardiac arrest patients often and increasingly receive protective ventilation. Optimization of ventilator settings and limiting exposure to modifiable factors of mechanical ventilation and in particular to high respiratory rate and driving pressure may improve patient's outcome after cardiac arrest.[35]

References

1. Kaul U, Bhatia V. Perspective on coronary interventions & cardiac surgeries in India. Indian J Med Res 2010;132(5): 543–548
2. Chiu KM. Modified parasternal approach is a good alternative for aortic valve surgery. Mini-invasive Surg 2017;1:81–88
3. Verbeek GL, Myles PS, Westall GP, et al. Intra-operative protective mechanical ventilation in lung transplantation: a randomised, controlled trial. Anaesthesia 2017;72(8):993–1004
4. Ranieri VM, Rubenfeld GD, Thompson BT, et al; ARDS Definition Task Force. Acute respiratory distress syndrome: the Berlin Definition. JAMA 2012;307(23):2526–2533
5. Wong JJ, Liu S, Dang H, et al; Pediatric Acute & Critical care Medicine Asian Network (PACCMAN). The impact of high frequency oscillatory ventilation on mortality in paediatric acute respiratory distress syndrome. Crit Care 2020;24(1):31
6. Brower RG, Matthay MA, Morris A, Schoenfeld D, Thompson BT, Wheeler A; Acute Respiratory Distress Syndrome Network. Ventilation with lower tidal volumes as compared with traditional tidal volumes for acute lung injury and the acute respiratory distress syndrome. N Engl J Med 2000;342(18):1301–1308
7. Wild M, Alagesan K. PEEP and CPAP. BJA CEPD Rev 2001;1: 89–92
8. Sud S, Sud M, Friedrich JO, et al. High-frequency oscillatory ventilation versus conventional ventilation for acute respiratory distress syndrome. Cochrane Database Syst Rev 2016;4:CD004085
9. Tung A. Critical care of the cardiac patient. Anesthesiol Clin 2013;31(2):421–432
10. Wiesen J, Ornstein M, Tonelli AR, Menon V, Ashton RW. State of the evidence: mechanical ventilation with PEEP in patients with cardiogenic shock. Heart 2013;99(24):1812–1817
11. Tripathi RS, Stein EJ, Crestanello JA, Papademas TJ. High frequency oscillatory ventilation after cardiac surgery: a treatment for all ages. Crit Care 2012;16:405
12. Finkielman JD, Gajic O, Farmer JC, Afessa B, Hubmayr RD. The initial Mayo Clinic experience using high-frequency oscillatory ventilation for adult patients: a retrospective study. BMC Emerg Med 2006;6:2
13. Landoni G, Zangrillo A, Cabrini L. Noninvasive ventilation after cardiac and thoracic surgery in adult patients: a review. J Cardiothorac Vasc Anesth 2012;26(5):917–922
14. Dres M, Teboul JL, Monnet X. Weaning the cardiac patient from mechanical ventilation. Curr Opin Crit Care 2014;20(5): 493–498
15. An-Hsun Chou, Ching Chang Chen, Yu-Sheng Lin, Ming-Shyan Lin, Victor Chien Wu et al. A population-based analysis of endovascular aortic stent graft therapy in patients with liver cirrhosis. Journal of Vascular Surgery 2019; 69(5):1395-1404
16. Badenes R, Jalvier Belda F, Aguilar G. Mechanical ventilation in cardiac surgery. Curr Anaesth Crit Care 2010;21:250–254
17. Napolitano LM. Postoperative respiratory failure: current surgical therapy. 11th ed. Elsevier, Saunders
18. Mehta Y. Is cardiac anaesthesiologist the best person to look after cardiac critical care? Invited Editorial. Ann Card Anaesth 2015;18:14–16
19. Panacek EA, Kirk JD. Role of noninvasive ventilation in the management of acutely decompensated heart failure. Rev Cardiovasc Med 2002;3(Suppl 4):S35–S40
20. Fredericks AS, Bunker MP, Gliga LA, Ebeling CG, Ringqvist JR, Heravi H, Manley J, Valladares J, Romito BT. Airway Pressure Release Ventilation: A Review of the Evidence, Theoretical Benefits, and Alternative Titration Strategies. Clin Med Insights Circ Respir Pulm Med. 2020 Feb 5;14:1179548420903297
21. Habashi NM. Other approaches to open-lung ventilation: airway pressure release ventilation. Crit Care Med 2005; 33(3, Suppl):S228–S240
23. Malbrain ML, Roberts DJ, Sugrue M, et al. The polycompartment syndrome: a concise state-of-the-art review. Anaesthesiol Intensive Ther 2014;46(5):433–450
22. Chauhan R, Mehta Y, Mishra M. Inverse ratio ventilation in a patient with pulmonary oedema. Indian J Anaesth 1992;40: 39–42
24. Schmidt M, Pellegrino V, Combes A, Scheinkestel C, Cooper DJ, Hodgson C. Mechanical ventilation during extracorporeal membrane oxygenation. Crit Care 2014;18(1):203
25. Park SY, Kim HJ, Yoo KH, et al. The efficacy and safety of prone positioning in adults patients with acute respiratory distress syndrome: a meta-analysis of randomized controlled trials. J Thorac Dis 2015;7(3):356–367
26. Firodiya M, Mehta Y, Juneja R, Trehan N. Mechanical ventilation in the prone position: a strategy for acute respiratory failure after cardiac surgery. Indian Heart J 2001;53(1):83–86
27. Maillet J-M, Thierry S, Brodaty D. Prone positioning and acute respiratory distress syndrome after cardiac surgery: a feasibility study. J Cardiothorac Vasc Anesth 2008;22(3):414–417
28. Brüssel T, Hachenberg T, Roos N, Lemzem H, Konertz W, Lawin P. Mechanical ventilation in the prone position for acute respiratory failure after cardiac surgery. J Cardiothorac Vasc Anesth 1993;7(5):541–546
29. Shekar K, Mullany DV, Thomson B, Ziegenfuss M, Platts DG, Fraser JF. Extracorporeal life support devices and strategies for management of acute cardiorespiratory failure in adult patients: a comprehensive review. Crit Care 2014;18(3):219

30. Sharma J, Mehta Y. Extracorporeal membrane oxygenation in cardiogenic schok. In Malhotra Kapoor P, ed. Manual of extracorporeal membrane oxygenation (ECMO) in the ICU. New Delhi: Jaypee Brothers Medical Publishers (P) Ltd.; 2013:193–6

31. Badenes R, Lozano A, Javier Belda F. Postoperative pulmonary dysfunction and mechanical surgery. Crit Care Res Pract 2015;420153:8AQ27

32. Zhu F, Gomersall CD, Ng SK, Underwood MJ, Lee A. A randomized controlled trial of adaptive support ventilation mode to wean patients after fast-track cardiac valvular surgery. Anesthesiology 2015;122(4):832–840

33. Regli A, De Keulenaer BL, Singh B, Hockings LE, Noffsinger B, van Heerden PV. The respiratory pressure-abdominal volume curve in a porcine model. Intensive Care Med Exp 2017;5(1):11

34. Pelosi P, Vargas M. Mechanical ventilation and intra-abdominal hypertension: 'Beyond Good and Evil'. Crit Care 2012;16(6):187

35. Robba C, Badenes R, Battaglini D, Ball L, Brunetti I, et al., Ventilator settings in the initial 72 h and their association with outcome in out-of-hospital cardiac arrest patients: a pre-planned secondary analysis of the targeted hypothermia versus targeted normothermia after out-of-hospital cardiac arrest (TTM2) trial. Intensive Care Med. 2022; 48(8):1024–1038

3

Noninvasive Ventilation in the ICU

Poonam Malhotra Kapoor, Sambhunath Das, Minati Choudhary,
Arindham Choudhary, and Rohan Magoon

Introduction

Noninvasive ventilation or NIV as it is commonly referred to is defined as the "Delivery of ventilator support to the lungs without the need for an invasive artificial airway." This artificial airway could be an endotracheal tube or a laryngeal mask airway or a tracheostomy tube.

Historical Perspective

In the late 1880s the term "iron lung" was first used (**Fig. 3.1a, b**). In the early 1900s the iron lungs were first used for the polio epidemic. This continued throughout the 20th century when in the 1960s invasive ventilation first became available (**Box 3.1**).

The iron tank was like a chest wrap, creating a negative pressure and thus patient's breathing was enabled. This noninvasive negative pressure became redundant in 2021.

What is, however, being used pervasively today is noninvasive positive pressure ventilation (NIPPV). NIV is used as an equivalent in most modern ventilators today to NIPPV. It is now an accepted mode of ventilation in the treatment of acute respiratory failure (ARF). So the three different types of NIV are enumerated in **Box 3.2**.

Continuous Positive Airway Pressure (CPAP)

In hypoxemia, the CPAP mode is preferred as it provides constant positive airway pressure throughout the respiratory cycle. It improves oxygen gently by decreasing the work of breathing by alveolar recruitment, thereby decreasing the elastic work and unloading the inspiratory muscles. CPAP decreases hypoxia and there is also reduction in intrapulmonary shunting. It is indicated in acute pulmonary edema and pneumonia.

Non-Invasive Ventilation

NIV scores over invasive ventilation in many ways (**Boxes 3.3** and **3.4**): it is cheaper, avoids secondary infections as hospital and ICU stay duration gets reduced, and overcomes the

Box 3.1 Negative-pressure ventilation
• Late 1880s—iron lungs first used
• Early 1900s—iron lungs used for polio epidemic
• This continued throughout the 20th century until the 1960s when invasive ventilation became available

Box 3.2 Types of NIV
• Negative-pressure ventilation (iron lung)
• Continuous positive airway pressure (CPAP) (not really NIV!)
• Bilevel positive airway pressure (BiPAP)

Abbreviation: NIV, noninvasive ventilation.

Box 3.3 Advantages of NIV over IMV
• Avoids the resistance due to an artificial airway: ETT, LMA, TT
• Avoids the complications of an artificial airway: local edema, bronchospasm, etc.
• Noninvasive mode allows easy application of implementation and removal
• Enhances patient comfort
• Reduces the need for sedation
• Maintains the oral patency (speech, cough reflex, and swallowing are all preserved)
• Prevents iatrogenic, secondary infections
• Avoids both early and late complications of intubation (e.g., aspiration, injury to hypopharynx, larynx, nosocomial infections)

Abbreviations: ETT, endotracheal tube; LMA, laryngeal mask airway; NIV, noninvasive ventilation; IMV, invasive mechanical ventilation; TT, tracheostomy tube.

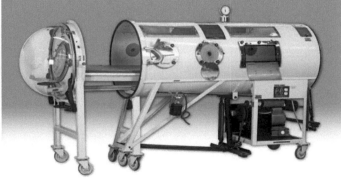

Fig. 3.1 (a, b) The Tron Seing ventilation.

Box 3.4 Ventilator setting: LVF

- CPAP at 5–8 and increase to 10–15 cm H_2O
- Mask is held gently on the patient's face
- Increase the pressure until adequate V_t (7 mL/kg), RR < 25/min, and patient comfortable
- Titrate FiO_2 to achieve SpO_2 > 90%
- Keep peak pressure <25–30 cm H_2O

COAD exacerbation: NIV

- Increase pH, reduces $PaCO_2$, reduces the severity of breathlessness in the first 4 h of treatment
- Decrease the length of hospital stay

Abbreviations: COAD, chronic obstructive airways disease; CPAP, continuous positive airway pressure; LVF, left ventricular failure; NIV, noninvasive ventilation.

Box 3.5 When to use NIV/CPAP

- Indication: APO, COAD
- Contraindications: exclude the assessment of the patient who should be:
  - Sick not moribund
  - Able to protect airway
  - Conscious/cooperative
  - Hemodynamically stable
- Premorbid state/ceiling of therapy?

Abbreviations: APO, acute cardiogenic pulmonary edema; COAD, chronic obstructive airways disease; CPAP, continuous positive airway pressure; NIV, noninvasive ventilation.

Box 3.6 Contraindications to NIV

- Impaired consciousness, confusion, agitation
- Inability to protect airway
- Excessive secretions or vomiting
- Hemodynamic instability
- Untreated pneumothorax
- Bowel obstruction, facial trauma, burns, recent surgery
- Fixed upper airway obstruction

Abbreviation: NIV, noninvasive ventilation.

Box 3.7 Complications of CPAP

- Hypoxia
- Pulmonary barotrauma
- Reduced cardiac output
- Vomiting and aspiration
- Pressure areas
- Gastric distension

Abbreviation: CPAP, continuous positive airway pressure.

Box 3.8 Disadvantages of NIV

- System of circuit
  - Slower correction of gas exchange abnormalities
  - Gastric distension (occurs in <2% patients)
- Mask
  - Air leakage
  - Eye irritation
  - Facial skin necrosis (most common complication)
- Lack of airways access and protection
  - Suctioning of secretions
  - Aspiration
- Compliance/Claustrophobia
- Work load and supervision needed all the time

Abbreviation: NIV, noninvasive ventilation.

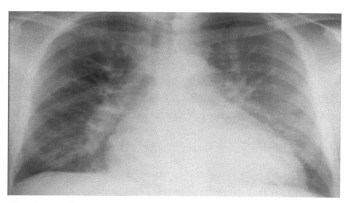

Fig. 3.2 Chest X-ray of a 70-year-old diabetic with signs of left ventricular (LV) failure who benefitted from continuous positive airway pressure (CPAP) at 5 to 8 cm H_2O.

are not cooperative for intubation or do not want an artificial airway (**Boxes 3.5–3.8**).

A Perfect Case for Non-Invasive Ventilation (NIV)

A 70-year-old diabetic lady, known case of ischemic heart disease (IHD) with a history of previous myocardial infarction (MI), came to the emergency ward with a BP of 130/95 mm Hg; HR of 120, and RR of 38/min with a SpO_2 of 87% on 15 liters of oxygen via a CPAP mask. Arterial blood gas (ABG) analysis showed a pH of 7.28 and a PCO_2 of 51 and PO_2 of 71 base excess (BE) of −32. Chest X-ray showed left ventricular failure (LVF) signs with cardiomegaly (**Fig. 3.2** and **Box 3.4**).

Which Mode of NIV to Use?

NIV brings about an improvement in gas exchange (**Box 3.9** and **Fig. 3.3**) by recruiting the alveoli and increasing the forced residual capacity to reverse hypoxia. In severe

complications of an artificial airway. In addition, NIV allows gradual weaning from ventilator. In this mode, the patient is awake and alert. It provides more efficacious nebulization and physiotherapy. Even mobilization of patient and expectoration are easier. NIV can be safely used in patients who

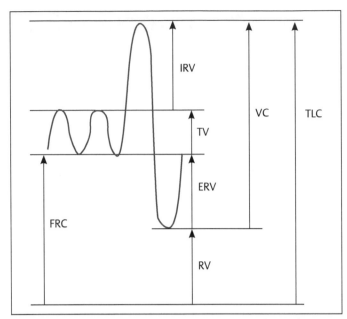

Fig. 3.3 Bilevel pressure support (BiPAP) is a combination of inspiratory positive airway pressure (IPAP) and expiratory positive airway pressure (EPAP). Abbreviations: ERV, expiratory reserve volume; FRC, functional residual capacity; IRV, inspiratory reserve volume; RV, residual volume; TLC, total lung capacity; TV, tidal volume; VC, vital capacity.

hypoxemia it is wise to choose the CPAP mode, but in hypercapnia with hypoxemia (e.g., chronic obstructive pulmonary disorder [COPD]), a bilevel NIV (bilevel positive airway pressure [BiPAP]) is preferred. In acute pulmonary edema and pneumonia CPAP is used, whereas in acute respiratory failure, asthma, and chronic respiratory exacerbations such as COPD, BiPAP is preferred.

NIV also reduces the work of breathing, as listed in **Box 3.10**, as it provides both EPAP and IPAP (expiratory & inspiratory positive airway pressure) ventilation. IPAP specially decreases work of breathing and also the oxygen demand.

Limitations of BiPAP

The limitation of BiPAP is the asynchrony among the trigger and cycle of respiration, decreased volume delivery, and tachypnea. Newer methods, such as adaptive servoventilation and neutrally adjusted ventilator assist (NAVA), have come into recent practice as NIV modes, overcoming the disadvantage of BiPAP.[1] Unlike invasive positive pressure ventilation (IPPV), NIV reduces the side effects of IPPV chiefly ventilator-associated pneumonia (VAP) and sinusitis sepsis, and decreases the rate of hospital admissions and mortality.[2]

CPAP and BiPAP

CPAP, a type of NIV, is used in acute congestive heart failure and obstructive sleep apnea (OSA). In OSA, CPAP is given

---

Box 3.9 Indications of BiPAP

- Exacerbation of COPD with respiratory acidosis
- Type II respiratory failure with chest wall deforming or neuromuscular disease
- Failure of CPAP
- Pneumonia with respiratory acidosis
- Therapeutic trial with a view to intubation if it fails
- Other (ARDS, postoperative respiratory failure to buy time for intubation)

Abbreviations: ARDS, acute respiratory distress syndrome; BiPAP, bilevel pressure support; COPD, chronic obstructive pulmonary disease; CPAP, continuous positive airway pressure.

Box 3.10 Bilevel pressure support

- Combination of IPAP and EPAP
  - Inspiratory PAP = Pressure support
  - Expiratory PAP = CPAP

Respiratory effects Bi-PAP

- EPAP
  - Provides PEEP
  - Increase functional residual capacity
  - Reduces FiO_2 required to optimize SaO_2
- IPAP
  - Decreases work of breathing + oxygen demand
  - Increases spontaneous tidal volume
  - Decreases spontaneous respiratory rate

Abbreviations: Bi-PAP, bilevel positive airway pressure; CPAP, continuous positive airway pressure; FiO_2, fraction of inspired oxygen; IPAP, inspiratory positive airway pressure; PEEP, positive end-expiratory pressure; SaO_2, oxygen saturation.

Box 3.11 Indications for Bi-level

- Acute respiratory failure
- Chronic airway limitation/COPD
- Asthma

Abbreviation: COPD, chronic obstructive pulmonary disease.

---

between 5 and 12 cm H_2O while patient is sleeping with the CPAP mask. BiPAP is the most commonly used NIV mode. Chiefly used in COPD (**Boxes 3.10** and **3.11**) and asthma, the mask setting is set at 3 to 5 cm H_2O as expiratory positive airway pressure (EPAP) and 5 to 15 cm H_2O as inspiratory positive airway pressure (IPAP). EPAP like positive end-expiratory pressure (PEEP) may later be also increased to 10 to 12 cm H_2O.

In case of hypercarbia or tachypnea, the IPAP can be increased to 20 to 25 cm of the pressure support which is calculated as the difference between IPAP and EPAP.

Monitoring During NIV

This should include monitoring of blood pressure, heart rate, respiratory rate, and ABGs showing PaO_2, $PaCO_2$, PH, and base excess. NIV is well maintained when above parameters are normal.[3-8] Both CPAP and BiPAP are not without limitations. Recommendations for using NIV for the treatment of ARF according to the recent ERS and ATS guidelines are mentioned in **Box 3.12**. **Box 3.13** enumerates some of the recent noninvasive ventilator modes which are being incorporated in the newer noninvasive positive pressure ventilator modes.

Interface

Positioning of the interface is very important. The anesthesia technique used for NIV is generally for overcoming anxiety and equipment fear (**Table 3.1**).

The commonest NIV modes are CPAP, BiPAP, and NIPSV, and PEEP remains the most frequently used NIV mode (**Box 3.14**).

Whatever modes are chosen, it is essential that the interface upped for a particular NIV mode is by a trained hospital personnel only. The personnel in an ICU should be well versed and trained in ABG monitoring also.
Interface can be:
- Mask.
- Nasal mask.
- Oronasal pillows.
- Mouth pieces.
- Helmet.
- Nasal total face.

Choice of Interface

The internal volume of masks is seen to have no short-term effect on either gas exchange or minute ventilator respiratory effect.[9] When the nasal mask was compared with the oronasal mask, more failure was seen with the nasal mask. Of all the four cited above, the nasal mask was tolerated best. The $PaCO_2$ was, however, best with oronasal pillows.[10] Less staff is required for mask and all complications of skin necroses; disrupted sleep with NIV failure occurs with an ill-fitting face mask. In case of latter, it is important to switch over to an alternative interface as soon as possible. Interface should be rotated frequently using different types and adjusting the headgears to prevent complications.[10]

The Face Mask or Mask

Mask application of interfaces in NIV is at 30 to 90 degrees upright position. The nasal mask fits just above the junction of nasal bridge and cartilage. Velcro straps are used to keep the interface well positioned over the patients' nose and mouth. To apply the nasal prongs, it is essential not to apply any lateral pressure on the septum and fill the nasal opening without stretching the skin or applying undue pressure on the nose (**Box 3.15** and **Fig. 3.4**). A comparison of the nasal pillows and face mask is done in **Table 3.2** and **Fig. 3.5**.

Box 3.12 Monitoring of NIV as per the recent ERS and ATS guidelines

- ABG
- RR
- Heart rate
- Continuous ECG recording during the first 12 h
- Repeat ABGs 1 h after initiation of NIV/change of settings, after 4 h in clinically nonimproving patients
- In acutely ill patients:
  - Every 15 min in the first hour
  - Every 30 min in 1–4 h period
  - Hourly in 4–12 h period
- Level of consciousness
- Patient comfort
- Chest wall movement, ventilator synchrony, and accessory muscle use

Abbreviations: ABG, arterial blood gas; ATS, American Thoracic Society; ECG, electrocardiography; ERS, European Respiratory Society; NIV, noninvasive ventilation; RR, respiratory rate.

Box 3.13 Other recent indications of noninvasive ventilation (NIV)

- Upper airway obstruction
- Mild to moderate hypoxemia
- Central apnea
- Hyperventilation syndrome
NIPPV NOT to be given in the following:
- Cardiac arrest
- Shock
- Hemodynamic instability
- Dangerous arrhythmias
- Non-cooperative patients
- Patient with increased discharge
- Airway surgery

Abbreviation: NIPPV, noninvasive positive pressure ventilation.

Box 3.14 Effects of PEEP

PEEP causes the following:
- Increase in FRC, tidal volume, lung compliance, and improved oxygenation
- Increase dead space and reduced compliance
- Increase peripheral reduced compliance
- Decreased cardiac output, renal blood flow with a decrease in GFR and urine output

Abbreviations: FRC, final residual capacity; GFR, glomerular filtration rate; positive end-expiratory pressure; PEEP, positive end-expiratory pressure.

The nasal pillows may cause a lot of drying. Thus, learning about interface troubleshooting is essential (**Table 3.3**).

Whatever the nature of the machine type used, it is all dependent on available facilities and cost which can be afforded.

Box 3.15   Interface positioning

- Nasal prong application
- Fill the nasal openings without stretching the skin or undue pressure on the nares
- No lateral pressure on the septum

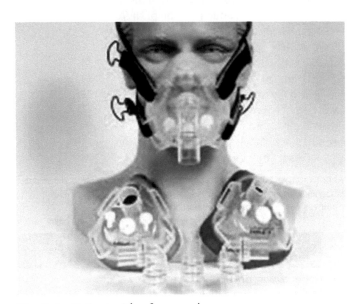

Fig. 3.4 Patient with a face mask.

Table 3.1   Interface choice in NIV

Disease type	Type of mask
1. Non-cooperative patient	Use full mask
2. Acute short-term diseases	Use oronasal mask
3. Chronic prolonged cases	Use a nasal mask

Table 3.2   Comparison of nasal pillows and face mask

Nasal pillows	Face mask
• Pressure range of 3–20 cm H_2O	• Tight seal
• Significant leak from mouth	• Advantage: good seal
• Advantage: comfort and patience compliance	• Disadvantages:

• Disadvantage: gas leak, nasal dryness, or discharge	➢ Patient noncompliance
	  ➢ Potential dangers of regurgitation and aspiration
	  ➢ Asphyxiation
	  ➢ Alarm and monitor are necessary

Table 3.3   Troubleshooting with interface

Problem	Resolution
Air leaks	• Adjust head gear • Try chin strap • Try spacers or foam pads • Try different masks
Pressure points, sore or dry eyes	• Adjust head gear • Change spacers or foam pads • Try different masks
Nasal congestion or discharge	• Adjust positive pressure setting • Add filter • Add humidity
Nasal airway drying	• Increase fluid intake • Increase room humidity • Try nasal saline- or water-based lubricant
Skin break down irritation	• Adjust or try another head gear • Use spacers, foam pad • Resize mask • Change to different cleaning solutions
Sensitive front teeth	• Adjust head gear
Head gear problem	• Try smaller or different masks • Try disposable head gears • Try larger head gear which also has a range from 2 to 20 cm H_2O

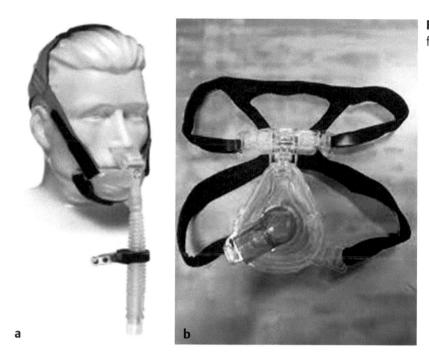

Fig. 3.5 Images showing nasal pillows **(a)** and face mask **(b)**.

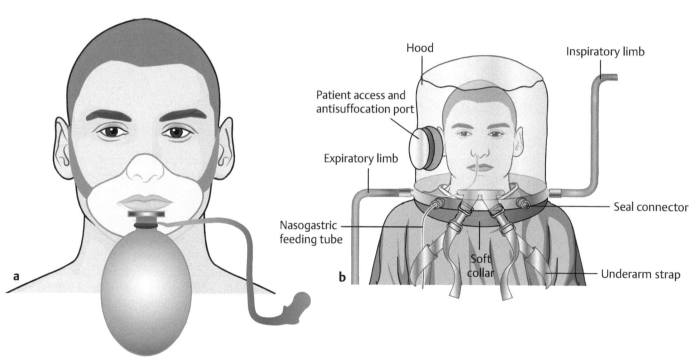

Fig. 3.6 **(a)** Nasal mask with nonrebreathing bag; **(b)** noninvasive ventilation (NIV) helmet.

An oxygen hood (**Fig. 3.6a, b**) providing an FiO$_2$ of up to 50% to the patient (**Fig. 3.6b**) shows another NIV interface called the nonrebreathing mask, which has a flap-type valve between the bag and the mask to ensure oxygen-enriched air to enter the patient during inspiration with good oxygen flow. Reservoir bag should be full during inspiration. This can generate an FiO$_2$ of up to 0.6 with flows up to 10 L/min. It has been extensively used during the COVID pandemic period to save many lives. Others as shown in **Fig. 3.7** deliver oxygen

to the patients at different rates. NIV can be used well for assessing the extubation potential with synchromised inermittent minute ventilation (SIMV) and CPAP.

Nasal Mask

They are available in various sizes and shapes and consists of a small transparent device, which covers patients' nose and is secured to their head by straps. A nasal mask offers several advantages over a full-face mask and is better tolerated by

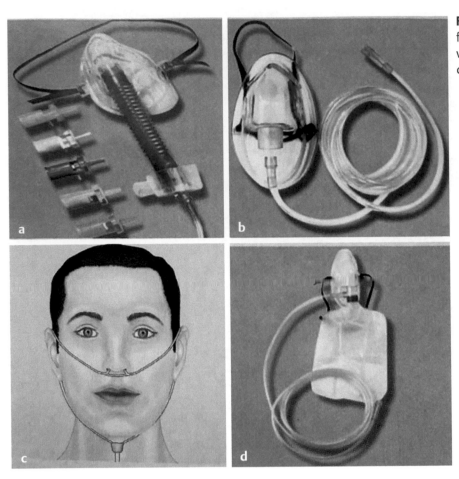

Fig. 3.7 (a–d) Showing different interfaces for noninvasive ventilation (NIV) delivery with different oxygen concentration delivery.

claustrophobic patients. It allows patients to cough and they can clear respiratory secretions. Patients can speak, eat, and drink while on nasal mask. Due to their small size they have less dead space.

The main problems with nasal mask are skin irritation and air leaks, especially in mouth breathers. The most common site of skin irritation is over the nasal bridge. To avoid skin irritation, the operator must ensure that the strap is not too tight, and the straps should be loose enough to pass one finger between the strap and the patient's face. Newer masks have features which minimize skin irritation such as forehead spacers so the gap between forehead and mask can be varied accordingly. Another important feature is gel-filled cushions (usually silicon) around mask to avoid leakage and minimize skin trauma. For prevention of air leak in mouth breathers a chin strap may be used to hold mouth closed during NIV administration. Nasal minimasks with head gear are also available which avoids contact with nasal bridge. Nasal pillows and nasal cushions consist of soft silicon or rubber pledges which can fit into patient's nostrils and help in better compliance.

Nasal masks and other interfaces are less commonly used in acute care settings as most acutely sick patients tend to breath from mouth, thus making the ventilation less effective. However, these are the most commonly used interfaces for domiciliary NIV.

Oronasal Mask

Also known as full-face mask, it covers nose and mouth, thus helping patients who have high oral leak through nasal masks. It is the most common type of interface used in acutely ill patients. It has problems of claustrophobia, poor communication and feeding, and risk of aspiration if vomiting occurs. Earlier, there used to be risk of asphyxia if ventilator malfunction occurred but these days most masks have a release valve to allow room air breathing if ventilator dysfunction happens.

Other Interfaces

There may be an entire face mask like a hood or helmet which is comfortable and causes no pressure necrosis and is evenly distributed around the face; lip seals/mouthpieces are used in patients with neuromuscular disorders.

Portable NIV Machine

It is mandatory as an intensivist to learn how to set up an NIV machine with all precautions (**Box 3.16**).

Choosing the Correct NIV Ventilator

Depending upon many factors, the correct NIV ventilator is indicated for each patient. The availability and familiarity of the NIV ventilator by the intensivist, along with the cast,

---

Box 3.16   Machine setup

- Humidifier with 1 L bag of water, adequate humidity prevents drying of secretions
- Oxygen flow: 6–10/L min which help in washing out carbon dioxide, compensates leak, generates adequate pressure
- Occlude the pressure line connection port with the white plug provided
- For CPAP, default pressure is 4–6 cm H_2O
- Pressure up to 10 cm H_2O can be used
- For BiPAP-IPAP 15 cm H_2O, EPAP 5 cm H_2O pressure is set

Abbreviations: BiPAP, bilevel positive airway pressure; CPAP, continuous positive airway pressure; IPAP, inspiratory positive airway pressure.

Box 3.17   BiPAP (pressure limited ventilation)

- IPAP: 15 cm H_2O—controls peak inspiratory pressure during inspiration
- EPAP: 5 cm H_2O—controls end expiratory pressure, PEEP when IPAP > EPAP
- Provides IPAP and EPAP
- CPAP when IPAP = EPAP
- Predetermined aspiratory pressure is delivered
- This causes different tidal volumes, depending on the resistance of the respiratory system
- Leak compensation

Abbreviations: BiPAP, bilevel positive airway pressure; CPAP, continuous positive airway pressure; EPAP, expiratory positive airway pressure; IPAP, inspiratory positive airway pressure.

Box 3.18   Continuous positive airway pressure (CPAP) monitoring 3/3

- After setting CPAP—pulse oximetry and the number of apnea episodes are monitored
- Polysomnography is used to fine-tune CPAP level
- Autotitration
- RAMP—gradually increases pressure
- C-FLEX—provides pressure relief during exhalation
- Provided breath to breath basis

---

and the level of ventilator support required by the patient are all factors pointing toward choosing the correct equipment. Choice depends upon the use of portable or stationary bigger NIV equipment as well.

The Portable Bilevel NIV Ventilators

Commonly referred to as the BiPAP ventilators are pressure targeted with a single system gas delivery port which permits intentional leakage to facilitate patient exhalation, this BiPAP machine is pressure limited, time and flow cycled and triggered. It has a IPAP ranging from 2 to 30 cm H_2O and an EPAP of 5 cm H_2O setting.

BiPAP: It is a pressure-limited ventilation mode. When the IPAP is equivalent to the EPAP, then BiPAP can function as CPAP. BiPAP provides leak compensation breath (one-third CPAP) and is used as a treatment modality in OSA and when two-thirds CPAP is applied then it is used for some oral applications such as prosthetic mandibular advancements, tonsillectomy, etc. (**Box 3.17**).

CPAP mode: The patient in this mode breathes spontaneously, so the rate and tidal volume are set as per the patient's efforts (**Box 3.18** and **Table 3.4**).

Pressure Support Ventilation

In this mode of NIV, the pressure is set during inspiration. In the pressure support ventilation (PSV) mode, the IPAP and EPAP are set by the intensivist, with a gap between the two, with a certain level of support given at each breath. Since the tidal volume required by the patient is set to some extent, in PSV the flow generally reduces usually to prefixed value of nearly 40 to 60% of the peak flow. In another mode called the noninvasive S/T mode, the intensivist has to present the optimal respiratory rate, IPAP, and EPAP. So, a breath is then triggered by the patient and the PSV mode then ensues. In case the patients fail to trigger the breath, then it is similar to PSV. This PSV mode has a backup option; thus it is great for patients with congestive heart failure because of rise time that the ventilator makes (**Fig. 3.8a**). This machine is appropriate for making the patient comfortably and maintain the oxygenation by reducing the work of breathing to better oxygen monitoring (**Fig. 3.8a, b**).

Table 3.4   Continuous positive airway pressure monitoring 2/3

Apnea-hypoapnea index	Desaturation index	Risk factors	Treatment	Surgical
Average number of apnea in each hour of sleep during the test	Average number of oxygen desaturation of 4% or more from baseline	History of snoring, obesity, increased neck circumference, hypertension, and family history	Oral applications, prosthetic mandibular advancement	Tonsillectomy and uvulopalatopharyngoplasty

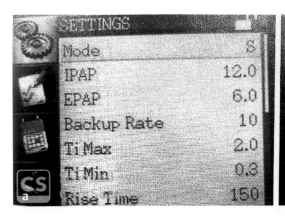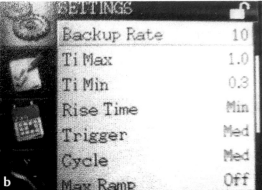

Fig. 3.8 (a, b) Ventilator screenshot showing rise time and back-up rate in pressure support ventilation (PSV) mode.

These ventilators have advantages of delivering a better H_2O monitoring; CPAP and PSV can be combined together with volume controlled ventilation (VCV) and PSV, if needed in some patients; it allows for leak compensation in most models available. The disadvantages are in case an NIV model does not have leak compensation, then patient's ventilator asynchrony may occur with increase in work of breathing (WOB) and decrease in PaO_2 (**Box 3.19**).

Indications of Noninvasive Ventilation

The use of NIV is indicated in various diseases associated with acute and chronic respiratory failure.

Acute Respiratory Failure

NIV is considered life-saving in ARF as it has several advantages over invasive mechanical ventilation. The goal of NIV is to improve gas exchange by unloading the respiratory muscles and thus improving ventilation. Application of EPAP helps offset auto-PEEP and thus reduces the work required to initiate ventilation. The IPAP helps in inspiration and thus increasing tidal volume.

Acute Hypercapnic Exacerbation of COPD

Hyperinflation is the hallmark of COPD and leads to auto-PEEP and alveolar hypoventilation. The main role of NIV in acute exacerbations of COPD (AECOPD) is to help patients increase their tidal volumes without loading the respiratory muscles. This is achieved by improving alveolar ventilation and reducing respiratory muscle overload. This one indication of NIV has strongest evidence to support its use as it reduces need for intubation, ICU stay, and mortality. The presence of respiratory acidosis and arterial pH between 7.25 and 7.35 in a COPD patient is a definite indication for NIV. In addition, evidence of benefit of NIV even in drowsy

---

Box 3.19 Three Modes of PSV

- Pressure support: set pressure during inspiration
- Pressure control: set the number of breaths per minute at set pressure
- Bilevel positive airway pressure: delivers different pressures during inspiration and expiration
- Main indications are:
  - ➤ Acute respiratory failure
  - ➤ COPD exacerbation
  - ➤ Not improving on CPAP: provides increased airway pressure during expiration, but it may add inspiratory assistance, thereby reducing WOB

Abbreviations: COPD, chronic obstructive pulmonary disease; CPAP, continuous positive airway pressure; PSV, pressure support ventilation; WOB, work of breathing.

---

patients with severe acidemia (pH < 7.25) has been demonstrated, albeit under strict monitoring settings.

Asthma

Acute severe asthma is not considered as a classical recommended indication for NIV. However, a few cohort studies have shown beneficial effects of NIV in asthma patients who have continued to worsen despite optimal medical management present. There are no specific recommendations for NIV use. It may also be used in ICU setting to prevent intubation.

NIV for Nonintubated Patients

NIV is primarily used in those patients who are difficult or not-to-intubate, old, severely debilitated and frail, and with advanced malignancy. These are some of the conditions which are managed well with NIV. NIV may be a life changer in advanced malignancy as a palliative measure. The prognosis of NIV depends upon the primary underlying disease, rather than NIV alone (**Boxes 3.20–3.22**).

Box 3.20 Noninvasive ventilation (NIV) for weaning from intubation

NIV used in three special categories:
- Extubation to NIV in which standard weaning criteria are not followed. However, NIV in this category does not show any benefit.
- NIV for extubation when standard weaning criteria is followed. This is used to prevent reintubation in sick patients like COPD and asthma who have high $PaCO_2$ at extubation.
- NIV for postextubation respiratory failure. This mode of NIV is not practiced commonly today, as it increases the hospital length of ICU stay and mortality.

Abbreviations: COPD, chronic obstructive pulmonary disease, PaCO2, partial pressure of carbon dioxide.

Box 3.21 Predictors of success in NPPV

- Young age
- Low acuity of illness
- Able to cooperate
- Able to coordinate breathing with ventilator
- Less air leaking, intact dentition
- Hypercarbia >45 but <92 mmHg
- Acidemia, pH 7.1–7.35
- Improvement of HR, RR, and gas exchange within the first 1 h

Abbreviations: HR, heart rate; NPPV, noninvasive positive pressure ventilation; RR, respiratory rate.

Box 3.22 Criteria for failure of NPPV

Major criteria
- Respiratory arrest
- LOC
- Psychomotor agitation requiring sedation
- Hemodynamic instability: HR < 50/min with loss of alertness

Minor criteria
- RR > 35/min and higher than as recorded on admission
- Arterial pH < 7.3
- PaO_2 < 45 despite oxygen supplementation
- Presence of weak cough

Notes: Presence of one major criterion is an indication of immediate intubation. Presence of two minor criteria after 1 h of treatment is considered an indication of intubation.

Abbreviations: LOC, location of care; NPPV, noninvasive positive pressure ventilation; RR, respiratory rate.

Noninvasive Ventilation in Bronchoscopy

Bronchoscopy procedure in severely ill may cause further deterioration and lead to hypoxemia and intubation. NIV may be useful in sick patients during bronchoscopy, but more data is needed for same.

Box 3.23 Indications for noninvasive ventilation (NIV) for not-to-intubate patients

Following patients who cannot be intubated benefit with NIV:
- Extremely difficult to intubate patient
- Advanced malignancy
- High frailing index patient
- Old age

Box 3.24 Indications for domiciliary noninvasive ventilation (NIV)

- Obesity
- COPD
- Neuromuscular diseases
- Hypoventilation syndrome

Abbreviation: COPD, chronic obstructive pulmonary disease.

Box 3.25 Noninvasive ventilation (NIV) and neuromuscular diseases

This is a class I indication for NIV

NIV → ↑ gas exchange:
- Improves respiratory muscle function
- Improved quality of life and psychosocial function

For restrictive disorders like:
- Chest wall deformities
- Neuromuscular diseases
- Weakness in respiratory muscles
- Hypoventilation

Noninvasive Ventilation Before Intubation

In a patient with bag and mask, if preoxygenation using a mask with high FiO_2 and hypoxemia persists, then NIV may help in achieving good oxygenation, just before intubation (**Box 3.23**).

Noninvasive Ventilation in Chronic Respiratory Failure

At home settings, NIV is used as BiPAP or CPAP with increasing ease and comfort to the patient because of sleek and portable NIV machines and better interfaces. The indications for domiciliary NIV are listed in **Box 3.24** and include obesity, COPD, neuromuscular diseases, and hypoventilation syndromes.

Neuromuscular Diseases

NIV is essential in patients with neuromuscular disorders too (**Box 3.25**). NIV improves the patients' psychosocial function and quality of life.

Initiation of Noninvasive Ventilation

After careful patient and interface selection, the process of NIV initiation should be explained in detail to the patient in simple language. This improves patient compliance with NIV attachments. The initial set pressure must be low to improve patient comfort, usually an EPAP of 2 to 4 cm H_2O and IPAP of 6 to 8 cm H_2O. Patient or operator should hold the mask to face before tying the straps so that he/she may become familiar with the mask and air pressure. When patient becomes comfortable then straps should be tied and it should be loose enough to allow finger insertion between strap and cheek (**Fig. 3.9a**). We should also check for leaks from mask and try to minimize it while not compromising patient comfort (**Fig. 3.9b**). Gradually, pressure may be increased as per patient's requirement.

Not all patients with neuromuscular diseases or OSA or chronic COPD will require NIV. Although CPAP remains the number one treatment of choice for OSA, titration of therapy to the individual patient's condition is imperative. Murphy et al[4] have emphasized the timely access to overnight eagle-eyed monitoring, and titration of NIV may be a challenge in some difficult situations as was found in COVID-19 patients recently.[5]

NIV Complications and Side Effects

Use of noninvasive mechanical ventilation (NIMV) has increased during the past few years. In acute exacerbation of COPD, it is now considered the ventilator mode of first choice. For treatment of acute pulmonary edema, CPAP alone is very effective. NIMV reduces the chances of end tracheal intubation in hypoxemic respiratory failure. It is also used to facilitate weaning from invasive ventilation (**Box 3.26**). NIMV is the first choice in patients with neuromuscular diseases and chest wall deformity.

NIV is a safe method of treating respiratory failure and most of the complications are related to the mask and inadequate monitoring. Serious complications like aspiration pneumonia and pneumothorax are uncommon. Complications of NIV are also many and every intensivist should be aware of it. Aerophagia and gastric distension may occur especially when high pressures are used. Aspiration pneumonia may occur, especially in patients who vomit while on oronasal mask. Ryles tube insertion is beneficial to prevent gastric distension and thus preventing aspiration but it may lead to increased leak from the mask. Sometimes due to inadequate humidification mucus plugging causing lung atelectasis may occur in patients with poor cough reflex. Finally, hypotension and respiratory arrest may develop if not monitored carefully.

Most of the complications of NIV are preventable and manageable if detected in time, which makes NIV a safe therapeutic option in carefully selected patient population.

Box 3.26 Side effects of noninvasive ventilation (NIV)
• Air leak
• Skin necrosis: particularly over the bridge of nose
• Retention of secretions due to decreased clearance
• Gastric distention due to aerophagia and aspiration
• Failure to ventilate
• Sleep fragmentation
• Upper airway obstruction

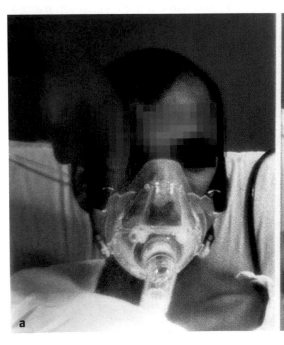
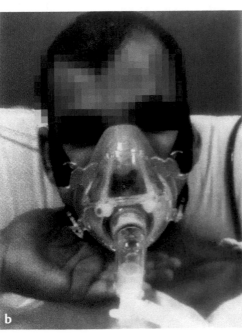

Fig. 3.9 (a, b) Noninvasive well-fitting mask to tackle hypercapnea in the ICU.

> **Box 3.27** Weaning from noninvasive ventilation (NIV)
> - Based on clinical improvement and stability of patient's condition
> - Studies show RR < 24/min
> - HR < 110/min
> - Compensated pH > 7.5
> - SpO_2 > 90% on FiO_2 < 4 L/min

Weaning from Noninvasive Ventilation

The duration of NIV therapy depends on the primary illness and its clinical course. In the absence of clear guidelines, NIV weaning is dependent primarily upon the physician's assessment (**Box 3.27**). There are mainly three methods of weaning:

- Immediate withdrawal.
- Gradual reduction of IPAP and EPAP to a minimum level before discontinuation.
- Gradual day-by-day reduction of duration of NIV before discontinuation. None of the methods is deemed superior to another. While keeping patients off NIV, supplemental oxygen should be given wherever required. Patients should be closely monitored for respiratory distress and fatigue. Some patients with hypoventilatory disorders, such as chronic hypercapnia due to COPD or obesity hypoventilation syndrome, may require nocturnal NIV for a longer period.

Conclusion

NIV can be used both in hospital and at home. NIV provides improved patient outcomes in both acute and chronic respiratory failure. The net of the underlying pathological disease, enhancing the patient comfort, seems the best strategy to improve the NIV rate of success, especially when NIV is administered for a prolonged period of time, also in combination with APP as rescue therapy. Accordingly, a strict comfort assessment with the "ad hoc" corrective measures is mandatory to prevent NIV discontinuation related to poor patient's tolerance.[11]

References

1. Seyfi S, Amri P, Mouodi S. New modalities for non-invasive positive pressure ventilation: A review article. Caspian J Intern Med 2019;10(1):1–6
2. Newsome AS, Chastain DB, Watkins P, Hawkins WA. Complications and Pharmacologic Interventions of Invasive Positive Pressure Ventilation During Critical Illness. J Pharm Technol 2018;34(4):153–170
3. Murphy PB, Suh ES, Hart N. Non-invasive ventilation for obese patients with chronic respiratory failure: Are two pressures always better than one? Respirology 2019;24(10):952–961
4. Masa JF, Mokhlesi B, Benítez I, et al; Spanish Sleep Network. Long-term clinical effectiveness of continuous positive airway pressure therapy versus non-invasive ventilation therapy in patients with obesity hypoventilation syndrome: a multicentre, open-label, randomised controlled trial. Lancet 2019; 393(10182):1721–1732
5. Marin JM, Soriano JB, Carrizo SJ, Boldova A, Celli BR. Outcomes in patients with chronic obstructive pulmonary disease and obstructive sleep apnea: the overlap syndrome. Am J Respir Crit Care Med 2010;182(3):325–331
6. Wang Z, Wang Y, Yang Z, et al. The use of non-invasive ventilation in COVID-19: a systematic review. Int J Infect Dis 2021;106:254–261
7. Praud J-P. Long-term non-invasive ventilation in children: current use, indications, and contraindications. Front Pediatr 2020;8:584334
8. Amaddeo A, Khirani S, Frapin A, Teng T, Griffon L, Fauroux B. High-flow nasal cannula for children not compliant with continuous positive airway pressure. Sleep Med 2019;63:24–28
9. Samannan R, Holt G, Calderon-Candelario R, Mirsaeidi M, Campos M. Effect of Face Masks on Gas Exchange in Healthy Persons and Patients with Chronic Obstructive Pulmonary Disease. Ann Am Thorac Soc 2021;18(3):541–544
10. Patel BK, Wolfe KS, Pohlman AS, Hall JB, Kress JP. Effect of Noninvasive Ventilation Delivered by Helmet vs Face Mask on the Rate of Endotracheal Intubation in Patients With Acute Respiratory Distress Syndrome: A Randomized Clinical Trial. JAMA 2016;315(22):2435–2441
11. Cammarota G, Simonte R, De Robertis E. Comfort during Noninvasive Ventilation. Front Med (Lausanne). 2022; 9:874250

4

Ventilation-Associated Pneumonia

Poonam Malhotra Kapoor, Sumit Aggarwal, and Rashmi Singh

Introduction

Critically ill patients in the intensive care unit are moribund and vulnerable. They often succumb to virulent infections. The main organs chiefly infected are the lungs, urinary tract, and soft tissues and skin. The commonest site besides the oral cavity to be infected remains the lung. A common manifestation of this is infection from the ventilators leading to ventilator-associated pneumonia or VAP as it is commonly called by most physicians. VAP has adverse outcomes; if not diagnosed and treated early it remains part of hospital-acquired pneumonia (HAP) which is chiefly iatrogenic (**Fig. 4.1**).

of a viral pandemic like COVID-19, that we globally witnessed in 2020–2022) also results in VAP.[1] The literature showed COVID-19 to be associated with a higher risk of VAP. The COVID viremia causes a pulmonary dysbiosis, which brings in secondary infections like bacterial activation as well.[2] So viral infection makes patients susceptible to develop VAP. Definition of VAP as given by the European CDC criteria (**Box 4.1**) is now universally followed by most intensivists: any significant growth with colony forming unit (CFU) of >104/mL (on bronchoalveolar lavage [BAL]) or >105/mL endotracheal aspirate (ETA) on mass spectrometry with microbiological and bacteriological criteria as defined in **Box 4.1**.[3–5]

Types of VAP

As enumerated in **Table 4.1**, VAP is of two types: early and late onset VAP whether it is accruing within or after 4 days.

Organisms Causing VAP

Organisms causing VAP are generally bacteria, but other pathogens like fungi and virus (especially after the outbreak

Table 4.1 Types of ventilation-associated pneumonia (VAP)

	Prognosis	Onset	Organism
Good	Early onset VAP	Onset within 4 d	Sensitive organism
Worst	Late onset VAP	After 5 d or more	Multidrug-resistant (MDR) organism

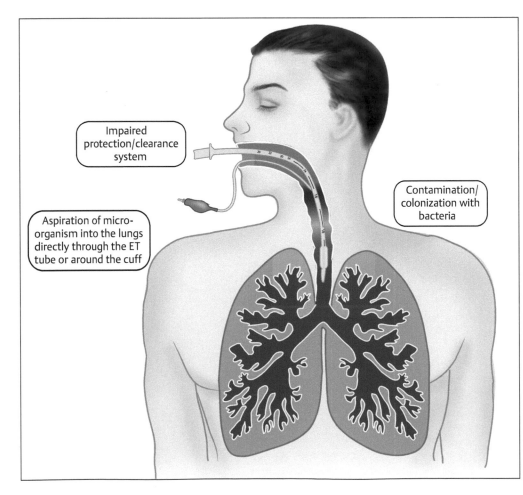

Fig. 4.1 Ventilator-associated pneumonia (VAP), observed from the endotracheal (ET) tube to the upper and lower respiratory tract. So the mouth and lungs are commonest culprits.

Impaired protection/clearance system

Contamination/ colonization with bacteria

Aspiration of microorganism into the lungs directly through the ET tube or around the cuff

Box 4.1 Ventilator-associated pneumonia (VAP) case definition—adapted from European Centre for Disease Control (EDC)

- A combination of radiological and microbiological criteria for patients who have been receiving mechanical ventilation for at least 48 h

Radiological
- New or worsening infiltrates on chest X-ray or CT thorax

Clinical
AND at least one of the following:
- Fever (>38°C or 100.4°F) with no recognized cause
- Leukopenia (<4000 WBC/mm³) or a leukocytosis (>12,000 WBC/mm³)

AND at least one of the following:
- New onset of purulent sputum, or change in character of sputum (color, odor, quantity, consistency)
- Suggestive auscultation (rales or bronchial breath sounds), rhonchi, wheezing
- Worsening gas exchange (e.g., PaO_2/FiO_2, $\leq$240), increased oxygen requirement, increased ventilator demand

Microbiological
Bacteriologic diagnostic performed by:
a) Positive quantitative culture from minimally contaminated lower respiratory tract (LRT) specimen (PN1)
- Bronchoalveolar lavage (BAL) with a threshold of >10 colony forming units (CFU)/mL
- Detection by TaqMan array with Ct <32
OR
- Positive quantitative culture from possibly contaminated LRT specimen (PN2)
- Quantitative culture of LRT specimen (e.g., endotracheal aspirate) with a threshold of 10 CFU/mL

Adapted from the European Centre for Disease Control definitions to meet local thresholds for quantitative culture of endotracheal aspirate and for the inclusion of molecular detection of pathogens (measured in Ct-cycles to threshold by quantitative PCR).[6]

Incidence of VAP in Cardiac ICU

The clinically defined pneumonia based on clinical and radiological criteria of VAP is for those patients who are on mechanical ventilation (MV) for more than or equal to 48 hours. This definition by CDC,[7] as described earlier too, does not take into consideration the methods of sample (e.g., tracheal aspirate procurement, from the lower respiratory tract, or using a nonbronchoscopy BAL).[8] Besides the clinical and radiological study, we also studied critically the organisms involved in the pneumonia etiology. The incidence of VAP is widely based as it depends on the definition of VAP and the timing of population studied, ranging from 9 to 27%. The highest incidence is in the phase of early ICU stay. As the duration of MV increases, the incidence of VAP increases. This increase in VAP incidence is shown in **Table 4.2**. There is an average increase in incidence by 1% by day, as days of MV increase.

Table 4.2 Incidence of VAP in ICU

% per day	Number of days
3% per day	First 5 d
2% per day	5–10 d of ICU stay
1% per day	After 10 d
Maximum VAP	First 4 d
35–70% of ARDS patients develop VAP	

Abbreviations: ARDS, acute respiratory distress syndrome; ICU, intensive care unit; VAP, ventilation-associated pneumonia.

Box 4.2 Indicators for ventilation-associated pneumonia (VAP)

- Primary diagnosis of trauma
- CNS, respiratory, or cardiac illness
- Witnessed aspiration
- Use of paralytic agents
- Diabetic, alcoholic, hypotensive, azotemia patients on enteral feeding
- Surgery in supine position
- Malignancy
- Severe illness (APACHE > 18)
- Older age of patient
- Presence of comorbidities such as influenza and pneumo-coccus in OR, pseudomonas and S. aureus are all prone to cause VAP with the staph aureus in bronchiectasis and MRSA in diabetics and alcoholics
- Inappropriate antibiotics
- Excessive antacids
- Steroid therapy
- Routine change of ventilator

Abbreviations: APACHE, Acute Physiology and Chronic Health Evaluation; CNS, central nervous system; MRSA, methicillin-resistant *Staphylococcus aureus*; OP, oropharynx.

Box 4.3 Etiology of ventilation-associated pneumonia (VAP)

- Aspiration of oral or esophageal content
- Direct inoculation of lower airways during intubation
- Infected aerosol inhalation
- Endotracheal tube (ETT) infection
- Bloodstream infection

There are indicators of VAP as MV days increase. These predictors are enlisted in **Box 4.2**. These predilections are generally associated with the occurrence of aspiration of oropharyngeal and/or esophageal contents. A direct attack by the virulent pathogens in the lower airways such as during intubation or presence of infected aerosol inhalation and spread through blood are all predictions of VAP development (**Box 4.2**) as are certain risk factors which when present predispose the patients to the development of VAP.

Besides the factors causing increased incidence and the etiology of VAP (**Box 4.3**) in mechanically ventilated, ICU

> **Box 4.4** Risk factors increasing the incidence of ventilation-associated pneumonia (VAP)
>
> - Concurrent steroid therapy
> - Inappropriate antibiotic use
> - Sedatives and use of gastroprotective agents
> - Chronic dialysis patients
> - Immunosuppressive therapy
> - Chronic hospitalization for greater than 2 d in the last 90 d
> - Current hospitalization for more than 5 d
> - Antibiotic resistance high in ICU

> **Box 4.5** Commonest microorganisms implicated in ventilation-associated pneumonia (VAP)
>
> **Early onset VAP bacteria:**
> - *Streptococcus pneumoniae* (and other *Streptococcus* species)
> - *Haemophilus influenza*
> - Methicillin-resistant *Staphylococcus aureus* (MRSA)
> - Antibiotic-sensitive gram-negative bacteria
> - *Escherichia coli*
> - *Klebsiella pneumonia*
> - *Enterobacter* species
> - *Proteus* species
>
> **Late onset VAP typical microorganisms:**
> - Multi-drug resistant (MDR) bacteria
> - Methicillin-resistant staphylococcus aureus (MRSA)
> - Acinetobacter
> - *Pseudomonas aeruginosa*
> - Extended spectrum beta-lactamase-producing organisms (ESBL)
>
> **Organisms in the lower respiratory tract causing VAP:**
> - *Streptococcus viridians*
> - *Corynebacterium* spp. and coagulase-negative staphylococcus spp. aureus (CNS)
> - *Neisseria species*
>
> **VAP due to polymicrobial infection:**
> - Aspergillosis and influenza virus
> - Fungal and viral infection mixed with MDR bacteria

> **Box 4.6** Sources causing lower ventilator-associated pneumonia (VAP)
>
> - Microaspiration during intubation
> - Endotracheal tube (ETT) site biofilm development which is full of bacteria (gram-negative bacteria and fungi)
> - Pooling of secretions around ETT
> - Impairment of mucociliary removal of secretions with gravity due to ongoing mechanical ventilation

patients, there are many other risk factors (**Box 4.4**) which precipitate VAP. Multidrug resistance pathogens emerge and are the toughest organisms to treat. The increased risk of mortality in VAP patients remains high. VAP may not be implicated as the sole cause of severe illness.

Iatrogenic cause in the ICU can be pathogens reaching the lung from various sites like tracheal aspirate, hands of caregivers, ventilator circuits, and endotracheal tube (ETT) biofilms especially around the cuff of the tube. Polymicrobial microorganisms cause nearly 25 to 40% of VAP in the cardiac ICU. The common microorganism causing VAP are enlisted in **Box 4.5**. The commonest of them all are *Pseudomonas aeruginosa*, *Staphylococcus aureus*, and *Klebsiella pneumoniae*.[8,9]

Approximately 50% of the antibiotics given in the ICU are for the development of VAP; it seems VAP has grave prognosis in intubation patients, as both early (within 4 d) and late implicated VAP (multidrug resistance [MDR] bacteria; beyond 4 d), from around the ETT site (**Box 4.6**). VAP when prolonged not only has adverse outcomes, but also is a healthcare burden in terms of cost.

The commonest organisms implicated remain the gram-negative bacteria, which include *K. pneumoniae*, *P. aeruginosa*, *Acinetobacter*, and *E. coli*. The gram-positive bacteria like methicillin-resistant *Staphylococcus aureus* (MRSA) are also common, leading to polymicrobial infection. The presence of a particular species varies among heterogenic population and ICU to ICU. The mixed and MDR infections leading to antibiotic resistance are a disaster in VAP prognosis. The commonest organism causing VAP in cardiac ICUs and in neuro ICU is the methicillin resistant *Staphylococcus aureus* (MRSA).

Pathogenesis of VAP

The mechanically ventilated patient in the ICU is (1) moribund, (2) supine, (3) lacks cough reflex, thus having no mucociliary clearance physiological mechanisms, (4) has no innate humoral or cellular immunity intact, (5) has poor mental sensorium due to sedation, and (6) remains on heavy doses of antibiotics. All above factors predispose to increased mortality in MV patients, but the incidence of VAP today has beneficial preventive strategies.[10]

The attributable mortality of VAP would be 33 to 50% but its incidence and pathogenesis vary, depending on the etiology of the underlying disease causing VAP.[11,12,13]

It is the mixed airway gastrointestinal tract which gets infested with pathogenic organisms (**Flowchart 4.1**) with aspiration, ETT contamination, biofilm, etc., which are the culprits for VAP formation.

Diagnosis of VAP

There is still a lack of consensus for gold standard diagnostic criteria for VAP today. There are clinical and radiological criteria that help diagnose a VAP, but every sick patient in the ICU is not a VAP either, according to the American Thoracic Society (ATS) guidelines. ATS recommends a third diagnostic criteria, which is the microbiology sampling of the lower airways using a BAL or a protected specimen brush (PSB; **Boxes 4.7–4.9**).[14]

VAP is generally suspected when an individual develops a new or progressive infiltrate on a chest radiograph

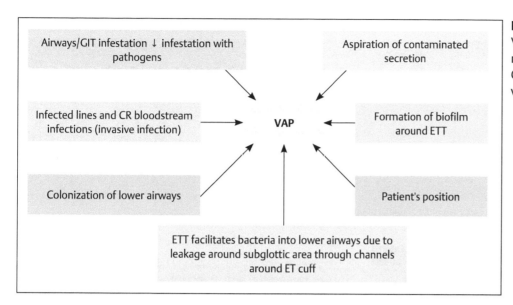

Flowchart 4.1 Pathogenesis of VAP. Abbreviations: CR, catheter-related; ETT, endotracheal tube; GIT, gastrointestinal tract; VAP, ventilator-associated pneumonia.

Box 4.7 Clinical diagnosis of ventilator-associated pneumonia (VAP) according to American College of Chest Physicians (ACCP) and Centers for Disease Control (CDC)

- Ventilator-associated pneumonia definition by ACCP: presence of new, persistent pulmonary infiltrates not otherwise explained appearing on chest radiographs at least of the following criteria are also required as a part of the clinical diagnosis:
  ➢ Temperature of more than 38°C
  ➢ Leukocytosis of more than 10,000 cells/mm³
  ➢ Purulent respiratory secretions
  ➢ Gas exchange degradation
- Pneumonia is VAP when:
  ➢ It occurs postintubation
  ➢ Never due to preintubation preincubation of pathogens in the airways

Box 4.8 Centers for Disease Control (CDC) radiological criteria for ventilator-associated pneumonia (VAP)

- On two or more chest X-rays, it is VAP
- New or progressive or persistent infiltration
- Consolidation
- Cavitations

Box 4.9 Criteria used to delineate the clinical and ABG diagnosis of ventilator-associated pneumonia (VAP)

- Device-associated module:
  ➢ Bloodstream infection (CLABSI—central line-associated bloodstream infection)
  ➢ Central line insertion practice (CLIP) adherence
  ➢ Urinary tract infection (CAUTI—catheter-associated urinary tract infection)
  ➢ Pediatric ventilator-associated events (PedVAE) (NICU and pediatric locations of plane only)
  ➢ Ventilator-associated events (VAE) (adult locations only)
  ➢ Pneumonia (VAP—ventilator-associated pneumonia): in pediatric locations (in-plane and off-plane), or NICU and adult locations (off-plane only)[15]
- Procedure-associated module:
  ➢ Surgical site infection (SSI)
- Antimicrobial use and resistance module (AUR)
- Coronavirus Infections Disease 2019 (Covid-19) module (off-plane only):
  ➢ Patient impact and hospital capacity pathway
  ➢ Healthcare worker staffing pathway
  ➢ Healthcare supply pathway
- Multidrug-resistant organism and clostridium difficile infection (MDRO/CDI) module

Abbreviation: ABG, arterial blood gas.

with endocytosis and purulent tracheobronchial secretions. The accepted clinical criteria (**Box 4.7**) were found to be of limited value and thus other criteria such as radiological, microbiological, and analytical have been added to make it a complete and thorough diagnostic criteria (**Boxes 4.7, 4.9, 4.10**).

The CDC definition of VAP involves the radiological definition which requires at least two or more serial chest X-rays, which satisfy at least one of the radiological criteria listed in **Box 4.8**.

The criteria in **Box 4.9** delineate the clinical and arterial blood gas (ABG) criteria for VAP. Ideally the presence of at least two of the total four criteria is needed to make a final diagnosis of VAP. The clinical criteria include (1) fever, (2) leukopenia or leukocytosis, and (3) at least one of the previous two. The second criteria include at least one of the following parameters:[1] purulent or change in character of infection (e.g., sputum or[2] on auscultation rales or bronchial breath sounds), rhonchi or wheezing, or[3] worsening of gas exchange with desaturation due to increased oxygen requirement or

Table 4.3 Clinical pulmonary infection score

Variable	Points		
	0	**1**	**2**
Temperature, °C	≥36.1 to ≤38.4	≥38.5 to ≤38.9	≥39 to ≤36
WBC count, µL	≥4000 to ≤11000	<4000 to >11000	
Secretions	Absent	Present, nonpurulent	Present, purulent
PaO_2/FiO_2	240 or ARDS		≤240 and no ARDS
Chest radiography	No infiltrate	Diffuse or patchy infiltrate	Localized infiltrate
Microbiology	No or light growth	Moderate or heavy growth	

Abbreviations: ARDS, acute respiratory distress syndrome; WBC, white blood count.

Box 4.10 VAP diagnostic criteria

- *Radiological criteria:* New or progressive infiltrates, cavitations, consolidation, or pneumatoceles
- *Clinical criteria:* Worsening of gas exchange; and three of the following criteria:
  - ➤ Temperature instability
  - ➤ White blood cell count <4000/mm³ or >15,000/mm³
  - ➤ New onset in purulent sputum or increase in respiratory secretion, apnea or tachypnea, wheezing or rales or rhonchi
  - ➤ Cough: heart rate <100 bpm or >170 bpm³
- *Analytical criteria:* Positive culture of alveolar lavage using a blind-protected catheter (>10³ CFU/mL)

---

increased ventilation demand, requiring greater oxygen.[2,3] **Table 4.3** sums up the entire clinical, radiological, and arterial blood gas criteria, as laid down by the CDC and ACCP (combined with microbiological criteria as well).

Microbiological Methods for VAP Diagnosis

Most intensivists feel the need to adopt the microbiological criteria to optimize the use of the right antibiotic therapy. Literature has shown that specimens procured by bronchoscopy or even without bronchoscopy, but taken from the lower RT, should be procured and then sent for culture, to facilitate best results (**Flowchart 4.2**). The PSB from diseased site is generally dependent upon an X-ray image with samples from the image sites showing maximum endobronchial abnormality. The BAL and PSB samples should be cultured so that the right treatment choices are adopted in a narrow spectrum.[16]

Most studies, however, conclude about BAL culture being the most common microbiological method for diagnosing VAP, with a sensitivity of 71% and specificity of 79.6%. The latter value does suggest that the BAL culture report does not correlate well with the histopathological examination,[17,18] knowing fully well that the diagnostic techniques can alter the rate of diagnosis. Thus, careful

---

1. Ventilator-associated condition (VAC): After 2 days of stability or improvement on the ventilation, patient has at least one of following:
   a. Increase in daily minimum FiO_2, 20% for at least 2 days
   b. Increase in daily minimum PEEP 3 cm H_2O for at least 2 days

↓

2. Infection-related ventilator-associated complication (IVAC): After at least 3 days of mechanical ventilation and within 2 days of worsening oxygenation, the patient has:
   a. Body temperature 38°C or <36°C
   b. WBC count <4000 or >12,000

↓

3. Probable ventilator-associated pneumonia: After at least 3 days of mechanical ventilation and within 2 days of worsening oxygenation, the patient has one of the following:
   A: Purulent secretions and one of the following:
   a. Positive culture of endotracheal aspirate at 10 CFU/mL
   b. Positive culture of BAL at 10 CFU/mL
   c. Positive culture of lung tissue at 10 CFU/mL
   d. Positive culture of protected specimen brush at 10 CFU/mL
   B: One of the following:
   a. Positive pleural fluid culture
   b. Positive lung histopathology
   c. Positive diagnostic test for *Legionella*
   d. Positive diagnostic test on respiratory secretions for influenza virus, adenovirus, respiratory syncytial virus, rhinovirus, human metapneumovirus, or corona virus

Flowchart 4.2 National Health Safety Network algorithm for the diagnosis of VAP.

---

sampling of the RT lavage and trying best to decrease the contamination rate from the upper to lower RT is essential. Also, it is important to adopt sensitive diagnostic tests such as Tachman Array Test (TAQ). Such tests lower the rate of false-negative cultures and help in choosing the right antimicrobial treatment for VAP patients.[19] According to the January 2021 National Healthcare Safety Network (NHSN) guidelines identifying microorganisms from central lines and devices and calculating bloodstream infections (CLABSI)

Table 4.4 Various methods for microbiologic diagnosis and their yield

Methods	Quantitative culture	Sensitivity	Specificity
Endotracheal aspirate	$\geq 10^5$ CFU/mL	76 ± 28%	75 ± 28%
Bronchoscopy BAL PSB	$\geq 10^4$ CFU/mL $\geq 10^3$ CFU/mL	73 ± 18% 66 ± 19%	82 ± 19% 90 ± 15%
Blind mini BAL	$\geq 10^4$ CFU/mL	63 – 100%	66 – 96%
Nonbronchoscopically (NB) obtained (blind) specimens NB-BAL NB-PSB	 $\geq 10^4$ CFU/mol $\geq 10^3$ CFU/mL		

Abbreviations: BAL, bronchoalveolar lavage; PSB, protected specimen brush.

Box 4.11 VAP rate and device utilization ratio

VAP Rate

The VAP rate per 1000 ventilator days is calculated by dividing the number of VAPs by the number of ventilator days and multiplying the result by 1000 (ventilator days).

$$\text{VAP Rate per 1000 ventilator days} = \frac{\text{Number of VAPs}}{\text{Number of ventilator days}} \times 1000$$

Device Utilization Ratio

The ventilator utilization ratio is calculated by dividing the number of ventilator days by the number of patient days. These calculations will be performed separately for the different types of ICUs, SCAs, and other locations in the institution.

$$\text{DUR} = \frac{\text{Number of ventilator days}}{\text{Number of patient days}}$$

and surgical site infections (SSI), etc., by using the standardization utilization ratio (SUR) and the device utilization ratio (DUR) are also wise to be adopted for VAP (**Box 4.11** and **Table 4.4**).

Evaluating the accuracy of sampling to estimate central line-days and having a CLABSI analysis report help determine and analyze the data on the number of devices, tracking device use over shorter periods of time and for internal trend analysis, as well as for initiating and maintaining right therapy,[15,20] when pneumonia occurs in a ventilated patient after 1 or 2 days of ventilation.

For the purpose of clinical testing, organisms are tested either bronchoscopically or nonbronchoscopically. Bronchoscopy experts are adept at performing a mini-BAL as well (**Box 4.9**) wherein a thin catheter is passed through a larger catheter, like a sheath protection, which minimizes antibiotic-related toxicity and any contamination from the proximal airways.

The nonbronchoscopic techniques include mini-BAL, and blind PSB. The advantage of these techniques is that they can be performed by individuals qualified to do bronchoscopy.

Mini-BAL involves insertion of one thin catheter through a large catheter.

Potential Pathogens Implicated in VAP

This can broadly be divided into two categories. VAP develops about 48 hours postintubation. The two categories are (1) those without the risk of developing MDR pathogens and (2) patients who are at a high risk of developing MDR (**Table 4.5**). So, accordingly the guidelines enumerate the appropriate antibiotic required for a particular microorganism that is being isolated.[24,25] Common organisms in VAP are both gram-positive and gram-negative, such as *Streptococcus pneumonia*, *H. influenza*, *Pseudomonas*, *Klebsiella* sp., *Acinetobacter*, and MSRA. The antibiotic regime may vary from ICU to ICU, depending on the local flora (**Flowchart 4.3**). Invasive aspergillosis causing VAP needs an integrative diagnosis with serum galactomannan of the BAL fluid. These patients are in severe respiratory failure. Definitive antibiotic treatment in bacterial VAP should be given for at least 7 days. A few studies have found the male gender to be at a potential risk factor for VAP.[26]

Prevention of VAP

VAP can be prevented by improving the ICU infrastructure. As VAP has a dismissal prognosis, its prevention is of utmost importance, in each ICU. The infection control policy should be known to all in the ICU. Strict adherence to infection control should be followed. Adequate resources and regular surveillance are essential for improved outcomes as an essential communication in the whole ICU staff.[27] Hemodynamic filters and reducing circuit changes is cost-effective and reduces the incidence of VAP. Pharmacological interventions such as decontamination with chlorhexidine in the oral cavity decreases VAP incidence. Having strict protocols for right nutrition (**Boxes 4.12–4.14**) and stress ulcer prophylaxis are other bundles to be adopted, in ICU to reduce VAP.

Table 4.5 Potential pathogens and recommended antibiotics for VAP

For patients with no risk factors for MDR pathogens	
Pathogens	**Recommended antibiotic**
Streptococcus pneumoniae *Haemophilus influenza* MSRA Antibiotic-sensitive gram-negative bacilli: *E. coli*, *Klebsiella*, *Proteus*	Ceftriaxone Levofloxacin, moxifloxacin Ciprofloxacin Ampicillin/sulbactam Ertapenem
For patients with risk factors for MDR pathogens	
Pathogens	**Recommended antibiotic**
Pseudomonas *Klebsiella pneumoniae* *Acinetobacter*	Antipseudomonal cephalosporin (Cefepime/ceftazidime) Antipseudomonal Carbapenem (Meropenem/imipenem) Piperacillin–tazobactam plus antipseudomonal fluroquinolone (Ciprofloxacin/levofloxacin) Aminoglycoside (Amikacin/gentamicin) Linezolid or vancomycin

Abbreviations: MDR, multidrug resistance; MRSA, methicillin-resistant *Staphylococcus aureus*; VAP, ventilator-associated pneumonia.

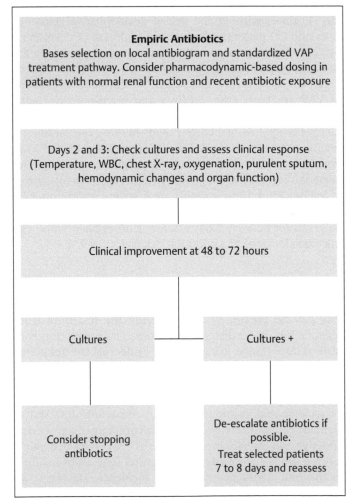

Flowchart 4.3 Use of empiric antibiotics and culture timing in VAP. Abbreviation: VAP, ventilator-associated pneumonia.

Box 4.12 VAP prevention bundle strategies

- Healthcare professional training
- Adherence to hand hygiene guidelines and correct use of sterile gloves prior to the management of ventilation equipment/supplies
- Sterile management of airway
- Avoiding reintubations
- Oral care
- Positioning
- Feeding
- Care of the ventilator circuit
- Checklist

Abbreviation: VAP, ventilator-associated pneumonia.

Box 4.13 Importance of head elevation in neonatal VAP

- Elevation of head of bed to reduce gastric microaspiration is found in most of the studies
- A disparity in grades of elevation from 10 to 45 degrees is noted in several articles on neonates[21,22]
- The highest elevation is of 12 degrees because it is the maximum elevation that the design of incubators allows. This is in accordance with the study by Azab et al[23]

Abbreviation: VAP, ventilator-associated pneumonia.

Treatment of VAP

The treatment of VAP always involves a multitude of antibiotics over a prolonged period of time. Thus, treatment of VAP involves a deeper knowledge of antibiotic types for different organisms, in a staged manner. Local antibiotic sensitivity

> **Box 4.14**   Nutrition in VAP
>
> - Bolus feeding has been related to gastric distension which could facilitate the microaspiration of gastric content to the pharynx and reach the lower respiratory airways
> - Continuous feeding, however, induces changes in gastric pH which can promote gram-negative microorganism proliferation[24,25]
> - Authors decided to standardize feeding rhythm using 60- to 120-min gastroschisis

Abbreviation: VAP, ventilator-associated pneumonia.

> **Box 4.15**   Different stages for the treatment of VAP with antibiotics
>
> - **Stage 1:** Initiate or start the use of broad-spectrum antibiotics
> - **Stage 2:** Stop the antibiotics if no infection is seen
> - **Stage 3:** Once the microorganism is known, start the narrow-spectrum antibiotics
> - **Stage 4:** Optimize the treatment
> - **Stage 5:** Day 3–5 start immunotherapy
> - **Stage 6:** Decrease the antibiotic therapy treatment period to 7–8 d

levels in an institute, with different antibiotic resistances and cross-infection, should be known to all intensivists. It involves different antibiotics given over a prolonged period in different stages as shown in **Box 4.15**. Thus, an in-depth knowledge of giving the right antibiotic in an individualistic manner is important.

If appropriate therapy is not initiated at an appropriate time, mortality due to VAP occurs easily. Today, MDR to antibiotics is found frequently. Organisms such as *P. aeruginosa*, *K. pneumonia*, and *Acinetobacter* are found in VAP cases, as does the gram-positive MRSA; thus, the initial treatment with broad-spectrum antibiotics (Stage 1) is recommended for VAP. The antibiotics taken prior to VAP should be taken into consideration in choosing the same over next few days followed by blood culture and sensitivity to isolate the etiologic agent. Now, the sensitive antibiotic only is given (Stages 2 to 4). De-escalation of antibiotic and shortening its duration is most imperative (Stages 5 and 6). All this involves multiple clinical, microbiological, and radiological assessments at timely intervals. Prolonged antibiotic therapy of 14 to 21 days is essential only for care as VAP may coexist with comorbidities of malnutrition, cavitations, multilobar consolidation, gram-negative necrotizing pneumonia, and isolation of MDR *Pseudomonas* and *Acinetobacter*.

Conclusion

Focusing on preventive period measures such as hand hygiene has been included in all of bundle VAP card

described, since it has been shown to be the most important measure to reduce nosocomial infections and thus VAP. The incidence and density of VAP can be controlled by strict implementation of right infrastructure in the cardiac ICU and communication among the ICU staff for adopting the VAP bundles for prevention of VAP. The incidence of multi-drug-resistant pathogens in VAP can be high, but it has a multi-factorial cause. Initial clinical severity presentation is not associated with multi-drug resistance.[28]

References

1. Maes M, Higginson E, Pereira-Dias J, et al. Ventilator-associated pneumonia in critically ill patients with COVID-19. Crit Care 2021;25(1):25
2. Kollef MH. Is antibiotic cycling the answer to preventing the emergence of bacterial resistance in the intensive care unit? Clin Infect Dis 2006;43(Suppl 2):S82–S88
3. Grasselli G, Zangrillo A, Zanella A, et al; COVID-19 Lombardy ICU Network. Baseline characteristics and outcomes of 1591 patients infected with SARS-CoV-2 admitted to ICUs of the Lombardy Region, Italy. JAMA 2020;323(16):1574–1581
4. Navapurkar V, Bartholdson-Scott J, Maes M, et al. Development and implementation of a customised rapid syndromic diagnostic test for severe pneumonia. medRxiv. 2020. 1–21
5. Chastre J, Fagon J-Y. Ventilator-associated pneumonia. Am J Respir Crit Care Med 2002;165(7):867–903
6. Plachouras D, Lepape A, Suetens C. ECDC definitions and methods for the surveillance of healthcare-associated infections in intensive care units. Intensive Care Med 2018;44(12):2216–2218
7. Vincent J-L, Sakr Y, Singer M, et al; EPIC III Investigators. Prevalence and outcomes of infection among patients in intensive care units in 2017. JAMA 2020;323(15):1478–1487
8. Álvarez-Lerma F, Palomar-Martínez M, Sánchez-García M, et al. Prevention of ventilator-associated pneumonia. Crit Care Med 2018;46(2):181–188
9. Goyal P, Choi JJ, Pinheiro LC, et al. Clinical characteristics of covid-19 in New York City. N Engl J Med 2020;382(24):2372–2374
10. Kalanuria AA, Ziai W, Mirski M. Ventilator-associated pneumonia in the ICU. Crit Care 2014;18(2):208
11. Zolfaghari PS, Wyncoll DL. The tracheal tube: gateway to ventilator-associated pneumonia. Crit Care 2011;15(5):310–317
12. Melsen WG, Rovers MM, Koeman M, Bonten MJM. Estimating the attributable mortality of ventilator-associated pneumonia from randomized prevention studies. Crit Care Med 2011;39(12):2736–2742
13. American Thoracic Society; Infectious Diseases Society of America. Guidelines for the management of adults with hospital-acquired, ventilator-associated, and healthcare-associated pneumonia. Am J Respir Crit Care Med 2005;171(4):388–416
14. Koenig SM, Truwit JD. Ventilator-associated pneumonia: diagnosis, treatment, and prevention. Clin Microbiol Rev 2006;19(4):637–657
15. https://www.cdc.gov/nhsn/pdfs/pscmanual/pcsmanual_current.pdf January 2021
16. Klompas M, Kulldorff M, Platt R. Risk of misleading ventilator associated pneumonia rates with use of standard clinical and microbiological criteria. Clin Infect Dis 2008;46(9):1443–1446

17. Fernando SM, Tran A, Cheng W, et al. Diagnosis of ventilator-associated pneumonia in critically ill adult patients: a systematic review and meta-analysis. Intensive Care Med 2020;46(6):1170–1179

18. Rea-Neto A, Youssef NCM, Tuche F, et al. Diagnosis of ventilator-associated pneumonia: a systematic review of the literature. Crit Care 2008;12(2):R56

19. Asri AK, Pan WC, Lee HY, Su HJ, Wu CD, Spengler JD. Spatial patterns of lower respiratory tract infections and their association with fine particulate matter. Sci Rep 2021;11(1):4866

20. Thrompson ND, et al. Simplication of NHSN surveillance methods: infection control. Hospital Epidemiol 2013;34(3): 221–228

21. Gokce IK, Kutman HGK, Uras N, Canpolat FE, Dursun Y, Oguz SS. Successful implementation of a bundle strategy to prevent ventilator-associated pneumonia in a neonatal intensive care unit. J Trop Pediatr 2018;64(3):183–188

22. Weber CD. Applying adult ventilator-associated pneumonia bundle evidence to the ventilated neonate. Adv Neonatal Care 2016;16(3):178–190

23. Azab SFA, Sherbiny HS, Saleh SH, et al. Reducing ventilator-associated pneumonia in neonatal intensive care unit using "VAP prevention Bundle": a cohort study. BMC Infect Dis 2015;15:314

24. Parker LA, Weaver M, Murgas Torrazza RJ, et al. Effect of gastric residual evaluation on enteral intake in extremely preterm infants: a randomized clinical trial. JAMA Pediatr 2019;173(6):534–543

25. Lin Y, Sun Z, Wang H, Liu M. The effects of gastrointestinal function on the incidence of ventilator-associated pneumonia in critically ill patients. Open Med (Wars) 2018;13:556–561

26. Wu D, Wu C, Zhang S, Zhong Y. Risk factors of ventilator-associated pneumonia in critically ill patients. Front Pharmacol 2019;10:482

27. Jacobs Pepin B, Lesslie D, Berg W, Spaulding AB, Pokora T. ZAP-VAP: a quality improvement initiative to decrease ventilator-associated pneumonia in the neonatal intensive care unit, 2012–2016. Adv Neonatal Care 2019;19(4):253–261

28. Ranzani OT, Niederman MS, Torres A. Ventilator-associated pneumonia. Intensive Care Med. 2022; 48(9):1222–1226

5

Decompensated Heart Failure

Ajmer Singh and Yatin Mehta

Introduction

Heart failure (HF) is a major cardiovascular disease because of its ever-increasing prevalence, substantial morbidity, high mortality, and increasing healthcare costs. It is a major community health issue, responsible for most of the emergency hospital admissions in patients aged 65 years or more. The incidence of HF rises with age, increasing from about 20 per 1,000 persons of 65 to 69 years of age, to more than 80 per 1,000 persons ≥85 years of age.[1] Prevalence of HF is about 5.1 million individuals in the United States, 8 to 10 million individuals in India, and approximately 23 million persons worldwide.[2] The mean age of presentation is lower in India compared to western countries (53 y vs. 65–73 y). The prevalence of HF is on the rise due to improved survival from the comorbid conditions and an overall increase in lifespan.

Definition and Classification

HF is a complex clinical disorder that results from any structural or functional impairment of ventricular filling or ejection of blood. The heart either fails to pump blood at a rate proportionate with the metabolic demand of tissues or is able to pump blood at an elevated diastolic filling pressure. The primary features of HF comprise of shortness of breath, fatigue, and fluid retention, with pulmonary/splanchnic congestion and peripheral edema. While many individuals with HF develop symptoms due to left ventricular (LV) myocardial dysfunction, about 50% of the patients with HF have normal LV size and have preserved ejection fraction (EF).

2013 American College of Cardiology Foundation (ACCF)/American Heart Association (AHA) guidelines for the management of HF have categorized HF into two major classes: (1) HF with reduced (≤40%) EF (HFrEF), and (2) HF with preserved (≥50%) EF (HFpEF).[3] HFrEF is also called systolic HF, and efficacious therapies based on randomized controlled trials (RCTs) have been demonstrated in these groups of patients. HFpEF is referred to as diastolic HF, and its diagnosis is largely based on excluding all possible noncardiac causes of HF. HFpEF group is further divided into (a) HFpEF borderline with EF 41 to 49%, and (b) HFpEF improved with EF >40%, a subgroup of patients who earlier had HFrEF.[3] European Society of Cardiology (ESC) guidelines (2016) have classified HF into three categories based on EF: HFpEF, HFrEF, and HFmrEF (HF midrange with EF 40–49%).[4] Patients suffering from HFpEF normally do not have LV dilatation, but rather have an increased LV wall thickness, and increased left atrial (LA) size due to increased filling pressures. Classification of patients based on EF is essential due to divergent etiologies, comorbid conditions, and therapeutic modalities.

Acute decompensated heart failure (ADHF) manifests as unexpected or gradual worsening of signs and symptoms of HF requiring unintended emergency room visit or hospital admission. It is a fatal medical disorder that requires immediate assessment, stabilization, and management. The cardinal feature of decompensated heart failure (DHF), irrespective of underlying etiology, is pulmonary or systemic congestion resulting from high right- and/or left-sided filling pressure. A preliminary observation from the first 100,000 cases in acute decompensated heart failure national registry (ADHERE) indicates that in-patient and postdischarge mortality rates after HF are 5 and 10%, respectively.[5] More recent study has concluded that the hospitalization for DHF is a strong indicator for repeat admission and postdischarge mortality as high as 20%.[6] It is estimated that only half of the HF patients survive after 5 years of diagnosis.

Precipitating Factors

Approximately 80 to 85% of patients with DHF requiring hospital admission have acute exacerbation of chronic HF, the remaining present with de novo diagnosis of HF. Patients with DHF usually present with pulmonary edema or cardiogenic shock, while those with chronic HF have milder symptoms such as worsening dyspnea or orthopnea. In patients with HF, coronary artery disease (CAD) is seen in 60% of patients, hypertension in 70%, diabetes mellitus in 40%, and renal impairment in 20 to 30% patients.[5] Other comorbid conditions seen with DHF include atrial fibrillation (AF) or atrial flutter (30–46%), valvular heart disease (44%), and dilated cardiomyopathy (25%). The common precipitating factors for DHF requiring hospitalization are listed in **Box 5.1**.[7]

Etiological Factors

HFrEF results mostly from cardiovascular causes, in the form of poor contractile function, whereas HFpEF is caused by noncardiovascular comorbid conditions resulting in impaired

---

Box 5.1 Precipitating factors for decompensated heart failure

- Noncompliance with dietary restrictions
- Noncompliance with medications
- Inadequate medical regimen
- Excessive physical exertion
- Uncontrolled hypertension
- Arrhythmias, myocardial ischemia/infarction
- Initiation of negative inotropic agents
- Nonsteroidal anti-inflammatory drugs
- Alcohol intake
- Infection (e.g., pneumonia)
- Toxins (e.g., ethanol, anthracycline)
- Pulmonary thromboembolism, hypoxemia
- Renal failure, pregnancy
- Cardiac surgery, valvular catastrophe

relaxation and passive stiffness of the LV in majority of the patients. Dilated or restrictive cardiomyopathies, and structural abnormalities of the myocardium, pericardium, valves, or circulatory system, form the majority of causative factors. Etiology of systolic and diastolic HF is shown in **Boxes 5.2** and **5.3**, respectively.

Clinical Manifestations

The clinical manifestations of DHF include dyspnea (due to pulmonary vascular congestion), orthopnea, paroxysmal nocturnal dyspnea, nocturnal angina, and easy fatigability due to low cardiac output (CO). Physical examination may reveal tachycardia, narrow pulse pressure, S_3 gallop, fine pulmonary crackles, tachypnea, peripheral edema, ascites, congestive hepatomegaly, jugular venous distension, hepatojugular reflux, peripheral cyanosis, poor capillary refill, and cold extremities.

Admission to the hospital should be considered in the event of:
- Worsened congestion even without dyspnea.
- Pulmonary or systemic congestion.
- Electrolyte imbalance.
- Coexisting disorders like pneumonia, pulmonary embolism, diabetic ketoacidosis, transient ischemic attack, or stroke.
- Repeated implantable cardioverter defibrillator (ICD) firings.

Hospitalization and intensive care unit (ICU) admission is advised for patients with DHF who have:
- Signs and symptoms of DHF including hypotension, low CO, renal dysfunction, or altered sensorium.
- Dyspnea associated with tachypnea, or oxygen saturation <90% (impending respiratory failure).
- Hemodynamically significant arrhythmia including atrial fibrillation (AF) of new onset.

Box 5.2 Etiology of systolic heart failure

- Left ventricular systolic dysfunction
  - Ischemic cardiomyopathy
  - Dilated cardiomyopathy (idiopathic, viral, familial)
  - Valvular heart disease
  - Hypertensive heart disease
  - Toxin-induced cardiomyopathy
  - Chagas disease
  - Congenital heart disease
  - High output failure
- Right ventricular systolic dysfunction
  - Secondary to left ventricular dysfunction
  - Right ventricular infarction
  - Pulmonary hypertension
  - Chronic severe tricuspid regurgitation
  - Arrhythmogenic right ventricular dysplasia (ARVD)

- Acute coronary syndrome (ACS).
- Need for continuous vasodilator/inotropic support.

Initial Evaluation

For patients presenting for the first time, the possibility of HF should be suspected based on history (hypertension, use of diuretics, CAD), presenting symptoms, physical examination, and resting electrocardiogram (ECG). Physical examination will reveal whether the patient has symptoms/signs of congestion (dry or wet, if absent or present) or hypoperfusion (warm or cold, if absent or present), to guide appropriate therapy (**Table 5.1**).

The tests that are recommended to identify the etiology of HF are: hemoglobin, white blood count, serum electrolytes, renal and hepatic function tests, glucose, glycosylated hemoglobin, lipid profile, and thyroid function test. A 12-lead ECG provides information about heart rate, rhythm, QRS morphology, and QRS duration. The ECG nomenclature for Q, R, and S wave signify ventricular depolarization phase of the cardiac cycle. If ECG and all laboratory parameters are within normal limits, HF is unlikely and if at least one element is abnormal, plasma natriuretic peptides (NPs) should be measured. B-type natriuretic peptide (BNP) is a small peptide secreted by the heart to regulate BP and fluid balance. It is stored in the ventricles in its pro form (proBNP) and released from the heart as N-terminal (NT-proBNP) piece. The upper limit of BNP in the nonacute setting is 35 pg/mL, and for NT-proBNP it is 125 pg/mL. Higher values (BNP < 100 pg/mL,

---

Box 5.3 Etiology of diastolic heart failure

- Myocardial
  - Impaired relaxation
    - Epicardial or myocardial ischemia
    - Myocyte hypertrophy
    - Hypertension
    - Cardiomyopathies
    - Aging
    - Hypothyroidism
  - Increased passive stiffness
    - Diffuse fibrosis
    - Postinfarct scarring
    - Infiltrative myocyte hypertrophy such as amyloidosis and hemochromatosis
- Endocardial
  - Fibroelastosis
  - Mitral stenosis, tricuspid stenosis
  - Pericardial constriction, tamponade
  - Coronary microcirculation impairment
  - Capillary compression
  - Venous engorgement
- Others
  - fluid overload, extrinsic compression by tumor

Table 5.1 Signs and symptoms of congestion

	Congestion (−)	Congestion (+)
Hypoperfusion (−)	Warm, dry	Warm, wet
Hypoperfusion (+)	Cold, dry	Cold, wet

Note: (−) denotes absence while (+) denotes presence.

NT-proBNP < 300 pg/mL) should be used in acute settings. The cut-off values are similar in both HFpEF and HFrEF, although they are lower for HFpEF than for HFrEF.[8,9] Patients with BNP values <100 pg/mL are less likely to have HF, whereas HF is likely if the value is >500 pg/mL. Similarly, HF is likely if NT-proBNP values are >450, >900, and >1,800 pg/mL in patients <50 years, 50 to 75 years, and >75 years of age, respectively. At these cut-off values, the negative predictive values are high (0.94–0.98), but the positive predictive values are lower (0.66–0.67). Therefore, NP estimation is recommended to rule out HF, but not to confirm the diagnosis of HF. Plasma NP levels may be disproportionately high in individuals with AF, old age, and renal failure, and low in obese patients.

An abnormal ECG is commonly seen in patients with HF, but has low specificity. An ECG may provide clue to the etiology (e.g., myocardial infarction [MI]), and it may also provide information about indications for therapy (e.g., anticoagulation for AF, pacing for bradycardia, cardiac resynchronized therapy [CRT] if broadened QRS complex). It is very unlikely for a patient of HF to have normal ECG. ECG has a sensitivity of about 89%; therefore, the routine use of an ECG is recommended to exclude HF. Chest X-ray may show florid alveolar edema, interstitial edema, basal pleural effusions, or pulmonary venous congestion in patients with DHF. Common respiratory conditions leading to HF, such as chronic obstructive lung disease/interstitial lung disease, are better diagnosed with spirometry and computed tomography scan.

Two-dimensional echocardiography with Doppler is the most commonly used modality in patients with suspected HF to confirm the diagnosis. It provides information about chamber size, systolic and diastolic ventricular function, regional and global wall motion abnormalities, EF, wall thickness, valvular function, and pulmonary hypertension.[10,11] While transthoracic echocardiography (TTE) is the preferred technique for the evaluation of ventricular function, transesophageal echocardiography (TEE) may be required when TTE imaging is suboptimal, or in clinical conditions such as infective endocarditis, suspected aortic dissection, intracardiac thrombi, and congenital heart diseases. Doppler echocardiography is useful for evaluation of anatomic and flow abnormalities across valves. Mitral annular velocity, mitral valve inflow pattern, and pulmonary venous inflow pattern provide information about LV filling pressure and LA pressure and help in the diagnosis of HFpEF.

Further Evaluation

A comprehensive echocardiographic examination is recommended for the evaluation of systolic and diastolic function of LV, RV function, and pulmonary artery pressure (PAP) measurement. Assessment of diastolic function of LV is important in patients with HFpEF and HFmrEF, and echocardiography is the best modality to assess diastolic dysfunction. The key echocardiographic findings are LA enlargement (LA volume index > 34 mL/m²) and LV hypertrophy (LV mass index > 115 g/m² for males, >95 g/m² for females). E/e' (ratio between early mitral inflow velocity and mitral annular early diastolic velocity) ratio is the most useful and reproducible method of estimating LV filling pressure. The functional alterations seen in diastolic HF are E/e' >14, septal e' velocity <7 cm/s, lateral e' velocity <10 cm/s, and tricuspid regurgitation systolic jet velocity >2.8 m/s.[12] RV function is assessed by measurement of RA/RV dimensions, PAP, an estimation of tricuspid annular plane systolic excursion (TAPSE), and tricuspid lateral annular systolic velocity (s'). A TAPSE of <17 mm and an s' wave velocity <9.5 cm/s indicate RV systolic dysfunction. Stress echocardiography may be helpful for the diagnosis of inducible myocardial ischemia, myocardial viability, dynamic mitral regurgitation, and low-flow low-gradient aortic stenosis.

Cardiac catheterization criteria for the diagnosis of HFpEF include: an increase in LV end diastolic pressure (LVEDP) <16 mmHg with preserved LV systolic function and normal ventricular volumes. Cardiac magnetic resonance (CMR) is considered gold standard for the assessment of ventricular volume, mass, and EF. CMR can differentiate between ischemic and nonischemic etiologies of HF and assessment of myocardial structure and function in patients with congenital heart diseases, myocarditis, cardiomyopathy, amyloidosis, sarcoidosis, Chagas disease, etc. Coronary angiography is advocated in patients who suffer from unstable angina despite medical therapy, ventricular arrhythmia or who have had cardiac arrest. It is also recommended in patients with intermediate to high likelihood of CAD on noninvasive stress test, to confirm the diagnosis and severity of CAD. Right heart study with pulmonary artery catheter (PAC) is advocated for severe HF patients, being considered for cardiac surgery, heart transplantation, or mechanical circulatory support (MCS). Invasive monitoring should be considered in selected patients admitted to ICU with persistent symptoms refractory to standard therapies or those who require parenteral vasoactive medications.

Treatment

DHF is a life-threatening disease, occurring with rapid onset or aggravation of symptoms and signs of HF. It requires urgent admission to the hospital, thorough evaluation, initiation of appropriate therapy to facilitate early discharge, and to prevent rehospitalization. Echocardiography is helpful in patients with hemodynamic instability to rule out acute mitral regurgitation, ventricular septal rupture, pulmonary embolism, or aortic dissection. It is recommended to monitor the arterial oxygen saturation (SpO_2) by pulse oximetry. Oxygen therapy is advocated for patients with SpO_2 of <90% or PaO_2 of <60 mmHg. Noninvasive positive pressure ventilation (NIPPV) either as continuous positive airway pressure (CPAP) or bilevel positive pressure ventilation (BiPAP) should be considered in patients with respiratory rate >25/min, SpO_2 < 90%, pulmonary edema, and acidemia to improve minute ventilation. Mechanical ventilation with endotracheal intubation is recommended in patients with respiratory failure, that is, those with PaO_2 < 60 mmHg, $PaCO_2$ > 50 mmHg, pH < 7.35, reduced consciousness, and physical exhaustion who cannot be managed noninvasively.

Intravenous loop diuretics (20–40 mg of furosemide or 10–20 mg of torasemide) are recommended for patients of DHF admitted with features of hypervolemia. Diuretics administered intermittently or via continuous infusion increase renal salt and water excretion and provide symptomatic relief in these patients. Intravenous vasodilators (nitroglycerine, isosorbide dinitrate, nitroprusside, and nesiritide) are the second commonest group of drugs used in DHF for symptomatic relief. They act by reducing preload/afterload and by increasing stroke volume. Vasodilators are useful in hypertensive HF, but should be used with caution in patients with stenotic valvular lesions. For vasodilators, the recommended doses are: Nitroglycerine @ 10–20 µg/min to 100 µg/min, Isosorbide dinitrate @ 1–10 mg/h, nitroprusside @ 0.3–5 µg/kg/min, nesiritide @ 2 µg/kg bolus followed by 0.01 µg/kg/min. Inotropes are generally used for patients with hypotensive HF with severe reduction in cardiac output and perfusion (cardiogenic shock). Patients with cardiogenic shock should be referred to a tertiary care center which has a facility of cardiac catheterization, cardiac ICU, and short-term mechanical circulatory shock (MCS). The commonly used inotropes include: dobutamine (2–20 µg/kg/min), dopamine (3–5 µg/kg/min), epinephrine (0.05–0.5 µg/kg/min), milrinone (0.375–0.75 µg/kg/min after a bolus of 50 µg/kg), levosimendan (0.05–0.2 µg/kg/min). Dobutamine is the most commonly used agent, while phosphodiesterase (PDE) III-inhibitor may be a suitable alternative in nonischemic patients. Levosimendan, in combination with vasopressors, may be used to improve cardiovascular hemodynamics without risk of producing hypotension. Vasopressors (commonly used agent norepinephrine @ 0.2–1 µg/kg/min) can be considered in patients with cardiogenic shock to increase BP and vital organ perfusion. Vasopressin antagonist such as tolvaptan may be helpful in patients with fluid overload and hyponatremia. Thromboprophylaxis with heparin or low-molecular-weight heparin (LMWH) is recommended unless contraindicated to minimize the chances of deep vein thrombosis and pulmonary embolism in patients who are not anticoagulated.[4]

Chronic care for ADHF includes a number of nonpharmacologic, pharmacologic, and invasive methods to limit the disease process and reverse its clinical effects. Depending on the severity of the disease, nonpharmacologic modalities include sodium restriction (2–3 g/day) and fluid restriction (2 L/day), appropriate physical activity, and avoidance of weight gain. Pharmacologic therapies consist of diuretics, vasodilators, anticoagulants, beta-blockers, digoxin, and inotropic agents. Ivabradine, an $I_{(f)}$ inhibitor, is recommended in patients with symptomatic HF with LVEF ≤ 35%, who are in sinus rhythm with HR ≥ 70 per minute.[13] A combination of sacubitril and valsartan, an angiotensin receptor neprilysin inhibitor (ARNI), has shown a reduction in risk of cardiovascular death and hospitalization in patients with NYHA class III–IV and HFrEF.[14] Invasive therapies for HF include cardiac resynchronization therapy (CRT), pacemakers, and ICDs. Additional therapies include revascularization procedures such as coronary artery bypass grafting (CABG) and percutaneous coronary intervention (PCI), valve replacement or repair, and ventricular restoration. Heart transplantation has been the gold standard for progressive end-stage HF patients on maximal medical therapy. MCS devices recommended for short-term use include intra-aortic balloon pump (IABP), extracorporeal membrane oxygenator (ECMO), Impella, Transcore, and Centrimag, etc. Ventricular assist devices (VADs) and total artificial hearts (TAHs) can be used as bridge to transplantation, although VADs are increasingly being used as permanent therapy.[15]

Conclusion

Hospitalizations for DHF and prevalence of HF are on the rise due to an increased number of older patients, as well as due to refinement in therapeutic modalities that have enabled patients to live longer with cardiovascular disease. Optimal treatment for DHF is based on the precise diagnosis of underlying etiology. The goals of therapy for hospitalized patients are to promote diuresis, restore normal volume status and electrolyte balance, and minimize the complications. Treatment with nonpharmacological, modern pharmacological, and surgical therapies can substantially reduce the morbidity and mortality associated with DHF. New technologies can be challenging from the beginning because the precise indication for use and the success and failure criteria are not completely defined. Likewise, medical societies should be agile enough to introduce those criteria with new technologies before their approval and integration into clinical practice.[16]

References

1. Curtis LH, Whellan DJ, Hammill BG, et al. Incidence and prevalence of heart failure in elderly persons, 1994–2003. Arch Intern Med 2008;168(4):418–424

2. Chaturvedi V, Parakh N, Seth S, et al. Heart failure in India: The INDUS (INDia Ukieri Study) study. J Pract Cardiovasc Sci 2016;2:28–35

3. Yancy CW, Jessup M, Bozkurt B, et al. 2013 ACCF/AHA guideline for the management of heart failure: a report of the American College of Cardiology Foundation/American Heart Association Task Force on Practice Guidelines. Circulation 2013;128:1810–1852

4. Ponikowski P, Voors AA, Anker SD, et al; ESC Scientific Document Group. 2016 ESC guidelines for the diagnosis and treatment of acute and chronic heart failure: the task force for the diagnosis and treatment of acute and chronic heart failure of the European Society of Cardiology (ESC)Developed with the special contribution of the Heart Failure Association (HFA) of the ESC. Eur Heart J 2016;37(27):2129–2200

5. Adams KF Jr, Fonarow GC, Emerman CL, et al; ADHERE Scientific Advisory Committee and Investigators. Characteristics and outcomes of patients hospitalized for heart failure in the United States: rationale, design, and preliminary observations from the first 100,000 cases in the Acute Decompensated Heart Failure National Registry (ADHERE). Am Heart J 2005;149(2):209–216

6. Ahmed A, Allman RM, Fonarow GC, et al. Incident heart failure hospitalization and subsequent mortality in chronic heart failure: a propensity-matched study. J Card Fail 2008;14(3):211–218

7. Fonarow GC, Abraham WT, Albert NM, et al; OPTIMIZE-HF Investigators and Hospitals. Factors identified as precipitating hospital admissions for heart failure and clinical outcomes: findings from OPTIMIZE-HF. Arch Intern Med 2008;168(8):847–854

8. Roberts E, Ludman AJ, Dworzynski K, et al; NICE Guideline Development Group for Acute Heart Failure. The diagnostic accuracy of the natriuretic peptides in heart failure: systematic review and diagnostic meta-analysis in the acute care setting. BMJ 2015;350:h910

9. Maisel A, Mueller C, Adams K Jr, et al. State of the art: using natriuretic peptide levels in clinical practice. Eur J Heart Fail 2008;10(9):824–839

10. Paulus WJ, Tschöpe C, Sanderson JE, et al. How to diagnose diastolic heart failure: a consensus statement on the diagnosis of heart failure with normal left ventricular ejection fraction by the Heart Failure and Echocardiography Associations of the European Society of Cardiology. Eur Heart J 2007;28(20):2539–2550

11. Lang RM, Badano LP, Mor-Avi V, et al. Recommendations for cardiac chamber quantification by echocardiography in adults: an update from the American Society of Echocardiography and the European Association of Cardiovascular Imaging. Eur Heart J Cardiovasc Imaging 2015;16(3):233–270

12. Nagueh SF, Smiseth OA, Appleton CP, et al. Recommendations for the evaluation of left ventricular diastolic function by echocardiography: an update from the American society of echocardiography and the European association of cardiovascular imaging. J Am Soc Echocardiogr 2016;29(4):277–314

13. Swedberg K, Komajda M, Böhm M, et al; SHIFT Investigators. Ivabradine and outcomes in chronic heart failure (SHIFT): a randomised placebo-controlled study. Lancet 2010;376(9744):875–885

14. McMurray JJ, Packer M, Desai AS, et al; PARADIGM-HF Investigators and Committees. Angiotensin-neprilysin inhibition versus enalapril in heart failure. N Engl J Med 2014;371(11):993–1004

15. Stewart GC, Givertz MM. Mechanical circulatory support for advanced heart failure: patients and technology in evolution. Circulation 2012;125(10):1304–1315

16. de Oliveira Cardoso C, Elgalad A, Li K, Perin EC. Device-based therapy for decompensated heart failure: An updated review of devices in development based on the DRI2P2S classification. Front Cardiovasc Med. 2022; 9:962839

6

Hyponatremia in Heart Failure

Poonam Malhotra Kapoor, Archana Malhotra Jain, and Pranav Kapoor

Introduction

Heart failure (HF) is emerging as one of the major causes of mortality in the developed and the developing world. Studies have shown that low serum sodium is associated with increased mortality in patients with HF.

Hyponatremia is defined as serum Na concentration below 135 mmol/L or mEq/L. Mild hyponatremia is defined as a serum sodium concentration between 130 and 135 mEq/L, and moderate hyponatremia as sodium concentration between 125 and 129 mEq/L or less.

Hyponatremia is the most common electrolyte abnormality encountered in patients hospitalized with HF. The hyponatremia occurring in HF is mostly hypotonic hyponatremia where the plasma osmolality is less than 280 mOsm/kg H_2O.

Mechanisms of Hyponatremia in HF

Mechanisms of hyponatremia in HF are manifold:
- Nonosmotic release of arginine vasopressin (AVP) due to reduced cardiac output, decreased renal blood flow and baroreceptor stimulation mediated by low arterial blood pressure. This is the most important mechanism of hyponatremia in HF.
- Renal vasoconstriction will reduce glomerular filtration rate (GFR) and will enhance sodium and water reabsorption.
- Potent thirst stimulation mediated by both low cardiac output and angiotensin II.
- HF therapy-related diuretics, including thiazides, rid the body of salt and water.

All these will lead to relative excess of water to solute in the extracellular fluid.

Drug-Induced Hyponatremia

Diuretics are one of the most common causes of drug-induced hyponatremia especially in patients with HF. Diuretics causing hyponatremia fall in the category (**Table 6.1**) of drug-induced hyponatremia, with maximal incidence caused by thiazides (73%) and least by furosemide (2%). The thiazide

Table 6.1 Incidence of type of diuretics-induced hyponatremia in heart failure[1]

Diuretic name	Incidence
Thiazides	73%
Thiazide potassium-sparing diuretics	20%
Furosemide	2%

diuretics do not interfere with any urinary concentration and act through the distal convoluting tubules only, unlike the loop diuretics which act through concentrating and diluting mechanisms; thus, loop diuretics do not generally cause hyponatremia, whereas thiazide diuretics cause worst hyponatremia in HF patients.[1] More diuretics use in newly initiated users than in long-term users and all types of diuretics except thiazides have been discussed by Holland-Bill et al[2] as a negative prognostic factor in patients admitted with hyponatremia. The absolute risk of an HF patient for the development of hyponatremia, which demands patient hospitalization, however, was found by Mannheimer et al to be modest.[3]

The combination of hydrochlorothiazide and amiloride confers an increased risk of hyponatremia. Amiloride causes enhanced sodium loss, as it has a direct effect on the collecting tubule. Also, it has a potassium-sparing effect, wherein, in the distal convoluting tubule of the nephron, potassium is exchanged for sodium thus causing greater sodium loss. Indapamide administration too has been implicated in diuretic-induced hyponatremia. Hyponatremia with thiazides occurs more just on initiation and more so within one month of the thiazide initiation.[4] It has been suggested to have a detailed list of absolute risk factors and time course of thiazide initiation, with good communication within the treating team. This is a prerequisite to prevent this drug-induced hyponatremia. While dealing with hyponatremia in COVID-19 patients, a U-shaped pattern was found in the relationship between admission serum sodium level and the hospital mortality, despite all compensations and treatment for illness severity, comorbidity, and demographics (**Fig. 6.1**). Both hyponatremia and hypernatremia were associated with increased mortality. A serum sodium value of 140 mEq/L was used as a reference value (**Table 6.2**). Patients with moderate-to-severe hyponatremia in COVID-19 showed greater mortality. **Flowchart 6.1** highlights the steps involved in therapy of diuretic-induced hyponatremia.

Clinical Features of Hyponatremia in Heart Failure

The clinical manifestations of hyponatremia are mainly due to central nervous system (CNS) dysfunction which is secondary to cerebral edema. Symptoms of hyponatremia vary according to the duration and severity of hyponatremia. For example, at a serum sodium concentration of ≤120 mEq/L, patients present with seizures and coma, while patients with chronic hyponatremia may tolerate these low sodium levels and can remain asymptomatic.[5]

Usually in patients with decompensated HF or chronic HF, hyponatremia is a relatively slowly evolving process. In such patients, gastrointestinal symptoms (nausea and vomiting)

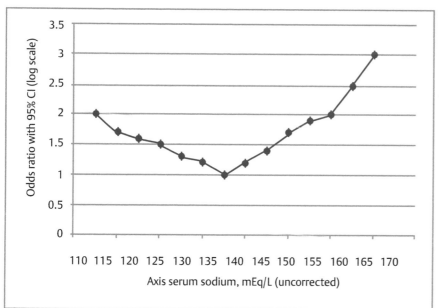

Fig. 6.1 The association of serum sodium at hospital presentation and mortality demonstrated a U-shaped pattern. Both hyponatremia and hypernatremia were significantly associated with mortality, which was more pronounced at the extremes of serum sodium, even after adjustment for demographic, comorbid conditions and illness severity.

Table 6.2 Types of hyponatremia

Types of hyponatremia	Na⁺ levels (in mEq/L)
Normonatremia	136–144
Moderate/severe hypernatremia	≥150
Mild hypernatremia	145–149
Moderate/severe hyponatremia	<130
Mild hypernatremia	130–135

and disorientation are the most frequent symptoms. Motor and gait disturbances along with attention-deficit problems leading to falls are reported to be common in patients with even mild hyponatremia (**Box 6.1**).[6]

Consequences of Hyponatremia in Heart Failure

Hyponatremia is a powerful determinant of mortality in patients with HF regardless of ventricular function. Severity of hyponatremia parallels the severity of cardiac dysfunction. Na level less than 125 mmol/L is usually associated with end-stage HF. It has been shown that hyponatremia is relatively common in HF patients with left ventricular (LV) dysfunction and is independently associated with increased risk factor and it is reported that low sodium at hospital admission is predictive of longer hospital stay and increased mortality (**Box 6.2**).[7,8]

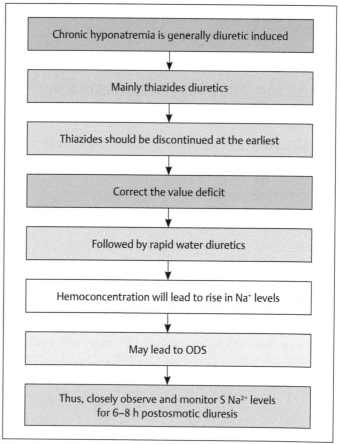

Flowchart 6.1 Therapy for diuretics induced hyponatremia. Abbreviations: ODS, osmotic demyelination syndrome; S Na, serum sodium.

Box 6.1 Clinical features of hyponatremia in heart failure

- Nausea, vomiting
- Headache
- Confusion
- Fatigue; loss of energy
- Insufficient urine production
- Mental confusion
- Restlessness, irritability
- Muscle weakness
- Spasms or cramps
- Seizures, coma

Box 6.2 Consequences of persistent hyponatremia in heart failure

- Higher rates of heart failure
- Osteoporosis and fractures with persistent hyponatremia
- Higher rates of hospitalization
- Decreased neurological function
- Increased risks of adverse events
- Cerebral edema
- Decreased mental function

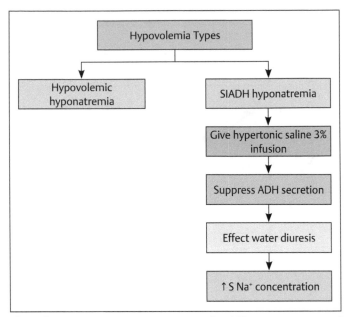

Flowchart 6.2 Management of different types of hypovolemia. Abbreviations: ADH, antidiuretic hormone; S Na, serum sodium; SIADH, syndrome of inappropriate secretion of antidiuretic hormone.

Management of Hyponatremia in Heart Failure

The treatment of hyponatremia depends on the following factors:

- Duration—whether it is acute hyponatremia or chronic.
- Severity of hyponatremia.
- Neurological status—acute (<48 h) symptomatic hyponatremia warrants urgent treatment.[7]

Hyponatremia in patients with chronic HF is mainly due to the effect of AVP.

Fluid Restriction

Fluid is restricted to less than 800 to 1000 mL/d in order to achieve a negative water balance. However, many patients with HF have increased feeling of thirst, which reduces the compliance to this mode of therapy. But this modality should be tried in all patients.

Loop Diuretic Therapy

Loop diuretics act by bringing about salt-free water excretion, which is termed as "water diuresis," which is very beneficial in fluid overloaded (positive balance) HF patients. Loop diuretic therapy alone may lead to worsening; also secondary to renin-angiotensin-aldosterone (RAA) stimulation in the HF patient. A combination of furosemide and

angiotensin-converting enzyme inhibitor (ACEI) has shown to be effective in correcting chronic hyponatremia associated with HF.[9]

Hypertonic Saline

Repletion of the extracellular volume by infusion of saline corrects the hypovolemia and removes the volume stimulus for vasopressin release in the circulation. Osmolality in hyponatremia due to syndrome of inappropriate secretion of antidiuretic hormone (SIADH) is decreased. Vasopressin release remains under the influence of osmolality which is low (**Flowchart 6.2**). Infusion of hypertonic saline (3% NaCl) is the mainstay of treatment of acute symptomatic hyponatremia (**Box 6.3** and **Flowchart 6.3**). The concern regarding infusion of hypertonic saline is that the sudden volume expansion achieved can acutely worsen HF. The other concern is the neurological side effects associated with rapid correction of sodium levels. There are few reports of combination of hypertonic saline and loop diuretic therapy, which reported efficacy and also safety in patients with HF.[10]

Vasopressin Receptor Antagonists

Recent addition to the treatment of hyponatremia is a group of drugs called vasopressin receptor antagonists. These agents bring about an increase in the solute-free exertion by the kidneys and thus enhance sodium levels. This group of agents blocks the activation of the endogenous AVP by

Box 6.3 Uses of hypertonic saline 3%

- Increases blood pressure in hypovolemia shock (Grade A)
- Resuscitates in nonobstructive cardiogenic shock (Grade C)
- Can cause hypernatremic shock as in cardiopulmonary resuscitation (CPR) when given with hypertonic saline sodium bicarbonate
- Inadvertent IV hypertonic saline is used for therapeutic purposes
- Therapy for cerebral edema with head trauma patients
- Helpful in postoperative edema post head trauma

Abbreviation: IV, intravenous.

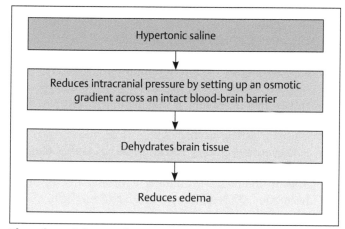

Flowchart 6.3 Mechanism of action of hypertonic saline.

Box 6.4 Antidiuretic hormone (ADH) receptors, their subtypes, placement, and actions

- ADH receptors are the G protein coupled cells present on membrane receptors
- There are two cell types (V1 and V2) of ADH receptors
- V1 receptors are further divided into two types: V1a and V1b receptors
- V1a receptors are present on vascular smooth muscles
- V1b receptors (present on anterior pituitary and pancreas) release calcium (Ca_{2+}) from intracellular stores
- Actions of ADH receptors are:
  - ➤ Vasoconstriction
  - ➤ Visceral smooth muscle contraction
  - ➤ Glycogenolysis
  - ➤ Platelet aggregation
  - ➤ ACTH release arachidonic acid leading to generation of prostaglandins
- The result of persistent V1 effect is growth of vascular smooth muscles

Abbreviation: ACTH, adrenocorticotropic hormone.

Box 6.5 Types of vaptans used in hyponatremia

Vaptans are a class of drugs having various components with selective affinity for the vasopressin receptors.
Unselective (Mixed) (VlA and V2 RA):
- Conivaptan

VlA selective (V2 RA):
- Relcovaptan

VlB selective (V2RA):
- Nelivaptan

V2 selective (V2 RA):
- Lixivaptan
- Mozavaptan
- Satavaptan
- Tolvaptan

Demeclocycline and Lithium:
- Antidote to vasopressin used in SIADH to block the action of AVP
- Lithium carbonate is similar in action

Abbreviations: AVP, arginine vasopressin; SIADH, syndrome of inappropriate secretion of antidiuretic hormone.

binding to the V2R receptors in the body. This leads to a process called "aquarists" or solute-free water excretion. The examples of some of these drugs are listed in **Box 6.4** and include conivaptan, tolvaptan, sataptan, and lixivaptan to be used for oral and intravenous use. Conivaptan blocks both V1a and V2 receptors and thus can be given intravenously, whereas the other three are oral agents, which block only V2 receptors (**Box 6.4**).[11]

Vaptans are only to be used for euvolemic or hypervolemic hyponatremia and not for hypovolemic and hypervolemic type of hypernatremia, wherein isotonic saline 0.9% is given (**Box 6.5**).

Tolvaptan is the drug which is available in India. The starting dose is 15 mg on day 1, and the dose titrated to 30 and 60 mg at 24-hour intervals. The dose titration is based on the very frequent Na estimations (6–8 hourly). Up titration of the dose is recommended if the Na levels remain below 135 mmol/L or the 24-hour rise in Na levels is below 5 mmol/L.

One of the limitations of vaptans is increase in thirst which may prevent rise in sodium, which again can be controlled to certain extent by combining with ACEI/angiotensin receptor blockers (ARBs).

One of the major side effects of tolvaptan is liver toxicity. The Food and Drug Administration (FDA) recommends that treatment should be limited to less than 30 days and patients with underlying liver disease including cirrhosis should avoid tolvaptan therapy (**Box 6.6**).[12]

For resistant symptomatic HF with persistent hyponatremia, intermittent or continuous ultrafiltration is also occasionally found to be effective.

Box 6.6 Major side effects of vaptans
Gastrointestinal symptoms:
• Increased thirst or urination
• Dry mouth
• Loss of appetite
• Constipation
• Weakness
• Fruity breath odor
• Drowsiness
• Dry skin
• Feeling confused, mood change
• Dehydration symptoms
• Liver problems may go into liver failure
Metabolism and nutritional symptoms:
• Hyperglycemia
• Anorexia
Renal and urinary disorders:
• Polyuria

Box 6.7 Risk factors that may precipitate an osmotic demyelination syndrome
• Serum Na^{2+} levels <105 mEq/L
• Hypokalemia
• Alcoholism
• Malnutrition
• Advanced liver disease
• Rapid 3% NaCl transfusion

Treatment of Acute Symptomatic Hyponatremia in Patients with Heart Failure

Urgent treatment protocols are mandatory when symptoms like seizures, confusion, or drowsiness exist due to hyponatremia. A sign of acute hyponatremia is herniation of brain, a fatal complication.

Correction Should be Done Slowly

It is imperative, while correcting the low sodium levels, to correct the same in an hourly manner, that is, using hypertonic saline (3% NaCl) to increase serum sodium by 1 to 2 mEq/L per hour, till all neurological symptoms improve. It has been seen that 4 to 6 mmol/L increase in sodium is adequate to a bolus of 100 mL of 3% NaCl. The latter increases sodium by 2 mEq/L.[13]

Osmotic Demyelination Syndrome

When hyponatremia is corrected very rapidly, the brain's ability to recapture lost osmolytes is outpaced leading to osmotic demyelination. The osmotic demyelination present clinically as a bimodal pattern, with initial improvement in neurological symptoms followed by development of severe and even permanent neurological deficits. It is observed that when rapid correction of hyponatremia is done, then neurological symptoms persist in the first 48 to 72 hours itself, then residual sequelae such as locked-in syndrome

and spastic quadriparesis are observed. **Box 6.7** shows the factors that place a hyponatremia patient at a greater risk of developing the osmotic demyelination syndrome (ODS).

The recommendations of the Third International Consensus Development Conference in California in 2015 still holds true.

- The rate of infusion of saline need not be restricted in patients with true acute hyponatremia.
- For patients with severe symptoms, the first days' correction can be done in the first 6 hours of therapy and subsequent treatment platooned to the next day. This strategy is described as "rule of sixes," six a day makes sense for safety, so six in 6 hours and stop.
- For severe symptoms, 100 mL of 3% NaCl infused intravenously over 10 minutes +3 as required.
- Mild-to-moderate symptoms with low risk of brain herniation, 3% NaCl infused at 0.5 to 2 mL/kg/h.

It is recommended that the rate of sodium correction should not exceed beyond a limit. In chronic hyponatremia, it is recommended that the correction limits should not exceed 8 mmol/L in any 24-hour period in those who are at high risk of ODS. In patients who are at normal risk of ODS, the proposed limits are 10 to 12 mmol/L in any 24-hour period and 18 mmol/L in any 48-hour period.

It is a common practice to withhold loop diuretics in patients with HF when they develop hyponatremia. This can worsen outcomes of patients as persistent clinical congestion is associated with poor outcomes in patients with HF.

Since vaptans can be used as concomitant therapy along with loop diuretics in patients with HF, this becomes an attractive therapeutic option. Tolvaptan is the most studied molecule among vaptans in patients with HF. Post-hoc analysis of trials like acute and chronic therapeutic impact of vasopressin (ACTIV) and efficacy of vasopressin antagonism in HF outcome study with tolvaptan (EVEREST) have shown that there is benefit by captain therapy in HF, with tolvaptan being the captain of low sodium levels treatment.

There are other reasons which favor the therapy with vaptans in HF as listed in **Box 6.8**.

As recommended in the expert panel report, the overall approach to treat hyponatremia in HF is as follows:

- Severely symptomatic patients: Hypertonic saline combined with loop diuretics.

Box 6.8 Factors that favor therapy with vaptans in heart failure

In that vaptans:
- Do not cause much intravascular volume depletion
- Cause no neurohumoral activation, so no worsening of heart failure
- No depletion of magnesium

- Mild-to-moderate symptoms: Fluid restriction, if volume overload—loop diuretics with ACEI/ARB.
- If Na levels do not reach the desired level, lift fluid restriction and start on vaptans.
- Tolvaptan: start with 15 mg up-titrate to 30 to 60 mg/d till the desired Na levels are achieved.
- Continue therapy until serum sodium levels has normalized and symptoms have improved.
- The limits of correction recommended for chronic hyponatremia should be observed.
- Tolvaptan therapy is usually recommended for 30 days. Liver function needs to be monitored.
- If a patient again becomes symptomatic after stopping tolvaptan after 30 days, it is suggested that the drug may be restored if other measures fail. It is of utmost importance to monitor liver function on chronic therapy.

Renal Insufficiency in Acute Heart Failure: Old Habits We Need to Let Go?

Renal dysfunction in HF has been shown to be an independent prognostic in detecting systolic and diastolic dysfunction. As blood through the kidneys decrease, there is oliguria, and factors to define diuretic resistance leading to hyponatremia must be checked (**Box 6.9**).[14-16]

Conclusion

Hyponatremia is the most common electrolyte abnormality encountered in patients with HF. Hyponatremia is associated with increased mortality and morbidity in patients with HF. Treatment of hyponatremia includes fluid restriction, loop diuretics, ACEI/ARBs, hypertonic saline infusion, and vaptans. Rapid correction of Na levels can lead to the catastrophic complication of ODS, so controlled correction of Na is recommended. Vaptans have varied unique features which will help patients with HF and hyponatremia and are increasingly utilized in the treatment of this electrolyte abnormality associated with HF. Most patients should be managed by treating their underlying disease and according

Box 6.9 Parameters to define diuretic resistance

Ambulatory patient:
- Weight gain: 2–3 kg/wk
- Water (<1 L/d) and sodium restriction (<3 g/d)
- Furosemide 250 mg
- Antialdosterone 6 thiazide

In-hospital patient:
- Inadequate weight loss
- Urine output <1000 mL/24 h
- Water (<750 mL/d) and sodium restriction
- Furosemide 40 mg/h infusion
- Metolazone 5–10 mg/d 6 acetazolamide 250 mg b.i.d.
- Antialdosterone

to whether they have hypovolemic, euvolemic, or hypervolemic hyponatremia. Urea and vaptans can be effective in managing the syndrome of inappropriate antidiuresis and hyponatremia in patients with heart failure; hypertonic saline is reserved for patients with severely symptomatic hyponatremia.[17]

References

1. Yamazoe M, Mizuno A, Kohsaka S, et al; West Tokyo Heart Failure Registry Investigators Tokyo, Japan. Incidence of hospital-acquired hyponatremia by the dose and type of diuretics among patients with acute heart failure and its association with long-term outcomes. J Cardiol 2018;71(6):550–556
2. Holland-Bill L, Christiansen CF, Ulrichsen SP, Ring T, Lunde Jørgensen JO, Sørensen HT. Preadmission diuretic use and mortality in patients hospitalized with hyponatremia: a propensity score-matched cohort study. Am J Ther 2019; 26(1):e79–e91
3. Mannheimer B, Bergh CF, Falhammar H, Calissendorff J, Skov J, Lindh JD. Association between newly initiated thiazide diuretics and hospitalization due to hyponatremia. Eur J Clin Pharmacol 2021;77(7):1049–1055
4. Hirsch JS, Uppal NN, Sharma P, et al; Northwell Nephrology COVID-19 Research Consortium. Prevalence and outcomes of hyponatremia and hypernatremia in patients hospitalized with COVID-19. Nephrol Dial Transplant 2021;36(6):1135–1138
5. Ambrosy A, Goldsmith SR, Gheorghiade M. Tolvaptan for the treatment of heart failure: a review of the literature. Expert Opin Pharmacother 2011;12(6):961–976
6. Farmakis D, Filippatos G, Parissis J, Kremastinos DT, Gheorghiade M. Hyponatremia in heart failure. Heart Fail Rev 2009;14(2):59–63
7. Harikrishnan S, Sanjay G, Anees T, et al; Trivandrum Heart Failure Registry. Clinical presentation, management, in-hospital and 90-day outcomes of heart failure patients in Trivandrum, Kerala, India: the Trivandrum Heart Failure Registry. Eur J Heart Fail 2015;17(8):794–800
8. Klein L, O'Connor CM, Leimberger JD, et al; OPTIME-CHF Investigators. Lower serum sodium is associated with increased short-term mortality in hospitalized patients with worsening

heart failure: results from the Outcomes of a Prospective Trial of Intravenous Milrinone for Exacerbations of Chronic Heart Failure (OPTIME-CHF) study. Circulation 2005;111(19): 2454–2460

9. Sonnenblick M, Friedlander Y, Rosin AJ. Diuretic-induced severe hyponatremia. Review and analysis of 129 reported patients. Chest 1993;103(2):601–606

10. Sterns RH, Cappuccio JD, Silver SM, Cohen EP. Neurologic sequelae after treatment of severe hyponatremia: a multicenter perspective. J Am Soc Nephrol 1994;4(8):1522–1530

11. Greenberg A, Verbalis JG. Vasopressin receptor antagonists. Kidney Int 2006;69(12):2124–2130

12. Schrier RW, Gross P, Gheorghiade M, et al; SALT Investigators. Tolvaptan, a selective oral vasopressin V2-receptor antagonist, for hyponatremia. N Engl J Med 2006;355(20):2099–2112

13. Verbalis JG, Goldsmith SR, Greenberg A, et al. Diagnosis, evaluation, and treatment of hyponatremia: expert panel recommendations. Am J Med 2013; 126(10, Suppl 1):S1–S42

14. Cice G. Renal insufficiency in acute heart failure: old habits we need to let go? Eur Heart J Suppl 2019;21(Suppl B):B38–B42

15. Hew-Butler T, Rosner MH, Fowkes-Godek S, et al. Statement of the Third International Exercise-Associated Hyponatremia Consensus Development Conference, Carlsbad, California, 2015. Clin J Sport Med 2015;25(4):303–320

16. McAlister FA, Ezekowitz J, Tonelli M, Armstrong PW. Renal insufficiency and heart failure: prognostic and therapeutic implications from a prospective cohort study. Circulation 2004;109(8):1004–1009

17. Adrogué HJ, Tucker BM, Madias NE. Diagnosis and Management of Hyponatremia: A Review. JAMA. 2022;328(3):280–291

7

Dyselectrolytemia in ICU

Rohan Kapur, Naveen Garg, and K. K. Kapur

Introduction

Abnormalities in fluid and electrolyte balance are very commonly observed problems in the intensive care unit (ICU). Several recent studies have shown that these imbalances are associated with increased morbidity and mortality. Therefore, to provide optimal care, the ICU personnel should be familiar with the principles of fluid and electrolyte pathophysiology. In several critical conditions such as burns, heart failure, brain damage, sepsis, and trauma, there is associated derangement of fluid and electrolyte homeostasis. The underlying mechanism includes diminished renal perfusion due to hypovolemia or hypotension or activation of renin–angiotensin–aldosterone system as well as release of vasopressin. In addition, ischemic or nephrotoxic insult to the kidney also results in dyselectrolytemia. This is compounded by a multitude of medications used in the critical care setting. Inappropriate administration of fluids and electrolytes could be deleterious and prompt recognition is essential to provide for corrective measures.[1]

Although volume resuscitation is a sine-qua-non of hypovolemic shock or sepsis, aggressive fluid administration leads to fluid overload, tissue hypoxia, and increased mortality in the critical care setting. Early institution of targeted therapies, together with judicious use of fluids and electrolytes, has been shown to improve survival and outcomes in ICUs.[2] Meticulous monitoring of input and output as well as considerations of third-space losses should be performed. In this chapter, authors intend to provide basic principles of management of various electrolyte imbalances that occur in the ICU.

Hyponatremia

Hyponatremia can be defined as sodium level <135 mmol/L.[3] It is divided into mild (Na levels 130–135 mmol/L), moderate (Na levels 125–130 mmol/L), and severe (Na levels <125 mmol/L). It is the single, most common electrolyte imbalance observed in the ICU, involving almost 25% of such patients.[4] Many of the hyponatremias occur after admission into the ICU and the presence of this electrolyte abnormality is associated with a poor prognosis.[5-7] Hyponatremia can be acute (developing in <48 h) or chronic (developing in >48 h). Lethal neurological complications can result when sodium level falls below 120 mmol/L, or even at higher sodium levels when the hyponatremia is acute in nature. Moreover, rapid correction of hyponatremia can also result in additional neurological complications.

Hyponatremia represents a relative water excess together with impaired ability of kidney to excrete electrolyte free water. Urinary dilution is severely compromised in a large proportion of patients in the ICU who are in sepsis, shock, multiorgan dysfunction, and heart failure. The problem is compounded by the use of diuretics and tubulointerstitial pathologies, which compromise the ability of the kidney to reabsorb sodium and chloride.

Etiology

Causes of hyponatremia are summarized in **Table 7.1**. Hypovolemic hyponatremia results because of the loss of both solutes and water, with greater loss of solutes compared to water. This could occur in patients taking diuretics. Euvolemic hyponatremia occurs in psychogenic polydipsia, syndrome of inappropriate antidiuretic hormone (SIADH) secretion, and hypothyroidism. Hypervolemic hyponatremia occurs when both water and sodium are retained in the body but water is retained to a greater extent and this could be related to severe cardiac, liver, or renal dysfunction. Hyperglycemia can cause a hyperosmolar hyponatremia by transfer of water from intracellular compartment to the extracellular compartment.

Spurious hyponatremia also termed as pseudohyponatremia arises due to a major increase in lipid or protein fraction of the plasma. Associated neurological symptoms are not related to low-sodium levels but to hyperviscosity.[3]

Table 7.1 Causes of hyponatremia

Plasma osmolality	Extracellular volume (volume status)	Causes
Low (<275 mOsm/kg)	Hypovolemic (depletional hyponatremia)	• Renal salt loss: diuretics, primary adrenal insufficiency • Nonrenal salt loss: diarrhea, vomiting, dehydration
	Euvolemic (dilutional hyponatremia)	SIADH, psychogenic polydipsia, beer potomania, hypothyroidism
	Hypervolemic (dilutional hyponatremia)	Cirrhosis, congestive heart failure, nephrotic syndrome
Normal High (>290 mOsm/kg)	Variable	• Pseudohyponatremia (e.g., paraproteinemia, hyperlipidemia) • Hyperglycemia, exogenous solutes (mannitol)

Abbreviation: SIADH, syndrome of inappropriate antidiuretic hormone.

Clinical Features

The clinical manifestations are primarily neurological and their pattern correlates with both the level of hyponatremia and the rapidity of its development. There is graded symptomatology depending upon the level of plasma sodium. Mild hyponatremia is usually asymptomatic; symptoms, if present, are restricted to fatigue and mild cognitive impairment. In moderate hyponatremia, in addition to symptoms of mild hyponatremia, there may be nonspecific symptoms including headache, nausea, and abdominal cramps. In severe hyponatremia, there could be greater restlessness, lethargy, confusion, and delirium, and lethal neurological complications such as coma, seizures, and brain herniation could occur as a result of cerebral edema.[8] Hyponatremia is one of the top causes for development of new-onset seizures in the ICU. Risk factors for development of acute cerebral edema include elderly women on thiazide diuretics, marathon runners, children, and polydipsic patients.[9] However, the course of the symptoms may be unpredictable and the patients' clinical condition may rapidly worsen even when there is a moderate decline in plasma sodium.

Extraneurological manifestations of hyponatremia includes neurogenic respiratory failure and this has been observed mainly in premenopausal women especially in the postoperative setting.[10]

Symptoms of hyponatremia may not be apparent in sedated patients who may develop brain herniation leading to respiratory herniation. Brain herniation may also cause sudden death in ventilated patients.

Management

Management of hyponatremia is summarized in **Table 7.2**. The mode of treatment and management of hyponatremia is guided by the presence or absence of symptoms, rapidity of development, and the level of plasma sodium. In other words, if the plasma Na levels are below 120 mmol/L even in asymptomatic patients, urgent treatment is essential. Moreover, in acutely developing symptomatic hyponatremia, emergency treatment can be initiated with higher sodium levels (between 120 and 130 mmol/L).

Emergency treatment involves intravenous infusion of hypertonic sodium chloride (3% NaCl) with or without a loop diuretic, usually initiated at a rate of 1.5 to 2 mL/kg/h in the first 3 to 4 hours so as to raise the sodium concentration by 1 to 2 mEq/L/h. A single bolus dose of 2 mL/kg of 3% NaCl increases the plasma sodium by almost 2 mmol/L.

The overall correction should not exceed plasma sodium level by 8 to 10 mmol/L in the first 24 hours and 18 mmol/L in the first 48 hours because these are associated with risks for osmotic demyelination syndrome. A correction by 4 to 6 mmol/L/d is sufficient to alleviate symptoms associated with hyponatremia and is also protective against cerebral edema and is the recommended correction.[1,3] The anticipated rise in plasma sodium following the administration of 1 L of hypertonic saline can be computed by Madias and Adrogue equations.[11] Although this equation is quite accurate in predicting plasma sodium changes in most clinical changes, there is a tendency to underestimate the achieved plasma sodium in some patients and hence needs to be used with caution.

$$\text{Change in plasma [Na] concentration} = \frac{\text{Infusate [Na]} - \text{plasma [Na]}}{\text{Total body water} + 1}$$

Asymptomatic hyponatremia with plasma Na levels >120 mmol/L does not require emergent therapy and can be managed by fluid restriction and identification as well as removal of reversible causes. In hypovolemic hyponatremia, withdrawal of diuretics and replacement of volume deficit should be undertaken. Loop diuretics can be used in patients with hypervolemic hyponatremia. In some patients with hypervolemic hyponatremia (heart failure, cirrhosis) V2-receptor antagonists could be used. Only conivaptan is available for intravenous use while tolvaptan, lixivaptan, and satavaptan are available orally but are more selective V2 receptor antagonists. However, the use of these agents in the intensive care setting is limited by their high cost and sometimes a risk of rapid rise of plasma sodium. These agents have not been shown to improve survival.[8,12,13]

Osmotic Demyelination Syndrome

Osmotic demyelination syndrome (ODS) occurs after a lucid interval of 1 to 7 days (occasionally up to 2 weeks) of the rapid correction of sodium. The classical pathology is central pontine myelinolysis. Classical signs of ODS include ataxia, nystagmus, dysarthria, ophthalmoplegia, dysphagia, pseudobulbar palsy, and spastic quadriparesis. In addition, various extrapyramidal symptoms have been described including rigidity, choreoathetosis, and myoclonic jerks. In the full-blown form, osmotic demyelination is characterized by a locked-in syndrome (preserved cortical function with

Table 7.2 Treatment of hyponatremia

Emergent treatment	Nonemergent treatment
Hypertonic saline (3%) 1.5–2 mL/kg/h for the first 3–4 h. Recommended correction up to 4–6 mmol/d, do not go beyond 8–10 mmol/d. Use diuretics depending on volume status	Fluid restriction, treat reversible causes like withdrawing diuretics, V2 receptor antagonists can be used in fluid overload like heart failure

inability to move (viz., spastic quadriparesis), along with brainstem signs such as nystagmus, dysarthria, dysphagia, and ophthalmoplegia as described above. Clinical symptoms depend on the region of the brain compromised by ODS. Patients at a greater risk for developing ODS include alcoholics, malnourished, hypokalemic patients, burn patients, elderly women on thiazides, and patients with plasma sodium <105 mmol/L.[14–16]

Treatment of osmotic demyelination includes withdrawal of sodium infusion as well as supportive treatment.[3] Occasionally V2-receptor agonists like desmopressin can be used in this condition with variable results. The prognosis is generally unfavorable with a mortality rate reported between 31 and 50%.[17–19]

Hypernatremia

Hypernatremia is defined as a sodium concentration more than 145 mmol/L. It can develop either as a result of sodium gain, loss of free water, or a combination of both. It is always associated with hyperosmolality.[20,21]

In nonsedated, conscious, healthy patients, development of thirst is a major defense mechanism against hypernatremia. Even slight elevations of osmolality result in development of thirst and increased secretion of antidiuretic hormone. Therefore, hypernatremia usually occurs in the ICU setting where the patients are usually sedated, intubated, and often unconscious. It is rarely seen in nonhospitalized patients with a prevalence of 0.2% on admission and 1% during the hospital stay.[22] However, in contrast, among the critically ill patients being managed in the ICUs, 2 to 6% are hypernatremic on admission.[6,23] During their ICU stay between 6 and 26% of the patients in the medical ICU and 4 to 10% of the patients in the surgical ICU develop hypernatremia.[23–27] Usually this electrolyte disturbance develops during the first week of admission in the ICU and could be related to administration of large amounts of fluid which may be relatively hypertonic or containing potassium for hypokalemia (potassium administration can trigger the development of hypernatremia).[28]

Etiology

The causes of hypernatremia can be due to either excess sodium administration or loss of free water.[29] Etiopathogenesis is summarized in **Table 7.3**. A major cause of sodium excess in ICU patients is the infusion of hypertonic solutions, such as overcorrection of hyponatremia using hypertonic saline or correction of metabolic acidosis using 8.4% sodium bicarbonate. However, in patients with multiorgan failure, excess use of isotonic solutions over several days (e.g., 0.9% NaCl), Ringer's lactate is a common cause of hypernatremia.

Clinical Features

Major clinical manifestations of hypernatremia are neurological including lethargy, irritability, confusion, and somnolence. These are due to hyperosmolality leading to shift of free water from intracellular to extracellular space and thus causing brain cell shrinkage.[30] Other effects include neuromuscular effects such as muscle weakness or cramps.[31] Occasionally, cerebral demyelination (not related to overcorrection of hyponatremia) has also been noted.[32–34] The severity of symptoms of hypernatremia depends upon rapidity of development. Hypernatremia is a potentially lethal condition which, in part, could be due to the severity of the underlying disease in hypernatremic ICU patients. Most studies have reported mortality rates between 30 and 48% for patients with sodium levels exceeding 150 mmol/L.[23,24,29] However, even in slightly elevated sodium levels, mortality rates are increased in comparison to normonatremic controls (30% vs. 15%).[24]

Management

Management of hypernatremia is summarized in **Table 7.4**. The first step in the management of hypernatremia is to assess whether this electrolyte disorder is due to sodium gain (hypervolemic hypernatremia) or loss of free water (hypovolemic hypernatremia) or a combination of the two. The rate of development is also important; classified

Table 7.3 Causes of hypernatremia

Loss of free water	Gain of sodium
• Polyuria including diabetes insipidus • Diarrhea • Increased sweating during pyrexia • Drainage from open wounds • Nasogastric suction	• Administration of hypertonic solutions, e.g., sodium bicarbonate (8.4%) and hypertonic saline • Acute renal failure • Accidental ingestion in infants • Sodium-rich IV antibiotics such as fosfomycin, ciprofloxacin, fluconazole, voriconazole

Abbreviation: IV, intravenous.

as acute (<48 h) and chronic (>48 h). In the case of hypovolemic hypernatremia, volume resuscitation is undertaken by administration of isotonic solutions like Ringer's lactate and normal saline. It is recommended that half the water deficit be replaced in 12 to 24 hours, during which the neurological status is monitored.[28] The remaining deficit is corrected over the next 48 hours. The rate of plasma sodium correction should not exceed 2 mmol/h or 8 to 12 mmol/L/d. Frequent estimation of sodium levels every 2 hours and the rate of correction can be modified accordingly.[28] In chronic hypernatremia, too rapid a correction may result in cerebral edema with catastrophic cerebral herniation.

Euvolemic/hypervolemic hypernatremia is generally iatrogenic and treatment requires removal of excess sodium from the body. Loop diuretics should be administered by replacing free water with sodium-free solutions like 5% dextrose. In this situation, usually the renal function is compromised and renal replacement therapy (RRT) may be required.

Hypokalemia

Hypokalemia is an extremely common electrolyte abnormality observed in the critical care setting. Hypokalemia is classified into mild (serum potassium 3–3.4 mEq/L), moderate (2.5–2.9 mEq/L), and severe (serum potassium <2.5 mEq/L). The prevalence of severe hypokalemia in hospitalized patients varies from 2.6 to 5.2%.[35,36] Mortality rate varies between 20 and 30% depending on the severity of hypokalemia.

Etiology

The etiology of hypokalemia is summarized in **Table 7.5**[1,37–39] and can be divided into low dietary potassium intake, shifting potassium inside the cell, renal potassium loss, and extra-renal potassium loss.[1] Among the medications administered in the ICU causing hypokalemia, catecholamines and other sympathomimetics, aminophylline and other methylxanthines, cause intracellular shift by stimulating Na/K adenosine triphosphatase (ATPase). On the other hand, diuretics increase the renal potassium loss by inhibiting sodium reabsorption in renal tubules. Amphotericin B disrupts the functioning of the collecting ducts causing renal tubular acidosis, potassium loss, and nephrogenic diabetes insipidus.

Clinical Features

Mild hypokalemia does not result in significant signs and symptoms. Moderate-to-severe hypokalemia can result in neuromuscular features affecting skeletal, smooth, and respiratory muscles. Features such as fatigue, weakness, myalgia, muscle cramps, flaccid paralysis with absent tendon jerks, and paralytic ileus may be present.[38,39] Severe hypokalemia can result in respiratory muscle weakness and rhabdomyolysis. However, the most feared complications are the cardiac manifestations. Predisposing factors for cardiac complications include hypertension, coronary artery disease, and heart failure. Earliest cardiac manifestations are observed in the electrocardiogram (ECG). These changes include ST depression, T-wave flattening, T-wave inversion, and appearance of U-waves[37] (**Fig. 7.1**).

Table 7.4 Management of hypernatremia

Hypervolemic hypernatremia	Hypovolemic hypernatremia
Loop diuretics with sodium-free solutions like 5% dextrose	Volume resuscitation with isotonic fluids like Ringer's lactate and normal saline. Correction should not exceed 2 mmol/h or 8–12 mmol/L/d. Check sodium every 2 h

Table 7.5 Causes of hypokalemia

Criteria	Conditions
Low dietary potassium intake	Starvation, malnutrition, IV fluids without potassium
Shifting potassium inside the cell	Insulin, beta-agonists, hypo-osmolarity, alkalosis
Renal potassium loss	Diuretics: loop diuretics, thiazide diuretics, renal tubular damage, primary hyperaldosteronism (Conn's syndrome)
Extrarenal potassium loss	Vomiting, diarrhea, burns
Drugs	Diuretics, sympathomimetics, insulin, methylxanthines, penicillin, and dobutamine, amphotericin B, glucocorticoids, laxatives
Hypomagnesemia	Causes refractory hypokalemia
Genetic renal transport defects	Bartter and Gitelman syndromes

Abbreviation: IV, intravenous.

These ECG changes could portend significant and often life-threatening arrhythmias including high-grade ventricular and supraventricular ectopics, ventricular and supraventricular tachycardia, and torsades de pointes. These arrhythmias could result in sudden cardiac death.[38-40]

Management

Management of hypokalemia is summarized in **Table 7.6**. Management of hypokalemia is determined by the urgency of the clinical scenario. In patients with respiratory paralysis, ECG changes or in cases with potassium levels <2.5 mEq/L (severe hypokalemia) immediate emergent therapy should be instituted. However, in the absence of any clinical urgency and potassium levels >2.5, hypokalemia treatment can be planned according to causative or aggravating factors.

Using thiazide/loop diuretics, and when the etiology is not obvious, the estimation of potassium deficit can be calculated based on the following formula:

$$\text{K-deficit (mmol)} =$$
$$(\text{K-normal lower limit} - \text{K-measured}) \times \text{body weight (kg)} \times 0.4^{41}$$

Further insight into the etiological mechanisms by assessing the rate of urinary potassium excretion is required. If it is appropriately low (<20 mEq/d or random urine potassium/urine creatinine of <15mEq/g) then suspect transcellular shifts or extrarenal loss. However, if the urinary potassium excretion is high (>20 mEq/d or random urine potassium/urine creatinine >15 mEq/g) then various causes of renal potassium loss have to be considered. In such a situation, transtubular potassium concentration gradient (TTKG) can be calculated as follows:

$$\text{TTKG} - (\text{Urine potassium/serum potassium}) \text{ divided by}$$
$$(\text{Urine osmolality/serum osmolality})$$

In hypokalemia, TTKG should be <2. If TTKG >4, it suggests increased potassium secretion in cortical collecting duct (i.e., a high potassium concentration in the cortical collecting duct which suggests an increased renal potassium loss). TTKG, together with acid-base status and presence or absence of hypertension, is helpful to differentiate the causes of hypokalemia due to renal potassium loss.

In the nonemergent settings, oral administration of potassium is preferred to parenteral replacement. Oral tablets of 600 mg/750 mg can be used twice a day or equivalent doses of KCl syrup can be given according to the potassium deficit calculated.[1,42,43] In patients with resistant hypokalemia not improving with potassium supplements, hypomagnesemia should be considered.

In cases where emergent treatment is required (i.e., hypokalemia leading to arrhythmias, respiratory failure, ECG changes), rapid infusion of potassium of about 10 to 20 mEq/h may be required via a central venous catheter.[42,43] Infusion via a peripheral line could cause phlebitis and vein injury. However in an urgent situation a dose of <10 mEq/h could be infused via the peripheral vein. In severe cases, the initial dose should be in the range of 40 to 80 mEq/h and then subsequently tapered according to potassium levels.[1] Total dose should not exceed 240 to 400 mEq/d. If high doses

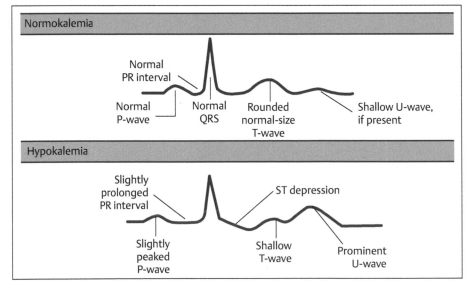

Fig. 7.1 Electrocardiogram (ECG) changes during hypokalemia. Shallowing of T-wave and prominent U-wave can be appreciated in hypokalemia as compared to normal ECG.

Table 7.6 Management of hypokalemia

Mild-to-moderate, asymptomatic hypokalemia	Severe (<2.5 mEq/L) or symptomatic hypokalemia
Correction of reversible causes, oral administration of potassium with either tablets or syrup	Rapid infusion of potassium 10–20 mEq/h via central venous catheter, can go up to 40–80 mEq/h. Do not exceed 240–400 mEq/d

of 40 to 80 mEq/h are being used, then cardiac monitor needs to be placed. Monitoring of serum potassium levels is essential and should be carried out at least 6 hourly.[43]

Guidelines for giving intravenous (IV) KCl infusion are:

- Never give potassium intramuscular (IM) or as rapid IV push.
- KCl infusion should be given in the form of dextrose-free solutions as dextrose infusion induces insulin secretion and therefore prevents rapid correction of extracellular potassium deficit.
- Use central line for high-dose infusions (>10–20 mEq/h).
- Do not add KCl solution to hanging fluid bag. The fluid bag should be fully inverted multiple times to ensure proper mixing.

Hyperkalemia

Hyperkalemia is a potentially lethal electrolyte aberration that frequently occurs in hospitalized patients, especially in the critical care setting. According to European Resuscitation Council, hyperkalemia is defined as a plasma level more than 5.5 mmol/L and severe hyperkalemia is a potassium level of more than 6.5 mmol/L.[44] This electrolyte abnormality is generally associated with poor outcomes in many different clinical settings including the acutely ill patient in ICUs.[45,46]

Etiology

The causes for hyperkalemia are summarized in **Table 7.7**. They can be divided into increased dietary intake, altered renal clearance of potassium as in chronic renal failure, and acute kidney injury as well as sepsis. Release of potassium from intracellular space and decreased transfer into intracellular space are also common mechanisms that cause hyperkalemia in the critical care setting.[47] Several medications can cause hyperkalemia including potassium-sparing

diuretics, inhibitors of renin–angiotensin–aldosterone system, nonsteroidal anti-inflammatory drugs (NSAIDs), β-blockers, heparin and its derivatives, and trimethoprim.[1,48] Succinylcholine, a depolarizing muscle relaxant commonly used in critical care, should be avoided in patients at risk for hyperkalemia.[49]

Clinical Features

Patients with hyperkalemia are usually asymptomatic, but can rarely present with neuromuscular weakness and paresthesia. On examination, tendon reflexes may be depressed and flaccid paralysis may be appreciated. However, elevation of extracellular potassium alters the myocardial electrophysiology leading to conduction disturbances which can cause arrhythmias. These conduction disturbances cause several ECG abnormalities which occur in a stepwise fashion according to severity of hyperkalemia as shown in **Fig. 7.2**. Prolonged PR interval and peaked T-waves are the initial manifestations which occur between potassium levels of 6 to 7 mmol/L. Loss of P-waves, ST-segment elevation (pseudo-Brugada syndrome), bradycardia, and terminally a sine-wave pattern occur with progressive increase in serum potassium levels between 7 and 8 mmol/L. However, the correlation between potassium elevation and ECG changes is rather poor.[50] The ECG manifestations occur due to development of a potassium gradient across the myocardial membrane and are also influenced by underlying cardiac disease.[51] The mortality from hyperkalemia increases in patients showing abnormal ECG findings.[52]

Management

Management of hyperkalemia is summarized in **Table 7.8**. The management strategy depends on the potassium level and presence or absence of ECG changes as well as other cardiac manifestations of hyperkalemia. When such changes are present or potassium level is >6.5 mmol/L, immediate

Table 7.7 Causes of hyperkalemia

Criteria	Conditions
Increased dietary intake	Excess intake of potassium supplements
Altered renal clearance of potassium	Renal failure (chronic kidney disease, acute kidney injury). Acute kidney injury due to hypovolemia, sepsis
Release from intracellular space	Hemolysis, rhabdomyolysis, tissue injury, tumor lysis syndrome
Decreased transfer into intracellular space	Acidosis, insulin deficit/resistance, β-blockers, hyperosmolarity
Drugs	Digitalis, succinylcholine, aldosterone antagonists, ACE inhibitors, ARBs, β-blockers, calcineurin inhibitors like cyclosporine, NSAIDs, potassium-sparing diuretics, trimethoprim, pentamidine, heparin
Iatrogenic	Blood transfusions, excessive correction of hypokalemia
Falsely elevated as a result of hemolysis due to storage of blood sample	Pseudohyperkalemia

Abbreviations: ACE, angiotensin-converting enzyme; ARB, angiotensin receptor blocker; NSAID, nonsteroidal anti-inflammatory drugs.

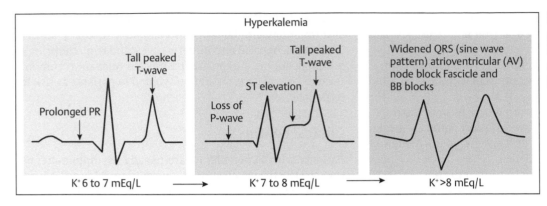

Fig. 7.2 Electrocardiogram (ECG) changes in hyperkalemia. ECG changes correspond to increased blood potassium levels.

Table 7.8 Treatment of hyperkalemia

Mechanism of treatment	When to treat	How to treat
Cardiac membrane stabilization	Within 10 min	10% Calcium gluconate IV, hypertonic sodium if calcium is contraindicated
Intracellular shift of potassium	Within 30 min	Insulin with dextrose, inhaled beta-2 agonists, hypertonic sodium bicarbonate in select patients
Removal of potassium from the body	Hours-days	Diuretics, potassium-binding agents like sodium polystyrene sulfonate, patiromer, renal replacement therapy, if indicated

Abbreviation: IV, intravenous.

attention is given to myocardial protection. This includes immediate injection of 10 to 20 mL of 10% calcium salt (calcium gluconate or calcium chloride).[48] This reverses the ECG changes almost instantaneously and is potentially lifesaving. In cases of contraindication to calcium administration, infusion of hypertonic sodium (either as chloride, lactate, or bicarbonate) can be considered.[48]

Once the ECG changes are stabilized, the next step is facilitation of shift of potassium into the intracellular compartment. This can be achieved by the following.

Insulin–Dextrose Combination

A combination of insulin and dextrose given as intravenous infusion causes a transfer of potassium from the extracellular compartment to the intracellular compartment. Usually 5 to 10 units of regular insulin are combined with 25 g of dextrose in 25% dextrose solution. To limit hypoglycemia, insulin may be administered according to body weight[53] (0.1 U/kg body weight up to a maximum of 10 units) and using up to 50 to 60 g of dextrose in 25% dextrose solution.[54] Using a rapid rate of infusion (limiting the infusion time to 30 min) leads to a faster decrease in potassium and less hypoglycemia as compared to a slower continuous infusion.[55] Blood sugar should be measured at an hourly basis for the first 2 hours. Insulin–dextrose combination is recommended for all patients with potassium greater than 6 mmol/L.[48]

Beta-2 Agonists

Drugs like salbutamol are preferably administered via nebulization.[56,57] About 10 mg of nebulized salbutamol can

be considered as a first-line therapy in nonsevere hyperkalemia in spontaneously breathing patients without tachycardia.[48]

Hypertonic Sodium Bicarbonate

Although sodium bicarbonate causes intracellular shift of potassium, its effect is less effective than patients given insulin–dextrose or salbutamol.[58] The recommended dose of hypertonic sodium bicarbonate is 100 to 250 mL of 8.4% sodium bicarbonate over 20 minutes, used only in patients with metabolic acidosis with pH levels <7.2.[48] Routine use of hypertonic sodium bicarbonate could lead to fluid overload and alkalosis.

The third step involves increased potassium excretion from the body, which can be done via urinary excretion or intestinal excretion. Urinary excretion involves the use of loop diuretics, especially in patients with acute kidney injury. Furosemide can be used for this purpose at a dose of 1 to 1.5 mg/kg. Urinary output should be closely monitored to avoid additional kidney insult resulting from iatrogenic hypovolemia.

For gastrointestinal excretion, sodium polystyrene sulfonate (SPS) can be given orally, although no studies on the efficacy of SPS in the acute setting are available. Therefore, it is not recommended in acutely ill patients as several gastrointestinal complications can occur including intestinal perforation.[59] Newer alternatives for SPS such as patiromer[60,61] and sodium-zirconium cyclosilicate[61,62] are emerging treatments for hyperkalemia, and their efficacy in critically ill patients is currently being investigated.

Renal Replacement Therapy

Although medical treatment for hyperkalemia could avoid or delay RRT, in severe hyperkalemia (>6.5 mmol/L) when the patient is not appropriately responsive to medical treatment, RRT is mandated.[63] This includes the following modalities of RRT:

- **Diffusive (hemodialysis):** Extremely efficient method for rapid reduction of serum potassium, but requires a high flow and is not suitable for patients with hypotension and shock.
- **Convective (hemofiltration):** Entails a continuous filtration and is the most frequently used modality in ICU. This technique causes a slower but continuous decrease in serum potassium levels.
- **Mixed (hemo-diafiltration):** Entails both diffusive transfer and a continuous low-flow hemofiltration. Potassium drops at a faster rate than hemofiltration alone.

Hypocalcemia

Hypocalcemia is one of the most frequent electrolyte derangements in patients requiring intensive care. Normal values of total serum calcium are 8.6 to 10.3 mg/dL. Normal values of ionized calcium are 1.1 to 1.3 mmol/L. Mild-to-moderate hypocalcemia is 0.9 to 1.1 mmol/L of ionized calcium or 7.5 to 8.5 mg/dL of total calcium. Severe hypocalcemia is <0.9 mmol/L of ionized calcium or <7.5 mg/dL[64] as given in **Table 7.9**. There is a wide variation in the reported prevalence of hypocalcemia in the ICU with figures ranging from 15 to 88% depending on the cut-off values used.[65,66]

Etiology

The causes of hypocalcemia are explained in **Table 7.10**. Briefly, these can be divided into parathyroid dependent (low parathyroid hormone [PTH] levels) and parathyroid independent (high PTH levels).[67–70] Parathyroid-dependent etiology encompasses the various causes of hypoparathyroidism. Among the parathyroid-independent causes, trauma, acute and chronic renal failure, sepsis, and low albumin levels are some of the common causes. Use of citrated blood or infusion of albumin or phosphate causes complexing of ionized calcium leading to hypocalcemia. Septic state causes hypocalcemia due to intracellular transfer of calcium ions as well as due to depressed PTH secretion. Although the exact cause of association of hypocalcemia with hypomagnesemia is not clearly known, it is hypothesized that magnesium deficiency may impair the release or activity of PTH.[67–70]

Clinical Features

The primary manifestations of acute hypocalcemia are neuromuscular. Paresthesias of the extremities (tingling, numbness in the fingertips and toes) and also the perioral region are common symptoms of neuromuscular irritability. Mild muscle cramps could progress to carpopedal spasm or tetany and in severe hypocalcemia, bronchospasm with laryngospasm and stridor may also occur. Occasionally, the muscular symptoms resemble those of polymyositis with elevated CK levels. Clinical signs of tetany can be elicited in Chvostek sign (ipsilateral contracting of facial muscles on tapping the skin over facial nerve) and Trousseau sign (carpopedal spasm—flexion of wrist and metacarpophalangeal

Table 7.9 Normal values of calcium in blood

	Ionized calcium (mmol/L)	Total calcium (mg/dL)
Mild-to-moderate hypocalcemia	0.9–1.1	7.5–8.5
Severe hypocalcemia	<0.9	<7.5

Table 7.10 Causes of hypocalcemia

Parathyroid dependent	Parathyroid independent
Surgical: parathyroidectomy, thyroidectomy, radical neck surgery	Common causes: low albumin levels (pseudohypocalcemia), blood transfusion, drugs (cisplatin, loop diuretics), trauma
Infiltrative disease: metastatic cancer, Wilson disease, hemochromatosis	Metabolic: CKD, vitamin D deficiency, hypomagnesemia
Genetic: PTH gene, or calcium sensing receptor gene mutations	Inflammatory: sepsis, pancreatitis
Autoimmune destruction of parathyroid	Oncology: tumor lysis syndrome
	PTH resistance: pseudohypoparathyroidism
	Spurious hypocalcemia due to gadolinium contrast used in MRI

Abbreviations: CKD, chronic kidney disease; MRI, magnetic resonance imaging; PTH, parathyroid hormone.

[MCP] joints and extension of interphalangeal [IP] joints on inflating the BP cuff 20 mmHg above systolic BP).[71,72]

Cardiac manifestations of acute hypocalcemia include prolongation of QT-interval and lengthening of the ST-segment on the ECG with nonspecific T-wave abnormalities, as shown in **Fig. 7.3**. These ECG changes can be associated with significant ventricular arrhythmias and sudden cardiac death. Pattern of anteroseptal myocardial injury on ECG[73,74] without actual infarction may also occur, especially with associated hypomagnesemia. Rarely, congestive cardiac failure[75,76] and reversible cardiomyopathy[77] could occur.

Chronic hypocalcemia as seen in idiopathic hypoparathyroidism may present with extrapyramidal symptoms like tremor and rigidity as well as focal or generalized seizures due to calcification in the basal ganglia. Increased intracranial pressure (ICP) and papilledema are also seen. It can also present with dermatological manifestations such as brittle nails and hair loss.[78–81]

Management

Management of hypocalcemia is summarized in **Table 7.11**. Acute, symptomatic hypocalcemia requires intravenous slow-bolus infusion of calcium which can be given as calcium gluconate or calcium chloride. Calcium gluconate is the preferred IV calcium salt over calcium chloride (less irritant). One ampoule of 10 mL calcium gluconate contains 90 mg of elemental calcium and usually 1 to 2 ampoules (180 mg of elemental calcium) diluted in 50 to 100 mL of 5% dextrose is infused over 10 minutes. However with persistent hypocalcemia, administration of calcium gluconate drip is required over a longer period of time. In such situations, the rate of infusion should be 0.5 to 2 mg/kg/h of elemental calcium. Ionized calcium concentration should be raised to a low-normal range of 1.0 to 1.1 mmol/L.[71,72]

Chronic, asymptomatic, mild-to-moderate hypocalcemia does not warrant IV calcium therapy. This can be managed with oral calcium with/without vitamin D. If concomitant hyperphosphatemia is present then phosphorus-lowering therapy also needs to be administered. Hypocalcemia is also accompanied by other electrolyte abnormalities like hypomagnesemia and also with acidosis which need to be managed. When metabolic acidosis is present, first the hypocalcemia should be corrected and then the acidosis treated. Treatment of acidosis first can decrease the concentration of ionized calcium and precipitate tetany. In this respect, bicarbonate solution and calcium salt should not be administered in the same IV line so as to avoid precipitation of calcium carbonate.[71,72]

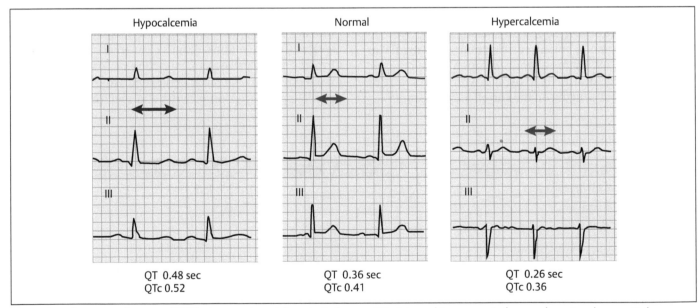

Hypocalcemia	Normal	Hypercalcemia
QT 0.48 sec	QT 0.36 sec	QT 0.26 sec
QTc 0.52	QTc 0.41	QTc 0.36

Fig. 7.3 Electrocardiogram (ECG) changes in calcium imbalance. QTc interval increases in hypocalcemia whereas it decreases in hypercalcemia.

Table 7.11 Management of hypocalcemia

Acute, symptomatic hypocalcemia or severe hypocalcemia	Chronic, asymptomatic, mild-to-moderate hypocalcemia
1–2 ampoules of 10 mL calcium gluconate diluted in 50–100 mL of 5% dextrose infused over 10 min. If infusion is required for longer, recommended rate of infusion is 0.5–2 mg/kg/h	Oral calcium with/without vitamin D. Correct concomitant electrolyte abnormalities like hypomagnesemia and hyperphosphatemia as well as acid-base abnormality, if present

Hypomagnesemia

Magnesium is an essential element to maintain life because it is critical for many physiological and biochemical processes in the body. It is the fourth most abundant cation in the body and second most abundant intracellular cation.[82] Only 0.3% of the total magnesium in the body is in the serum. Normal serum levels of magnesium vary between 1.5 and 1.9 mEq/L.[83] Mild hypomagnesemia is defined as magnesium levels between 1 and 1.5 mEq/L and severe hypomagnesemia is defined as magnesium levels <1 mEq/L. Hypomagnesemia is a common cause of hypokalemia and hypocalcemia in the critical care setting, and should be suspected in patients with resistant hypocalcemia and hypokalemia. Hypomagnesemia is common in hospitalized patients with a prevalence of 7 to 11%[84,85] and is more frequent when other electrolyte abnormalities coexist.[86] In critically ill patients the prevalence of hypomagnesemia is as high as 50%[87] and is associated with increased mortality and prolonged hospitalization.[88,89]

Etiology

Etiological factors for the genesis of hypomagnesemia in critically ill patients are mainly a result of gastrointestinal and renal losses.[82] Causes of hypomagnesemia are summarized in **Table 7.12**. These include prolonged nasogastric suction, malabsorption syndromes, protein-calorie malnutrition, sepsis, burns, osmotic diuresis as in diabetic ketoacidosis, and chronic parenteral fluid therapy. Certain medications including diuretics, amphotericin B, aminoglycosides, cisplatin, and cyclosporine cause excessive renal loss of magnesium. Drugs like proton-pump inhibitors cause gastrointestinal loss of magnesium by decreasing the intestinal absorption of magnesium.[90]

Clinical Features

Neuromuscular hyperexcitability is often the first manifestation of hypomagnesemia.[91] This is enhanced in patients with concomitant calcium deficiency. Neuromuscular features include muscle spasms, cramps, muscle irritability, and tetany with positive Chvostek and Trousseau signs. In severe cases, coma and seizures may also occur and extrapyramidal features in the form of choreoathetoid movements may be present.[92]

Magnesium levels influence myocardial excitability because magnesium is an essential cofactor for the sodium-potassium adenosine triphosphate (ATP) pump which controls the movement of sodium and potassium across cell membranes.[93] Typical ECG changes (**Fig. 7.4**)[94] include widening of QRS complex and peaking of T-waves in mild-to-moderate magnesium deficiency. In severe magnesium deficiency, there is prolongation of PR interval, further widening of QRS complex and diminution of the T-wave.[95,96] These ECG changes are associated with relatively benign arrhythmias including atrial fibrillation[95] and ventricular

Table 7.12 Causes of hypomagnesemia

Gastrointestinal loss	Renal loss
• Prolonged nasogastric suction • Malabsorption disorders • Extensive bowel resection • Acute and chronic diarrhea • Intestinal and biliary fistulae • Malnourishment and starvation • Parenteral nutrition • Refeeding syndrome • Drugs: proton pump inhibitors	• Chronic parenteral fluid therapy • Osmotic diuresis (high glucose, mannitol, urea) • Hypercalcemia • Alcohol abuse • Drugs: loop and thiazide diuretics, amphotericin B, aminoglycosides, cisplatin, calcineurin inhibitors like tacrolimus • Renal diseases: chronic pyelonephritis, interstitial nephritis, glomerulonephritis, renal tubular acidosis, postrenal transplantation

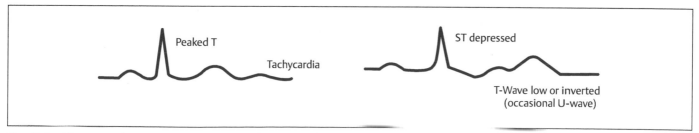

Fig. 7.4 Electrocardiogram (ECG) changes during moderate and severe hypomagnesemia. In moderate hypomagnesemia T-waves are peaked with widening of QRS complex, whereas in severe hypomagnesemia T-wave is low in amplitude with widening of QRS and PR intervals.

premature beats as well as life-threatening arrhythmias like torsades de pointes and ventricular fibrillation.[97,98] Intracellular magnesium depletion may be present even with normal serum magnesium levels and could be a potential factor for these arrhythmias.

Management

Management of hypomagnesemia is summarized in **Table 7.13**. Mild, asymptomatic hypomagnesemia (magnesium levels between 1 and 1.5 mEq/L) does not require urgent parenteral treatment and oral supplementation with 400 mg of magnesium oxide or 500 mg if magnesium gluconate may be sufficient.[99] Concomitant treatment of other associated electrolyte abnormalities is important. Although the serum magnesium levels show improvement with oral magnesium therapy, there is insufficient data with regard to the improvement of outcomes.

Indications for urgent parenteral magnesium therapy include patients with symptomatic hypomagnesemia, that is, those having neuromuscular and other neurological manifestations or cardiac arrhythmias as well as patients with severe hypomagnesemia (serum magnesium <1 mEq/L) with or without symptoms. In these patients 2 g of magnesium sulfate (16 mEq of magnesium) in 100 mL of 5% dextrose is administered urgently followed by a continuous infusion of 4 to 6 g/d for 3 to 5 days if renal function is relatively normal.[100] Maintenance therapy with oral magnesium oxide may also be used for prolonged treatment rather than parenteral maintenance therapy.

Patients with renal failure are at risk for developing hypermagnesemia, and parenteral magnesium therapy should be given with caution. If features of hypermagnesemia like somnolence, respiratory depression, areflexia, and cardiac arrest develop, magnesium therapy needs to be stopped and emergent treatment with calcium gluconate needs to be administered.

Hypophosphatemia

Phosphate is an important anion for numerous cellular mechanisms including glycolysis, oxidative phosphorylation, and synthesis of ATP. The normal level of serum phosphate is 2.5 to 4.5 mg/100 mL. Hypophosphatemia is therefore defined as a serum phosphate concentration <2.5 mg/dL. Hypophosphatemia can be mild (phosphorus level, 2–2.5 mg/dL), moderate (1–1.9 mg/dL), or severe (<1 mg/dL). The prevalence of hypophosphatemia is up to 5% of hospitalized patients but it is more common in critically ill patients (26–28%[6]). Severe hypophosphatemia is much less common.

Etiology

The etiology of hypophosphatemia in the ICU is summarized in **Table 7.14**. Critical care patients have multiple risk factors that may lower phosphate levels. There are four mechanisms by which hypophosphatemia can occur in critical care patients: internal redistribution, decreased absorption in gastrointestinal tract (GIT), increased renal loss, and RRT.[101–103]

Clinical Features

Symptomatic hypophosphatemia usually occurs when the phosphate levels are below 1 mg/dL or 0.32 mmol/L. Symptoms are generally due to impaired metabolism. Acute

Table 7.13 Management of hypomagnesemia

Severe hypomagnesemia or symptomatic hypomagnesemia	Mild, asymptomatic hypomagnesemia
• Urgent infusion of 2 g of magnesium sulfate in 100 mL of 5% dextrose followed by a continuous infusion of 4–6 g/d for 3–5 d. Caution in patients with renal failure • Monitor magnesium levels frequently	Oral magnesium oxide 400 mg twice a day

Table 7.14 Causes of hypophosphatemia

Mechanism	Causes
Internal redistribution: intracellular shift of phosphate	Major surgeries: cardiac surgery, hepatic surgery; hormonal triggers: insulin, glucagon; infusion of carbohydrates like dextrose; drugs: beta-agonists, steroids, xanthine derivatives; respiratory alkalosis: sepsis, mechanical ventilation, anxiety; treatment of diabetic ketoacidosis; refeeding syndrome in patients with malnutrition: chronic alcoholics, anorexia nervosa
Decreased absorption of GIT	Poor phosphate diet, malabsorption syndromes, phosphate-binding antacids, chronic diarrhea, vitamin D deficiency
Increased renal loss	Use of diuretics, drugs: tenofovir, imatinib
Renal replacement therapy	Continuous renal replacement therapy

Abbreviation: GIT, gastrointestinal tract.

respiratory failure and failure to wean off from mechanical ventilation, decreased myocardial contractility with increased inotropic requirement, supraventricular as well as ventricular cardiac arrhythmias, altered mental status, delirium, seizures, coma, and skeletal muscle weakness going on to rhabdomyolysis are some of the severe manifestations of hypophosphatemia.[101,104-108] Due to the life-threatening nature of these symptoms, emergent therapy is required.

Management

Treatment depends upon severity of hypophosphatemia. Management of hypophosphatemia is summarized in **Table 7.15**. It can be enteral as well as parenteral replacement. In asymptomatic patients with mild hypophosphatemia (serum phosphate 1–2.5 mg/dL), oral or enteral replacement is given in the form of phosphate effervescent tablets as well as increased phosphate in the diet. Oral tablets such as Phosphate Sandoz can be given which contain phosphate, sodium, and potassium. Up to 6 tablets can be taken. Tablets should be dissolved in 1/3 to 1/2 of a tumblerful of water. Reversible causes like diuretics, insulin, and other drugs should be corrected.[101]

Severe, symptomatic hypophosphatemia requires emergent therapy, given in the form of intravenous phosphate: 2 to 5 mg/kg of inorganic phosphate is dissolved in 0.45% saline and given over 6 to 12 hours and repeated if required.[101,102] Sodium phosphate is preferred over potassium phosphate in patients with potassium levels greater than 4 to prevent hyperkalemia.[109,110] Patients on continuous renal replacement therapy (CRRT) require higher initial dosage as the amount of phosphate removed by CRRT can be enormous.

Hypermagnesemia

Hypermagnesemia is an uncommon clinical condition especially in the critical care setting, although it can result from overzealous treatment of hypomagnesemia which is a common condition in the ICU. Symptomatic hypermagnesemia occasionally occurs because of excessive magnesium ingestion, especially taken as laxatives, particularly in elderly individuals with constipation and renal failure.[111-115] Hypermagnesemia is defined as serum Mg levels >2.5 mg/dL. Signs and symptoms of mild hypermagnesemia (serum Mg levels 2.5–6 mg/dL) may be nonspecific and include flushing, nausea, headache, and lightheadedness. Severe

hypermagnesemia (serum Mg concentrations >6 mg/dL) is characterized by ECG changes (**Fig. 7.5**) including prolonged QRS interval, increased QRS duration, prolonged QT interval, and increased height of the T-wave similar to hyperkalemia, which is a reason why hypermagnesemia can be mistaken for hyperkalemia in the ICU. Very high levels of serum magnesium lead to sinoatrial and atrioventricular block as well as ventricular arrhythmias including ventricular fibrillation. Neurological manifestations include somnolence, areflexia, muscle paralysis, hypoventilation, coma, and respiratory arrest.[116]

Treatment of hypermagnesemia consists of discontinuation of the source of magnesium and administration of calcium gluconate IV in cases of severe, symptomatic hypermagnesemia. Calcium gluconate reverses the cardiac and neurologic complications of hypermagnesemia by its antagonistic action as well as by increasing renal excretion of magnesium. Close monitoring of ECG, BP, and neurological function is also important. Along with calcium gluconate IV normal saline at 150 mL/h should also be started. Hemodialysis may be required when kidney function is impaired.[116]

Hypercalcemia

Hypercalcemia is common in patients who are hospitalized, it is responsible for approximately 0.6% of all acute medical admissions[117] and its prevalence in the general population is 1 per 1,000. Hypercalcemia is classified into mild (serum calcium 10.3–12 mg/dL), moderate (serum calcium 12–14 mg/dL), and severe (serum calcium >14 mg/dL) hypercalcemia.

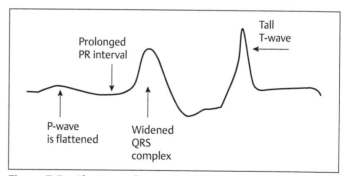

Fig. 7.5 Electrocardiogram (ECG) changes during hypermagnesemia. Changes are very similar to those depicted in hyperkalemia.

Table 7.15 Management of hypophosphatemia

Asymptomatic patients with mild hypophosphatemia	Severe or symptomatic hypophosphatemia
Phosphate effervescent tablets dissolved in water	2–5 mg/kg of inorganic phosphate dissolved in 0.45% saline given over 6–12 h and repeated, if required

The two commonest causes of hypercalcemia are primary hyperparathyroidism and nonparathyroid malignancy.[118] Causes for hypercalcemia in malignancy include release of PTHrP (as in small cell carcinoma of the lung; renal cell carcinoma), increased formation of vitamin D in macrophages (as in lymphomas), and also because of osteolytic metastases (as in multiple myeloma). Approximately 20% of all malignancies are associated with hypercalcemia. Other causes of hypercalcemia include tertiary hyperparathyroidism (autonomous secretion of PTH in secondary parathyroidism), sarcoidosis, thyrotoxicosis, and drugs: thiazides, lithium, milk-alkali syndrome, and overingestion of vitamin D.

Hypercalcemia is usually asymptomatic and detected on lab testing. Mild-to-moderate symptoms are classically described as moans (due to abdominal pain and constipation), bones (referring to bone pain), stones (referring to renal colic), and psychiatric overtones (referring to depressed mood and other psychiatric symptoms). Severe symptoms include nausea, vomiting, confusion, and coma, and physical signs related to etiology of hypercalcemia. Band keratopathy is a rare manifestation of severe hypercalcemia. ECG manifestations include short QT- and ST-segment elevation mimicking myocardial infarction.[119]

Emergency management is indicated in severe, symptomatic hypercalcemia. Intravenous hydration with normal saline is the recommended treatment to restore calciuresis. If the hypercalcemia does not correct adequately, the next step is intravenous bisphosphonate therapy using zoledronate and pamidronate.[120] Other options for emergency treatment that have been used include calcitonin, dialysis, and mithramycin. The most recently introduced adjunctive treatment is antiresorptive agent—denosumab.[121,122] Mild-to-moderate, asymptomatic hypercalcemia could be treated with oral bisphosphonates.

Hyperphosphatemia

Hyperphosphatemia is defined as a phosphate level of more than 4.5 mg/dL. There are four different etiopathogenic mechanisms of hyperphosphatemia. These include acute phosphate load, cellular shifts, decreased renal clearance, and pseudohyperphosphatemia.[123]

Acute phosphate load can be exogenous load or endogenous load. Exogenous load is relatively uncommon; it is observed in patients taking high-dose laxatives[124] or fosphenytoin (used in treatment of status epileptics). Endogenous phosphate load is seen in rhabdomyolysis and tumor-lysis syndrome. Acute cellular shift from intracellular to extracellular compartments is another cause and is usually seen in diabetic ketoacidosis as well as in lactic acidosis.

Decreased renal clearance includes chronic kidney disease, as glomerular filtration is a major mechanism of phosphate excretion. In chronic kidney disease, compensatory mechanisms come into play as increased PTH levels decrease the reabsorption of phosphorous and thus lead to increased excretion of phosphorous. However in advanced renal insufficiency, this mechanism is insufficient and at a creatinine clearance of <25 mL/min, hyperphosphatemia ensues. Increased tubular reabsorption includes drugs like bisphosphonates and excess use of vitamin D. Pseudohyperphosphatemia is caused by hyperglobulinemia, hyperlipidemia, hemolysis, hyperbilirubinemia, and administration of amphotericin B, heparin, tissue plasminogen activator (tPA).[123]

Clinical features of acute hyperphosphatemia occur as a result of concomitant hypocalcemia which can lead to muscle cramps, tetany, along with perioral numbness, or tingling. Bone pain, rash with pruritus, as well as fractures also occur. Life-threatening arrhythmias can also occur due to myocardial depressant action. In addition, there is increased calcification in the myocardium, heart valves, as well as in the vessels.[125]

Management of hyperphosphatemia includes three-pronged approach which includes a decreased dietary intake, use of phosphate-binding agents, and dialysis. Foods which are rich in phosphorous include poultry and dairy products. Phosphate-binders decrease the GI absorption of phosphate and include calcium carbonate or acetate, sevelamer carbonate or hydroxychloride, and lanthanum carbonate. Calcium compounds may lead to hypercalcemia, and therefore sevelamer carbonate and lanthanum carbonate are preferred in patients at risk of developing hypercalcemia. Dialysis is indicated in patients with acute rise in phosphate levels leading to life-threatening symptoms of hyperphosphatemia mentioned above. This usually occurs in patients with rhabdomyolysis and tumor lysis syndrome, especially in patients with preexisting renal dysfunction.[126]

Conclusion

Hyponatremia affects approximately 5% of adults and 35% of patients who are hospitalized. Most patients should be managed by treating their underlying disease and according to whether they have hypovolemic, euvolemic, or hypervolemic hyponatremia. Urea and vaptans can be effective in managing the syndrome of inappropriate anti-diuresis and hyponatremia in patients with heart failure; hypertonic saline is reserved for patients with severely symptomatic hyponatremia. Risk factors for osmotic demyelination include extreme chronic hyponatremia (serum sodium level <110mEq/L), alcohol use disorder, liver disease or transplant, potassium depletion, and malnutrition.[127]

References

1. Lee JW. Fluid and electrolyte disturbances in critically ill patients. Electrolyte Blood Press 2010;8(2):72–81
2. Rivers E, Nguyen B, Havstad S, et al; Early Goal-Directed Therapy Collaborative Group. Early goal-directed therapy in the treatment of severe sepsis and septic shock. N Engl J Med 2001;345(19):1368–1377
3. Rafat C, Flamant M, Gaudry S, Vidal-Petiot E, Ricard JD, Dreyfuss D. Hyponatremia in the intensive care unit: how to avoid a Zugzwang situation? Ann Intensive Care 2015;5(1):39
4. DeVita MV, Gardenswartz MH, Konecky A, Zabetakis PM. Incidence and etiology of hyponatremia in an intensive care unit. Clin Nephrol 1990;34(4):163–166
5. Vandergheynst F, Sakr Y, Felleiter P, et al. Incidence and prognosis of dysnatraemia in critically ill patients: analysis of a large prevalence study. Eur J Clin Invest 2013;43(9):933–948
6. Funk GC, Lindner G, Druml W, et al. Incidence and prognosis of dysnatremias present on ICU admission. Intensive Care Med 2010;36(2):304–311
7. Sakr Y, Rother S, Ferreira AM, et al. Fluctuations in serum sodium level are associated with an increased risk of death in surgical ICU patients. Crit Care Med 2013;41(1):133–142
8. Spasovski G, Vanholder R, Allolio B, et al. Clinical practice guideline on diagnosis and treatment of hyponatraemia. Intensive Care Med 2014;40(3):320–331
9. Thurman JM, Berl T. Therapy in Nephrology and hypertension, a companion to Brenner & Rector's the kidney. 3rd ed. Philadelphia: Saunders; 2008. Therapy of dysnatremic disorders; pp. 337–352
10. Ayus JC, Arieff AI. Pulmonary complications of hyponatremic encephalopathy. Noncardiogenic pulmonary edema and hypercapnic respiratory failure. Chest 1995;107(2):517–521
11. Adrogué HJ, Madias NE. Hyponatremia. N Engl J Med 2000;342(21):1581–1589
12. Verbalis JG, Goldsmith SR, Greenberg A, et al. Diagnosis, evaluation, and treatment of hyponatremia: expert panel recommendations. Am J Med 2013;126(10, Suppl 1):S1–S42
13. Palmer BF. The role of V2 receptor antagonists in the treatment of hyponatremia. Electrolyte Blood Press 2013;11(1):1–8
14. Laubenberger J, Schneider B, Ansorge O, et al. Central pontine myelinolysis: clinical presentation and radiologic findings. Eur Radiol 1996;6(2):177–183
15. de Souza A. Movement disorders and the osmotic demyelination syndrome. Parkinsonism Relat Disord 2013;19(8):709–716
16. Odier C, Nguyen DK, Panisset M. Central pontine and extrapontine myelinolysis: from epileptic and other manifestations to cognitive prognosis. J Neurol 2010;257(7):1176–1180
17. Gocht A, Colmant HJ. Central pontine and extrapontine myelinolysis: a report of 58 cases. Clin Neuropathol 1987;6(6):262–270
18. Louis G, Megarbane B, Lavoué S, et al. Long-term outcome of patients hospitalized in intensive care units with central or extrapontine myelinolysis. Crit Care Med 2012;40(3):970–972
19. Kallakatta RN, Radhakrishnan A, Fayaz RK, Unnikrishnan JP, Kesavadas C, Sarma SP. Clinical and functional outcome and factors predicting prognosis in osmotic demyelination syndrome (central pontine and/or extrapontine myelinolysis) in 25 patients. J Neurol Neurosurg Psychiatry 2011;82(3):326–331
20. Rose BD. Clinical physiology of acid-base and electrolyte disorders. 5th ed. New York, NY: Mcgraw-Hill; 2001
21. Kumar S, Berl T. Sodium. Lancet 1998;352(9123):220–228
22. Palevsky PM, Bhagrath R, Greenberg A. Hypernatremia in hospitalized patients. Ann Intern Med 1996;124(2):197–203
23. Lindner G, Funk GC, Schwarz C, et al. Hypernatremia in the critically ill is an independent risk factor for mortality. Am J Kidney Dis 2007;50(6):952–957
24. Darmon M, Timsit JF, Francais A, et al. Association between hypernatraemia acquired in the ICU and mortality: a cohort study. Nephrol Dial Transplant 2010;25(8):2510–2515
25. Lindner G, Funk GC, Lassnigg A, et al. Intensive care-acquired hypernatremia after major cardiothoracic surgery is associated with increased mortality. Intensive Care Med 2010;36(10):1718–1723
26. Stelfox HT, Ahmed SB, Khandwala F, Zygun D, Shahpori R, Laupland K. The epidemiology of intensive care unit-acquired hyponatraemia and hypernatraemia in medical-surgical intensive care units. Crit Care 2008;12(6):R162
27. O'Donoghue SD, Dulhunty JM, Bandeshe HK, Senthuran S, Gowardman JR. Acquired hypernatraemia is an independent predictor of mortality in critically ill patients. Anaesthesia. 2009 May;64(5):514-520
28. Lindner G, Funk GC. Hypernatremia in critically ill patients. J Crit Care 2013;28(2):216.e11–216.e20
29. Hoorn EJ, Betjes MG, Weigel J, Zietse R. Hypernatraemia in critically ill patients: too little water and too much salt. Nephrol Dial Transplant 2008;23(5):1562–1568
30. Adrogué HJ, Madias NE. Hypernatremia. N Engl J Med 2000;342(20):1493–1499
31. Knochel JP. Neuromuscular manifestations of electrolyte disorders. Am J Med 1982;72(3):521–535
32. Chang L, Harrington DW, Milkotic A, Swerdloff RS, Wang C. Unusual occurrence of extrapontine myelinolysis associated with acute severe hypernatraemia caused by central diabetes insipidus. Clin Endocrinol (Oxf) 2005;63(2):233–235
33. van der Helm-van Mil AH, van Vugt JP, Lammers GJ, Harinck HI. Hypernatremia from a hunger strike as a cause of osmotic myelinolysis. Neurology 2005;64(3):574–575
34. AlOrainy IA, O'Gorman AM, Decell MK. Cerebral bleeding, infarcts, and presumed extrapontine myelinolysis in hyper-natraemic dehydration. Neuroradiology 1999;41(2):144–146
35. Paice BJ, Paterson KR, Onyanga-Omara F, Donnelly T, Gray JM, Lawson DH. Record linkage study of hypokalaemia in hospitalized patients. Postgrad Med J 1986;62(725):187–191
36. Janko O, Seier J, Zazgornik J. Hypokalemia: incidence and severity in a general hospital. Wien Med Wochenschr 1992;142(4):78–81
37. Elliott TL, Braun M. Electrolytes: potassium disorders. FP Essent 2017;459:21–28
38. Marti G, Schwarz C, Leichtle AB, et al. Etiology and symptoms of severe hypokalemia in emergency department patients. Eur J Emerg Med 2014;21(1):46–51
39. Kardalas E, Paschou SA, Anagnostis P, Muscogiuri G, Siasos G, Vryonidou A. Hypokalemia: a clinical update. Endocr Connect 2018;7(4):R135–R146
40. Papademetriou V. Diuretics, hypokalemia, and cardiac arrhythmia: a 20-year controversy. J Clin Hypertens (Greenwich) 2006;8(2):86–92
41. Gumz ML, Rabinowitz L, Wingo CS. An integrated view of potassium homeostasis. [published correction appears in N

Engl J Med. 2015 Sep 24;373(13):1281] N Engl J Med 2015; 373(1):60–72

42. Ashurst J, Sergent SR, Sergent BR. Evidence-based management of potassium disorders in the emergency department. Emerg Med Pract 2016;18(11):1–24

43. Sterns RH. Treatment of severe hyponatremia. Clin J Am Soc Nephrol 2018;13(4):641–649

44. Truhlář A, Deakin CD, Soar J, et al; Cardiac Arrest in Special Circumstances Section Collaborators. European Resuscitation Council Guidelines for Resuscitation 2015: Section 4. Cardiac arrest in special circumstances. Resuscitation 2015;95: 148–201

45. Khanagavi J, Gupta T, Aronow WS, et al. Hyperkalemia among hospitalized patients and association between duration of hyperkalemia and outcomes. Arch Med Sci 2014;10(2): 251–257

46. Phillips BM, Milner S, Zouwail S, et al. Severe hyperkalaemia: demographics and outcome. Clin Kidney J 2014;7(2):127–133

47. Kovesdy CP, Appel LJ, Grams ME, et al. Potassium homeostasis in health and disease: a scientific workshop cosponsored by the National Kidney Foundation and the American Society of Hypertension. J Am Soc Hypertens 2017;11(12):783–800

48. Dépret F, Peacock WF, Liu KD, Rafique Z, Rossignol P, Legrand M. Management of hyperkalemia in the acutely ill patient. Ann Intensive Care 2019;9(1):32

49. Blanié A, Ract C, Leblanc P-E, et al. The limits of succinylcholine for critically ill patients. Anesth Analg 2012;115(4):873–879

50. Aslam S, Friedman EA, Ifudu O. Electrocardiography is unreliable in detecting potentially lethal hyperkalaemia in haemodialysis patients. Nephrol Dial Transplant 2002;17(9): 1639–1642

51. Burchell HB. Electrocardiographic changes related to disturbances in potassium metabolism. J Lancet 1953;73(6):235–238

52. Durfey N, Lehnhof B, Bergeson A, et al. Severe hyperkalemia: can the electrocardiogram risk stratify for short-term adverse events? West J Emerg Med 2017;18(5):963–971

53. Wheeler DT, Schafers SJ, Horwedel TA, Deal EN, Tobin GS. Weight-based insulin dosing for acute hyperkalemia results in less hypoglycemia. J Hosp Med 2016;11(5):355–357

54. Coca A, Valencia AL, Bustamante J, Mendiluce A, Floege J. Hypoglycemia following intravenous insulin plus glucose for hyperkalemia in patients with impaired renal function. PLoS One 2017;12(2):e0172961

55. Harel Z, Kamel KS. Optimal dose and method of administration of intravenous insulin in the management of emergency hyperkalemia: a systematic review. PLoS One 2016;11(5): e0154963

56. Allon M, Dunlay R, Copkney C. Nebulized albuterol for acute hyperkalemia in patients on hemodialysis. Ann Intern Med 1989;110(6):426–429

57. Mandelberg A, Krupnik Z, Houri S, et al. Salbutamol metered-dose inhaler with spacer for hyperkalemia: how fast? How safe? Chest 1999;115(3):617–622

58. Ngugi NN, McLigeyo SO, Kayima JK. Treatment of hyperkalaemia by altering the transcellular gradient in patients with renal failure: effect of various therapeutic approaches. East Afr Med J 1997;74(8):503–509

59. Harel Z, Harel S, Shah PS, Wald R, Perl J, Bell CM. Gastrointestinal adverse events with sodium polystyrene sulfonate (Kayexalate) use: a systematic review. Am J Med 2013;126(3):264.e9–264. e24

60. Bushinsky DA, Williams GH, Pitt B, et al. Patiromer induces rapid and sustained potassium lowering in patients with

chronic kidney disease and hyperkalemia. Kidney Int 2015; 88(6):1427–1433

61. Meaney CJ, Beccari MV, Yang Y, Zhao J. Systematic review and meta-analysis of patiromer and sodium zirconium cyclosilicate: a new armamentarium for the treatment of hyperkalemia. Pharmacotherapy 2017;37(4):401–411

62. Kosiborod M, Peacock WF, Packham DK. Sodium zirconium cyclosilicate for urgent therapy of severe hyperkalemia. N Engl J Med 2015;372(16):1577–1578

63. Kellum JA, Lameire N, Aspelin P, et al. Work group membership. Kidney Int 2012;2:1

64. Steele T, Kolamunnage-Dona R, Downey C, Toh CH, Welters I. Assessment and clinical course of hypocalcemia in critical illness. Crit Care 2013;17(3):R106

65. Zaloga GP. Hypocalcemia in critically ill patients. Crit Care Med 1992;20(2):251–262

66. Zivin JR, Gooley T, Zager RA, Ryan MJ. Hypocalcemia: a pervasive metabolic abnormality in the critically ill. Am J Kidney Dis 2001;37(4):689–698

67. Kelly A, Levine MA. Hypocalcemia in the critically ill patient. J Intensive Care Med 2013;28(3):166–177

68. Zaloga GP, Chernow B. The multifactorial basis for hypocalcemia during sepsis. Studies of the parathyroid hormone-vitamin D axis. Ann Intern Med 1987;107(1):36–41

69. Buckley MS, Leblanc JM, Cawley MJ. Electrolyte disturbances associated with commonly prescribed medications in the intensive care unit. Crit Care Med 2010;38(6, Suppl): S253–S264

70. Lind L, Carlstedt F, Rastad J, et al. Hypocalcemia and parathyroid hormone secretion in critically ill patients. Crit Care Med 2000;28(1):93–99

71. Cooper MS, Gittoes NJ. Diagnosis and management of hypocalcaemia. BMJ 2008;336(7656):1298–1302

72. Schafer AL, Shoback DM. Hypocalcemia: diagnosis and treatment. [Updated 2016 Jan 3]. In: Feingold KR, Anawalt B, Boyce A, et al., eds. Endotext [Internet]. South Dartmouth, MA: MDText.com, Inc.; 2000

73. Rallidis LS, Gregoropoulos PP, Papasteriadis EG. A case of severe hypocalcaemia mimicking myocardial infarction. Int J Cardiol 1997;61(1):89–91

74. Lehmann G, Deisenhofer I, Ndrepepa G, et al. ECG changes in a 25-year-old woman with hypocalcemia due to hypoparathyroidism: Hypocalcemia mimicking acute myocardial infarction. Chest 2001;119:668–669

75. RuDusky BM. ECG abnormalities associated with hypocalcemia. Chest 2001;119(2):668–669

76. Kudoh C, Tanaka S, Marusaki S, et al. Hypocalcemic cardiomyopathy in a patient with idiopathic hypoparathyroidism. Intern Med 1992;31(4):561–568

77. Suzuki T, Ikeda U, Fujikawa H, Saito K, Shimada K. Hypocalcemic heart failure: a reversible form of heart muscle disease. Clin Cardiol 1998;21(3):227–228

78. Shoback D. Clinical practice. Hypoparathyroidism. N Engl J Med 2008;359(4):391–403

79. Bilezikian JP, Khan A, Potts JT Jr, et al. Hypoparathyroidism in the adult: epidemiology, diagnosis, pathophysiology, target-organ involvement, treatment, and challenges for future research. J Bone Miner Res 2011;26(10):2317–2337

80. Illum F, Dupont E. Prevalences of CT-detected calcification in the basal ganglia in idiopathic hypoparathyroidism and pseudohypoparathyroidism. Neuroradiology 1985;27(1): 32–37

81. Mitchell DM, Regan S, Cooley MR, et al. Long-term follow-up of patients with hypoparathyroidism. J Clin Endocrinol Metab 2012;97(12):4507–4514

82. Hansen BA, Bruserud Ø. Hypomagnesemia in critically ill patients. J Intensive Care 2018;6:21

83. Jahnen-Dechent W, Ketteler M. Magnesium basics. Clin Kidney J 2012;5(Suppl 1):i3–i14

84. Wong ET, Rude RK, Singer FR, Shaw ST Jr. A high prevalence of hypomagnesemia and hypermagnesemia in hospitalized patients. Am J Clin Pathol 1983;79(3):348–352

85. Hayes JP, Ryan MF, Brazil N, Riordan TO, Walsh JB, Coakley D. Serum hypomagnesaemia in an elderly day-hospital population. Ir Med J 1989;82(3):117–119

86. Whang R, Oei TO, Aikawa JK, et al. Predictors of clinical hypomagnesemia. Hypokalemia, hypophosphatemia, hyponatremia, and hypocalcemia. Arch Intern Med 1984; 144(9):1794–1796

87. Reinhart RA, Desbiens NA. Hypomagnesemia in patients entering the ICU. Crit Care Med 1985;13(6):506–507

88. Rubeiz GJ, Thill-Baharozian M, Hardie D, Carlson RW. Association of hypomagnesemia and mortality in acutely ill medical patients. Crit Care Med 1993;21(2):203–209

89. Soliman HM, Mercan D, Lobo SS, Mélot C, Vincent JL. Development of ionized hypomagnesemia is associated with higher mortality rates. Crit Care Med 2003;31(4):1082–1087

90. Hanna S. Plasma magnesium in health and disease. J Clin Pathol 1961;14:410–414

91. Nadler JL, Rude RK. Disorders of magnesium metabolism. Endocrinol Metab Clin North Am 1995;24(3):623–641

92. Flink EB. Magnesium deficiency. Etiology and clinical spectrum. Acta Med Scand Suppl 1981;647:125–137

93. Skou JC, Butler KW, Hansen O. The effect of magnesium, ATP, P i, and sodium on the inhibition of the (Na++ K+)-activated enzyme system by g-strophanthin. Biochim Biophys Acta 1971;241(2):443–461

94. Khan AM, Lubitz SA, Sullivan LM, et al. Low serum magnesium and the development of atrial fibrillation in the community: the Framingham Heart Study. Circulation 2013;127(1):33–38

95. Agus ZS. Hypomagnesemia. J Am Soc Nephrol 1999;10(7): 1616–1622

96. Sueta CA, Clarke SW, Dunlap SH, et al. Effect of acute magnesium administration on the frequency of ventricular arrhythmia in patients with heart failure. Circulation 1994; 89(2):660–666

97. Tsuji H, Venditti FJ Jr, Evans JC, Larson MG, Levy D. The associations of levels of serum potassium and magnesium with ventricular premature complexes (the Framingham Heart Study). Am J Cardiol 1994;74(3):232–235

98. Efstratiadis G, Sarigianni M, Gougourelas I. Hypomagnesemia and cardiovascular system. Hippokratia 2006;10(4):147–152

99. Yamamoto M, Yamaguchi T. Causes and treatment of hypomagnesemia. Clin Calcium 2007;17(8):1241–1248

100. Martin KJ, González EA, Slatopolsky E. Clinical consequences and management of hypomagnesemia. J Am Soc Nephrol 2009;20(11):2291–2295

101. Geerse DA, Bindels AJ, Kuiper MA, Roos AN, Spronk PE, Schultz MJ. Treatment of hypophosphatemia in the intensive care unit: a review. Crit Care 2010;14(4):R147

102. Suzuki S, Egi M, Schneider AG, Bellomo R, Hart GK, Hegarty C. Hypophosphatemia in critically ill patients. J Crit Care 2013;28(4):536.e9–536.e19

103. Amanzadeh J, Reilly RF Jr. Hypophosphatemia: an evidence-based approach to its clinical consequences and management. Nat Clin Pract Nephrol 2006;2(3):136–148

104. Aubier M, Murciano D, Lecocguic Y, et al. Effect of hypophosphatemia on diaphragmatic contractility in patients with acute respiratory failure. N Engl J Med 1985;313(7):420–424

105. Gravelyn TR, Brophy N, Siegert C, Peters-Golden M. Hypophosphatemia-associated respiratory muscle weakness in a general inpatient population. Am J Med 1988;84(5): 870–876

106. Schwartz A, Gurman G, Cohen G, et al. Association between hypophosphatemia and cardiac arrhythmias in the early stages of sepsis. Eur J Intern Med 2002;13(7):434

107. Ognibene A, Ciniglio R, Greifenstein A, et al. Ventricular tachycardia in acute myocardial infarction: the role of hypophosphatemia. South Med J 1994;87(1):65–69

108. Singhal PC, Kumar A, Desroches L, Gibbons N, Mattana J. Prevalence and predictors of rhabdomyolysis in patients with hypophosphatemia. Am J Med 1992;92(5):458–464

109. Charron T, Bernard F, Skrobik Y, Simoneau N, Gagnon N, Leblanc M. Intravenous phosphate in the intensive care unit: more aggressive repletion regimens for moderate and severe hypophosphatemia. Intensive Care Med 2003;29(8): 1273–1278

110. Perreault MM, Ostrop NJ, Tierney MG. Efficacy and safety of intravenous phosphate replacement in critically ill patients. Ann Pharmacother 1997;31(6):683–688

111. Birrer RB, Shallash AJ, Totten V. Hypermagnesemia-induced fatality following epsom salt gargles(1). J Emerg Med 2002; 22(2):185–188

112. Harker HE, Majcher TA. Hypermagnesemia in a pediatric patient. Anesth Analg 2000;91(5):1160–1162

113. Onishi S, Yoshino S. Cathartic-induced fatal hypermagnesemia in the elderly. Intern Med 2006;45(4):207–210

114. Kontani M, Hara A, Ohta S, Ikeda T. Hypermagnesemia induced by massive cathartic ingestion in an elderly woman without pre-existing renal dysfunction. Intern Med 2005;44(5): 448–452

115. Vissers RJ, Purssell R. Iatrogenic magnesium overdose: two case reports. J Emerg Med 1996;14(2):187–191

116. Cascella M, Vaqar S. Hypermagnesemia. [Updated 2020 Jul 4]. In: StatPearls [Internet]. Treasure Island (FL): StatPearls Publishing; 2020 Jan

117. Dent DM, Miller JL, Klaff L, Barron J. The incidence and causes of hypercalcaemia. Postgrad Med J 1987;63(743):745–750

118. Goltzman D. Approach to hypercalcemia. In: De Groot LJ, Chrousos G, Dungan K, et al., eds. Approach to hypercalcemia. South Dartmouth, MA: MDText.com, Inc.; 2000

119. Turner JJO. Hypercalcaemia: presentation and management. Clin Med (Lond) 2017;17(3):270–273

120. Walsh J, Gittoes N, Selby P; Society for Endocrinology Clinical Committee. Society for Endocrinology Endocrine Emergency Guidance: emergency management of acute hypercalcaemia in adult patients. Endocr Connect 2016;5(5):G9–G11

121. Karuppiah D, Thanabalasingham G, Shine B, et al. Refractory hypercalcaemia secondary to parathyroid carcinoma: response to high-dose denosumab. Eur J Endocrinol 2014; 171(1):K1–K5

122. Adhikaree J, Newby Y, Sundar S. Denosumab should be the treatment of choice for bisphosphonate refractory hypercalcaemia of malignancy. BMJ Case Rep 2014;2014: bcr2013202861

123. Wadsworth RL, Siddiqui S. Phosphate homeostasis in critical care. BJA Educ 2016;16(9):305–309

124. Tan HL, Liew QY, Loo S, Hawkins R. Severe hyperphosphataemia and associated electrolyte and metabolic derangement following the administration of sodium phosphate for bowel preparation. Anaesthesia 2002;57(5):478–483

125. Albaaj F, Hutchison A. Hyperphosphataemia in renal failure: causes, consequences and current management. Drugs 2003;63(6):577–596

126. Shaman AM, Kowalski SR. Hyperphosphatemia management in patients with chronic kidney disease. Saudi Pharm J 2016;24(4):494–505

127. Horacio J Adrogue, Bryan M Tucker, Nicolaos E Madias. Diagnosis and Management of Hyponatremia: A Review. JAMA 2022, 328 (3): 280–291

8

STEMI: Complications and Management

Naveen Garg, Rohan Kapur, and K. K. Kapur

Introduction

Globally, acute coronary syndrome (ACS) is the number one cause of death, disability, and human suffering. Mortality due to ACS outnumbers that due to any other disease. In developed countries, ACS presents mostly in older age group whereas in developing countries it affects young, economically productive age groups. ACS is identified as a lifestyle disease with risk profiles including hypertension, obesity, diabetes, dyslipidemia, smoking, and sedentary lifestyle. The pathophysiological changes of ACS occur in the myocardium and so its management is time dependent, and therefore patients are often unable to afford the specified medical facility. Globally, annual mortality cases due to ACS are about 17 million per year, which is one-third of all-cause mortality. Early recognition, awareness, and approachable facilities in some developed countries are the major reasons for the decline in ACS deaths in recent years.[1,2]

ACS is an umbrella term which comprises the clinico-pathological changes that occur after the occlusion of blood supply to the myocardium, whereas myocardial infarction (MI) is the last consequence of ACS leading to myocardial cell death due to prolonged ischemia induced by occlusion of blood supply.[3-5] ACS is diagnosed with the help of electro-cardiogram (ECG) and cardiac enzymes (troponins). Based on these interpretations, ACS is further classified into different groups, as listed in **Table 8.1**.

Thus, ECG and troponins help in deciding the further management of ACS (**Flowchart 8.1**).

STEMI

Acute MI is commonly defined as a cardiomyocyte death due to a prolonged ischemia resulting from an acute imbalance between oxygen supply and demand.

ST-elevation myocardial infarction (STEMI) is a clinical presentation involving ECG changes and chest pain (angina). As depicted in **Flowchart 8.1**, the ECG changes in the form of ST elevation with clinical symptoms of angina are indicative of myocardial injury. Myocardial enzymes, troponins, are elevated after acute insult and are indicative of myocardial necrosis. These tests in critical care help in formulating immediate treatment strategy and management of disease in process.

Table 8.1 Classification of acute coronary syndrome

ACS class	ECG	Troponins
UA	No ST elevation	Absent
NSTEMI	No ST elevation	Present
STEMI	ST elevation	Present

Abbreviations: ACS, acute coronary syndrome; ECG, electrocardiogram; NSTEMI, non-ST-elevation myocardial infarction; STEMI, ST-elevation myocardial infarction; UA, unstable angina.

Pathophysiology of STEMI

STEMI involves a complete occlusion of coronary artery with thrombus formed due to rupture of atherosclerotic plaque or dissection of the artery. This results in ischemia and later myocardial cell death in the region of arterial supply distal to occlusion. This ischemic "wave" spreads from endocardium to epicardium and involves the whole full thickness of cardiac tissue. Whole of infarcted region is later replaced by fibrotic tissue. This remodeling affects cardiac contractility which could lead to heart failure (HF).[6-11]

The atherosclerotic plaques in arterial lumen were thought to be the culprit spots causing thrombus formation and then ACS. This was demonstrated by many newer imaging techniques like intra-arterial ultrasound, optical coherence tomography (OCT), micro-positron emission tomography (PET), etc. It is now proposed that microcalcifications within the plaques create cutting edges that burst with sheer stress of circulating luminal blood. These plaques are called vulnerable plaques in contrast to "stable plaques" wherein these microcalcifications progressively aggregate to form sheets (loss of cutting edges). The core of these plaques is made up of necrotic tissue from apoptosis of macrophages and other cells. This necrotic tissue on rupture leads to platelet aggregation and thrombus formation.[12-16]

Experimental molecular imaging modalities such as micro-PET, micro-computed tomography (CT), etc., have shown vulnerability of these plaques (**Fig. 8.1**).

STEMI versus NSTEMI/UA

The basic pathophysiology of plaque formation in STEMI or NSTEMI/UA is same; however, their clinical presentation and treatment strategies are different. STEMI is managed aggressively, and fibrinolytic therapy is must within

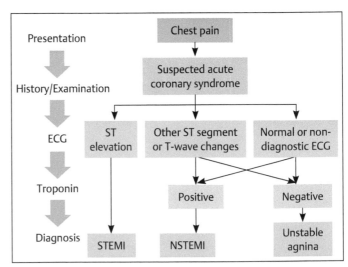

Flowchart 8.1 Depicting pathways of chest pain in diagnosing acute coronary syndrome (ACS). Abbreviations: ECG, electrocardiogram; NSTEMI, non-ST-elevation myocardial infarction; STEMI, ST-elevation myocardial infarction.

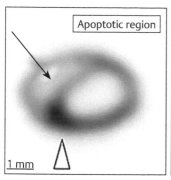
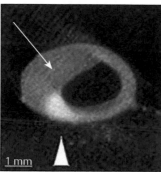

Fig. 8.1 18F-ApoPep1 positron emission tomography (PET) and fusion imaging with micro-CT (computed tomography) clearly imaged apoptotic process occurring in the vulnerable plaque on PET imaging. *Arrows show the apoptotic region, near the plaque.*

30 minutes of its presentation, whereas NSTEMI is managed less aggressively with antithrombotic medications. Invasive intervention in both cases is essential for risk identification and treatment. Thrombus in STEMI is known as "red thrombus" as it is rich in RBCs and fibrin, whereas thrombus in NSTEMI is known as "white thrombus" or platelet plug. This difference in composition defines the variation in treatment strategies for different types of ACS. Cardiac mortality and major adverse cardiac events (MACE) are higher in patients with red thrombus as compared to white thrombus.[17-20] However, some studies indicate that white thrombus over a period of time could change over to red thrombus. As imaged by intravascular ultrasound (IVUS), morphology of plaques in STEMI versus NSTEMI shows that STEMI-associated plaques have:

1. Greater plaque burden (calculated as area of plaque).
2. Less severe calcification.
3. More lipid-pool like image (more hypoechoic plaque).
4. Higher incidence of multiple plaque rupture.

Unlike STEMI or NSTEMI, in unstable angina (UA), blood flow in the coronary artery becomes sluggish and patients develop angina at rest (known as preinfarct angina). Total coronary occlusion does not usually occur. Thus, the primary aim of therapy in UA is to prevent MI. In NSTEMI/UA, the occlusive thrombus is rich in platelet and has less fibrin; therefore, fibrinolytic agents are contraindicated in NSTEMI/UA patients.[20-23]

Acute Complications of AMI (STEMI)

Acute complications of STEMI[24-27] are as follows:

1. *Left ventricular dysfunction:* This is the most frequent consequence of STEMI. Left ventricular ejection fraction (LVEF) reduces after myocardial injury. This occurs due to loss of healthy myocardium or ischemic injury (stunning effect). Other causes of LV dysfunction include mechanical complications, valvular dysfunctions, or arrhythmias. Dysfunctional LV progresses to HF. Diagnostic imaging especially noninvasive cardiac ultrasound (echocardiography) is frequently used for its detection and monitoring.

2. *LV aneurysm:* Large transmural infarct undergoes adverse remodeling leading to LV wall aneurysm. Owing to low-flow state in the aneurysm, there is a potential for thrombus formation. Less than 5% of STEMI patients develop LV aneurysm. Patients with LV aneurysm often develop HF and arrhythmias. Treatment strategies may include surgical repair, depending upon the size of the aneurysm.

3. *LV thrombus:* It is most commonly seen in anterior wall infarctions. Echocardiography is the best modality to diagnose thrombus and monitoring the therapy.

4. *Free-wall rupture:* LV free-wall rupture is a devastating complication which could occur within one week of the episode of STEMI. The incidence is less than 1% and is decreasing due to prompt revascularization therapy (thrombolysis, percutaneous coronary intervention [PCI], or combination of both). Risk factors include delayed reperfusion and old age. Myocardial free-wall rupture often leads to hemopericardium and tamponade resulting in cardiogenic shock (CS). Echocardiography, if available at the time of this complication, helps in its diagnosis. Urgent surgical repair, if possible, could salvage such patients as otherwise mortality is extremely high (up to 75%).

5. *Ventricular septal rupture:* Septal rupture leading to left-to-right shunt with hemodynamic instability occurs suddenly after STEMI. It follows within 24 hours to a week after STEMI. A loud systolic murmur with deteriorating condition of the patient and congestive HF are often the first signs which alert the treating physician to this complication. Color Doppler echocardiography clinches the diagnosis by demonstrating apical turbulence and left-to-right shunt in anterior STEMI and turbulence across the inferobasal interventricular septum (IVS) in inferior STEMI. This complication is associated with high mortality and usually is managed with intra-aortic balloon pump (IABP), and urgent surgical repair should be planned. However, owing to fragile necrotic myocardium around the ventricular septal defect (VSD), direct patching of the VSD is challenging. Excluding the apical region with Dorr repair is a viable option in such a setting. In extremely high-risk patients with multiple comorbidities, percutaneous device closure of post-MI-VSD should be considered. However, this is often hampered because of the failure of the implanted device to hold on to the edges of the VSD owing to necrotic myocardial tissue.

6. *Papillary muscle rupture:* Rupture of papillary muscle leads to acute onset of mitral regurgitation (MR) within few days of STEMI. The papillary muscle tear could occur at the chordal end or a massive rupture of the entire papillary muscle itself could occur. Posteromedial papillary muscles (PMPM) are more often (>60%) affected due to single coronary artery

supply (right coronary artery [RCA] or left circumflex artery [LCX]). It results in sudden development of pulmonary edema or CS. Once diagnosed, prompt valve replacement surgery is required. However, there are few reports of percutaneous Mitraclip insertion in patients with CS following acute papillary muscle rupture. In addition, there are few reports of percutaneous papillary muscle suturing with some initial observational studies showing a relatively high mortality (20–25%).[28]

7. *Ischemic mitral valve regurgitation:* This occurs usually 1 week to 10 days after apical or inferolateral STEMI. Owing to post-STEMI fibrosis, remodeling occurs which causes apical tethering and traction of the papillary muscles in case of anterior STEMI and tethering and displacement of chordae and papillary muscles toward the basal lateral wall in case of posteroinferior STEMI. This causes incomplete coaptation of mitral leaflets leading to significant mitral regurgitation (Ischemic-MR).

8. *Right ventricular infarct:* RV infarction occurs in approximately 30–40% of patients with inferior wall MI. Clinically, a triad of features including hypotension, distended jugular veins, and clear lung fields are indicative of RV involvement in STEMI. Echocardiography allows a prompt diagnosis of RV involvement with inferior wall MI and thus facilitates appropriate management strategy.

9. *Cardiogenic shock (CS):* It is clinically diagnosed as hypotension not responding to fluids with pulmonary congestion and association with systemic hypoperfusion. Hypotension is defined as systolic BP <90 mmHg lasting for more than 30 minutes after an episode of MI or failure to maintain a systolic BP of 90 mmHg or more without the support of mechanical or pharmacological agents. Systemic hypoperfusion can be recognized by any one of the following symptoms: altered mental status, cool extremities, and decreased urine output (<30 mL/h). On investigative work-up, there could be an increased serum lactate (>2 mmol/L), decreased cardiac output (<2.2 L/min/m²), as well as increased pulmonary capillary wedge pressure (PCWP) of >18 mmHg. If RV infarction is associated with it, then there will be elevation of right ventricular end-diastolic pressure (RVEDP >15 mmHg).[28–34]

This hemodynamic instability occurs due to acute myocardial injury (AMI, pump failure) or as a consequence of other mechanical complications or conduction disorders (arrhythmias) resulting from MI. Low cardiac output resulting from depressed LV contractility leads to low perfusion of myocardium itself and thus causing further myocardial and tissue ischemia. This vicious cycle if not interrupted may lead to death[35,36] (**Flowchart 8.2**).

Clinical hallmark of CS is low cardiac index (<2.2 L/min/m²), but pulmonary congestion could be variable according to Forrester classification,[36] as listed in **Table 8.2**:

1. *Cold and wet type:* This is the classic form of CS, where low cardiac output is associated with pulmonary congestion due to increased pulmonary capillary wedge pressure (PCWP) and with compensatory peripheral vasoconstriction. This phenotype is about 70 to 75% MI-associated CS. This phenotype often has history of previous MI or chronic kidney disease (CKD).

2. *Cold and dry type:* This "euvolemic" phenotype is about 25 to 28% of MI-associated CS. It is recognized as cold extremities without pulmonary congestion.

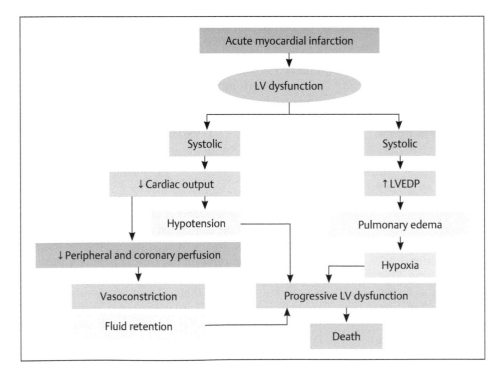

Flowchart 8.2 Showing sequel of events leading to progressive left ventricular (LV) dysfunction and death after acute myocardial infarction. Abbreviation: LVEDP, left ventricular end-diastolic pressure.

Table 8.2 Depicting clinical scenario in shock syndrome and Forrester classification

PCWP
18 mmHg

	Wet	**Dry**
Cold	Classic cardiogenic shock Forrester Class-VI Mortality-51%	Euvolemic shock Forrester Class-III Mortality-23%
Warm	Mixed shock Forrester Class-II Mortality-9%	Non-cardiac shock Forrester Class-I Mortality-3%

CI 2.2 L/min/m²

Abbreviation: PCWP: pulmonary capillary wedge pressure.

This phenotype is less likely to have a history of previous MI. The use of diuretic drugs by patients prior to the development of CS could also have a role in this phenotype.

3. *Wet and warm type:* This CS is of mixed type and is associated with systemic inflammation resulting from cytokine cascade and increased nitric oxide (NO) generation. This systemic inflammation causes vasodilatory response.

4. *Warm and dry type:* This particular category is controversial because it includes acute STEMI with shock due to other etiology (associated sepsis). Therefore, this entity should not be included in the discussion related to CS.

However, there are other two types of CS which have been recognized:

5. *"Normotensive" CS:* The so-called "Normotensive" CS actually implies "relative hypotension" in patients with acute STEMI who have pre-existing hypertension. Signs of hypoperfusion in this subset are likely to be less obvious than those in patients with classical CS. The systolic BP may be more than 90 mmHg despite the patient being in CS. This entity is relatively rare, occurring in less than 5% of patients. The SVR (systemic vascular resistance) in this group is higher than that in patients with classical CS while the other indices like CO LVEDP are similar.

6. *RV dysfunction:* In some patients with inferior wall infarction (owing to occlusion of proximal RCA), there is infarction of the RV diaphragmatic wall with/without additional involvement of RV anterolateral wall. Since the RV function is crucial to maintain the cardiac output, low CO, hypotension, and shock occur in some patients with RV infarction. Another mechanism for RV dysfunction could occur in patients with septal MI and RV ischemia. Involvement of both the septum and RV free wall could result in significant RV dysfunction despite absence of associated RV-MI. The latter

Table 8.3 Factors associated with development of CS after STEMI

Variables	Points
Age	2
Previous stroke/TIA	2
On admission cardiac arrest	3
Anterior MI	1
Delay to PCI >90 min	2
Killips Class II on admission	2
Killips Class III on admission	6
HR >90	3
SBP <125 or DBP <45 mmHg	4
Glycemia >10 mmol	3
Left main lesion	5
TIMI <3	5

Risk category/score	Incidence of CS
Low 0–7	1.3%
Low–intermediate 8–10	6.6%
Intermediate–high 11–12	11.7%
High >13	31.8%

Abbreviations: CS, cardiogenic shock; HR, heart rate; MI, myocardial infarction; PCI, percutaneous coronary intervention; PP, pulse pressure; SBP, systolic blood pressure; STEMI, ST-elevation myocardial infarction; TIA, transient ischemic attack; TIMI, thrombolysis in myocardial infarction.

group of patients are usually younger and have no history of previous insult but show symptoms/signs of RV failure (central venous pressure [CVP]:PCWP ≥0.8).

Risk Stratification

CS is associated with high mortality, is twice as common in STEMI as in non-STEMI, and occurs in about 5 to 10% of all STEMI cases. Old age, female gender, and Asian ethnicity are more prone for CS after STEMI.[37–42]

The risk factors that could be predictive of CS after STEMI have been studied and some scoring system has been devised. One such scoring system is listed in **Table 8.3**.

Some other identifiable risk factors are:
- Left bundle branch block.
- HF on admission.
- Multivessel coronary artery disease.
- Medications such as beta-blockers, angiotensin-converting enzyme inhibitors (ACEIs), diuretics.
- Although the development of CS after STEMI is usually sudden, sometimes a gradual evolution of this entity from preshock stage to advanced CS could be discernible, as illustrated in **Fig. 8.2**.

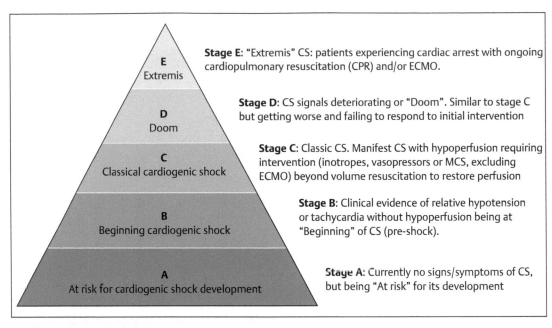

Stage E: "Extremis" CS: patients experiencing cardiac arrest with ongoing cardiopulmonary resuscitation (CPR) and/or ECMO.

Stage D: CS signals deteriorating or "Doom". Similar to stage C but getting worse and failing to respond to initial intervention

Stage C: Classic CS. Manifest CS with hypoperfusion requiring intervention (inotropes, vasopressors or MCS, excluding ECMO) beyond volume resuscitation to restore perfusion

Stage B: Clinical evidence of relative hypotension or tachycardia without hypoperfusion being at "Beginning" of CS (pre-shock).

Stage A: Currently no signs/symptoms of CS, but being "At risk" for its development

Fig. 8.2 Various stages of development of classic shock from preshock stage after ST-elevation myocardial infarction (STEMI). Abbreviations: CS, cardiogenic shock; ECMO, extracorporeal membrane oxygenation; MCS, mechanical circulatory support.

Table 8.4 Predictors of mortality (IABP-SHOCK-II trial)

Variables or predictors	Points	Risk category—mortality
Age	1	0–2—Low (<20%)
History of stroke	2	3–4—intermediate (<40%)
Blood glucose 191 mg/dL	1	5–9—high (40–80%)
Serum creatinine >1.5 mg/dL	1	
Arterial lactate >5 mmol/L	2	
TIMI grade <3 after PCI	2	

Abbreviations: IABP, intra-aortic balloon pump; PCI, percutaneous coronary intervention; SHOCK, should we emergently revascularize occluded coronaries for cardiogenic shock; TIMI, thrombolysis in myocardial infarction.

Various Factors Predicting Mortality in CS

Various factors which are predictive of mortality in CS have been systematically analyzed. The IABP-SHOCK trial[37] and the scoring system used in this study are given in **Table 8.4**.

STEMI versus Non-STEMI for CS

Non-STEMI patients develop CS less often as compared to STEMI, but mortality is same in both groups after the development of CS. A multicenter study "GUSTO-IIb trial" has shown that older, diabetic patients with multivessel disease and having low thrombolysis in myocardial infarction (TIMI) flow, who developed CS, usually had NSTEMI. On the other hand, STEMI patients developed CS earlier (median time 9.6 h) than NSTEMI patients (76.2 h). Thus, most STEMI patients had CS prior to hospitalization whereas NSTEMI patients developed CS during hospital stay. However, 30-day mortality is higher in NSTEMI than in STEMI (approximately 10% higher).[43,44]

Investigations in Patients with CS

1. Laboratory biomarkers: These include the following:
   - **Troponins:** Increased cardiac enzymes indicate extent of myocardial necrosis.
   - **Natriuretic peptides:** Elevated levels predict mortality in CS associated with MI or HF.
   - **Arterial lactic acid:** Serial measurement of arterial lactate levels is a reliable prognostic indicator.
   - **Serum creatinine:** Elevated levels of creatinine is an adverse prognostic marker.
2. Noninvasive investigations:
   - **ECG:** The various ECG patterns in STEMI and NSTEMI are shown in **Fig. 8.3**.
   - **Chest X-ray:** Despite its limitations, still a good tool to indicate pulmonary venous congestion (**Fig. 8.4**).
   - **Echocardiography:** Echocardiography is a robust bedside tool to evaluate various cardiac pathologies. Almost all causes of CS can be diagnosed by echocardiography. Point-of-care ultrasound (POCUS) of heart in the emergency room or ICU can rapidly differentiate CS from other shock syndromes. Other etiologies of chest pain resulting in CS (i.e., aortic dissection and pulmonary embolism) can be readily diagnosed. Moreover, this technique can easily assess the pathophysiological mechanisms underlying CS, which is, mechanical complications of STEMI (e.g., VSD, papillary muscle rupture) (causing severe MR), free-wall rupture, as well as

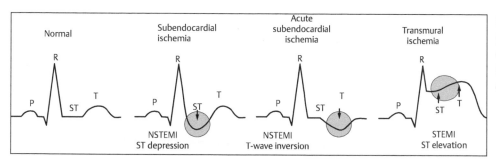

Fig. 8.3 Depicting electrocardiogram (ECG) changes in non-ST-elevation myocardial infarction (NSTEMI) and ST-elevation myocardial infarction (STEMI).

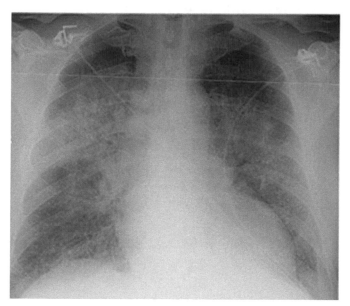

Fig. 8.4 Chest X-ray showing pulmonary edema.

pump failure. The use of Doppler hemodynamic for cardiac output and filling pressures is extremely helpful in monitoring and guiding therapy in CS.

Both STEMI and NSTEMI result in regional or global wall motion abnormalities which can be easily detected by echocardiography. However, in some instances wall motion abnormality could be subtle and speckle tracking echocardiography with strain analysis could help in evaluation of such patients. Global LVEF which is readily assessed and is variably affected is an important parameter in the evaluation of CS. Moreover, associated LV aneurysms and/or thrombus as well as pericardial effusion including cardiac tamponade are easily detected (**Fig. 8.5a–f**).

Management Strategies

Early Reperfusion

Early reperfusion/revascularization is the mainstay in the initial management of STEMI. CS can thus be prevented by early intervention. PCI is also the treatment of choice in patients with CS.[45-51] Various fibrinolytic agents including streptokinase and tissue plasminogen activator (tPA: alteplase, rateplase) are shown in **Table 8.5**.

The often-quoted SHOCK (*Should We Emergently Revascularize Occluded Coronaries for Cardiogenic Shock*) trial[51] has conclusively shown that invasive therapy in CS, if feasible (preferably PCI or if not possible CABG), has significantly lower mortality both in short term and long term as compared to noninvasive strategy (**Fig. 8.6**).

However, according to the *AHA guidelines*, fibrinolytic therapy should be instituted in the management of CS due to STEMI if within the window period of 0 to 4 hours and if the patient cannot be moved to PCI facility.[52-57]

Inotrope/Vasopressor Support

Inotropes are an important part of management of CS. These increase cardiac contractility and thus initially help in increasing the cardiac output (**Tables 8.6** and **8.7**). Inotropes can be divided into three groups:

1. Adrenergic receptor agonists (β-agonists)—dopamine (inotrope + vasopressor), dobutamine (inodilator), epinephrine (inotrope + vasopressor) and norepinephrine (vasopressor).
2. PDE-3 inhibitors—milrinone, amrinone (inodilators).
3. Calcium sensitizers—levosimendan (inodilator).

Beta-agonists cause release of sarcoplasmic calcium via increased synthesis of cAMP by stimulation of sarcolemmal beta-1 adrenergic receptors.

Phosphodiesterase III inhibitors (PDE-III) inhibit sarcoplasmic-associated PDE-III enzyme and increase intracellular cAMP which in turn increase calcium in the cells.

Levosimendan sensitizes cardiac troponin proteins (troponin-c) to calcium, thus increasing cardiac contractility without affecting cardiac relaxation.

Inotropes and vasopressor are extremely useful in the initial management of CS. However, prolonged use of inotropes leads to development of resistance to their efficacy. Inotropes help in temporarily tiding over the critical phase in CS, but are not the mainstay in the overall management.[58-64]

Management of CS

Dobutamine is used as a first-line drug during systolic blood pressure of less than 100 mmHg in the absence of signs and symptoms of shock; however, dopamine is preferred in the presence of symptoms of shock. Both these agents in moderate doses help in improving the hemodynamics and avoiding end-organ ischemia by maximizing the cardiac contractility

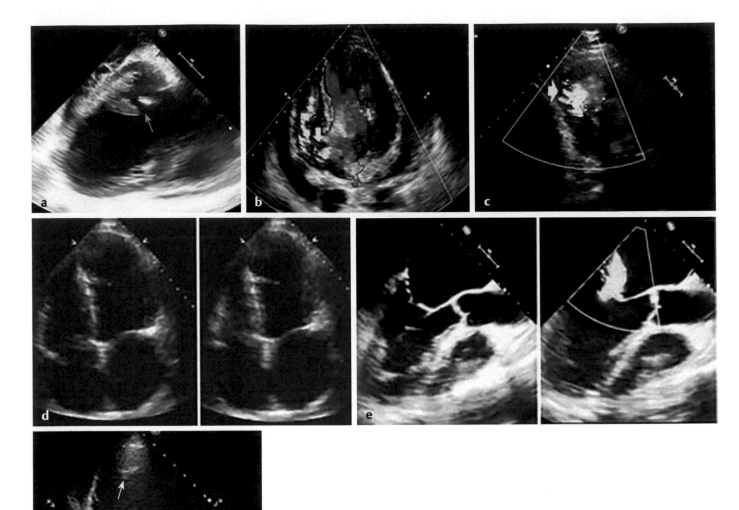

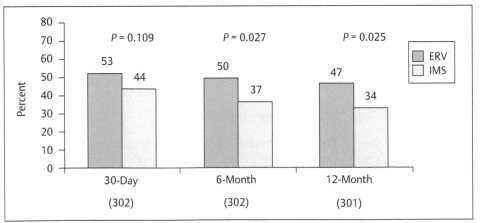

Fig. 8.5 **(a–f)** Various myocardial complications observed by echocardiographic studies after ST-elevation myocardial infarction (STEMI). **(a)** Showing rupture of papillary muscle after STEMI (*arrow*). **(b)** Color Doppler study depicting ventricular septal defect (VSD) at basal septum after inferolateral STEMI. **(c)** Color Doppler showing VSD at apical septum after anterior wall STEMI. **(d)** 2D-echocardiography depicting global left-ventricular (LV) dysfunction after STEMI. **(e)** Showing tethering of mitral valve (seagull sign) due to inferolateral myocardial infarction (MI). **(f)** Showing marked LV dilatation with apical thrombus after STEMI.

Fig. 8.6 Overall survival at 1, 6, and 12 months of follow-up. Abbreviations: ERV, early revascularization (PCI); IMS, initial medical stabilization (includes thrombolysis).

Table 8.5 Various fibrinolytic agents

Name	Dose	Source	Fibrin specificity
Streptokinase	1.5 MU in 30–60 min	Bacterial	Indirect (Plasminogen)
Alteplase	60 + 20 + 20 mg over 3 h	Recombinant DNA	Fibrin +
Reteplase	10 + 10 MU after 30 min	Recombinant DNA	Fibrin +
Tenecteplase	40 mg single dose	Tissue type	Fibrin +++
Lanoteplase	120 kU/kg single dose	Tissue type	Fibrin +
Staphylokinase	20 mg single dose	Bacterial	Fibrin ++++

Table 8.6 Properties of inotropes mainly used in CS or heart failure

	Mechanism of action	Inotropic action	Vasoconstriction	Vasodilator	Dose
Dopamine	D > B	++	++	+	3–5 µg/kg/min
Dobutamine	B1 > B2 > A	++	–	+	1–20 µg/kg/min
Norepinephrine	A > B1 > B2	+	++	–	0.02–10 µg/kg/min
Epinephrine	B1 = B2 > A	++	–	–/+	0.05–0.5 µg/kg/min
Milrinone	PDE-III Inhibitor	+	–	+++	0.375–0.75 µg/kg/min
Levosimendan	Ca sensitizer	+	–	++	0.05–0.2 µg/kg/min
Vasopressin	V1 agonist	–/+	+++	–	0.01–0.04 U/min
Phenylephrine	A1 agonist	–	+++	–	50–200 µg/kg/min

Abbreviations: CS, cardiogenic shock; PDE, phosphodiesterase.

Table 8.7 Effects of inotropes mainly used in CS or heart failure

	CO	HR	MAP/SVR	PVR
Dopamine	↑	↑	↑	↔
Dobutamine	↑	↑	↓↔	↓
Norepinephrine	↔	↔	↑	↑
Epinephrine	↑	↑	↑	↔
Milrinone	↑	↑	↓	↓↓
Levosimendan	↑	↔	↓↑	↓
Vasopressin	↔	↔		↔
Phenylephrine	↔	↓	↑	↑↑

Abbreviations: CO, cardiac output; HR, heart rate; MAP, mean arterial pressure; PVR, pulmonary vascular resistance; SVR, systemic vascular resistance.

and avoiding excess vasoconstriction. The stronger vasopressor action of norepinephrine makes it a preferable first-line agent in marked hypotension with CS.

Vasopressin is introduced in norepinephrine-resistant vasodilatory shock. It improves mean arterial pressure (MAP) without increasing cardiotoxicity and arrhythmias. The use of levosimendan in CS, however, is controversial. Recent trials on use of levosimendan in CS have shown improvement in hemodynamics but no significant survival benefit as compared to dobutamine.

A combination of moderate doses of inotropes likely complement each other especially when excessive

vasodilatory/vasoconstrictive actions of different inotropes need to be finely balanced. Use of very high doses of one particular inotrope can thus be avoided.

Limitations of Inotropes in Management of CS

Inotropes provide a critical support during the initial management of CS, but their prolonged use can cause several adverse effects.

1. They could cause increase in myocardial oxygen demand, which could be detrimental in the management of ischemic ventricle.
2. They could lead to systemic inflammatory response syndrome, which could complicate the treatment of CS.
3. Ultimately, they could lead to resistance to inotropes.
4. Therefore, treatment of CS only with inotropes associated with high mortality.

Role of Diuretics

The use of intravenous diuretics (furosemide, torsemide) is extremely important to relieve pulmonary venous congestion in patients with CS. These agents act by reducing the using their venodilator properties and thus are associated management of pulmonary edema which is often associated with CS. Furthermore, because of their diuretics help help in reducing intravascular volume. These diuretics help in reducing pulmonary venous pressure as well as LVEDP, which are markedly elevated in CS, while maintaining the urinary output which otherwise is often significantly reduced due to hypotension and vasoconstriction.[65–67]

However, diuretics should only be used in combination with inotropes, so that blood pressure is kept above 95 to 100 mmHg. The addition of mineralocorticoids could enhance the action of loop diuretics as well as prevent hypokalemia. However, the use of diuretics is often associated with hyponatremia, which can be both depletional and dilutional. If hyponatremia is mainly dilutional, addition of vasopressin antagonist could be useful in maintaining normal sodium levels. Indiscriminate use of vasopressin antagonist in patients with CS and hyponatremia should be discouraged.

Mechanical Circulatory Support (MCS) Devices

Although the use of inotropes and diuretics in patients with CS is extremely crucial in the initial management, patients with CS often become resistant to the use of these agents. The addition of MCS devices (**Table 8.8**) is often necessary to maintain cardiac output as well as unload the heart. It is recommended that MCS devices should be introduced early in the treatment of CS after initial management with pharmacological agents. However, the outcome of patients in CS is often dependent on the amount of functional myocardium, which can recover by early intervention. Therefore, the long-term results of MCS are crucially dependent on the amount of myocardial damage and its recovery with the use of appropriate therapy.[68–73]

8.8   Various MCS options

taneous	Surgical MCS–ventricular-assist devices; implanted surgically within thorax
	HeartMate I, II, III
a	HeartWare
m Heart	

tions: ECMO, extracorporeal membrane oxygenation; IABP, ic balloon pump; MCS, mechanical circulatory support.

Intra-Aortic Balloon Counter Pulsation (IABP)

The earliest MCS and still the most commonly used MCS device is IABP. The intra-aortic balloon is inserted via the transfemoral route into the descending thoracic aorta just distal to the origin of left subclavian artery. This balloon deflates during systole causing unloading of the left ventricle and inflates during diastole, which helps in coronary perfusion. The use of IABP should be instituted early in the management of CS while the appropriate interventional therapy is being planned (myocardial revascularization, repair of myocardial rupture, or mitral valve replacement in patients with ruptured papillary muscle). Although the use of IABP could provide immediate benefit to patients in CS, long-term results of this therapy are often dependent on the degree of recovery of functional myocardium in pump failure and surgical management in patients with mechanical complications. There is a small increase in cardiac output with the use of IABP (about 500–800 mL/min/m²). Thus, although IABP-shock-II trial did not show any long-term benefit in patients with CS due to pump failure, the use of this device is still widely practiced especially in centers where advanced MCS devices are not available.[53,74,75]

Impella

Impella is a continuous pump device which propels blood from ventricle to the major artery (LV to aorta or RV to pulmonary artery). This device is inserted transfemorally (for LV to aorta pump) and positioned into LV cavity and across the aortic valves as shown in **Fig. 8.7**. It contains battery-operated motor which pumps blood from LV to proximal aorta (also known as percutaneous ventricular-assist device [pVAD]). Unlike IABP, Impella does not require synchronization with cardiac cycle. It pumps blood independent of ventricular activity. Thus, it effectively and continuously unloads the LV and both provides hemodynamic support and improves coronary circulation; and thus could help in the recovery of injured myocardium. Impella device is a short-term (few hours to maximum 10 d) support device with capacity of pumping blood about 2.5 to 5 L/min.

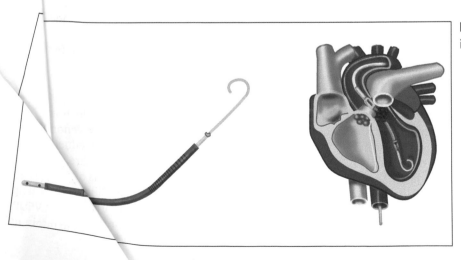

Fig.   8.7 Showing Impella device inserted near atrioventricular (AV) valve.

Although initial trials comparing IABP with Impella did not show mortality benefit with the placement of Impella device, recent trials such as Detroit Cardiogenic Shock Initiative Pilot Study have shown more than 76% survival at 30 days using this device. Therefore, Impella device is considered a significant advancement over the conventional inotrope as well as IABP management and it is recommended that it should be introduced early. If indicated, PCI could be performed with Impella support. A recent PROTECT-II study has shown that the combination of Impella device and PCI leads to 29% lower MACE as compared to IABP in patients with CS.[76-78]

Tandem Heart

This device unloads the LV by pumping blood from left atrium (LA) to aorta; thus, like the Impella device, it improves cardiac output and reduces ventricular filling pressures. It provides circulatory support by pumping blood from LA to aorta. It contains inflow/outflow catheters and a pump. Inflow catheter is positioned in LA by puncturing interatrial septum approaching from femoral vein and outflow catheter is kept at bifurcation of aorta advancing through contralateral femoral artery (**Fig. 8.8**). Thus, this device, as the name suggests, acts like ventricle (pVAD) and pumps continuously nonpulsatile oxygenated blood into abdominal aorta. Early randomized clinical trials had shown improvement in hemodynamics with use of tandem heart as compared to IABP; however, 30-day mortality had not shown any significant difference in patients with severe CS. Recent studies suggest that an early use of tandem heart in severe cases of CS show survival benefits as compared to IABP.[79-81]

Similar to Impella device, tandem heart can also be used for severe RV dysfunction. This is performed by cannulating the right atrium (RA) through right internal jugular vein (IJV) and pulmonary artery through femoral vein. Thus in cases of profound CS, biventricular tandem heart can be used.

Extracorporeal Membrane Oxygenation (ECMO)

This helps in enhancing oxygen supply to tissues, especially in patients with potentially reversible acute cardiac or respiratory failures. The extracorporeal pump withdraws blood from venous system, which is oxygenated in the membrane oxygenator and then pumped back into circulation via artery or vein. ECMO is thus categorized as venoarterial (VA) ECMO (blood is drawn from iliac vein or RA and pumped into femoral artery) or venovenous (VV) ECMO (blood is drawn from IJV and pumped into femoral vein). Usually in CS, which is resistant to inotropes as well as IABP and where facilities for Impella device or tandem heart are not available, VA-ECMO is used to tide over this critical situation. However, implantable VADs are usually required for long-term management. The use of VA-ECMO provides unloading of LV and delivers oxygenated blood into arterial circulation[82-85] (**Fig. 8.9**).

Surgical MCS

This is also known as implantable VADs and require surgery (sVAD). These devices also help in unloading the failing ventricles and provide high levels of cardiac output. These devices are indicated in those patients who cannot be weaned off pVAD. These devices generate more flow than pVAD and are used for long-term therapy. Recently, two types of sVADs are in use: HeartMate (**Fig. 8.10**) and HeartWare.

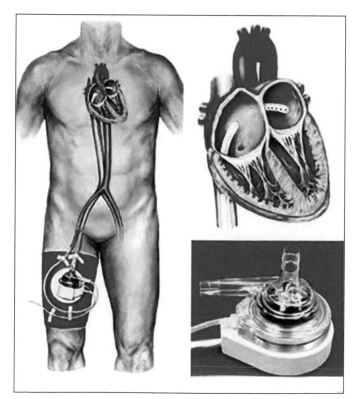

Fig. 8.8 Showing tandem heart insertion; cannula in left atrium (LA) and extracorporeal pump at thigh.

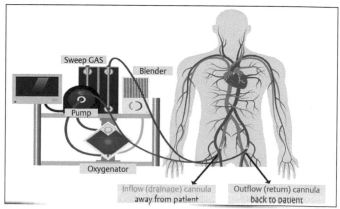

Fig. 8.9 Showing venoarterial extracorporeal membrane oxygenation (VA-ECMO) and its extracorporeal machinery.

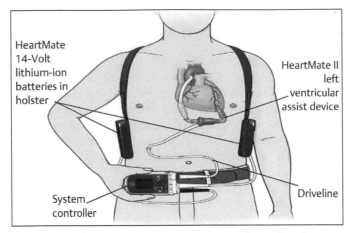

Fig. 8.10 Showing HeartMate device implanted in thorax.

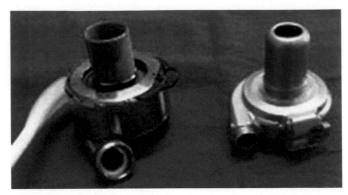

Fig. 8.11 HeartMate-III (*left*) and HeartWare (*right*).

HeartMate

HeartMate-III is a new, improved version of previous HeartMate devices I and II. It is an intrathoracic implantable device with magnetically levitated centrifugal motor having longer durable batteries (17 h) than its previous versions. It takes out blood from LV through inflow cannula and pumps out into ascending aorta, as depicted in **Fig. 8.11**. HeartMate-III is able to push more than 10 L/min blood by maintaining a mean pressure of 100 mmHg. The major benefits of HeartMate-III include:
- The highest survival rates for any LVAD in a randomized controlled trial.
- The lowest hemocompatibility-related adverse event (bleeding, stroke, etc.) rates of any LVAD.
- Immediate, significant, and sustained improvements in functional capacity and quality of life.

HeartWare

In comparison to HeartMate, HeartWare is less popular, probably due to its lower centrifugal power (2400 vs. 8000 rpm). It entails intrapericardial implantation and the reported incidence of cardiac arrhythmias and thrombosis is greater than HeartMate. However, there is no difference in quality of life and functional capacity between these two devices[86-88] (**Fig. 8.11**).

These surgical devices (sVAD) can be used for destination therapies (longest survival 12 y) or can be bridge to transplant or occasionally it could be a bridge to recovery.

Total Artificial Heart (TAH)

Although in majority of patients LVADs are used as bridge to transplant or destination therapies, in a very small set of patients with severe biventricular HF, TAH is used. These patients have increased central pressure (>18 mmHg) with reduced RV function (<20%). In comparison to BiVAD (biventricular-assist device—both LVAD and RVAD), TAH showed no significant benefit over mortality in one small retrospective study. However, the InterMedics Registry data

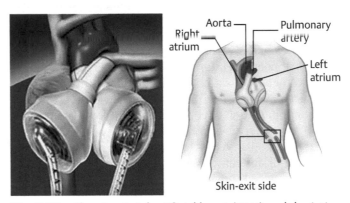

Fig. 8.12 Showing total artificial heart (TAH) and depicting its extracorporeal batteries.

shows a small benefit of TAH over BiVAD, although the quoted studies were too small to draw any conclusion. TAH includes two ventricles and two valves in each ventricle, with pumping stroke volume capacity of 70 mL. Both artificial ventricles are attached to an external battery[89] (**Fig. 8.12**).

Though many companies are trying to make a durable TAH, *SynCardia* is the only one approved as yet. Nurullah, a 61-year-old Turkish man, has been having a fair quality of life for more than 4.5 years using SynCardia.

Heart Transplant

Heart transplant is the last possible treatment in a patient refractory to HF treatment.[90-92] Brain dead donor must fulfil traditional criteria for heart transplant (**Box 8.1**).

Apart from the traditional criteria provided in **Box 8.1**, many other factors are under scrutiny (including diabetes mellitus, thyroid hormonal status, kidney profile, any chronic disease, etc.) to reduce the mortality and to increase the quality of life after transplant. There is an increased role of donor-recipient mismatch in transplantation due to antibodies against leukocyte antigens. Various methods including use of immunosuppressants as well as intravenous immunoglobulins and even plasmapheresis are used to reduce donor-recipient mismatch (desensitization).[93-99]

Box 8.1 Traditional criteria for heart transplant (donor)
• Age <55 y old
• No history of chest trauma or cardiac disease
• No prolonged hypotension or hypoxemia
• Appropriate hemodynamics
• Mean arterial pressure >60 mmHg
• Central venous pressure 8–12 mmHg
• Inotropic support less than 10 mg/kg/min (dopamine or dobutamine)
• Normal electrocardiogram
• Normal echocardiogram
• Normal cardiac angiography (if indicated by donor age and history)
• Negative serology (hepatitis B surface antigen, hepatitis C virus, and human Immunodeficiency virus)

Quality of life after transplant has improved over the past few years. After transplant, patients can resume their work without much difficulty. One-year survival rate is more than 90% and over 5 years is 70%, but only about 20% recipients live longer than 20 years. The maximum survival after cardiac transplant has been 34 years in a patient from Iowa, Richard Gullickson, who recently died at the age of 83. The leading causes of death after transplant are vasculopathy, graft rejection, HF, and malignancy.

Heart Failure

HF after STEMI can be defined as a clinical syndrome characterized by pulmonary or systemic venous congestion resulting from systolic and/or diastolic dysfunction. HF after STEMI is no more a very common event as there is widespread availability of early reperfusion therapies. The incidence of HF after AMI has drastically reduced from 40% in prethrombolysis era to less than 20% in postreperfusion era. The early introduction of PCI in STEMI patients has reduced the mortality from 20% to less than 5%. Early reperfusion improves LV function and hence mortality. In an analysis from the cohort of 3602 patients in HORIZONS-AMI study (2005–2007) treated with PCI, only 8.0% had HF in hospital, whereas at 1 month and after 2 years HF was only 4.6 and 5.1%, respectively. Spencer et al found that during 1994 to 2000, out of 123,938 AMI patients 20.4% presented with HF, whereas only 8.6% developed HF during hospital stay.[100–105]

However, STEMI patients presenting with HF still carry fivefold 1-year mortality risk than those presenting without HF.

Temporal profile of HF presentation after AMI has important management and prognostic implications. This temporal profile can be classified into:

1. HF at the index MI presentation.
2. During the stay in hospital.
3. After discharge.

Box 8.2 Signs/Symptoms of HF after STEMI
HF at the index MI presentation/in hospital:
• Dyspnea—pulmonary rales
• Peripheral edema
• Jugular venous distention
• S3 gallop
• Tachycardia
• Hepatojugular reflux/increased JVP
• Pulmonary capillary wedge pressure >18 mmHg or cardiac output <2.2 L/min/m²
HF after discharge:
• Appearance of more than two signs as above
• Increase in NYHA class
• Increase in dose titration of oral therapies for HF
• Initiation of intravenous diuretic, inotrope, or vasodilator therapy
• Need for any MCS or surgical intervention

Abbreviations: HF, heart failure; MI, myocardial infarction; JVP, jugular venous pressure; MCS, mechanical circulatory support ; NHYA, New York Heart Association; STEMI, ST-elevation myocardial infarction.

Table 8.9 Killips classification

Killips class	Clinical characters	Mortality %
I	No signs of congestion	6
II	Basal rales S3	17
III	Acute pulmonary edema	38
IV	Cardiogenic shock	81

Box 8.2 lists few clinical signs which may be used to define the HF in STEMI.

Dyspnea is often present and is classified as Killips classification[35] (**Table 8.9**).

Risk Stratification for HF after MI

Although many clinical, biochemical, echocardiographic, and angiographic parameters are used for HF risk stratification following MI, only a few are in routine clinical use (**Table 8.10**).[106,107]

Treatments for Myocardial Infarction Complicated by Heart Failure

• **Beta-blockers:** The use of β-blockers is recommended in STEMI patients without HF or without high risk of HF. In a meta-analysis of 31 randomized trials with a total of about 25,000 patients with MI, the use of β-blockers was found to reduce the risk of reinfarction and mortality in 2 years of follow-up. Although use of β-blockers is a recommended treatment, as per the guidelines, for HF, their use in acute HF post-STEMI is interdicted owing to potentially harmful effects (pulmonary congestion and progression to CS).

Table 8.10 Risk factors for developing HF after STEMI

Age	Door to PCI time	LVEF	Cardiac troponin
Male sex	LAD artery involvement	WMAS	CRP
Killips class	TIMI flow grade	Cardiac chamber size	BNP/NTpro-BNP
NYHA class		MR/TR	CKMB
Comorbidities		E/Ea × Sa >2 (systolo-diastolic index)	

Abbreviations: BNP, B-type natriuretic peptide; CKMB, creatine kinase MB; CRP, C-reactive protein; HF, heart failure; LAD, left anterior descending; LVEF, left-ventricular ejection fraction; MR, mitral regurgitation; NYHA, New York Heart Association; PCI, percutaneous coronary intervention; STEMI, ST-elevation myocardial infarction; TIMI, thrombolysis in myocardial infarction; TR, tricuspid regurgitation; WMAS, wall motion abnormality and stenosis.

- **ACEI/ARBs:** ACEI and angiotensin receptor blockers (ARBs) are strongly recommended in patients with STEMI having LV dysfunction or HF without hypotension or other contraindications. A meta-analysis of more than 100,000 randomized patients has conclusively demonstrated that early oral ACEIs are beneficial with an anterior infarct in elderly patients. ACEI not only reduces the production of angiotensinogen-II which is a potent vasoconstrictor but also upregulates beta-receptor density. ACEIs increase vasodilator bradykinin levels and help in positive remodeling of ventricles. ARBs may be used as an alternative to ACEIs in order to avoid unwanted effects of ACEIs (viz., angioedema and cough).[108-110]
- **Diuretics:** Diuretics are recommended in patients with HFrEF (heart failure with reduced ejection fraction) with STEMI having evidence of fluid retention. Loop diuretics are preferred in most patients with HF. Loop diuretics also help in synthesis of prostaglandins, which result in renal and venous dilatation. This explains its action of decongestion of vascular as well as pulmonary beds. This class includes furosemide and torsemide.

Aldosterone antagonists, also known as mineralocorticoid receptor antagonists (MRAs) or potassium-sparing diuretics including spironolactone or eplerenone, are useful additive to loop diuretics. Aldosterone levels remain elevated in patients with HF despite the use of ACEIs/ARBs or β-blockers. Increased aldosterone levels are associated with cardiorenal dysfunction and increased mortality. The MRAs should be used in conjunction with ACEIs/ARBs.[111,112]

- **Angiotensin receptor neprilysin inhibitors (ARNIs):** Neprilysin inhibitors in combination with ARBs (sacubitril + valsartan) are one of the latest agents in the pharmacotherapy of HF. While the neprilysin inhibition increases the level of natriuretic peptides (NPs), the addition of ARBs prevents the increase in angiotensin-II levels, which are associated with elevated levels of NPs as well as HF itself.

  This combination is a potential "game-changer" in the management of HF following STEMI. ARNI (sacubitril + valsartan) should not be used in conjunction with ACEI/ARB or renin inhibitor because of the risk of hypotension, angioedema, renal dysfunction, or hyperkalemia. Thus, ARNI must be started after discontinuation of ACEIs/ARBs for at least 36 hours.[113-115]

- **Hydralazine and isosorbide dinitrate:** The use of this combination is recommended in patients with STEMI (HFrEF having NYHA-III/IV) who do not tolerate ACEI or ARNI (ACEI/ARB-induced cough). However, such patients are less than 10% and mostly are of African-American race. The compliance of this combination is also very less among these patients. This combination has a potential to reduce 3-year mortality of HF as compared to placebo (36 vs. 46%).
- **Digoxin:** As per the current guidelines for management of HF after STEMI, digitalis is not the recommended therapy. However, some clinicians prefer adding digoxin to the HF treatment regimen in patients with HFrEF even in sinus rhythm. Digoxin could have a more beneficial effect in patients with atrial fibrillation (AF) post-STEMI. However, it must not be given with other drugs (β-blockers) that slow the heart rate or cause AV blockage. Digoxin toxicity occurs with serum digoxin levels >2 ng/mL; hence, it needs to be monitored.

Future Directions

The advent of primary PCI has been monumental in the management of STEMI. However, owing to lack of adequate logistics for timely transportation to PCI centers, many patients fail to receive timely PCI. If delay in transportation is likely, prompt administration of modern thrombolytics (reteplase, alteplase) followed by referral to a PCI center is a practical solution. Patients who develop mechanical or pump failure complications have a high mortality unless timely surgical or interventional management in tertiary care centers is given. Mechanical complications such as papillary muscle rupture requires emergency treatment usually with surgical mitral valve replacement (MVR); however, with the recent introduction of percutaneous mitral valve/Mitraclip implantation, such high surgical risk patients could be subjected to this interventional treatment. Percutaneous closure of post-STEMI-VSD, although feasible, is hampered by the lack of adequate viable muscle which is essential for providing support to the closure device. This could cause significant residual shunt around the device. Therefore, surgical repair especially using the Dorr technique is the preferred choice. Free-wall rupture is a surgical emergency associated with high mortality unless immediate repair is undertaken.

The management of pump failure causing CS or refractory HF is challenging. Use of various inotropes followed by MCS devices including IABP, Impella, tandem heart, and LVAD/BiVAD is the standard of care in carefully selected patients. However, use of such advanced devices is limited even in tertiary care centers due to their nonavailability. If available, LVAD/BiVAD can be used as bridge to recovery or bridge to cardiac transplant. The facility for TAH, if available, is the ultimate option for patients who are candidates of cardiac transplant but are waiting for a suitable donor. Patients could survive several years on TAH. Although cardiac transplantation has a high short-term and long-term success rate, limited availability of donor is a major limitation besides the challenges associated with transplant rejection and vasculopathy.

Conclusion

The management of pump failure causing CS or refractory HF is challenging. Use of various inotropes followed by MCS devices including IABP, Impella, tandem heart, and LVAD/BiVAD is the standard of care in carefully selected patients. However, use of such advanced devices is limited even in tertiary care centers due to their nonavailability. If available, LVAD/BiVAD can be used as bridge to recovery or bridge to cardiac transplant. The facility for TAH, if available, is the ultimate option for patients who are candidates of cardiac transplant but are waiting for a suitable donor. Patients could survive several years on TAH. Although cardiac transplantation has a high short-term and long-term success rate, limited availability of donor is a major limitation besides the challenges associated with transplant rejection and vasculopathy. Today in 2022, NIRS is the most frequently brain monitor used and it has been adopted as the endpoint in many algorithms for hemodynamic and respiratory management during cardiac surgery to improve patient outcomes.[116]

References

1. Sanchis-Gomar F, Perez-Quilis C, Leischik R, Lucia A, et al. Epidemiology of coronary heart disease and acute coronary syndrome. Ann Transl Med 2016;4(13):256
2. Khan MAB, Hashim MJ, Mustafa H, et al. Global epidemiology of ischemic heart disease: results from the Global Burden of Disease Study. Cureus 2020;12(7):e9349
3. Munguti CM, Akidiva S, Wallace J, Farhoud H. ST-segment elevation is not always myocardial infarction: a case of focal myopericarditis. Case Rep Cardiol 2017;2017:3031792
4. Wang K, Asinger RW, Marriott HJ. ST-segment elevation in conditions other than acute myocardial infarction. N Engl J Med 2003;349(22):2128–2135
5. Thygesen K, Alpert JS, Jaffe AS, et al; Executive Group on behalf of the Joint European Society of Cardiology (ESC)/American College of Cardiology (ACC)/American Heart Association (AHA)/World Heart Federation (WHF) Task Force for the Universal Definition of Myocardial Infarction. Fourth universal definition of myocardial infarction. Circulation 2018;138(20):e618–e651
6. Lee KY, Chang K. Understanding vulnerable plaques: current status and future directions. Korean Circ J 2019;49(12):1115–1122
7. Konstantinidis K, Whelan RS, Kitsis RN. Mechanisms of cell death in heart disease. Arterioscler Thromb Vasc Biol 2012;32(7):1552–1562
8. Libby P, Tabas I, Fredman G, Fisher EA. Inflammation and its resolution as determinants of acute coronary syndromes. Circ Res 2014;114(12):1867–1879
9. Ahmadi A, Leipsic J, Blankstein R, et al. Do plaques rapidly progress prior to myocardial infarction? The interplay between plaque vulnerability and progression. Circ Res 2015;117(1):99–104
10. Bentzon JF, Otsuka F, Virmani R, Falk E. Mechanisms of plaque formation and rupture. Circ Res 2014;114(12):1852–1866
11. Montecucco F, Carbone F, Schindler TH. Pathophysiology of ST-segment elevation myocardial infarction: novel mechanisms and treatments. Eur Heart J 2016;37(16):1268–1283
12. Kumar A, Thompson EW, Lefieuxet A, et al. High coronary shear stress in patients with coronary artery disease predicts myocardial infarction. JACC 2018;72(16):1926–1935
13. Yang Y, Li J, Xu W, et al. Thrombus aspirated from patients with ST-elevation myocardial infarction: clinical and angiographic outcomes. J Int Med Res 2016;44(6):1514–1523
14. Uchida Y, Uchida Y, Sakurai T, Kanai M, Shirai S, Morita T. Characterization of coronary fibrin thrombus in patients with acute coronary syndrome using dye-staining angioscopy. Arterioscler Thromb Vasc Biol 2011;31(6):1452–1460
15. Quadros AS, Cambruzzi E, Sebben J, et al. Red versus white thrombi in patients with ST-elevation myocardial infarction undergoing primary percutaneous coronary intervention: clinical and angiographic outcomes. Am Heart J 2012;164(4):553–560
16. Hong YJ, Jeong MH, Choi YH, et al. Differences in intravascular ultrasound findings in culprit lesions in infarct-related arteries between ST segment elevation myocardial infarction and non-ST segment elevation myocardial infarction. J Cardiol 2010;56(1):15–22
17. Sia C-H, Zheng H, Ho AF, et al. The lipid paradox is present in ST-elevation but not in non-ST-elevation myocardial infarction patients: insights from the Singapore Myocardial Infarction Registry. Sci Rep 2020;10(1):6799
18. Montalescot G, Dallongeville J, Van Belle E, et al; OPERA Investigators. STEMI and NSTEMI: are they so different? 1 year outcomes in acute myocardial infarction as defined by the ESC/ACC definition (the OPERA registry). Eur Heart J 2007;28(12):1409–1417
19. Cohen M, Visveswaran G. Defining and managing patients with non-ST-elevation myocardial infarction: sorting through type 1 versus other types. Clin Cardiol 2020;43:242–250
20. van 't Hof AWJ, Badings E. NSTEMI treatment: should we always follow the guidelines? Neth Heart J 2019;27(4):171–175
21. Amsterdam EA, Wenger NK, Brindis RG, et al. 2014 AHA/ACC guideline for the management of patients with non-ST-elevation acute coronary syndromes: a report of the American College of Cardiology/American Heart Association Task Force on Practice Guidelines. J Am Coll Cardiol 2014;64(24):e139–e228

22. Sheridan PJ, Crossman DC. Critical review of unstable angina and non-ST elevation myocardial infarction. Postgrad Med J 2002;78(926):717–726

23. Roffi M, Patroo C, Collet J-P, et al. 2015 ESC Guidelines for the management of acute coronary syndromes in patients presenting without persistent ST-segment elevation. Eur Heart J 2016;37:267–315

24. Bajaj A, Sethi A, Rathor P, Suppogu N, Sethi A. Acute complications of myocardial infarction in the current era: diagnosis and management. J Investig Med 2015;63(7):844–855

25. Hasin Y, Ghanim D. Mechanical complications of acute myocardial infarction (AMI): an article from the e-journal of the ESC Council for Cardiology Practice. ESC 2005;3(35)

26. Bahlmann E, Frerker C, Kreidel F, et al. MitraClip implantation after acute ischemic papillary muscle rupture in a patient with prolonged cardiogenic shock. Ann Thorac Surg 2015;99(2): e41–e42

27. Armstrong PW, Fu Y, Chang WC, et al. Acute coronary syndromes in the GUSTO-IIb trial: prognostic insights and impact of recurrent ischemia. The GUSTO-IIb Investigators. Circulation 1998;98(18):1860–1868

28. Papadopoulos K, Chrissoheris M, Nikolaou I, Spargias K. Edge-to-edge mitral valve repair for acute mitral valve regurgitation due to papillary muscle rupture: a case report. Eur Heart J Case Rep 2019;3:1–4

29. Kurmani S, Squire I. Acute heart failure: definition, classification and epidemiology. Curr Heart Fail Rep 2017;14(5):385–392

30. Chapman B, DeVore AD, Mentz RJ, Metra M. Clinical profiles in acute heart failure: an urgent need for a new approach. ESC Heart Fail 2019;6(3):464–474

31. Reynolds HR, Hochman JS. Cardiogenic shock: current concepts and improving outcomes. Circulation 2008;117(5):686–697

32. Thiele H, Allam B, Chatellier G, Schuler G, Lafont A. Shock in acute myocardial infarction: the Cape Horn for trials? Eur Heart J 2010;31(15):1828–1835

33. Kapur NK, Thayer KL, Zweck E. Cardiogenic shock in the setting of acute myocardial infarction. Methodist DeBakey Cardiovasc J 2020;16(1):16–21

34. Arrigo M, Parissis JT, Akiyama E, Mebazaa A. Understanding acute heart failure: pathophysiology and diagnosis. European Heart Journal Supplements 2016;18(Suppl_G):G11–G18

35. Mello BH, Oliveira GB, Ramos RF, et al. Validation of the Killip-Kimball classification and late mortality after acute myocardial infarction. Arq Bras Cardiol 2014;103(2):107–117

36. Madias JE. Killip and Forrester classifications: should they be abandoned, kept, reevaluated, or modified? Chest 2000;117(5):1223–1226

37. Pöss J, Köster J, Fuernau G, et al. Risk stratification for patients in cardiogenic shock after acute myocardial infarction. J Am Coll Cardiol 2017;69(15):1913–1920

38. Singh M, White J, Hasdai D, et al. Long-term outcome and its predictors among patients with ST-segment elevation myocardial infarction complicated by shock: insights from the GUSTO-I trial. J Am Coll Cardiol 2007;50(18):1752–1758

39. Lin M-J, Chen C-Y, Lin HD, Wu HP. Prognostic analysis for cardiogenic shock in patients with acute myocardial infarction receiving percutaneous coronary intervention. BioMed Res Int 2017;2017:8530539

40. Auffret V, Cottin Y, Leurent G, et al; ORBI and RICO Working Groups. Predicting the development of in-hospital cardiogenic shock in patients with ST-segment elevation myocardial infarction treated by primary percutaneous coronary intervention: the ORBI risk score. Eur Heart J 2018;39(22):2090–2102

41. Dangas G, Guedeney P. Prediction, staging, and outcomes of ischaemic cardiogenic shock after STEMI: a complex clinical interplay. Eur Heart J 2018;39(22):2103–2105

42. Acharya D. Predictors of outcomes in myocardial infarction and cardiogenic shock. Cardiol Rev 2018;26(5):255–266

43. Holmes DR Jr, Berger PB, Hochman JS, et al. Cardiogenic shock in patients with acute ischemic syndromes with and without ST-segment elevation. Circulation 1999;100(20):2067–2073

44. Ibanez B, Halvorsen S, Roffi M, et al. Integrating the results of the CULPRIT-SHOCK trial in the 2017 ESC ST-elevation myocardial infarction guidelines: viewpoint of the task force. Eur Heart J 2018;39(48):4239–4242

45. Holmes DR, Bates ER, Kleiman NS, et al. Contemporary reperfusion therapy for cardiogenic shock: the GUSTO-I trial experience. J Am Coll Cardiol 1995;26(3):668–674

46. Armstrong PW, Collen D. Fibrinolysis for acute myocardial infarction: current status and new horizons for pharmacological reperfusion, part 2. Circulation 2001;103(24):2987–2992

47. Picard MH, Davidoff R, Sleeper LA, et al; SHOCK Trial. SHould we emergently revascularize Occluded Coronaries for cardiogenic shocK. Echocardiographic predictors of survival and response to early revascularization in cardiogenic shock. Circulation 2003;107(2):279–284

48. Jacobs AK, Leopold JA, Bates E, et al. Cardiogenic shock caused by right ventricular infarction: a report from the SHOCK registry. J Am Coll Cardiol 2003;41(8):1273–1279

49. Thiele H, Ohman EM, de Waha-Thiele S, Zeymer U, Desch S. Management of cardiogenic shock complicating myocardial infarction: an update 2019. Eur Heart J 2019;40(32): 2671–2683

50. Menon V, Hochman JS. Management of cardiogenic shock complicating acute myocardial infarction. Heart 2002;88(5): 531–537

51. Adivitiya, Khasa YP. The evolution of recombinant thrombolytics: current status and future directions. Bioengineered 2017;8(4):331–358

52. Menon V, Fincke R. Cardiogenic shock: a summary of the randomized SHOCK trial. Congest Heart Fail 2003;9(1):35–39

53. Holger Thiele, Uwe Zeymer, et al. Intraaortic balloon pump in cardiogenic shock complicating acute myocardial infarction long-term 6-year outcome of the randomized IABP-SHOCK II trial. Circulation 2019;139(3):395–403

54. Ryan TJ, Anderson JL, et al. ACC/AHA guidelines for the management of patients with acute myocardial infarction: executive summary. A report of the American College of Cardiology/American Heart Association Task Force on Practice Guidelines (Committee on Management of Acute Myocardial Infarction)

55. Vahdatpour C, Collins D, Goldberg S. Cardiogenic shock. J Am Heart Assoc 2019;8(8):e011991

56. Wong GC, Welsford M, Ainsworth C, et al; Members of the Secondary Panel. 2019 Canadian Cardiovascular Society/ Canadian Association of Interventional Cardiology guidelines on the acute management of ST-elevation myocardial infarction: focused update on regionalization and reperfusion. Can J Cardiol 2019;35(2):107–132

57. Anbe Daniel T, Armstrong Paul Wayne, et al. ACC/AHA guidelines for the management of patients with ST-elevation myocardial infarction--executive summary: a report of the American College of Cardiology/American Heart Association Task Force on Practice Guidelines (Writing Committee to Revise the 1999 Guidelines for the Management of Patients With Acute Myocardial Infarction)

58. Farmakis D, Agostoni P, Baholli L, et al. A pragmatic approach to the use of inotropes for the management of acute and advanced heart failure: an expert panel consensus. Int J Cardiol 2019;297:83–90

59. Mebazaa A, Tolppanen H, Mueller C, et al. Acute heart failure and cardiogenic shock: a multidisciplinary practical guidance. Intensive Care Med 2016;42(2):147–163

60. Overgaard CB, Dzavík V. Inotropes and vasopressors: review of physiology and clinical use in cardiovascular disease. Circulation 2008;118(10):1047–1056

61. Pan J, Yang Y-M, Zhu JY, Lu YQ. Multiorgan drug action of levosimendan in critical illnesses. Biomed Res Int 2019;2019: 9731467

62. Manolopoulos PP, Boutsikos I, Boutsikos P, Iacovidou N, Ekmektzoglou K. Current use and advances in vasopressors and inotropes support in shock. J Emerg Crit Care Med 2020;4:20

63. Amado J, Gago P, Santos W, Mimoso J, de Jesus I. Cardiogenic shock: inotropes and vasopressors. Rev Port Cardiol 2016;35(12):681–695

64. Cholley B, Levy B, Fellahi JL, et al. Levosimendan in the light of the results of the recent randomized controlled trials: an expert opinion paper. Crit Care 2019;23:385

65. Bandak G, Sakhuja A, Andrijasevic NM, Gunderson TM, Gajic O, Kashani K. Use of diuretics in shock: temporal trends and clinical impacts in a propensity-matched cohort study. PLoS One 2020;15(2):e0228274

66. Vazir A, Cowie MR. Decongestion: diuretics and other therapies for hospitalized heart failure. Indian Heart J 2016;68(Suppl 1): S61–S68

67. Baliga RR. Diuretic therapy for heart failure patients. American College of Cardiology. JACC State-of-the-Art Review. J Am Coll Cardiol 2020;75:1178-1195

68. Wiedemann D, Haberl T, Riebandt J, Simon P, Laufer G, Zimpfer D. Ventricular assist devices: evolution of surgical heart failure treatment. Eur Cardiol 2014;9(1):54–58

69. Poulidakis E, Spaulding C. Cardiac assist devices in cardiogenic shock what you see is what you get? CirculationAHA 2019;139: 1259–1261

70. Naidu SS. Novel percutaneous cardiac assist devices: the science of and indications for hemodynamic support. Circulation 2011;123(5):533–543

71. Burkhoff D, Sayer G, Doshi D, Uriel N. Hemodynamics of mechanical circulatory support. J Am Coll Cardiol 2015;66(23): 2663–2674

72. Basir MB, Schreiber T, Dixon S, et al. Feasibility of early mechanical circulatory support in acute myocardial infarction complicated by cardiogenic shock: the Detroit cardiogenic shock initiative. Catheter Cardiovasc Interv 2018;91(3): 454–461

73. Combes A, Price S, Slutsky AS, Brodie D. Temporary circulatory support for cardiogenic shock. Lancet 2020;396(10245): 199–212

74. Hajjar LA, Teboul J-L. Mechanical circulatory support devices for cardiogenic shock: state of the art. Crit Care 2019;23(1):76

75. Fuernau G, Thiele H. Intra-aortic balloon pump (IABP) in cardiogenic shock. Curr Opin Crit Care 2013;19(5):404–409

76. Alushi B, Douedari A, Froehlig G, et al. Impella versus IABP in acute myocardial infarction complicated by cardiogenic shock. Open Heart 2019;6(1):e000987

77. Hemradj VV, Karami M, Sjauw KD, et al. Pre-PCI versus immediate post-PCI Impella initiation in acute myocardial infarction complicated by cardiogenic shock. PLoS One 2020;15(7):e0235762

78. Kumbhani DJ. A prospective randomized clinical trial of hemodynamic support with Impella 2.5 versus intra-aortic balloon pump in patients undergoing high-risk PCI—PROTECT II. American College of Cardiology; 2012

79. Gregoric ID, Loyalka P, Radovancevic R, Jovic Z, Frazier OH, Kar B. TandemHeart as a rescue therapy for patients with critical aortic valve stenosis. Ann Thorac Surg 2009;88: 1822–1827

80. Kar B, Adkins LE, Civitello AB, et al. Clinical experience with the TandemHeart percutaneous ventricular assist device. Tex Heart Inst J 2006;33(2):111–115

81. Sibai RE, Bachir R, Sayed ME. Outcomes in cardiogenic shock patients with extracorporeal membrane oxygenation use: a matched cohort study in hospitals across the United States. Biomed Res Int 2018;2018:2428648

82. Gokalp O, Donmez K, Iner H, et al. Should ECMO be used in cardiogenic shock? Crit Care 2019;23(1):174

83. Banfi C, Pozzi M, Siegenthaler N, et al. Veno-venous extracorporeal membrane oxygenation: cannulation techniques. J Thorac Dis 2016;8(12):3762–3773

84. Zavalichi MA, Nistor I, Nedelcu AE, et al. Extracorporeal membrane oxygenation in cardiogenic shock due to acute myocardial infarction: a systematic review. BioMed Res Int 2020;2020:6126534

85. Rao P, Khalpey Z, Smith R, Burkhoff D, Kociol RD. Venoarterial extracorporeal membrane oxygenation for cardiogenic shock and cardiac arrest. Circ Heart Fail 2018;11(9):e004905

86. Schroder JN, Milano CA. A tale of two centrifugal left ventricular assist devices. J Thorac Cardiovasc Surg 2017;154(3): 850–852

87. Chatterjee A, Feldmann C, Hanke JS, et al. The momentum of HeartMate 3: a novel active magnetically levitated centrifugal left ventricular assist device (LVAD). J Thorac Dis 2018; 10(Suppl 15):S1790–S1793

88. Mohamed I, Lau CT, Bolen MA, et al. Building a bridge to save a failing ventricle: radiologic evaluation of short- and long-term cardiac assist devices. Radiographics 2015;35(2):327–356

89. Cook JA, Shah KB, Quader MA, et al. The total artificial heart. J Thorac Dis 2015;7(12):2172–2180

90. Kilic A, Emani S, Sai-Sudhakar CB, Higgins RSD, Whitson BA. Donor selection in heart transplantation. J Thorac Dis 2014; 6(8):1097–1104

91. Harris C, Cao C, Croce B, Munkholm-Larsen S. Heart transplantation. Ann Cardiothorac Surg 2018;7(1):172

92. Kittleson MM. Recent advances in heart transplantation. F1000Research 2018;7:F1000 Faculty Rev-1008

93. Deng MC. Cardiac transplantation. Heart 2002;87(2): 177–184

94. Chih S, McDonald M, Dipchand A, et al. Canadian Cardiovascular Society/Canadian Cardiac Transplant Network Position Statement on heart transplantation: patient eligibility, selection, and post-transplantation care. Can J Cardiol 2020; 36(3):335–356

95. Markus J. Wilhelm. Long-term outcome following heart transplantation: current perspective. J Thorac Dis 2015;7(3): 549-551

96. de Jonge N, Kirkels JH, Klöpping C, et al. Guidelines for heart transplantation. Neth Heart J 2008;16(3):79–87

97. Jeevanandam V, Furukawa S, Prendergast TW, Todd BA, Eisen HJ, McClurken JB. Standard criteria for an acceptable donor heart are restricting heart transplantation. Ann Thorac Surg 1996;62(5):1268–1275

98. Alraies MC, Eckman P. Adult heart transplant: indications and outcomes. J Thorac Dis 2014;6(8):1120–1128

99. Kim I-C, Youn J-C, Kobashigawa JA. The past, present and future of heart transplantation. Korean Circ J 2018;48(7): 565–590

100. van der Meer P, Gaggin HK, Dec GW. ACC/AHA versus ESC guidelines on heart failure: JACC guideline comparison. J Am Coll Cardiol 2019;73(21):2756–2768

101. Eapen ZJ, Tang WHW, Felker GM, et al. Defining heart failure end points in ST-segment elevation myocardial infarction trials: integrating past experiences to chart a path forward. Circ Cardiovasc Qual Outcomes 2012;5(4):594–600

102. Cahill TJ, Kharbanda RK. Heart failure after myocardial infarction in the era of primary percutaneous coronary intervention: mechanisms, incidence and identification of patients at risk. World J Cardiol 2017;9(5):407–415

103. Gho JMIH, Postema PG, Conijn M, et al. Heart failure following STEMI: a contemporary cohort study of incidence and prognostic factors. Open Heart 2017;4(2):e000551

104. Stone GW, Witzenbichler B, Guagliumi G, et al; HORIZONS-AMI Trial Investigators. Heparin plus a glycoprotein IIb/IIIa inhibitor versus bivalirudin monotherapy and paclitaxel-eluting stents versus bare-metal stents in acute myocardial infarction (HORIZONS-AMI): final 3-year results from a multicentre, randomised controlled trial. Lancet 2011;377(9784):2193–2204

105. Spencer FA, Meyer TE, Gore JM, Goldberg RJ. Heterogeneity in the management and outcomes of patients with acute myocardial infarction complicated by heart failure: the National Registry of Myocardial Infarction. Circulation 2002;105(22):2605–2610

106. Cecilia Bahit M, Kochar A, Granger CB. Post-myocardial infarction heart failure. JACC Heart Fail 2018;6(3):179–186

107. Gerber Y, Weston SA, Enriquez-Sarano M, et al. Mortality associated with heart failure after myocardial infarction: a contemporary community perspective. Circ Heart Fail 2016;9(1):e002460

108. Evans M, Carrero J-J, Szummer K, et al. Angiotensin-converting enzyme inhibitors and angiotensin receptor blockers in myocardial infarction patients with renal dysfunction. J Am Coll Cardiol 2016;67(14):1687–1697

109. Davies MK, Gibbs CR, et al. ABC of heart failure Management: diuretics, ACE inhibitors, and nitrates. BMJ 2000;320:12

110. ACE Inhibitor Myocardial Infarction Collaborative Group. Indications for ACE inhibitors in the early treatment of acute myocardial infarction: systematic overview of individual data from 100,000 patients in randomized trials. Circulation 1998;97(22):2202–2212

111. Serenelli M, Jackson A, Dewan P, et al. Mineralocorticoid receptor antagonists, blood pressure, and outcomes in heart failure with reduced ejection fraction. JACC Heart Fail 2020;8(3):188–198

112. Patterson SJ, Reaves AB, Tolley EA, et al. Underutilization of aldosterone antagonists in heart failure. Hosp Pharm 2017;52(10):698–703

113. Jhund PS, McMurray JJ. The neprilysin pathway in heart failure: a review and guide on the use of sacubitril/valsartan. Heart 2016;102(17):1342–1347

114. Mann DL, Greene SJ, Givertz MM, et al; LIFE Investigators. Sacubitril/Valsartan in advanced heart failure with reduced ejection fraction: rationale and design of the LIFE trial. JACC Heart Fail 2020;8(10):789–799

115. McMurray JJ, Packer M, Desai AS, et al; PARADIGM-HF Investigators and Committees. Angiotensin-neprilysin inhibition versus enalapril in heart failure. N Engl J Med 2014;371(11):993–1004

116. Klamt JG, Garcia WNP, Carvalho M, Garcia LV, Menardi AC. Multimodal Neuro monitoring during pediatric cardiac surgery. Braz J Cardiovasc Surg. 2022;37(2):251–258

9

Central Nervous System Monitoring in Cardiac Surgery

Keshava Murthy and Muralidhar Kanchi

Introduction

Neurological impairment in cardiac surgery is a significant concern; most often hemodynamic monitoring takes precedence over neurological monitoring. It is presumed that the neurological function is preserved if hemodynamic function is maintained but this is not invariable. Neurologic dysfunction may occur despite apparent normal cardiovascular function which makes it difficult to detect cerebral insult under anesthesia. Cerebral dysfunction after cardiopulmonary bypass (CPB) represents deficits ranging from neurocognitive deficits, occurring in approximately 25 to 80% of patients, to overt stroke, occurring in 1 to 5% of patients.[1] Neurological injury ranges from incapacitating or lethal stroke or coma to encephalopathy, delirium, and neurocognitive decline. Although stroke after cardiac surgery is an important concern for both short-term and long-term disability, subtler neurological effects, such as encephalopathy and neurocognitive dysfunction, are associated with increased medical costs and decreased quality of life. This underlines the importance of central nervous system (CNS) monitoring during cardiac surgical procedures to identify abnormalities that may escape undetected. This allows for early application of corrective measures to overcome the cerebrovascular disturbance and aid improved neurological outcomes. This chapter deals with (i) illustrative cases of neurologic insult in patients undergoing cardiac surgery, (ii) incidence of CNS injury in cardiac surgery, (iii) etiopathogenesis and pathophysiology of CNS injury, (iv) modalities of CNS monitoring as applicable to cardiac surgery, and (v) CPB practices for good neurological outcomes.

Illustrative Cases

Case 1

A 68-year-old male, suffering from ischemic heart disease (IHD), underwent a triple coronary artery bypass grafting (CABG). He had a 50% carotid stenosis on both sides as revealed by carotid Doppler performed preoperatively. Biochemical investigations were normal except for a serum creatinine level of 2 mg/dL. Sequential reversed saphenous vein grafting (RSVG) was performed onto the proximal and distal left anterior descending (LAD) artery and free left internal mammary artery (LIMA) was anastomosed to the obtuse marginal (OM) artery. Intraoperative course was complicated, with myocardial ischemia at the end of the procedure needing revision of the graft to the distal LAD. Postoperatively, the patient woke up confused with right hemiplegia. Subsequently, tracheostomy was performed to maintain artificial respiration. His postoperative computerized tomography (CT) scan of the brain revealed extensive infarcts in the left frontal and parietal regions of the cerebrum (**Fig. 9.1**).

Case 2

A 52-year-old male with aneurysm of ascending aorta underwent Bental procedure. His preoperative CT of the chest showed a large aneurysm of the ascending aorta with intramural thrombosis (**Fig. 9.2**); this saccular aneurysm was eroding into the sternum from behind. After an uneventful anesthetic induction, the aneurysm was injured inadvertently during sternotomy necessitating institution of emergency CPB after systemic heparinization. The patient suffered severe hypotension with a systemic BP of 60 mmHg for about half an hour despite rapid fluid resuscitation. His cerebral oximetry (Nonin-Equinox 7600, Plymouth, MN, USA) during the period of hypotension and subsequent hour showed a sharp decline from a mean value of 67% to less than 50% indicating severe cerebral hypoxia secondary to hypoperfusion. This patient did not wake up from surgery and succumbed on the 7th day after surgery despite successful repair.

Case 3

A 71-year-old male, an ex-public works department employee, underwent an elective triple CABG. His preoperative magnetic resonance imaging (MRI) of neck showed diffuse narrowing of both carotid arteries, which did not warrant surgical treatment. He woke up after surgery with right hemiparesis and confusion; ventilatory support was continued for 2 days. He made a complete recovery neurologically

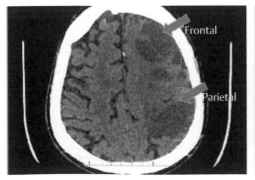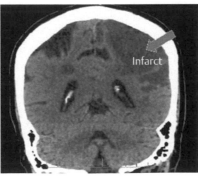

Fig. 9.1 Postoperative computerized tomography (CT) scan of the brain revealed extensive infarcts (*arrows*) in the left frontal and parietal regions of the cerebrum.

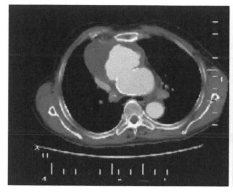 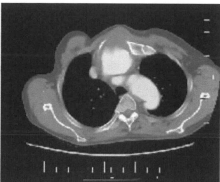

Fig. 9.2 Computerized tomography (CT) of the chest showing a large aneurysm of the ascending aorta with intramural thrombosis.

in 48 hours and was discharged from the hospital on the 8th postoperative day.

The above three cases are representative of the typical causes for neurological insult during cardiac surgery. Let us now focus a little more on the real issues involved and how we could ameliorate on the results of cardiac surgery from neurological point of view.

Incidence of CNS Injury in Cardiac Surgery

The CNS injury that may occur as a consequence of cardiac surgery has been classified into two major groups by Roach et al. Type I CNS injury includes focal neurological deficit, stupor, or coma at discharge while type II CNS injury is associated with deterioration in intellectual function, neuropsychiatric/neurobehavioral abnormality, recall/memory deficit, or seizures. In patients undergoing CABG, the American College of Cardiology Foundation/American Heart Association (ACCF/AHA) has categorized brain injury into cerebrovascular accident (stroke), encephalopathy (delirium), and cognitive dysfunction.[2] Assessment for cognitive decline is performed by application of standardized psychometric examinations administered prior to and after surgery.

A clinically detectable new focal sensory, motor, sensorimotor deficit that persists for longer than 24 hours is called stroke (CVA) whereas neurologic deficit of short duration that persists less than 24 hours is called *transient ischemic attack (TIA)*. The term reversible *ischemic neurologic deficit* is applied when the cerebral focal dysfunction lasts for greater than 24 hours but recovers within 72 hours. The following constitute the term *delirium*: transient impairment of intellectual function, decreased level of sensorium, profound alteration in sleep cycle, and attention anomalies. *Cognitive dysfunction* is defined as a decrease in score falling below some predetermined threshold, such as a decrease in postoperative score of magnitude 1 standard deviation or more derived from the preoperative performance of the study group as a whole. *Seizure* is categorized as either convulsive or nonconvulsive and may be related to overt CNS injury or alternatively may reflect transient biochemical or pharmacologically mediated neuroexcitation (**Flowcharts 9.1** and **9.2**).

There is a considerable disparity in the published literature regarding the incidence of these adverse cerebral outcomes due to the following reasons: (i) there exists a difference in definition of various types of neurological insult. Also there are numerous methodologic differences in the determination of neurological and neurocognitive outcomes, (ii) retrospective versus prospective assessment of neurologic deficits, (iii) experience and expertise of the examiner, and (iv) timing of postoperative testing, for example, the rate of cognitive deficits is as high as 80% for patients at discharge, between 10 and 35% at 6 weeks or longer after CABG, and 10 to 15% more than a year after surgery. **Flowchart 9.3** explains the pathophysiology of neuronal ischemia.

Various Modalities of CNS Monitoring

The various techniques of CNS monitoring may be broadly categorized, for the sake of convenience, into those that look at metabolic integrity and those looking at functional integrity. This classification is not mutually exclusive as metabolism and function are intimately interlinked (**Flowchart 9.4**).

Electroencephalography

A. **Physiological principle:** Electroencephalographic (EEG) waves are produced by potential differences that are caused by postsynaptic potentials in the cell membrane of cortical neurons. This potential difference is recorded on the surface by scalp electrodes. Each of the stages of human sleep-wakefulness cycle produces a characteristic electroencephalographic wave. The waveforms encompass four common frequency bands from the lowest frequency delta through theta and alpha to high-frequency beta (**Table 9.1**). The EEG waveforms are measured in cycles per second (cps) or Hertz (Hz). EEG detects voltage change with signal oscillations from synchronous excitation of neuronal population.

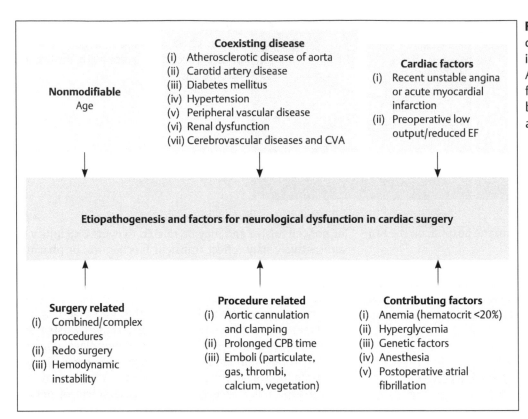

Flowchart 9.1 Factors associated with cerebral insult/injury in cardiac surgery. Abbreviations: EF, ejection fraction; CPB, cardiopulmonary bypass, CVA, cerebrovascular accident.

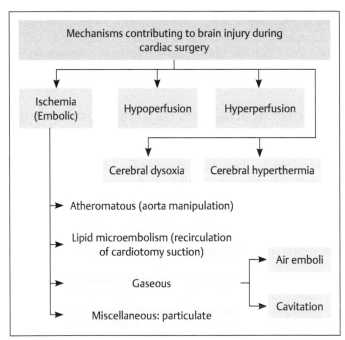

Flowchart 9.2 Algorithm explaining mechanisms of cerebral injury in cardiac surgery.

Modern EEG monitors have digital microprocessors with multichannel processed EEG that use computerized processing of EEG signals (**Fig. 9.3**).

Processed EEG works on the principle of power spectrum analysis: (i) compressed spectral array

Table 9.1 Various EEG waves and their clinical correlation

EEG waves	Frequency	Clinical interpretation
Delta wave	0.1–4 Hz	Deep coma, deepest sleep, hypoxia, ischemia
Theta wave	4–8 Hz	Progressive suppression
Alpha wave	8–14 Hz	Relaxed, drowsy state
Beta wave	14–25 Hz	Awake, mentally alert state
Gamma wave	25–55 Hz	Rarely found, highest frequency

(CSA):[3] enormous data compression occurs with high-amplitude bursts using Fourier transformation; (ii) density spectral array (DSA) is a 2D monochrome dot matrix plot of time as a function of frequency;[4] (iii) color DSA is also used; (iv) bispectral index (BIS) is most widely used for monitoring depth of anesthesia and intraoperative awareness during surgery.

The frequency descriptors used in EEG commonly are total power (TP), peak power frequency (PPF), mean dominant frequency (MDF), spectral edge frequency (SEF), and suppression ratio (SR).

B. Method: Standardized electrode placement is based on the International 10–20 system. Uniform spacing of electrodes in scalp region correlating with specific areas of cerebral cortex take into consideration four anatomical landmarks, namely, nasion, inion, and two preauricular points on either side. Through the intersecting lines

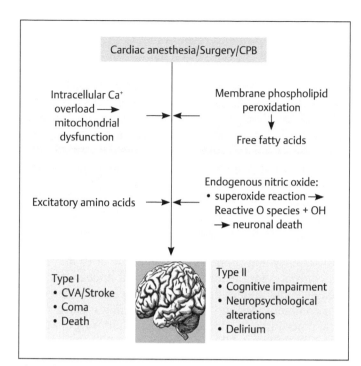

Cardiac anesthesia/Surgery/CPB

Intracellular Ca⁺ overload ——→ mitochondrial dysfunction

Membrane phospholipid peroxidation
↓
Free fatty acids

Excitatory amino acids ——→

Endogenous nitric oxide:
• superoxide reaction —→ Reactive O species + OH —→ neuronal death

Type I
• CVA/Stroke
• Coma
• Death

Type II
• Cognitive impairment
• Neuropsychological alterations
• Delirium

Flowchart 9.3 Algorithm depicting the pathophysiology of neuronal ischemia leading to cerebral injury in cardiac surgery. Abbreviations: CPB, cardiopulmonary bypass, CVA, cardiovascular accident.

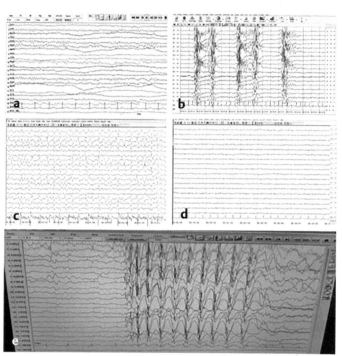

Fig. 9.3 Electroencephalographic (EEG) interpretation. **(a)** Normal EEG. **(b)** EEG showing generalized periodic complexes with burst suppression pattern. **(c)** EEG showing triphasic waves. **(d)** EEG showing electrocerebral inactivity. **(e)** EEG showing spike and wave pattern in an epileptic patient.

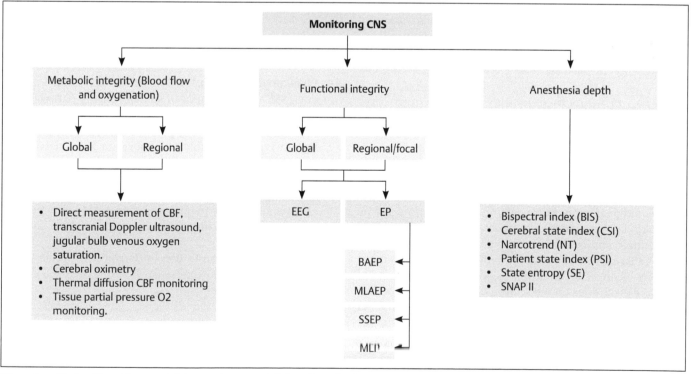

Monitoring CNS

Metabolic integrity (Blood flow and oxygenation)

Functional integrity

Anesthesia depth

Global   Regional

Global   Regional/focal

EEG   EP

• Direct measurement of CBF, transcranial Doppler ultrasound, jugular bulb venous oxygen saturation.
• Cerebral oximetry
• Thermal diffusion CBF monitoring
• Tissue partial pressure O2 monitoring.

BAEP ←

MLAEP ←

SSEP ←

MEP

• Bispectral index (BIS)
• Cerebral state index (CSI)
• Narcotrend (NT)
• Patient state index (PSI)
• State entropy (SE)
• SNAP II

Flowchart 9.4   Algorithm explaining various modalities of cerebral monitoring in cardiac surgery. Abbreviations: BAEP, brainstem auditory-evoked potential; CBF, cerebral blood flow; EEG, electroencephalography; EP, evoked potential; MEP, motor-evoked potential; MLAEP, middle-latency auditory-evoked potential; SSEP, somatosensory-evoked potential.

of the sagittal hemicircumference across the vertex and ipsilateral hemicircumference, the electrodes are placed in defined positions on the scalp, except the frontal (F3, F4) and parietal (P3, P4) electrodes which are placed halfway through circumferential ring and middle electrode. In the absence of disease, electroencephalographic amplitude and frequency are inversely related: Simultaneous decrease correlates with ischemia, anoxia, excessive hypnosis, hypothermia, while simultaneous increase correlates with seizure activity or artifact.

C. **Advantages:** EEG monitoring is a noninvasive technique that is useful in the identification of the following:
1. Preexisting electroencephalographic abnormality.
2. Level of hypnotic effect.
3. Cerebral ischemia and/or hypoxia.
4. Effects of head malposition.
5. Hypocarbia-induced cerebral ischemia.
6. Malperfusion syndrome.
7. Indirect effects of anemia on cerebral oxygen supply and hence need for blood replacement.
8. Determination of optimal cooling and rewarming for a given patient.
9. Occurrence of seizures.
10. Electrocortical silence.

D. **Disadvantages:**
1. EEG records signals from superficial layer of cerebral cortex and hence tracing is confounded by external factors such as anesthesia, temperature (hypo/hyperthermia), and roller pump artifacts. Recently, these concerns have been minimized with the use of fast-track anesthesia, normothermia or mild hypothermia during CPB, and centrifugal pumps.
2. EEG signals are cortical in origin; hence, these signals do not imply absence of subcortical sensory perception.

Auditory-Evoked Potentials

Auditory-evoked potential (AEP) is a simple and reproducible monitoring modality that is suitable for patients undergoing cardiovascular surgical procedures. It is an extremely useful method to evaluate specific areas of brainstem, midbrain, and auditory cortices.

A. **Physiological principles:** Neural response to acoustic stimuli is responsible for generation of early-latency potentials and middle-latency potentials. Biopotentials are generated at all levels of auditory system on application of an acoustic stimulus. With the placement of surface electrodes on the scalp, a dozen peaks can be recognized within the first 100 milliseconds after onset of the stimulus. Each peak is designated by its poststimulus latency and peak-to-peak amplitude. AEPs are designated as early- or middle-latency potentials. Early AEPs are generated from the auditory nerve and the brainstem and constitute sequence of wavelets recorded within the first 10 milliseconds after stimulus. These evoked responses have been designated as brainstem AEPs (BAEPs). Adult BAEPs are depicted as seven waves (I–VII). The origin of peaks I and II are from distal and proximal parts of the eighth nerve; peak III from cochlear nucleus; peak IV from the superior olivary complex, cochlear nucleus, and nucleus of the lateral lemniscus; peak V from both the lateral lemniscus and the inferior colliculus; and peak VI and VII may arise from the medial geniculate body and the acoustic radiations. The middle-latency AEPs (MLAEPs) are produced from the midbrain and primary auditory cortex and have a poststimulus latency between 10 and 100 milliseconds. In an awake adult subject, the MLAEPs usually consist of three main peaks: Na, Pa, and Nb, with respective latencies near 15, 28, and 40 milliseconds. Many agents with hypnotic effects prolong the latency and suppress the amplitude of Pa and Nb in a concentration-dependent manner. It appears that the latency and amplitude changes allow reliable detection of consciousness and nociception during cardiac surgical procedures. In addition, parallel monitoring of MLAEP and quantitative EEG descriptors (i.e., BIS) may permit distinction between the hypnotic and antinociceptive anesthetic components.[5]

B. **Advantages:** BAEPs are useful in assessing brainstem and subcortical function during surgical procedures, in part because of their relative resistance to the suppressant effects of most anesthetic agents.[6] BAEP is simple and reproducible and suitable for monitoring during cardiac surgical procedures, assessment of temperature effects on brainstem function, and evaluation of hypnotic effect. AEPs are technically speaking, noninvasive.

Somatosensory-Evoked Potentials

A. **Physiological principles:** Somatosensory-evoked potentials (SSEP) test integrity of somatosensory pathway and objectively measure ascending sensory pathway function. Electrical stimulus applied to peripheries, arms or legs, or both (preferably tibial nerve or facial nerve) and neuronal transmission via the spinal cord and subcortical structures are recorded.

B. **Advantage:** Very useful in thoracoabdominal aortic aneurysm surgery to monitor spinal cord function by objectively measuring integrity of ascending sensory pathways.

C. **Disadvantage:** Results are unreliable if volatile anesthetic agents or neuromuscular blockers are used during monitoring.

Motor-Evoked Potentials

A. **Physiological principle:** Motor-evoked potentials (MEPs) are produced by the application of high-intensity transcranial stimuli directly; this produces depolarization of cortical motor neurons. MEP tests integrity of descending motor pathways. Lower limb MEPs test functional integrity of motor pathways in thoracolumbar spinal cord, and upper limb MEPs provide information on MEP suppression which may be affected by anesthesia and hypothermia.

B. Advantages:

1. Most useful in open surgical or endovascular repair of descending aortic aneurysms/dissection.
2. There is no signal averaging in MEP; hence, it has more accuracy.

C. Disadvantages: Results are unreliable when used with volatile anesthetics and neuromuscular blockers; if used, should be monitored by train-of-four monitoring. Essential prerequisite is that correct interpretation of MEP amplitude needs precise monitoring and control of neuromuscular blockade.

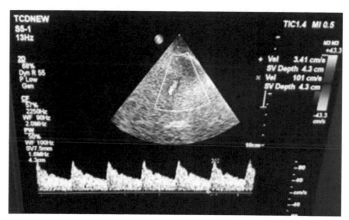

Fig. 9.4 Transcranial Doppler showing middle cerebral artery (MCA) velocity of 101 cm/s indicating mild vasospasm.

Transcranial Doppler (TCD)

A. Physiological principle: The principle of TCD is based on production of ultrasound by electrical activation of piezoelectric crystals. Ultrasonic waves of 1- to 2-MHz frequency are passed through the thinnest portion of temporal bone across the cranium into the cerebral tissue. Doppler principle is used to determine the direction and velocity of blood flow in the major cerebral arteries to derive the adequacy of cerebral perfusion. Blood (erythrocytes) acts as a medium for reflecting back ultrasonic waves.

B. Clinical use:

1. Blood flow across the middle cerebral artery (MCA) is monitored and a 50% reduction in cerebral blood flow (CBF) velocity with loss of diastolic velocity suggests cerebral ischemia.
2. TCD detects blood flow during antegrade cerebral perfusion and helps in detecting air and particulate matter emboli by high-intensity transit signals (HITS).[7]
3. A sudden decrease in the velocity of blood flow during CPB may indicate cannula malposition or dissection of the vessel.
4. **Lindegaard Ratio** is the relationship between mean velocity in the MCA and mean velocity in the ipsilateral extracranial internal carotid artery. High velocities in the MCA (>120 cm/s) represent hyperemia or vasospasm (**Fig. 9.4**). The Lindegaard Ratio helps distinguish these conditions (<3 = hyperemia; >3 = vasospasm: >3–6 mild; >6 severe).

C. Advantages:

1. It detects changes in intracranial blood flow noninvasively during cardiac anesthesia.
2. It is very helpful in detecting air or particulate emboli in cerebral circulation.

D. Disadvantages: Signal attenuation occurs on the skull and this can lead to artifact formation; tapping the ultrasound probe can help distinguish artifact from an embolus.

Jugular Venous Oxygen Saturation

A. Physiological principle: Oximeter catheters transmitting three wavelengths of light may be inserted into the cerebral venous circulation to measure jugular venous oxygen saturation ($SjvO_2$) directly and continuously. Commercially available devices are modifications of the oximetry catheter originally developed for determining mixed venous oxygen saturation in pulmonary artery. Physiologically speaking, clinical determination of $SjvO_2$ reflects the balance of cerebral oxygen supply and consumption.

Factors affecting $SjvO_2$ include CBF, cerebral oxygen consumption, arterial oxygen content, and hemoglobin concentration. Jugular vein is cannulated retrogradely using oximetry catheter inserted in jugular venous bulb, but a radiographic confirmation of correct precise placement is needed for accurate $SjvO_2$ readings. The normal $SjvO_2$ range is widely assumed to be between 55 and 70%.[8] However, a study using radiographically confirmed catheter placement observed a much wider 45 to 70% range in healthy subjects.[9]

B. Advantages:

1. Jugular bulb oximetry can be used as a trend monitor rather than absolute measurement.
2. $SjvO_2$ is helpful in the rewarming phase after hypothermic CPB where cerebral venous blood desaturation can be correlated with Hb concentration and depth of anesthesia.
3. $SjvO_2$ can be used as a transfusion trigger.
4. Deleterious effects of cerebral hyperthermia can be detected early.

C. Disadvantages:

1. $SjvO_2$ needs continuous flow postcatheter and hence not suitable during total circulatory arrest in cardiac surgical procedures.
2. Expertise and learning curve are needed for insertion of a jugular oximetry catheter.

3. Risk of intracranial infection.
4. Catheter kinking, temperature changes, and fibrin deposition on the catheter interfere with the measurement of oximetry.

Cerebral Oximetry

A. **Physiological principle:** The human skull is translucent to infrared light; hence, intracranial intravascular regional oxygen saturation (rSO_2) may be measured noninvasively with transcranial near-infrared spectroscopy (NIRS). Isosbestic point is at a level at which peak absorption is same for oxyhemoglobin and deoxyhemoglobin at an infrared wavelength of 810 nm. Infrared light penetrates bones, muscles, and other tissues when self-adhesive pads, containing light-emitting diodes and sensing optodes, are connected to forehead. Normal range of regional cerebral oxygen saturation (rSO_2) for adult cardiac surgery is 71 ± 6%.[10] Baseline values less than 50% represent reduced brain tolerance of ischemic insult. Clinically important decrease is 20% below baseline values (**Flowchart 9.5**). Cerebral oximetry index (COX index) is the correlation coefficient between cerebral perfusion pressure (CPP) and rSO_2. COX index is expressed between zero and negative value when in cerebral autoregulation range. COX index indicates low perfusion pressure earlier than NIRS.

Near-infrared light and some wavelengths of visible red light easily penetrate human tissue, including bone. Light is used noninvasively to interrogate gray matter in the frontal portion of the cerebral cortex. A light emitter is the source of the near-infrared light used to interrogate the tissue. There are two light detectors spaced at 1.5 cm from the light emitter, and one spaced at 5 cm from the light emitter. The light moves in an elliptical pathway from emitter to detector. The measurements taken by the near detector light path are used to eliminate superficial tissue readings which are not valuable in the calculation of cerebral tissue saturation. This includes the readings from the skin, the skull, and the dura mater of the brain. These values are subtracted from the deeper tissue readings as measured by the far detector. The depth of the light path is based on the separation of light source to detector and the strength of the light source.

B. **Cerebral autoregulation** as quoed by Silverman et al.[11] is the ability of the cerebral vasculature to maintain stable blood flow despite changes in cerebral perfusion pressure. Various etiology like myogenic, neurogenic,

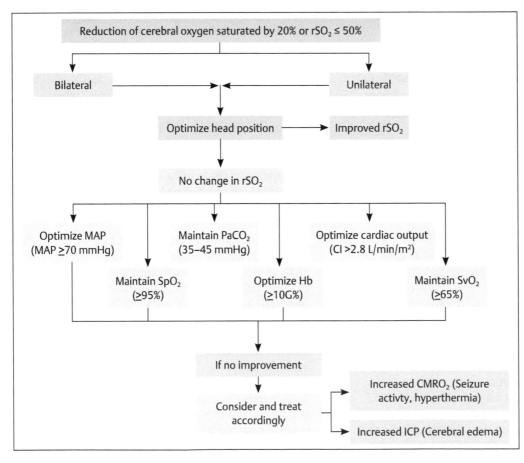

Flowchart 9.5 Algorithm for trouble shooting of reduced rSO_2 during cardiac surgery. Abbreviations: CI, cardiac index; $CMRO_2$, cerebral oxygen consumption; Hb, hemoglobin; ICP, intracranial pressure; MAP, mean arterial pressure; $PaCO_2$, partial pressure of carbon dioxide; rSO_2, regional cerebral oxygen saturation; SpO_2, oxygen saturation; SvO_2, mixed venous oxygen saturation.

metabolic response have been known as causative factors in the mediation of cerebral vasomotor reactions. It has both advantages and disadvantages as mentioned below.

C. Advantages:

1. Detects imbalance in oxygen supply and demand by noninvasive technique.
2. Cerebral oximetry correlates well with direct microprobe measurement technique of brain oxygen partial pressure.
3. Cerebral oximetry is useful to derive the cerebral autoregulatory curves for a given patient. Use of cerebral oximetry to determine autoregulation during cardiac surgery is depicted in **Fig. 9.5**.

D. Disadvantages:

1. The sensors are disposable and add to the cost of treatment.
2. Electrode placement is limited to glabrous skin.
3. Posterior infarcts may not be captured with traditional frontoparietal placement of the sensors.
4. rSO_2 values are device-dependent and are not interchangeable.[12]

Multimodal Neuromonitoring

Each of neurological monitoring methods described above assesses only a portion of the CNS. It is logical to apply a multimodal technique for wholesome monitoring of neurologic function. It is confusing to have multiple sources of information and plethora of display attempting to follow the neurologic events in a given anesthetic and surgical procedure. Considerable technological advances are necessary for the development of a comprehensive display format to effectively assimilate all the information provided to improve neurological safety during cardiac surgical procedures.

Key Points

- EEG can detect both cerebral ischemia or hypoxia and seizures and can measure hypnotic effect.
- Middle-latency auditory-evoked potentials objectively document inadequate hypnosis.
- Somatosensory-evoked potentials may detect developing injury in cortical and subcortical brain structures and peripheral nerves.
- Transcranial electric motor-evoked potentials monitor function of the descending motor pathways.
- Transcranial Doppler ultrasound examination assesses the direction and the character of the blood flow through large intracranial arteries and identifies microemboli.
- Cerebral oximetry, using spatially resolved transcranial near-infrared spectroscopy, provides a continuous measure of change in the balance of cerebral oxygen supply and demand.

Conclusion

Increasing evidence suggests that the use of brain monitoring–EEG, evoked potentials, TCD, and NIRS is gaining popularity even in non-neurocritical care settings, e.g., in the perioperative setting, ED, and ICU, to improve patient care. Neuromonitoring devices can be non-invasive, low-cost, safe tools available at the bedside, with a great potential for both diagnosis and monitoring of patients at risk of brain insult.[13,14]

Acknowledgment
We would like to express our heartfelt thanks Dr Gopal Dash for providing **Fig. 9.3**.

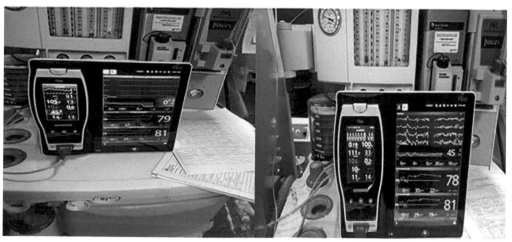

Fig. 9.5 Sideline monitor with integrated patient state index, with rSO_2 (regional cerebral oxygen saturation) being used during cardiac surgery.

References

1. Shetty V, Muralidhar K. Good CPB practices for prevention of cerebral injury in cardiac surgery. Indian J Extra-Corporeal Technol 2011;21(2):4-11

2. Blume WT, Sharbrough FW. EEG monitoring during carotid endarterectomy and open heart surgery. In: Niedermeyer E, Lopes Da Silva F, eds. Electroencephalography. 4th ed. Philadelphia, PA: Lippincott Williams & Wilkins; 1999: 797-808

3. Myers RR, Stockard JJ, Fleming NI, France CJ, Bickford RG. The use of on-line telephonic computer analysis of the E.E.G. in anaesthesia. Br J Anaesth 1973;45(7):664-670

4. Fleming RA, Smith NT. An inexpensive device for analyzing and monitoring the electroencephalogram. Anesthesiology 1979;50(5):456-460

5. Musialowicz T, Niskanen M, Yppärilä-Wolters H, Pöyhönen M, Pitkänen O, Hynynen M. Auditory-evoked potentials in bispectral index-guided anaesthesia for cardiac surgery. Eur J Anaesthesiol 2007;24(7):571-579

6. Sloan TB. General anesthesia for monitoring. In: Koht A, Sloan TB, Toleikis JR, eds. Monitoring the nervous system for anesthesiologists and other health care professionals. New York: Springer; 2012:319-336

7. Georgiadis D, Siebler M. Detection of microembolic signals with transcranial Doppler ultrasound. Front Neurol Neurosci 2006;21:194-205

8. Samra SK, Rajajee V. Monitoring of jugular venous oxygen saturation. In: Koht A, Sloan TB, Toleikis JR, eds. Monitoring the nervous system for anesthesiologists and other health care professionals. New York: Springer; 2012:255-277

9. Chieregato A, Calzolari F, Trasforini G, Targa L, Latronico N. Normal jugular bulb oxygen saturation. J Neurol Neurosurg Psychiatry 2003;74(6):784-786

10. Kim MB, Ward DS, Cartwright CR, Kolano J, Chlebowski S, Henson LC. Estimation of jugular venous O_2 saturation from cerebral oximetry or arterial O_2 saturation during isocapnic hypoxia. J Clin Monit Comput 2000;16(3):191-199

11. Silverman A, Petersen NH. Physiology, Cerebral Autoregulation. 2022 Feb 16. In: StatPearls [Internet]. Treasure Island (FL): StatPearls Publishing; 2022 Jan.

12. Kok WF, van Harten AE, Koene BM, et al. A pilot study of cerebral tissue oxygenation and postoperative cognitive dysfunction among patients undergoing coronary artery bypass grafting randomised to surgery with or without cardiopulmonary bypass. Anaesthesia 2014;69(6):613-622

13. Battaglini D, Pelosi P, Robba C. The Importance of Neuromonitoring in Non Brain Injured Patients. Crit Care. 2022;26(1):78

14. Klamt JG, Garcia WNP, Carvalho M, Garcia LV, Menardi AC. Multimodal Neuromonitoring During Pediatric Cardiac Surgery. Braz J Cardiovasc Surg. 2022 ;37(2):251-258

10

The Role of NIRS in Postoperative Pediatric Cardiac ICU

Manjula Sarkar and Sonali Kore

Introduction

The role of near-infrared spectroscopy (NIRS) in cardiac theater is well established, and its use for noncardiac surgeries in cardiac patients is picking up popularity, but its role in postsurgical pediatric cardiac ICU is not established. By understanding its role and importance of values of cerebral saturation, and its implementation in the treatment of critically ill patients, cerebral saturation monitoring in pediatric cardiac intensive care unit (ICU) during the postoperative period should help in diagnosing critical events and their management for a better outcome and early discharge.

Common postoperative complications in pediatric post-cardiac surgery patients are arrhythmias, hypotension, cardiac arrest, ST wave segment on ECG done, acute low cardiac output, pulmonary hypertension, diastolic dysfunction, valve dysfunction, residual shunts, or residual obstruction of ventricular outflow tracts, and brain injuries such as cerebral infarction, postoperative cognitive dysfunction where cerebral oxygen saturation is affected. It is important to note that the congenital cardiac complex may be associated with genetic abnormalities which can lead to cerebral dysfunction and is different from hypoxic cerebral dysfunction. If we notice a fall in cerebral saturation during the postoperative period, early and immediate intervention can be done.

Surgical treatment for congenital heart diseases is common. Around one-fourth of complex congenital heart diseases with different degrees of heart failure, or respiratory failure, experience postoperative complications. So close monitoring, timely intervention, and treatment are very critical to avoid occurrence of multiple complications.

Congenital cardiopathy (acyanotic and cyanotic heart disease) is the most common congenital anomalies, estimated recently at 6 to 10 for every 1,000 live births. These congenital diseases may or may not be associated with pulmonary artery hypertension (PAH).

A significant number of these babies need surgery to correct or relieve their heart defects, and many of them need surgery while still in the uterus.[1] Because of the issues of aortopulmonary shunts, the undeveloped cardiovascular system, and deep hypothermic circulatory arrest, there is a difference in cardiopulmonary (CP) bypass machines in infants. Prolonged CP bypass time causes overload on the systemic circulation, which may contribute to heart failure. CP bypass time, specific surgical technique, anesthesia, and different medications may result in the production of multisystemic complications in the postoperative period.[2] The focus of postoperative treatment is primarily on preserving CP homeostasis and preventing end-organ damage.[3] The postoperative period in children requires close observation. Children of complex congenital heart diseases with different degrees of heart failure, respiratory failure, or shock are at risk of multiple concomitant complications and mortality as they require complex surgeries. Although reported mortality in the modern era is around 6%, due to changes and advances in surgical treatment, early postoperative complications are still expected.

NIRS cerebral oximetry has been used in cardiovascular anesthesia, and regional cerebral oxygen saturation is applied on patients at risk of cerebral ischemia. Early detection and treatment of cerebral hypoperfusion can help to reduce the risk of avoidable brain injury. For the prevention of postoperative neurological damage in pediatric patients undergoing cardiovascular surgery, proper awareness and implementation of NIRS oxygenation monitoring are essential.

Hypoxia or hypoperfusion of the brain due to reduced cardiac activity, elevated central venous pressure due to intracardiac shunting, or cyanosis is normal in ICUs. Some cardiac operations have been known to cause ischemia and infarction in the middle cerebral artery, which can be identified by a drop in cerebral saturation. For the treatment of hypoplastic left heart syndrome, the Norwood technique is used.[4]

The Basics of NIRS Oxygenation and Principles of the Monitoring System

Literature has shown that postoperative NIRS oxygenation monitoring will increase the probability of detecting and preventing cerebral injury because of the high tissue permeability of near-infrared light that reaches body tissues and is absorbed by oxygenated and deoxygenated hemoglobin molecules, which have different absorption spectra. The noninvasive optical monitor of regional cerebral oxygen saturation (rSO_2) is NIRS. Although NIRS-dependent regional cerebral oximetry correlates with mixed venous oxygen saturation (SvO_2) obtained via invasive testing, absolute SvO_2 values cannot be predicted based on noninvasive rSO_2 measurements.

Practical Considerations in NIRS

Medical conditions, anatomical, physiological properties, anemia, cranial bone thickness, the cerebrospinal fluid layer, extracranial blood flow, and the subject's body location all affect oxygenation monitoring. The rSO_2 would be lower than the regional venous measure due to hyperbilirubinemia and excess melanin. The cerebral arterial/venous blood partitioning is a source of concern: individual arterial/venous ratios vary significantly. There is also a lot of difference in the blood's hemoglobin content.[5]

Points to Consider in Pediatric Cardiac Surgery

Variation in cerebral oximetry information during complex congenital surgeries will help us in ICU management. Cerebral oximetry monitoring in ICU in the postoperative period helps, where deep hypothermic circulatory arrest (DHCA) is used to achieve a bloodless operative field in many congenital complex surgeries, and fall in cerebral oxygen saturation is expected. In pediatric cardiac surgery, oxygenation control is used to assess the healthy length of DHCA and the possibility of hypoperfusion of the left hemisphere, which is less oxygenated than the right hemisphere during regional low-flow cerebral perfusion. The incidence of neurologic and other complications has been linked to a decrease in postoperative cerebral oxygen saturation. rSO_2 values in children undergoing cardiac surgery decreased to 60 to 70% of baseline throughout DHCA, hitting a nadir in 20 to 40 minutes.[6] The half-life of NIRS oxygenation saturation shift during DHCA was inversely related to age, with neonates having a half-life of 9 minutes (age 10%).[7]

The concepts of NIRS oxygenation monitoring is used to prevent surgically induced brain damage in clinical scenario to monitor brain oxygenation. Damage can be taken as a reference for the prevention of brain injury during postoperative pediatric ICU care, which needs further studies.

Discussion

In the coming years, NIRS is expected to play an increasingly important role in pediatric intensive care. NIRS is a noninvasive, compact technology that detects oxygenation in the brain, muscle, and other organs. It measures the capillary–venous oxygen saturation in the tissue immediately underneath the sensor to detect slight changes in tissue oxygenation in real time. It has been used by anesthesiologists in operating rooms in the past decade, but it is gaining popularity in the intensive care unit, especially among children with congenital heart disease.

History and Salient Points about the Evolution of Equipment

Sir Fredrick William Herschel discovered red-light radiation by mistake in 1800. In the manufacturing sector, NIRS was only produced in the 1950s. In 1977, the first medical article on NIRS was published. During the 1980s and 1990s, the equipment underwent significant growth, especially with the development of light fiberoptics and monochromatic detectors. Ferrari conducted the first human cerebral NIRS experiment in 1985, but it wasn't until 1993 that the US Food and Drug Administration (FDA) approved NIRS for medical and commercial use. The INVOS 3100, the first commercially available NIRS, was published in 1993.

Technical Aspects of NIRS

NIRS tracks the tissue bed underneath the sensor, which includes small gas-exchanging vessels, using infrared light

(700–900 nm) (arterioles, capillaries, and venules). This is the secret to comprehending the NIRS machine and its role in both the operating room and intensive care. NIRS was first developed as a system in the operating room that could calculate cerebral oximetry in real time during deep hypothermic circulatory arrests (DHCA) and cardiopulmonary bypass (CPB). For many years, there has been concern about neurological outcomes following cardiac surgery, especially in pediatric congenital cardiac surgery, and this system has been used as a proxy for SvO_2 (mixed venous saturations) in the operating room and allows direct cerebral oximetry readings.

NIRS can identify problems that can contribute to altered cerebral oxygenation in an operating theater, such as CPB cannulation issues, symptoms of deep hypothermia and low-flow CPB, effects of antegrade cerebral perfusion, and effects of ventilation or anesthetic strategies influencing cerebral blood flow. A recent study showed that a group of infants who underwent neonatal aortic arch repair with the use of NIRS to control regional cerebral perfusion had normal cognitive outcomes at 12 months.[8] NIRS may be useful in DHCA during cardiac surgery because it allows for continuous monitoring of cerebral perfusion regardless of changes in pH and temperature. Cardiovascular surgery, carotid endarterectomies, and neurosurgery are among the clinical uses of NIRS in the operating room.

NIRS and Its Role in Pediatric Intensive Care

Low cardiac output syndrome is characterized by a decline in cardiac output. It is well recognized that inadequate oxygen delivery occurs after congenital cardiac surgery. In the postoperative period, low cardiac output syndrome is linked to increased morbidity and mortality. Inflammatory response after CPB, the effects of a cross-clamp and myocardial ischemia, reperfusion injury, the effects of hypothermia, insufficient cardiac defense, and finally the effects of ventriculotomy are all factors that lead to low cardiac performance. After cardiac surgery, low cardiac output syndrome is normal in a percentage of children, and it can lead to late neurological dysfunction in survivors. In the ICU, simple monitoring of low cardiac output is required, which can be accomplished with the aid of cerebral oximetry. A recent review article found Class II level B evidence for NIRS as a hemodynamic control in critically ill patients.[9] Changes in regional oxygen saturation can reflect local changes rather than global hypoperfusion, which should be held in mind when interpreting the results from NIRS. No study has found a connection between low cardiac output and low cerebral saturation, so more research is needed. Poor regional cerebral oxygenation does not always imply a low cardiac output state or global cerebral perfusion impairment.

Advantages of the NIRS Monitor

Continuous monitoring of blood oxygen saturation in the internal jugular vein is a useful indicator for selective cerebral perfusion during aortic arch replacement,[10] but NIRS has several distinct advantages, including the fact that it is noninvasive, real time, and provides a continuous measurement of regional tissue oxygen saturation. It makes it possible to assess patterns and intervene promptly. There is a strong belief that NIRS monitoring will help pediatric cardiac surgery patients have a better outcome (**Table 10.1**).

The use of pulse oximetry to measure oxygen saturation is common in ICUs, but it has disadvantages. Pulsatile signal component reflecting arterial circulation is needed for pulse oximetry, whereas nonpulsatile signal component reflecting tissue circulation is monitored by cerebral oximetry (arterioles, capillaries, and venules). Cerebral saturation represents a greater real-time tissue circulation since it includes arterial, venous, and capillary components.[16]

Maintaining a sufficient cardiac performance in postoperative cardiac surgery patients is a vital determinant of outcome. Because of decreased tissue blood flow and increased oxygen extraction as cardiac production declines, mixed venous oxygen saturation drops (below the usual 65–70%) (increased arteriovenous [AV] oxygen difference).[17] The use of a pulmonary catheter to measure mixed venous oxygen saturation (SvO_2) is a common procedure that is used as a cardiac output predictor. SvO_2 can be measured directly in these postoperative patients, thanks to catheters inserted in the pulmonary artery. SvO_2 assessed invasively through a central venous catheter does not provide continuous monitoring, and acute SvO_2 declines may be missed. Furthermore, repeated blood sampling causes increased blood loss, colonization of the central venous catheter, contamination, and infection risk. Indwelling intracardiac catheter complications, on the other hand, include bleeding during removal, catheter breakage and entrapment during removal, inflammation, thrombus formation, and embolization,[18-20] all of which can be easily substituted by noninvasive technologies like NIRS.

Based on the foregoing findings, authors hypothesize that the two approaches would closely correlate, and that noninvasive cerebral rSO_2 would suffice for SvO_2 monitoring. The current clinical availability of many NIRS-based instruments represents a major improvement in the prevention, identification, and correction of oxygen delivery discrepancies to the brain and vital organs. In pediatric intensive care units (PICUs), treating cerebral ischemia is still a big concern. A significant number of clinical studies have been published on cerebral tissue oxygenation ($cStO_2$) and cerebral fractional tissue extraction (cFTOE).

In neonatology, noninvasive measurement of cerebral tissue oxygenation using NIRS is gaining popularity. NIRS provides continuous assessment of regional cerebral oxygenation ($cStO_2$) and cerebral tissue oxygen extraction (cFTOE).[21] Current NIRS-based system variability and definition of function in neonatology, clinical applications in continuous $cStO_2$ monitoring, drawbacks, disadvantages, and potential of current technology have all been extensively addressed.[22] In neonatal intensive care units (NICUs), it is not used as a routine brain monitoring tool.[23,24] $cStO_2$ has a strong connection to immediate postnatal adaptation, hypoxic-ischemic encephalopathy (HIE), patent ductus arteriosus (PDA), intraventricular hemorrhage (IVH), and respiratory distress syndrome (RDS). There is also clinical significance. Ferrari et al conducted NIRS-based human cerebral oximetry experiments in 1985.[25] The possibilities of NIRS monitoring have greatly improved since the first study of pediatric application of NIRS for monitoring cerebral oxygenation in sick preterm infants in 1986.[26] The use of NIRS to direct treatment decreased the severity of cerebral hypoxia without affecting the EEG or blood biomarkers.[27] In the premature infant, hemodynamically important PDA had a detrimental effect on cerebral oxygenation.[28,29] PDA can be detected using NIRS.[30] Cerebral oxygenation and peri/intraventricular hemorrhage have no clear association between the magnitude of the IVH and cerebral oxygenation, according to Sorensen et al.[31] According to Zhang et al, there is a connection between IVH and $cStO_2$ in preterm infants, with higher $cStO_2$ values in the first 3 hours after birth in neonates who later develop IVH.[32] Therefore, monitoring $cStO_2$ can help to protect the fragile preterm brain.

NIRS has been used in OR, but it is still being researched in critically ill patients with sepsis, inadequate perfusion, and neurological results linked to low cerebral oximetry in the ICU. The use of NIRS in the univentricular population has been proposed by Johnson and colleagues.[33] According to Bhalala and colleagues, postoperative cerebral rSO_2 and its association with long-term outcomes is used to detect and treat cerebral deoxygenation promptly.[34] NIRS should be linked for monitoring for prognosis of the patient to better long-term outcomes. Andropoulos and colleagues[8] reported magnetic resonance imaging (MRI) results and neurodevelopmental outcomes in children aged 12 months when regional cerebral perfusion was used during aortic arch reconstructions. Kussman and colleagues[35] looked at NIRS and long-term outcomes in over 100 children who had a biventricular repair and were monitored with NIRS. In infants undergoing cardiac surgery, perioperative cycles of decreased cerebral oxygen supply, as assessed by rSO_2, were related to 1-year PDI (Psychomotor and Developmental Indexes of the Bayley scales) and brain MRI abnormalities. These findings support the use of NIRS in this population for long-term cognitive sparing. To determine sensitive times, NIRS is used to assess regional cerebral oxygen saturation in children undergoing cardiac surgery.

Regional cerebral oxygenation was monitored using the INVOS 3100 cerebral oximeter and compared to hemodynamic parameters in authors' experience with pediatric cardiac surgery patients. Few patients in the ICU had a drop in

Table 10.1   Major pediatric cardiac surgery and its association between NIRS oxygenation and neurologic complications and outcomes

Author, Journal	Year published, volume, starting page	Number and subjects	Type of surgery	Device	Parameters indicating clinical abnormalities	Detection of abnormalities	Comments
Kurth et al,[11] Anesthesiology	1995 82:74	26; Neonates, infants, small children	VSD, SV, TOF, TGA	NIM	–	Three patients' postoperative neurologic condition was irregular	Three patients with abnormal postoperative neurologic status had a lower rSO_2 rise during DHCA and a shorter period to DHCA than other patients
Austin et al,[12] J Thorac Cardiovasc Surg	1997 114:707	250; Neonates, infants, small children	Congenital deficit	INVOS 3100	20% relative decrease from baseline in rSO_2	TCD flow velocity and NIRS oxygen desaturation were used to track neurophysiology	Neurophysiologic testing directed procedures lowered the frequency of postoperative neurologic sequelae from 24 to 6%, as well as the duration of hospital stay
Dent et al,[4] J Thorac Cardiovasc Surg	2006 131:190	22; Neonates	HLHS	INVOS 5100	rSO_2 <45% in >180 min	In 73% of patients, postoperative MRI revealed new or worsened ischemic lesions	A connection was discovered between prolonged low rSO_2 after surgery and the development of MRI lesions
McQuillen et al,[13] Stroke	2007 38:736	16 (52); Neonates	HLHS, TGA	NIRO 300	–	On postoperative MRI scans, six participants displayed signs of brain injury	On postoperative MRI scans, a lower mean total oxygen index during aortic clamping was related to brain injury
Phelps et al,[14] Ann Thorac Surg	2009 87:1490	50; Neonates	HLHS	INVOS	Mean rSO_2 Good outcome: 60.8%; Adverse outcome: 52.8%	Postoperative adverse events	Low rSO_2 levels were linked to postoperative complications
Andropoulos et al,[15] J Thorac Cardiovasc Surg	2010 139:543	68; Neonates	VSD, SV, TGA, HLHS	INVOS 5100A	rSO_2< 45%	New postoperative MRI brain injury	Sustained cerebral desaturation (total minutes of rSO_2)

Abbreviations: DHCA, deep hypothermic circulatory arrest; HLHS, hypoplastic left heart syndrome; MRI, magnetic resonance imaging; NIRS, near-infrared spectroscopy; rSO_2, regional cerebral oxygen saturation; SV, sinus venosus; TCD, transcranial Doppler; TGA, transposition of great arteries; TOF, tetralogy of Fallot; VSD, ventricular septal defect.

regional cerebral oxygenation; the cause was multifactorial, with a supply-demand imbalance playing a key role.[36] Cooling reduces cerebral metabolism and the cerebral metabolic rate falls exponentially as temperature decreases; profound hypothermia and CPB duration can cause cerebral saturation and become insufficient to meet metabolic demands, which can affect the postoperative period as well.[37-39] There may be times during the postoperative period when you are more vulnerable to hypoxic-ischemic injury.[40,41] On this basis, authors conclude that hypothermia and hypotension could be the cause of cerebral desaturation and inadequate oxygen supply for metabolism in the postoperative period. Any method that can evaluate the cerebral oxygen supply/demand relationship may be extremely useful in determining the most sensitive periods for ischemic damage following pediatric cardiac surgery.

Conclusion

The authors conclude that NIRS may be a useful technique for detecting periods of increased susceptibility to ischemic neurologic harm in the postoperative period following cardiac surgery due to a variety of factors such as hypothermia, bleeding, anemia, hypoxia, hypotension, and poor ventricular function. If jugular bulb oxygen saturation monitoring is not possible, then according to the authors NIRS can be a potential method for monitoring cerebral oxygenation. The cerebral metabolic rate will increase in the immediate postoperative period, but the ability to increase oxygen supply may be impaired. The use of NIRS in the environment of a pediatric cardiac ICU after congenital heart surgery is still a research tool. Sensitive times for neurological injury should be recognized and treated promptly using NIRS.

NIRS is the most frequently brain monitor used and it has been adopted as the endpoint in many algorithms for hemodynamic and respiratory management during cardiac surgery to improve patient outcomes.[42]

Acknowledgment
The authors would like to thank the Department of Cardiovascular and Thoracic Anesthesia, Seth GS Medical College and KEM Hospital for allowing the use of this tool for patient care and the Dean Dr. Deshmukh for his help and support. The authors are on the research path at Dr. DY Patil institution for further research on this subject of NIRS.

References

1. Krishnamurthy G, Ratner V, Bacha E. Neonatal cardiac care a perspective seminar in thoracic and cardiovascular surgery. Pediat Cardiac Surg Ann 2013;16:21–31
2. Beke DM, Braudis NJ, Lincoln P. Management of the pediatric postoperative cardiac surgery patient. Crit Care Nurs Clin North Am 2005;17(4):405–416, xi
3. Miletic KG, Spiering TJ, Delius RE, Walters HL III, Mastropietro CW. Use of a novel vasoactive-ventilation-renal score to predict outcomes after paediatric cardiac surgery. Interact Cardiovasc Thorac Surg 2015;20(3):289–295
4. Dent CL, Spaeth JP, Jones BV, et al. Brain magnetic resonance imaging abnormalities after the Norwood procedure using regional cerebral perfusion. J Thorac Cardiovasc Surg 2006; 131(1):190–197
5. Desmond FA, Namachivayam S. Does near-infrared spectroscopy play a role in paediatric intensive care? BJA Educ 2016; 16(8):281–285
6. Kussman BD, Wypij D, DiNardo JA, et al. Cerebral oximetry during infant cardiac surgery: evaluation and relationship to early postoperative outcome. Anesth Analg 2009;108(4): 1122–1131
7. Sakatani K. Basic principles (in Japanese). In: Japan Cerebral Metabolism Monitoring Research Group, ed. Near-infrared spectroscopy is made easy for clinicians. Tokyo: Shinkoh Igaku Shuppansha; 2002:1–9
8. Andropoulos DB, Easley RB, Brady K, et al. Neurodevelopmental outcomes after regional cerebral perfusion with neuro monitoring for neonatal aortic arch reconstruction. Ann Thorac Surg 2013;95(2):648–654, discussion 654–655
9. Ghanayem NS, Wernovsky G, Hoffman GM. Near-infrared spectroscopy as a hemodynamic monitor in critical illness. Pediatr Crit Care Med 2011;12(4, Suppl):S27–S32
10. Kuwabara M, Nakajima N, Yamamoto F, et al. Continuous monitoring of blood oxygen saturation of internal jugular vein as a useful indicator for selective cerebral perfusion during aortic arch replacement. J Thorac Cardiovasc Surg 1992; 103(2):355–362
11. Kurth CD, Steven JM, Nicolson SC. Cerebral oxygenation during pediatric cardiac surgery using deep hypothermic circulatory arrest. Anesthesiology 1995;82(1):74–82
12. Austin EH III, Edmonds HL Jr, Auden SM, et al. Benefit of neurophysiologic monitoring for pediatric cardiac surgery. J Thorac Cardiovasc Surg 1997;114(5):707–715, 717, discussion 715–716
13. McQuillen PS, Barkovich AJ, Hamrick SE, et al. Temporal and anatomic risk profile of brain injury with neonatal repair of congenital heart defects. Stroke 2007;38(2, Suppl):736–741
14. Phelps HM, Mahle WT, Kim D, et al. Postoperative cerebral oxygenation in hypoplastic left heart syndrome after the Norwood procedure. Ann Thorac Surg 2009;87(5):1490–1494
15. Andropoulos DB, Hunter JV, Nelson DP, et al. Brain immaturity is associated with brain injury before and after neonatal cardiac surgery with high-flow bypass and cerebral oxygenation monitoring. J Thorac Cardiovasc Surg 2010;139(3):543–556
16. Tortoriello TA, Stayer SA, Mott AR, et al. A noninvasive estimation of mixed venous oxygen saturation using near-infrared spectroscopy by cerebral oximetry in pediatric cardiac surgery patients. Paediatr Anaesth 2005;15(6):495–503
17. Roth SJ. Postoperative care. In: Chang AC, Hanley FL, Wernovsky G, Wessel DL, eds. Pediatric cardiac intensive care. 1st ed. Baltimore: Williams & Wilkins; 1998:163–188
18. Smith-Wright DL, Green TP, Lock JE, Egar MI, Fuhrman BP. Complications of vascular catheterization in critically ill children. Crit Care Med 1984;12(12):1015–1017
19. Petäjä J, Lundström U, Sairanen H, Marttinen E, Griffin JH. Central venous thrombosis after cardiac operations in children. J Thorac Cardiovasc Surg 1996;112(4):883–889
20. Damen J, Van der Tweel I. Positive tip cultures and related risk factors associated with intravascular catheterization in pediatric cardiac patients. Crit Care Med 1988;16(3):221–228
21. Schneider A, Minnich B, Hofstätter E, Weisser C, Hattinger-Jürgenssen E, Wald M. Comparison of four near-infrared

spectroscopy devices shows that they are only suitable for monitoring cerebral oxygenation trends in preterm infants. Acta Paediatr 2014;103(9):934–938

22. Gumulak R, Lucanova LC, Zibolen M. Use of near-infrared spectroscopy (NIRS) in cerebral tissue oxygenation monitoring in neonates. Biomed Pap Med Fac Univ Palacky Olomouc Czech Repub 2017;161(2):128–133

23. Kenosi M, Naulaers G, Ryan CA, Dempsey EM. Current research suggests that the future looks brighter for cerebral oxygenation monitoring in preterm infants. Acta Paediatr 2015;104(3): 225–231

24. Chock VY, Davis AS. Bedside cerebral monitoring to predict neurodevelopmental outcomes. Neoreviews 2009;10(3): e121–e129

25. Ferrari M, Giannini I, Sideri G, Zanette E. Continuous non-invasive monitoring of human brain by near infrared spectroscopy. Adv Exp Med Biol 1985;191:873–882

26. Brazy JE, Lewis DV. Changes in cerebral blood volume and cytochrome aa3 during hypertensive peaks in preterm infants. J Pediatr 1986;108(6):983–987

27. Plomgaard AM, van Oeveren W, Petersen TH, et al. The SafeBoosC II randomized trial: treatment guided by near-infrared spectroscopy reduces cerebral hypoxia without changing early biomarkers of brain injury. Pediatr Res 2016; 79(4):528–535

28. Nizarali Z, Marques T, Costa C, Barroso R, Cunha M. Ductus arteriosus: perinatal risk factors. J Neonatal Biol 2012; 1(3):109

29. Lemmers PMA, Toet MC, van Bel F. Impact of patent ductus arteriosus and subsequent therapy with indomethacin on cerebral oxygenation in preterm infants. Pediatrics 2008; 121(1):142–147

30. Underwood MA, Milstein JM, Sherman MP. Near-infrared spectroscopy as a screening tool for patent ductus arteriosus in extremely low birth weight infants. Neonatology 2007;91(2):134–139

31. Sorensen LC, Maroun LL, Borch K, Lou HC, Greisen G. Neonatal cerebral oxygenation is not linked to foetal vasculitis and predicts intraventricular haemorrhage in preterm infants. Acta Paediatr 2008;97(11):1529–1534

32. Zhang Y, Chan GS, Tracy MB, et al. Cerebral near-infrared spectroscopy analysis in preterm infants with intraventricular hemorrhage. Annu Int Conf IEEE Eng Med Biol Soc 2011; 2011:1937–1940

33. Johnson BA, Hoffman GM, Tweddell JS, et al. Near-infrared spectroscopy in neonates before palliation of hypoplastic left heart syndrome. Ann Thorac Surg 2009;87(2):571–577, discussion 577–579

34. Bhalala US, Nishisaki A, McQueen D, et al. Change in regional (somatic) near-infrared spectroscopy is not a useful indicator of clinically detectable low cardiac output in children after surgery for congenital heart defects. Pediatr Crit Care Med 2012;13(5):529–534

35. Kussman BD, Wypij D, Laussen PC, et al. Relationship of intraoperative cerebral oxygen saturation to neuro-developmental outcome and brain magnetic resonance imaging at 1 year of age in infants undergoing biventricular repair. Circulation 2010;122(3):245–254

36. Mange M, Sarkar M. Cerebral oxygenation during paediatric cardiac surgery: identification of vulnerable periods using near infrared spectroscopy. Res Innov Anesth Jan–June 2006; X(X):1–4

37. Kurth CD, Steven JM, Nicolson SC, Jacobs ML. Cerebral oxygenation during cardiopulmonary bypass in children. J Thorac Cardiovasc Surg 1997;113(1):71–78, discussion 78–79

38. Wernovsky G, Jonas RA, Hickey PR, duPlessis AJ, Newburger JW. Clinical neurologic and developmental studies after cardiac surgery utilizing hypothermic circulatory arrest and cardiopulmonary bypass. Cardiol Young 1993;3:308–316

39. Bracey VA, Greeley WG, Greibal JA, et al. Brain metabolism and cytochrome oxidation are impaired after hypothermic circulatory arrest in children. Circulation 1990;82(Suppl. III): III –412 abstract

40. Greeley WJ, Kern FH, Mault JR, Skaryak LA, Ungerleider RM. Mechanisms of injury and methods of protection of the brain during cardiac surgery in neonates and infants. Cardiol Young 1993;3:317–330

41. Cook DJ, Oliver WC Jr, Orszulak TA, Daly RC. A prospective, randomized comparison of cerebral venous oxygen saturation during normothermic and hypothermic cardiopulmonary bypass. J Thorac Cardiovasc Surg 1994;107(4):1020–1028, discussion 1028–1029

42. Klamt JG, Garcia WNP, Carvalho M, Garcia LV, Menardi AC. Multimodal Neuromonitoring During Pediatric Cardiac Surgery. Braz J Cardiovasc Surg. 2022;37(2):251–258

11

Cardiac Implantable Electronic Devices and Anesthesia

Raghu B., Deepak Padmanabhan, and Muralidhar Kanchi

Introduction

The first pacemaker implantation was performed in 1958.[1] Since then, the number of cardiac pacemaker implantations performed has seen an exponential rise with >3 million pacemakers in the United States alone. Over 700,000 new pacemakers are implanted worldwide annually. In addition, with the advent of implantable cardiac defibrillators (ICD), cardiac resynchronization therapy (CRT) devices, loop recorders, and subcutaneous defibrillators (SCDs), it is expected that a significant number of patients undergoing surgery will have a concomitant cardiac implantable electronic device (CIED) in situ. There is therefore a need to understand the perioperative management and care of these devices in patients undergoing surgery. Preoperative advisories driven by professional body statements are critical in guiding management in this regard (**Table 11.1**).

Pacemaker Codes

To indicate the modes of pacing, a five letter HRS/NASPE/BPEG (Heart Rhythm Society/North American Society of Pacing and Electrophysiology/British Pacing and Electrophysiology Group) pacemaker code is widely used.[2] The first and second positions indicate the chamber(s) paced and sensed, respectively. The third position indicates the response to sensing. T and I indicate triggered or inhibited responses, respectively.

The letter D in the third position indicates both inhibited and triggered responses (e.g., a sensed atrial event triggers ventricular simulation, unless a sensed ventricular event inhibits ventricular stimulation first). The fourth and fifth positions describe programmable and antitachyarrhythmia functions, but these letters are rarely used in practice, except for R (fourth position), which indicates a rate sensor (**Tables 11.2** and **11.3**).

Glossary of Terminology

The definitions of some of the terminologies used in CIED are as follows:

Sensitivity: The voltage (mV) above which the device detects a native electric deflection on electrocardiography (ECG) and perceives a chamber depolarization (either atrial or ventricular).

Threshold: The minimum current (mA) provided by device pacing that is required to elicit chamber depolarization.

Synchronous (demand) pacing refers to any pacing mode with a value of A, V, or D in position II (sensing chamber), which represents device pacing that is contingent on the native cardiac rhythm.

Asynchronous pacing refers to a pacing mode with O in position II, which represents device pacing irrespective of the native rhythm.

Table 11.1 Indications of pacemakers and ICDs

Indications for pacemaker	Indications for implantable cardioverter-defibrillator (ICD)
(a) Symptomatic sinus node disease (bradycardia with symptoms/signs) (b) Symptomatic atrioventricular node disease (c) Long QT syndrome (d) Hypertrophic obstructive cardiomyopathy (e) Dilated cardiomyopathy	(a) Ventricular fibrillation or ventricular tachycardia (VT) from nonreversible cause (b) Prophylactic ICD in ischemic cardiomyopathy, LVEF < 35% with nonsustainable VT inducible at EP study (c) Brugada syndrome (d) Arrhythmogenic right ventricular dysplasia (e) Long QT syndrome (f) Hypertrophic cardiomyopathy (g) Infiltrative cardiomyopathy

Abbreviations: EP, electrophysiology; LVEF, left ventricular ejection fraction.

Table 11.2 North American Society of Pacing and Electrophysiology/British Pacing and Electrophysiology Group (NASPE/BPEG) five position pacemaker codes

Pacemaker codes				
I—pacing	II—sensing	III—response	IV—programmability	V—tachycardia
O—None	O—None	O—None	O—None	O—None
A—Atrium	A—Atrium	I—Inhibited	C—Communicating	P—Pacing
V—Ventricle	V—Ventricle	T—Triggered	P—Simple programmable	S—Shocks
D—Dual (A+V)	D—Dual (A+V)	D—Dual (I+T)	M—Multiprogrammable	D—Dual (P+S)
S—Simple (A or V)	S—Simple (A or V)		R—Rate modulation	

Table 11.3 North American Society of Pacing and Electrophysiology/British Pacing and Electrophysiology Group [(NASPE/BPEG) Generic (NBG)] defibrillator codes

ICD codes			
Position I: shock chamber(s)	**Position II: antitachycardia pacing chamber(s)**	**Position III: tachycardia detection**	**Position IV: antibradycardia pacing chamber(s)**
O—None	O—None	E—Electrogram	O—None
A—Atrium	A—Atrium	H—Hemodynamic	A—Atrium
V—Ventricle	V—Ventricle		V—Ventricle
D—Dual (A+V)	D—Dual (A+V)		D—Dual (A+V)

Abbreviation: ICD, implantable cardioverter-defibrillator.

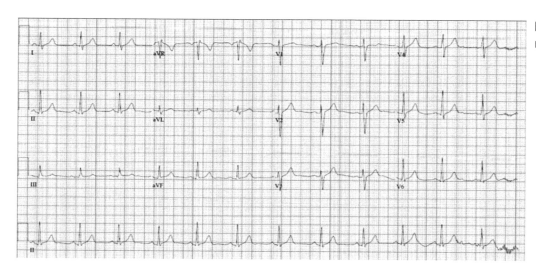

Fig. 11.1 Normal sinus rhythm.

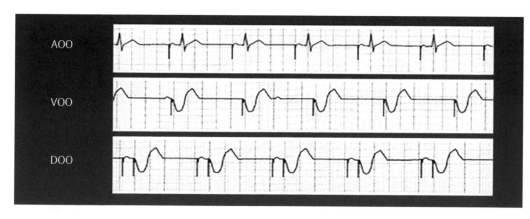

Fig. 11.2 Asynchronous modes. Abbreviations: AOO, asynchronous atrial pacing; middle panel: VOO, asynchronous ventricular pacing; DOO, asynchronous dual-chamber pacing.

Pacing Mode refers to which chamber(s) paced, chamber(s) sensed, sensing response, rate responsiveness, and antitachydysrhythmia function for a pacemaker system.

Paced Rhythms

Figs. 11.1 to **11.8** showcase the ECG tracing of various paced rhythms.

Preanesthetic Evaluation and CIED Reprogramming

Key information needed in these patients includes dependency on pacing, presence of an ICD, compatibility with use of a magnet, and finally the information regarding the functioning of the device. For pacemakers, device interrogation within the last 12 months, for ICDs 6 months, and for CRT 3 months is considered satisfactory. Magnet response for all

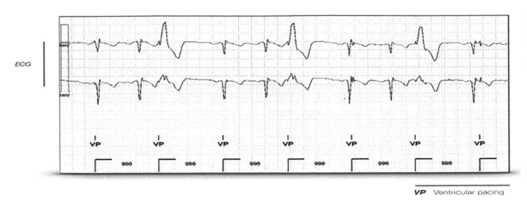

Fig. 11.3 VOO: asynchronous pacing. Abbreviation: VOO, asynchronous ventricular pacing.

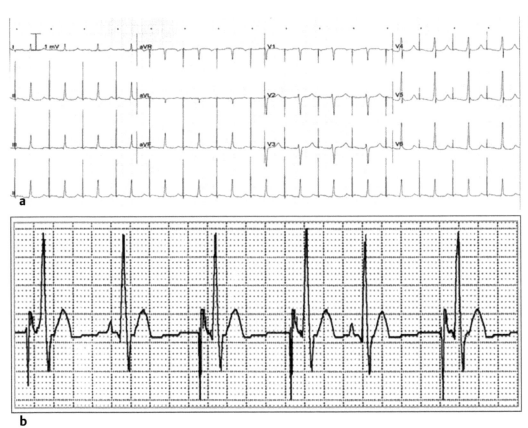

Fig. 11.4 (a, b) Atrial demand (AAI) pacing.

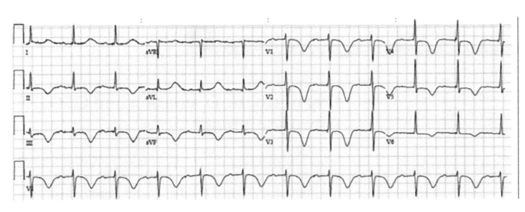

Fig. 11.5 Atrial paced rhythm.

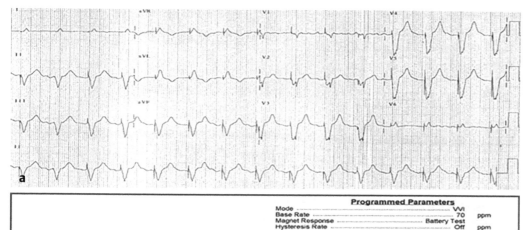

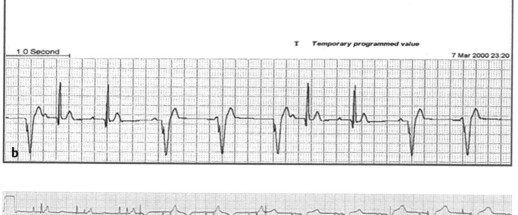

Fig. 11.6 (a, b) Ventricle (VVI) pacing.

Programmed Parameters

Mode VVI
Base Rate .... 70 ppm
Magnet Response .... Battery Test
Hysteresis Rate .... Off ppm

T   Temporary programmed value

1.0 Second

7 Mar 2000 23:20

Fig. 11.7 DDD AP-VP: Dual-chamber pacing, dual-chamber sensing, and dual response with atrial pacing (AP) and ventricular pacing (VP).

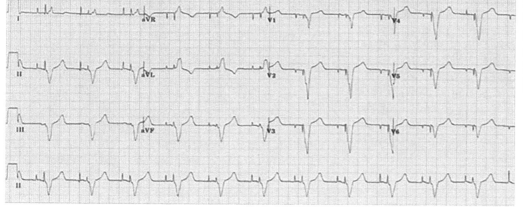

Fig. 11.8 DDD AS-VP: Dual-chamber pacing, dual-chamber sensing, and dual response with atrial sensing (AS) and ventricular pacing (VP).

AS Atrial sensing
VP Ventricular pacing

devices is different, and it is different based on the device make too. But, in general, magnet application switches the device to asynchronous pacing in pacemakers and inhibits antitachycardia pacing in patients with ICDs.

Pacemakers

Systemic examination and optimization of coexisting disease(s) forms the basic backbone of preoperative management of a patient with a pacemaker. Preoperative investigations should be dictated by the patient's underlying disease/s, medication/s, and planned intervention.

For programmable devices, interrogation with a programmer remains the only reliable method for evaluating lead performance and obtaining current program information. The anesthesiologist must review the patient's pacemaker history and follow-up schedule. In patients from countries where pacemakers might be reused, battery performance might not be related to the length of implantation in the current patient.[3,4] The safest way to avoid intraoperative problems is to reprogramme the pacemaker appropriately, especially if monopolar electrocautery is used. For lithotripsy, consideration should be given to programming the pacing function from an atrial paced mode, as some lithotripters are designed to fire on the R wave, and the atrial pacing stimulus could be misinterpreted as the contraction of the ventricle. Reprogramming a pacemaker to asynchronous pacing at a rate greater than the patient's underlying rate usually ensures that no oversensing or undersensing during electromagnetic interference (EMI) will take place, thus protecting the patient. Reprogramming a device will not protect it from internal damage or reset caused by EMI. A magnet can cause asynchronous pacing in patients with pacemaker; however, it does not cause inhibition of the rate response feature of the device. Unless turned off using a programmer, these patients may develop tachycardia (**Box 11.1**).

Implantable Defibrillators

Preoperative device programming for ICDs is critical. Inappropriate shocks increase mortality. Both manual and technician-based preoperative evaluations are available for these patients (**Box 11.2**). Manual magnet application disables antitachycardia therapies; however in patients with ICDs who are dependent on pacing, manual magnet application is not enough. The programming of ICDs to the asynchronous pacing mode is possible only via technician-based preoperative evaluation and the CIED programmer to set these parameters. Patients with ICDs made by Medtronic emit a loud tone when the magnet is placed and post removal antitachycardia therapy has to be restored. For patients having ICDs manufactured by Boston Scientific, there is a continuous intermittent tone indicating the inhibition of antitachycardia therapy. Some of the legacy devices

Box 11.1 Possible pacemaker behavior on application of magnet

- Asynchronous pacing without rate responsiveness
- Unexpected behavior
- No apparent rhythm or rate change
- Magnet mode permanently disabled by programming or temporarily suspended
- Program rate pacing in the patient who is already paced
- Improper monitor settings with pacing near the current heart rate
- No magnet sensor
- Brief (10–100 bpm) asynchronous pacing, then return to program values
- Continuous or transient loss of pacing
- Inadequate pacing output safety margin with failure to depolarize the myocardium
- Pacemaker enters diagnostic "Threshold Test Mode"
- Discharged battery (some pre-1990 devices)

Box 11.2 Preoperative evaluation

- Complete history and physical examination is mandatory
- Most have underlying cardiovascular disease. So, it is important to assess the following:
  - ➢ Functional status
  - ➢ Progression of disease
  - ➢ Associated disease (comorbid states, diabetics mellitus, and hypertension)
  - ➢ Current medication
  - ➢ Compliance with therapy (**Box 11.3**)
  - ➢ ECG—rhythm strip
  - ➢ Chest X-ray especially if cardiac disease/BiV pacemakers or AICD
- Pacemaker interrogation to evaluate performance[5]
- Reprogram to asynchronous mode (may be done in the OR just prior to start of anesthesia):
  - ➢ Reprogram pacemaker to a rate higher than the intrinsic rate
  - ➢ Suspend antitachycardia function
  - ➢ Rate-responsiveness is disabled[6–8]

Abbreviations: AICD, automated cardioverter defibrillator; BiV, biventricular; OR, operating room.

by Boston Scientific need reprogramming after magnet application since these devices do not switch back to restore antitachycardia function after the removal of the magnet. They need reprogramming with an analyzer to do so. Devices manufactured by Abbott and Biotronik do not emit any tone.

Cardiac Resynchronization Devices

Devices delivering CRT have two challenges to sort. These devices pace as well as deliver antitachycardia therapies and hence we need to be sure that there is programming that

> **Box 11.3** Hemodynamics of pacing: importance of atrial function
>
> - Properly timed atrial systole could enhance ventricular stroke volume by 50%
> - Atrial contribution to ventricular volume is divided into initial rapid ventricular filling, diastasis, atrial systole
> - Force and timing of atrial contraction and atrial compliance greatly influence the effect of atria on ventricular filling and contractility
> - Low atrial compliance restricts the increase in peak and mean atrial pressures during passive ventricular filling which occupies more than one-half of ventricular diastole, and pacing with nonsequential pacing modes results in low atrial compliance

targets safety in both of these therapies. It is important that the device programmer is used to reprogram the device to provide the appropriate settings in patients undergoing surgery. Use of a magnet may interfere with the atrioventricular (AV) synchrony and thereby cause the device to lose sensed ventricular pacing.

Radiographic images of various CIEDs are depicted in **Fig. 11.9**.

Intraoperative Management

Monitoring

Level and invasiveness of monitoring should be dictated by the patient's underlying disease(s), medication(s), and planned intervention.

- ECG: Continuous monitoring of ECG is obligatory to detect pacemaker discharges. The noise filtering on the ECG monitor must be changed to permit demonstration of the pacemaker discharge. Devices such as a nerve stimulator can interfere with detection and display of the pacemaker pulses.[9]
- Continuous monitoring must necessarily include the ability to ensure that myocardial activity is converted to mechanical systoles and pulsatile blood flow. The simplest method of monitoring the pulsatile blood flow is the "finger-on-the-pulse." However, clinically, mechanical systoles are best evaluated by pulse oximetry, plethysmography, or arterial waveform display.
- Arterial blood pressure monitoring, either noninvasive or invasive, is mandatory to assess the adequacy of tissue perfusion.
- Some patients might need an increased pacing rate during the preoperative period to meet an increased oxygen demand.
- An esophageal Doppler monitor or a transesophageal echocardiogram can be used to evaluate stroke volume, pacing frequency, and its relationship to

cardiac output. This may be considered necessary in high-risk surgery.

- Monitoring of arterial blood gases, serum electrolytes, and acid-base status will be needed if it is a major surgery and/or patient is at high risk for decompensation.
- A pulmonary artery catheter (PAC): presence of pacemaker by itself is not an indication for the insertion of a central venous pulmonary artery catheter. If central venous pressure (CVP) or PAC is indicated for other reasons, care should be taken during insertion of guidewire to not only prevent dislodgement of freshly placed pacing lead but also avoid arrhythmia.[10,11]

Anesthetic Technique

With respect to anesthetic technique, no studies have proved one technique superior to the other. The choice of anesthetic technique should be dictated by the physical condition of the patients and surgical need. Either of inhalational or narcotic technique can be used successfully. However, drugs that cause fasciculation (suxamethonium), myoclonic movements (etomidate, ketamine) may be avoided. Similarly shivering is not desirable in a patient with a pacemaker. A number of studies have reported prolongation of the QT interval with the use of isoflurane, desflurane, or sevoflurane, whereas halothane appears to reduce this interval. No interactions have been reported for enflurane. The pacemaker may interfere with the environment in the operating rooms as highlighted in **Table 11.4**.

Cautery

The use of electrocautery remains the major intraoperative issue for the patient with a pacemaker. The following guidelines are recommended regarding the use of cautery: (1) cautery tool and current return pad are positioned in a such a way that the current path does not pass through the CIED; (2) avoid proximity of cautery electric field to the pulse generator; (3) use short intermittent bursts at the lowest feasible energy level; (4) bipolar cautery is preferred during surgery in patients with implanted pacemakers; (5) use of an ultrasonic cutting device, commonly called a "harmonic scalpel," has been recommended to prevent EMI while providing the surgeon with the ability to both cut and coagulate tissue;[12-15] (6) "coagulation" electrocautery will likely cause more problems than no blended "cutting" electrocautery; (7) magnet placement during electrocautery might allow reprogramming of an older pulse generators; however, newer generators are relatively immune to such effects; (8) strong EMI can produce an electrical reset or a detection of battery depletion, which might change the programming mode, rate, or both, (9) if monopolar electrocautery is to be used, then the current return pad should be placed to ensure that the electrocautery current path does not cross the pacemaking system. For cases such as head and

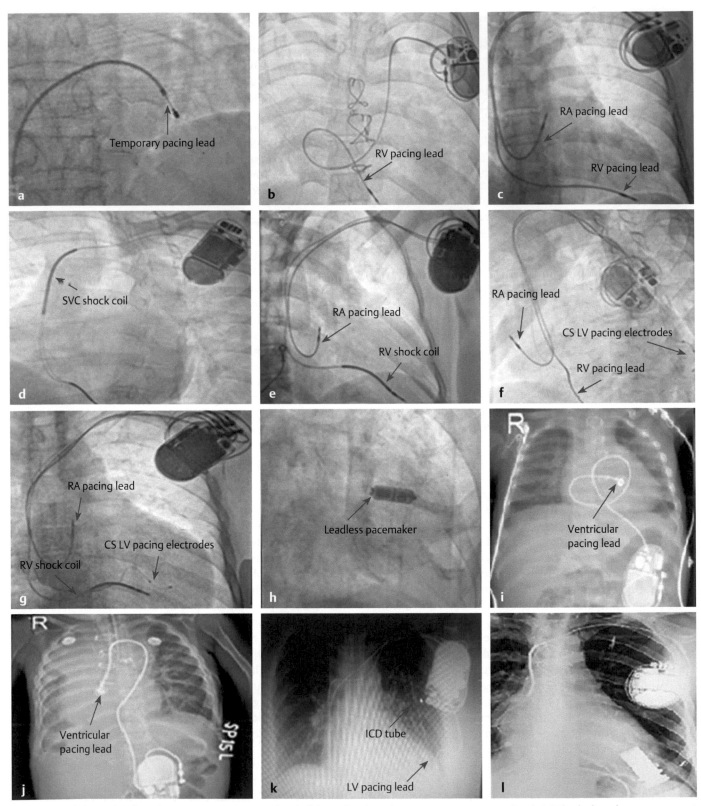

Fig. 11.9 **(a)** Single-chamber temporary pacing lead; **(b)** single-chamber permanent pacing lead; **(c)** dual-chamber permanent pacing lead; **(d)** AICD single chamber; **(e)** AICD dual chamber; **(f)** CRT pacing; **(g)** cardiac resynchronization with ICD (CRT-D); **(h)** leadless pacemaker; **(i, j)** post cardiac surgery with ventricular pacing; **(k)** LV lead placement intraoperatively for CRT; **(l)** pacemaker in a patient with LVAD. Abbreviations: AICD, automated cardioverter defibrillator; CRT, cardiac resynchronization therapy; ICD, implantable cardiac defibrillators; CS, coronary sinus; LV, left ventricle; LVAD, left ventricular assist device; RA, right atrium; RV, right ventricle, SVC, superior vena cava.

Table 11.4   Interference of pacemaker with the environment

Interference with pacemakers	Competing rhythms under anesthesia

• Electromagnetic interference (EMI)
• Mechanical and other interference
  ➤ Ventilators
  ➤ Cellular phones
  ➤ Whole-body vibrations
  ➤ Skeletal myopotentials
  ➤ Electroconvulsive therapy
  ➤ Scoline fasciculations
  ➤ Myoclonic movements
  ➤ Direct muscle stimulation
	• Myocardial ischemia
	• Electrolyte imbalance
	• Severe metabolic/physiologic disturbance
	• Digitalis toxicity
	• Exposure to high catecholamine levels
	• Long QT interval
	• Hypothermia

Box 11.4   How to minimize electromagnetic interference (EMI) with pacemakers

- Use bipolar cautery
- If unipolar, ground plate should be arranged in a path as far away as possible from pacemaker
- Monitor pulsatile flow of blood to detect pacemaker inhibition
- Request surgeon to reduce electrocautery time; not more than 1 second bursts every 10 seconds
- Program pacemaker to asynchronous operation: if this is not possible place a magnet over the device (caution!)
- Shield pulse generators from beams of ionizing radiation
- Do not place the cardioverter-defibrillator paddles directly over the pulse generator; use lowest possible energy shocks in the event of atrial/ventricular fibrillation
- Have the device checked for function after exposure to strong EMI
- Battery-powered cautery does not interfere with pacemaker function; have an alternative mode of temporary pacing available in the operating room (OR)

Box 11.5   Special procedures in patients with implantable generators

- Magnetic resonance imaging (MRI)—traditionally, MRI has been contraindicated in patients with CIED. However, MRI can be performed in patients with conditional CIEDs, whereas in patients with nonconditional CIEDs, certain imaging conditions need to be met. In both cases, device reprogramming must be done before and after MRI
- Lithotripsy—programming out of an atrial pacing mode is advised
- Transurethral resection (bladder, prostate) and uterine hysteroscopy—procedures using monopolar electrocautery that can be easily accomplished after device reprogramming
- Electroconvulsive therapy—requires asynchronous (nonsensing) mode
- Nerve stimulator testing/therapy—inappropriate detection of transcutaneous electrical nerve stimulation, neuromuscular, and chiropractic electrical muscle stimulation as ventricular tachycardia or fibrillation has been reported
- Radiofrequency (RF) ablation—during RF ablation the pacing function of a cardiac implantable electronic device is changed to an asynchronous pacing mode in the pacing-dependent patient and an implantable cardioverter-defibrillator's antitachycardia function is disabled; direct contact between the ablation catheter and the generator and leads should be avoided

neck surgery, the pad might be best placed on the shoulder contralateral to the implanted device. For breast and axillary cases, the pad might need to be placed on the ipsilateral arm with the wire prepped into the field by sterile plastic cover.

Competing Rhythms

At this time, magnetic resonance imaging (MRI) deserves special mention.[16,17] Guidelines from manufacturers define nonconditional CIEDs as those where either the pulse generator or the lead are not MRI-conditional. The presence of abandoned leads or fragments also makes the device nonconditional. Manufacturer guidelines still advise against performing MRI in these patients. However in patients with nonconditional CIEDs, there have been recent registry experiences that allow for MRI to be done for these patients when appropriate field conditions are met for patient safety.

Patients with MRI-conditional devices can be taken for an MRI after reprogramming the device to the MRI mode. Of all the manufacturers, Biotronik remains the only company where this is done automatically by detecting the gradient and static fields in the imaging chamber. The other patients do need preimaging reprogramming with an analyzer to allow for imaging. Recent societal guidelines from the Heart Rhythm Society have set up safety parameters for the same (**Boxes 11.4** and **11.5**; **Flowchart 11.1**).[18,19]

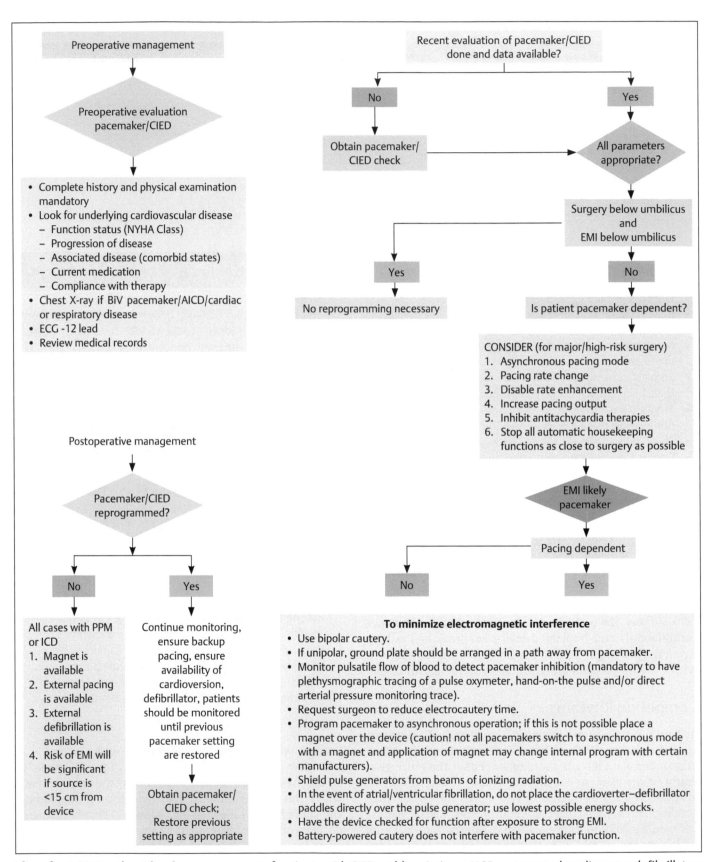

Flowchart 11.1 Algorithm for management of patients with CIEDs. Abbreviations: AICD, automated cardioverter defibrillator; CIED, cardiac implantable electronic device; ECG, electrocardiography; EMI, electromagnetic interference; ICD, implantable cardiac defibrillators; NYHA, New York Heart Association; PPM, posterior papillary muscle.

Conclusion

Aging population and patients presenting with complex cardiac disease states dictate that many patients with CIEDs will present for surgical services. Safe and efficient perioperative management of these patients depends on understanding pacing, indications for use, and techniques to monitor/maintain cardiac function during surgery. Perioperative management of patients with CIEDs can be challenging because electromagnetic interference (EMI) may cause device malfunction. To avoid CIED-related peri and intra-operative complications, it is of the utmost importance to assess indication to device implantation, evaluate current pacing dependency, check the device's last follow-up chart, and possibly contact patients' electrophysiologist or their device specialist. All this information will help implement the most convenient strategy for a safe surgical approach.[20]

References

1. Rozner MA. Cardiac pacing and defibrillation. In: Kaplan JA, Reich DL, Joseph S, eds. Savino, Kaplan's cardiac anesthesia: the echo era, 6th ed. St Louis, MO: Elsevier Saunders; 2011: 790–806

2. Bernstein AD, Daubert JC, Fletcher RD, et al; North American Society of Pacing and Electrophysiology/British Pacing and Electrophysiology Group. The revised NASPE/BPEG generic code for antibradycardia, adaptive-rate, and multisite pacing. Pacing Clin Electrophysiol 2002;25(2):260–264

3. Sethi KK, Bhargava M, Pandit N, et al. Experience with recycled cardiac pacemakers. Indian Heart J 1992;44(2):91–93

4. Panja M, Sarkar CN, Kumar S, et al. Reuse of pacemaker. Indian Heart J 1996;48(6):677–680

5. Rozner MA, Roberson JC, Nguyen AD. Unexpected high incidence of serious pacemaker problems detected by pre-and postoperative interrogations: a two-year experience. J Am Coll Cardiol 2004;43:A113

6. Augoustides JG, Fleisher LA. The future for B-type natriuretic peptide in preoperative assessment. Anesthesiology 2008; 108(2):332–333

7. Andersen C, Madsen GM. Rate-responsive pacemakers and anaesthesia. A consideration of possible implications. Anaesthesia 1990;45(6):472–476

8. Levine PA. Response to "rate-adaptive cardiac pacing: implications of environmental noise during craniotomy". Anesthesiology 1997;87(5):1261

9. Rozner MA. Peripheral nerve stimulators can inhibit monitor display of pacemaker pulses. J Clin Anesth 2004;16(2):117–120

10. Valls-Bertault V, Mansourati J, Gilard M, Etienne Y, Munier S, Blanc JJ. Adverse events with transvenous left ventricular pacing in patients with severe heart failure: early experience from a single centre. Europace 2001;3(1):60–63

11. Alonso C, Leclercq C, d'Allonnes FR, et al. Six year experience of transvenous left ventricular lead implantation for permanent biventricular pacing in patients with advanced heart failure: technical aspects. Heart 2001;86(4):405–410

12. Nandalan SP, Vanner RG. Use of the harmonic scalpel in a patient with a permanent pacemaker. Anaesthesia 2004;59(6):621

13. Epstein MR, Mayer JE Jr, Duncan BW. Use of an ultrasonic scalpel as an alternative to electrocautery in patients with pacemakers. Ann Thorac Surg 1998;65(6):1802–1804

14. Ozeren M, Doğan OV, Düzgün C, Yücel E. Use of an ultrasonic scalpel in the open-heart reoperation of a patient with pacemaker. Eur J Cardiothorac Surg 2002;21(4):761–762

15. Erdman S, Levinsky L, Strasberg B, Agmon J, Levy MJ. Use of the Shaw Scalpel in pacemaker operations. J Thorac Cardiovasc Surg 1985;89(2):304–307

16. Gimbel JR, Johnson D, Levine PA, Wilkoff BL. Safe performance of magnetic resonance imaging on five patients with permanent cardiac pacemakers. Pacing Clin Electrophysiol 1996;19(6):913–919

17. Gimbel JR, Kanal E. Can patients with implantable pacemakers safely undergo magnetic resonance imaging? J Am Coll Cardiol 2004;43(7):1325–1327

18. Practice advisory for the perioperative management of patients with cardiac implantable electronic devices: pacemakers and implantable cardioverter-defibrillators: an updated report by the American Society of Anesthesiologists Task Force on Perioperative Management of Patients with Cardiac Implantable Electronic Devices. American Society of Anesthesiologists. Anesthesiology. 2011 Feb;114(2):247–61

19. Cronin B, Essandoh MK. An update on cardiovascular implantable electronic devices for anesthesiologists. J Cardiothorac Vasc Anesth 2018;32(4):1871–1884

20. Özkartal T, Demarchi A, Caputo ML, Baldi E, Conte G, Auricchio A. Perioperative Management of Patients with Cardiac Implantable Electronic Devices and Utility of Magnet Application. J. Clin. Med., 691

12

Hemodynamic Monitoring in Cardiac Critical Care Units

*Poonam Malhotra Kapoor, Minati Choudhury, Mohit Prakash,
Pranav Kapoor, and Archana Malhotra Jain*

Introduction

Patients admitted in cardiac intensive care units (ICU) are critically ill and require continuous hemodynamic monitoring. Monitoring allows prompt detection of altered hemodynamics and result in appropriate changes in the management of the patient. The concept of accurate and continuous measurements of vital parameters evolved from operating rooms. Improved patient care and clinical outcomes in critically ill patients prompted the establishment of specialized ICUs in early 1950s. Initial monitoring tools were derived from miniaturized version of telemetry monitors for astronauts. Use of sphygmomanometer and invasive monitoring remained the mainstay of monitoring for long. The development of transcutaneous sensors, pulse oximetry, and end-tidal measurement of carbon dioxide in the 1980s added new dimension to monitoring. Recent advances in the field of noninvasive monitoring enabling insights into preload, afterload, and cardiac contractility allow timely detection of hemodynamic abnormalities.[1,2] However, more sensitive hemodynamic monitoring is by no means a replacement of carefully performed clinical assessment, and therefore careful correlation with the clinical status is mandatory to avoid misinterpretation of hemodynamic data.

Hemodynamic Monitoring

Principles

In modern-day practice of cardiology almost all the patients have diagnosis before reaching ICU. Nonetheless, hemodynamic assessment provides critical insights in clarifying the diagnostic dilemma in selected few. In a patient with known cardiac ailment hemodynamic monitoring guides the management by optimal utilization of various therapeutic options. The hemodynamic parameters to be monitored in a patient are directed by the underlying disease. For example, a central venous pressure (CVP) monitoring is useful in managing a patient with right ventricular (RV) myocardial infarction while noninvasive blood pressure (NIBP) monitoring alone is sufficient in a patient with acute coronary syndrome who is otherwise stable.

Methods

Although newer noninvasive tools allow assessment of various hemodynamic parameters conventionally, it is only the arterial blood pressure (BP) that is measured noninvasively with reasonable accuracy. A carefully interpreted invasive hemodynamic monitoring is unequivocally superior to any form of noninvasive monitoring, especially in patients with unstable hemodynamics.

Obtaining Accurate Measurements

The management of a patient with cardiac ailment is intricately related to the hemodynamic state. However, hemodynamic parameters are reliable only if the measurements are obtained with accuracy. The importance of recognizing various sources cannot be overemphasized.

Noninvasive Hemodynamic Monitoring

Clinical Assessment

Detailed assessment of clinical status of the patient is imperative. No form of advanced hemodynamic monitoring can replace good clinical evaluation. Measurement of vital signs—heart rate, respiratory rate, BP, and body temperature—sets the foundation while systemwise assessment provides insights into the underlying pathology and its hemodynamic consequences. Although many clinical parameters are subjective and suffer from high interobserver variables, most technical instruments work on guidelines which further guide the clinician as to what kind of monitoring is required. Further, in certain situations clinical parameters must be used as an essential adjunct to the hemodynamic parameters to avoid mismanagement. For example, adequate urine output which provides an estimate of end-organ perfusion indicates the efficacy of BP even if it remains below the 50th centile.

Assessment of Vital Parameters

The clinical evaluation, as in all other conditions, begins with the assessment of the vital parameters. Although the assessment of temperature and respiratory effort remains important, the assessment of BP and heart takes the precedence in cardiac ICU.

Heart Rate and Electrocardiogram

All monitors in modern day ICUs are equipped with modules for basic electrocardiogram (ECG) monitoring. Advances in computing have allowed advanced automated monitoring of heart rate as well as rhythm analysis in critically ill patients. The risk of rhythm abnormalities in almost all forms of cardiac diseases makes ECG monitoring an integral part of monitoring in cardiac ICUs. Modern-day monitors allow segment analysis of ECG, enabling treating physician to detect changes in ST segment and QT interval. All modern-day monitors are equipped with alarm function, which if set properly, can provide timely alerts to the health care professionals. The requirement of hemodynamic monitoring is different in all the patients and therefore alarm settings must be individualized. This is important to avoid unnecessary noise and for prompt detection of patient-specific hemodynamic abnormalities. The role of routine ECG monitoring for timely detection of life-threatening arrhythmias in patients with unstable hemodynamics is well known. Detailed discussion on ECG monitoring is beyond the scope of this chapter.

Noninvasive Blood Pressure (NIBP) Monitoring

BP is the most common hemodynamic parameter monitored in any ICU. Conventionally, sphygmomanometer is employed to measure arterial BP. Nevertheless, the reliability of sphygmomanometer is limited by inaccurate measurements both by the physicians and the nurses. Although multiple factors affect the accuracy, it is most commonly related to inappropriate cuff size. For proper measurement, bladder length should be at least 80% of the upper arm circumference and the width of the bladder should be at least 40% of the upper arm circumference.[4] Circumference of arm should be measured midway between the shoulder and elbow. If the bladder is too small, the pressure measurements will be falsely high. Conversely with inappropriately large cuff the BP measured is falsely low. Nevertheless, the errors are less if cuff bladder is inappropriately large compared to when it is smaller. Therefore, in the event of nonavailability of appropriate size, the health care professional should err on the side of larger cuff.[3]

With growing concern of environmental hazards, mercury sphygmomanometers are being rapidly replaced by newer oscillometric BP–measuring devices. These oscillometric-monitoring devices are the cornerstone of hemodynamic monitoring in modern-day cardiac ICUs with gated modules within the bedside monitors. Pulsatile arterial flow creates oscillations within the arterial wall, but only when the arteries are partially open. Using an inflatable bladder, pressure can be raised to a point where all the flow within the artery is impeded. Thereafter, pressure within the cuff is slowly reduced systematically while monitoring for the appearance and disappearance of pulse waves by the inbuilt sensors. The device thus determines the lowest pressure at which maximal returned amplitude of the pulse waves is measured, which corresponds to the mean arterial pressure (MAP). Mean pressure is the most precise measurement using oscillometric devices and correlates well with the mean pressure obtained by intra-arterial monitoring. The systolic and diastolic pressures, on the other hand, are calculated using predefined algorithm.

The accuracy of the BP measurements by oscillometry relies heavily on optimal positioning of the cuff.[5] In almost all monitoring devices the cuffs are marked for appropriate sensing of arterial pulsation by the device. However, even a well-placed cuff may get displaced after some time and result in inaccurate measurements. This is extremely important for patients in whom periodic measurements are done at regular interval. The BP cuff must be reapplied periodically to achieve optimal position. The presence of stiff arteries in elderly and low output state in critically ill patients interferes with reliable monitoring of BP by oscillometry.

Pulse Oximetry

Continuous pulse oximetry is yet another landmark advancement in monitoring of critically ill patients. Invented in 1972 by Japanese bioengineer Takuo Aoyagi, the oximeter came into widespread clinical use in the 1980s and has become essential to safe anesthetic and critical care practice. Using the principle of spectrophotometry, light of specific wavelengths when collected after traversing through a medium allows the concentration of a substance to be detected. According to the Lambert-Beer law, the absorption of light is proportionate to the concentration of the substance within the medium. Monochromate light emitted from the phototransmission is collected by the photodetector. Light waves passing through pulsating arteries develop phase shifts in intensity the amplified by the detector. Light passing through nonpulsating structures, veins, and tissues, on the other hand, is not detected, thus reducing sampling error created by deoxygenated hemoglobin (Hb) in the venous system. Hb absorbs red light in the visible region (660 nm) more effectively than HbO, while light in the infrared region (940 nm) is more intensely absorbed by HbO, compared to Hb. The amount of HbO detected can be expressed as typically at 660 nm and 940 nm, traverses the tissue, and is a function of total Hb detected in the patient:

$$\text{Fractional oxygen saturation (\%)} = (\text{OxyHb}(\text{OxyHb} + \text{DeoxyHb} + \text{COHb} + \text{MetHb})) \times 100$$

The hemoglobin variants, carboxy hemoglobin (COH) and Met hemoglobin (MetHb), if present, lead to errors. Significant skin pigmentation, certain shades of polish, and severe hypotension may produce sampling based errors.[8] Patients with reduced peripheral blood flow from vascular disease, sepsis, or pallor of the extremities may be monitored by ear probes or skin surface probes (reflectance spectrophotometry) or by central saturation measurements. Further, similar to other monitoring tools the readings obtained by pulse oximetry must be correlated with the prevailing clinical condition of the patient. One easy way is to ensure good plethysmography tracing while monitoring pulse oximetric oxygen saturation. Health care professionals must refrain from accepting oximetric saturation without confirming good quality plethysmography. Whenever in doubt, pulse oximetry must be confirmed by arterial blood gas (ABG) analysis. In addition, ABG is preferred over pulse oximetry in patients on ventilator.[6–8] Pulse oximetry is not only useful in initial assessment but is also important for continuous monitoring especially in patients with respiratory distress. The role of pulse oximetry in diagnosis and management of various cyanotic congenital heart diseases is well established.[9]

Invasive Hemodynamic Monitoring

The invasive hemodynamic monitoring system includes different components. The knowledge of the principles and basic mechanisms is essential for accurate measurement and troubleshooting.

Components

- *Indwelling intravascular catheter:* The invasive hemodynamic monitoring requires an indwelling catheter to be in arteries (typically the radial, brachial, femoral, or infrequently dorsalis pedis) or veins (most typically internal jugular, subclavian, and occasionally femoral). Long catheters can also be threaded from a peripheral site, such as the antecubital vein, into the central venous circulation. Catheters have single or multiple lumens and may be equipped with thermistors and/ or oxygen saturation sensors. Catheters with balloon-directed technology can be located from the venous circulation through the right heart into the pulmonary artery.
- *Pressure transducer and noncompliant fluid-filled connector:* Measurement of BP requires a closed system. The pressure transducer is usually a silicone diaphragm that is attached to a Wheatstone bridge. Currently available transducers have high natural frequency that reduces dependency on damping to some extent. The Wheatstone bridge converts mechanical arterial pulsations into electrical impulses which are then displayed by the monitoring system as waveforms. The pressure transducer is connected to the intravascular catheter via a fluid-filled noncompliant tubing of shortest possible length. The saline-filled column allows unimpeded transmission of pressure from vessels to the transducer.[10]
- *Monitor:* Most of the monitors in modern-day ICUs are equipped with in-built modules for various hemodynamic monitors. These monitors allow optimal representation of ECG, respiratory rate, pulse oximetry (including plethysmography), and various pressures. Almost all the monitors enable changes in the speed and scale of various hemodynamic parameters for easy visualization by the health care providers. In-built adjustable alarms have added to the ease with which a sick patient can be managed.[11] Nevertheless, the alarms can be source of unnecessary distraction if not used carefully in relation to the clinical requirement of the patient. For example, usual label of tachycardia at heart rate of 100 beats per minute is not appropriate for a child or a patient in heart failure in whom high heart rate is physiological or compensatory (**Box 12.1** and **Table 12.1**).

Box 12.1   CCO advantages over TDCO
- Earlier detection of hemodynamic crisis
- Better guidance to therapeutic approaches (Sasse Scott A, Chen Priscilla A, Berry Richard B, Sassoon Catherine SH, Mahutte CK. Variability of cardiac output over time in medical intensive care unit patients. Crit Care Med. 1994;22(2):225–232)
- Straightforward to implement, measures true volumetric flow, requires no user calibration, is independent of vascular geometry (Yelderman M. Continuous measurement of cardiac output with the use of stochastic system identification techniques. J Clin Monit. 1990;6(4):322–332)
- Is not operator-dependent—automatic CCO (Miyasaka K, Takata M, Miyasaka K. Flow velocity profile of the pulmonary artery measured by the continuous cardiac output monitoring catheter. Can J Anaesth. 1993;40(2):183–187)

Abbreviations: CCO, continuous cardiac output; TDCO, cardiac output by thermodilution.

Table 12.1   Complications of pulmonary artery catheter monitoring

Complications	Reasoning
- Arrhythmias - Transient RBBB - Complete heart block - Thrombus formation - Infection - Pulmonary infarction - Pulmonary artery rupture Others: Myocardial perforation; air embolism; catheter coiling or knotting; balloon rupture/embolism; misinterpretation of data	- Transient: 50%, sustained 3% - Incidence: 5% - Rare—pre-existing LBBB increases risk - Platelet aggregation begins within hours - Increased incidence after 3 d - Prolonged wedging of balloon or catheter tip - Incidence: 0.02–0.2%; mortality 50%

Abbreviations: LBBB, left bundle branch block; RBBB, right bundle branch block.

Almost all the monitoring stations are capable of providing recorded data for review. However, to maximize the benefits of the alarms and review facility of the monitors the patients must be admitted electronically in the monitor and various settings must be changed according to the patient's clinical condition and requirements.

Setting up the transducer: For meaningful measurement of pressures, it is mandatory to ensure accurate measurements by the transducer. This can be achieved by proper "leveling" and "zeroing" of the transducer.

Although commonly used interchangeably, these two terms are not the same. While "zeroing" exposes the transducer to the atmospheric pressure via an open air–fluid interface, "leveling" assigns this zero reference point to a specific position in the patient's body.

"Zeroing" the Transducer

"Zeroing" can be defined as "the use of atmospheric pressure as a reference standard against which all other pressures are measured." The device is zeroed when the air–fluid insert is opened to atmospheric pressure and the reading on the monitor is zero. In absence of "zeroing" the monitor would be at a risk of having a diastole pressure of 760 mmHg. There is a tendency of gradual drifting of zero, making the measurements unreliable; therefore, it is mandatory to perform "rezeroing" periodically.

"Leveling" the Transducer

"Leveling" can be defined as "the selection of a position of interest at which the reference standard, the zero is set." The system is conventionally "leveled" at the phlebostatic axis which corresponds roughly with the position of the right atrium. This level has generally been accepted as the ideal reference level for measuring the pressure of the blood returning to the heart, so it was therefore adopted as the reference level for CVP measurement. The specific reference point for the arterial transducer is actually the aortic root, but because it is very close to the right atrium the two reference levels are essentially the same. The transducer position above or below the phlebostatic axis results in under or overestimation of pressure, respectively. For every 10 cm change in the position there is change of 7.4 mmHg pressure.

Damping and Dynamic Response of the Measuring System

The accuracy of the pressure measurement is the function of natural frequency of the monitoring system and the input signal with optimal ratio being 5 or more. The fundamental frequency of the arterial system is 3 to 5 Hz and therefore the frequency of an ideal monitoring system should be greater than 20 Hz. Conventionally used fluid-filled monitoring system has a frequency of 10 to 20 Hz and therefore is at risk of amplification of the signals and inaccurate measurements. This excess amplification can be managed effectively by appropriate damping, a phenomenon whereby the amplitude of the oscillations is reduced, allowing accurate

measurement of the pressure. Nevertheless, both under- and overdamping are detrimental to pressure monitoring. An overdamping system results in underestimation while an underdamped system leads to overestimation of the systolic BP. For optimal damping the fluid column must be free of air bubbles, blood clots, and loose connections as all of these cause reductions in the amplitude of the oscillations and underdamping.

Before any meaningful measurements can be made by monitoring, it is mandatory to ensure proper damping of the fluid column. Nevertheless, the mean BP remains unchanged by damping since the area under the curve remains the same. Another important determinant of damping is length caliber of the tubing. Longer tubing counterintuitively results in underdamping since the natural frequency of a long tube approaches closer to the patient's pulse wave frequency. The short length of the tubing, on the other hand, allows optimal damping to be observed.

How to Check for Adequacy of Damping?

There are multiple ways to check for adequacy of damping but the most commonly used method is "fast flush test" or "square wave test." This is performed by briefly opening and closing the continuous flush line which produces a square wave displacement in the pressure waveform followed by a return to the baseline after few oscillations. Although damping coefficient and resonant frequency can be calculated, visual inspection of the waveforms is usually sufficient for evaluation of damping. "Fast flush test" in an optimally damped system results in one undershoot followed by small overshoot which then settles to the patient's waveform.

Arterial Blood Pressure Measurement

It requires placement of intra-arterial line in any of the peripheral artery. Radial artery is the most commonly used site. The arterial pressure wave travels much faster than the actual blood which is ejected. There is systolic amplification of BP as we move away from heart, and systolic BP in radial and femoral artery can be as high as 20 mmHg compared to proximal aorta. MAP is the principal determinant of blood flow and is calculated by area under the curve from BP recording and duration of cardiac cycle. Although systolic BP is monitored commonly, it is the mean BP that is most relevant. Any patient in circulatory shock requires monitoring of MAP, preferably by intra-arterial recording with a target of keeping it more than 65 mm.[12] The analysis of shape and various components of the arterial waveform is extremely useful in the diagnosis of various cardiac conditions.

Pulmonary Artery Catheterization

Pulmonary artery catheterization is a standard tool for measurement of right-sided pressures. In addition, capability of this catheter to measure both left-sided pressures and other derived indices and pressures makes it a lucrative choice (**Figs. 12.1–12.4**).

Providing pulmonary capillary wedge pressure (PCWP) allows hemodynamic assessment of left-sided cardiac chambers. Swan Ganz balloon floatation catheter with multisite assessment of pressure provides comprehensive hemodynamic assessment in a sick patient at the bedside.

Swan Ganz catheter is a balloon tipped catheter with two internal lumens: one opens 30 cm proximal to the tip allowing monitoring of the right atrial pressure, and the other at the tip with a length of 110 cm allows access to the distal branches of the pulmonary artery. The balloon at the tip when inflated allowed placement of the catheter without fluoroscopic guidance the jugular venous access without any fluoroscopic guidance (**Table 12.2**).

Appropriateness of the Wedging of the Pulmonary Artery Catheter

Swan Ganz catheter owing to its balloon at the tip allows wedging of the pulmonary capillaries which in turn allows assessment of the left-sided filling pressures. This measurement, however, is extremely dependent on the position of the catheter in the pulmonary arterial system (**Table 12.3**). The PAWP waveform is morphologically similar to the CVP trace. Due to the transmission delay from the LA to the wedged PAC, the pressure waves appear delayed in relation to the ECG. In general, CVP waveform components reflect right heart events, and PAWP waveforms reflect analogous left heart pathophysiology.

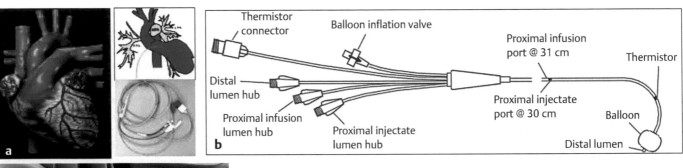

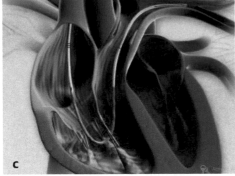

Fig. 12.1 **(a)** Assessment of left heart function (indirectly), pulmonary status, right heart function, oxygen delivery/demand balance, volumetric status (preload), and use of derived parameters. **(b)** Catheter ports: proximal port, VIP port, distal port, balloon port, and thermistor connector. **(c)** Continuous cardiac output (CCO) monitoring.

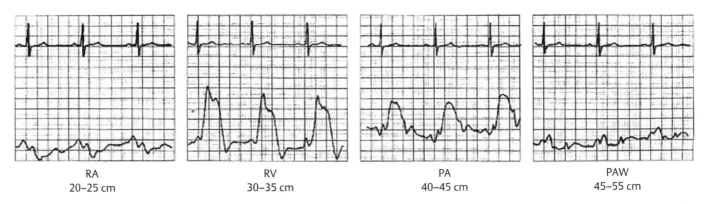

Fig. 12.2 A normal arterial pressure trace. Abbreviations: PA, pulmonary artery; PAW, pulmonary artery wedge; RA, right atrium; RV, right ventricle.

Table 12.2 Components and mechanical events of a CVP trace

Component	Cardiac phase	Mechanical event
a-wave	End-diastole	RA contraction
c-wave	Early systole	Isovolumic ventricular contraction; TV moving toward the RA
x-wave	Early/midsystole	RA relaxation; RV ejection
v-wave	Late diastole	RA filling
y-descent	Early diastole	Outflow from RA to RV

Abbreviations: CVP, central venous pressure; ECG, electrocardiogram; LA, left atrium; PAC, pulmonary artery catheter; PAWP, pulmonary artery wedge pressure; RA, right atrium; RV, right ventricle.

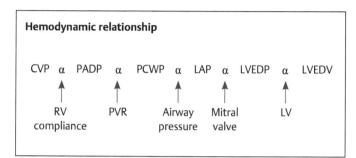

Fig. 12.3 Hemodynamic relationship with all relationships. Abbreviations: CVP, central venous pressure; LAP, left arterial pressure; LV, left ventricle; LVEDP, left ventricle end diastolic pressure; LVEDV, left ventricular end diastolic; PADP, pulmonary artery diastolic pressure; PCWP, pulmonary capillary wedge pressure; PVR, peripheral vascular resistance; RV, right ventricle.

Table 12.3 Pulmonary artery pressure

	Neonate	Child	Adult
PAS	30–60 mmHg	15–30 mmHg	15–25 mmHg
PAD	2–10 mmHg	5–10 mmHg	8–15 mmHg
PAM	13–15 mmHg	10–20 mmHg	10–20 mmHg

Abbreviations: PAD, pulmonary artery diastolic; PAS, pulmonary artery systolic; PAM, pulmonary artery mean.

Appropriate Position of the Catheter Tip

Position of the catheter tip on radiograph: Lung is divided into three zones on the basis of relative pressure in pulmonary circulation and alveoli. In zone 1, alveolar pressure is maximum and hence it compresses both arterial and venous pressure. In zone 2, pulmonary pressure is higher than alveolar pressure but venous pressure is lower than alveolar pressure. Zone 3 is the most dependent lung where capillary (venous) pressure exceeds alveolar pressure. PCWP is the reflection of left atrial pressure only when the pulmonary artery catheter is located in zone 3 of the lung. Fortunately, owing to the preferential flow with inflated balloon reaches zone 3 with ease. Nevertheless, it is important to ascertain the correct position of the catheter on chest radiograph. Generally, a catheter tip placed in the location below the level of left atrium on chest radiograph in anteroposterior view is optimal for measuring pulmonary artery wedge pressure (PAWP). Lateral chest radiograph is rarely required for this purpose (**Figs. 12.3** and **12.4**).

- **Pressure tracing:** The pressure obtained at the capillary wedge position reflects pressure in the pulmonary vein, which in turn equals left atrial pressure and diastolic left ventricular (LV) pressure in the absence of mitral stenosis. Similar to the pressure trace in the left atrium, there are "a" and "v" waves during early and late diastolic, respectively. In addition, the pressure trace shows respiratory variation with aspiratory decline in pressure. The absence of a well-seen waveform indicates inappropriate wedging and warrants repositioning of the catheter. Catheter positioned deep

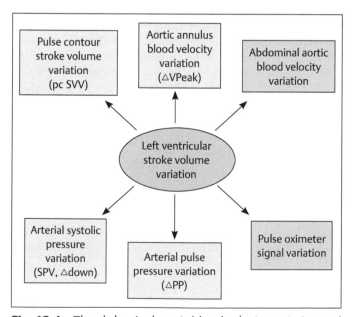

Fig. 12.4 The abdominal aortic blood velocity variation and the pulse oximeter signal variation have not been validated to predict fluid responsiveness.

within the branch of pulmonary artery and an overinflated balloon result in overwedging. An overwedged catheter gives inaccurate pressure reading but poses no risk of rupture of the pulmonary artery segment. A pressure trace with indistinct "a" and "v" waves indicates pulmonary wedged catheter. Underwedging, on the other hand, results in a pressure trace that is a hybrid of arterial and venous pressure traces.

- **Oxygen saturation of blood sample:** Although not possible all the time, a blood sample obtained from the wedge position represents pulmonary venous blood and therefore must have high oxygen saturation and PaO_2 as in pulmonary veins. Among all the methods it is the most confirmatory method.[10]

Measurement of Hemodynamic Parameters

Addition of thermostat to pulmonary artery catheter increases the capability of end diastolic area (EDA) catheter to measure multiple hemodynamic parameters. However, thermodilution method has drawbacks as it underestimates cardiac output in patients with tricuspid regurgitation while overestimation is common in patients with shock and low cardiac output states. Flicks method, using oxygen saturation, is more commonly used to calculate cardiac output and related hemodynamic variables.[10]

Current Indications of Pulmonary Artery Catheterization

The ease of assessing various hemodynamic parameters prompted wide use of the catheter during the end of the 20th century so much so that it became the standard of care in cardiac ICUs worldwide. This enhanced the ability of monitoring cardiac hemodynamics and guiding the therapy; however, it did not improve clinical outcomes. On the contrary, GUSTO IIb and III trials showed increased mortality with the use of pulmonary artery catheterization in patients with acute coronary syndromes.[13-16] At present, routine use of pulmonary artery catheterization has gone out of favor. It is currently used in only select clinical scenarios,[17] which are as follows:

- Refractory chronic heart failure when on a vasopressor with an inodilator.
- Cardiogenic shock on supportive therapy.
- Unexplained shock with hemodynamic instability.
- Treatment of potentially reversible cause of heart failures as fulminant myocarditis or peripartum cardiomyopathy.
- Awaiting cardiac transplantation.

Central Venous Catheterization

Unlike pulmonary artery catheterization, central venous catheterization is much more frequently practiced. In addition to providing real-time information regarding fluid status of the patient it allows reliable and speedy delivery of important medications such as inotropes. The central

veins, especially the superior vena cava considering its short length, reflect pressure within the right atrium. Further, in absence of significant stenosis or regurgitation of tricuspid valve it is equal to the RV filling pressure (i.e., end-diastolic pressure). Normal CVP is 0 to 6 mmHg and shows "a" and "y" waves similar to the right atrial pressure trace. Most of the transducers measure pressure in mmHg. However, water-filled manometers which are used occasionally to measure CVP record pressure in cm H_2O. As mercury is 13.6 times denser than water, value obtained in cm H_2O should be divided by 1.36 to obtain value in mmHg.

Interpreting Central Venous Pressure

Central venous catheter measures the difference between CVP and atmospheric pressure. However, our aim is to measure the transmural pressure, the difference in the right atrial pressure and intrathoracic pressure. The intravascular pressure is equal to the transmural pressure when thoracic pressure is zero (i.e., when it equalizes with the atmospheric pressure). Therefore, for accurate assessment of transmural pressure, CVP should be measured at end expiration. In patients on positive pressure ventilation with positive end-expiratory pressure (PEEP), the more you zero the CVP the less it reflect the transmural pressure. Nevertheless, this relationship is not linear and 10 PEEP of 10 mmHg CVP changes by −3 mmHg. The health care professionals must be aware of this change in CVP, especially in patients receiving ventilation with high PEEP.

Usefulness of CVP in Predicting the Fluid Status

The monitoring of CVP, therefore, is expected to provide a reasonable estimate of the intravascular volume status. This forms the basis of routine use of CVP monitoring in cardiac ICUs. Unfortunately, the changes in the CVP with the fluid boluses is not linear and depends upon various properties of the vascular system such as elasticity of central veins and compliance characteristics of the right ventricle. Further, contrary to the expectation, routine use of CVP monitoring is not shown to improve the clinical outcomes.[18] Nonetheless, in selected patients, CVP monitoring helps in adjusting the fluid being administered.

Assessing the Fluid Responsiveness

One of the most critical questions in ICU is whether a patient in cardiogenic shock will have improved cardiac output with fluid resuscitation.[19]

Dynamic Assessment of Preload Responsiveness

Conventionally only CVP was used for assessment of fluid responsiveness. Newer methods of assessment are based on the cyclical change in right atrial pressure with respiration. The changes in atrial pressure result in changes in ventricular filling. The resultant change in stroke volume and arterial pressure is measured and provides a useful insight into the fluid responsiveness of the patient. Stroke volume variation (SVV), systolic pressure variation (SPV), and pulse pressure variation (PPV) are the most commonly monitored dynamic parameters (**Figs. 12.5** and **12.6** and **Table 12.4**).[20,21] However for these methods to be used, the arterial tracing has to be good and continuous.

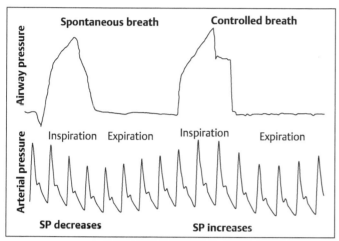

Fig. 12.5 Variation in systolic pressure (SPV) with respiration. Abbreviation: SP, systolic pressure.

The patient must be on ventilator controlled with tidal volume of at least 8 mL/kg. Further the utility is limited in patients with RV dysfunction, arrhythmia, and reduced pulmonary compliance.[21] PPV is defined as the maximal to minimal pulse pressure values over their mean three breaths or a fixed time interval. A >13% PPV predicts a >15% increase in cardiac output for a 500 mL volume bolus. While the assessment of PPV is easy by inspection of the arterial pressure trace the measurement of SVV requires calculation of stroke volume by echocardiography (**Box 12.2** and **Fig. 12.6**). Detailed discussion on dynamic assessment for fluid responsiveness is beyond the scope of this chapter.

Use of Echocardiography

Volume status of patient can be assessed using bedside echocardiography in cardiac ICU (**Box 12.3** and **Fig. 12.7**). This is easily achieved by the assessment of the diameter of inferior vena cava (IVC) and its collapsibility. The diameter and collapsibility correlates well with the right atrial pressure. However, these values have limited usefulness in patients on mechanical ventilation as IVC in these patients is often dilated to positive pressure ventilation.[23-25]

In addition, echocardiography is helpful in measuring left-sided filling pressure indirectly using mitral inflow velocities, tissue Doppler of the septal and lateral mitral annulus, and left atrial size. PCWP is likely to be elevated in

Table 12.4 Parameters for assessing fluid responsiveness

Parameter	Definition
Systolic pressure variation	Maximum minus minimum systolic arterial pressure over a full respiratory cycle Normal <10 mmHg
Pulse pressure variation	Maximum minus minimum pulse pressure (systolic–diastolic pressure) divided by the mean over a full respiratory cycle Normal approximately <13%
Stroke volume variation	Measured or calculated maximum minus minimum stroke volume divided by the mean over a full respiratory cycle Normal <15%

Box 12.2 Systolic pressure variation as a guide to fluid therapy in patients with sepsis-induced hypotension[22]

- The main value of the Δ down is that it is a reflection of the response of the LV output to fluid loading
- Offer information on a ventricular function curve
- Δ down component of the SPV was a sensitive indicator of the response of the left ventricle to volume infusion
- Pressure waveform analysis may be a valuable tool for hemodynamic assessment in patients requiring mechanical ventilation

Abbreviations: Δ, change; LV, left ventricle; SPV, systolic pressure.

Box 12.3 Esophageal Doppler (ED)

ED probe is approximately the size of nasogastric tube and is to be positioned at T5–T6 level (40 cm mark). Its specifications are:
- Unit: Height: 200 mm; Width: 250 mm; Depth: 300 mm; Weight: 4 kg
- Probe: Diameter of flexible section: <7 mm
- Length of flexible section: 610 mm
- Power: Voltage: 90–130 Vac, 180–270 Vac; Frequency: 50/60 Hz
- Power consumption: 100 VA Max
- Frequency: Doppler: 5 MHz Echo: 10 MHz

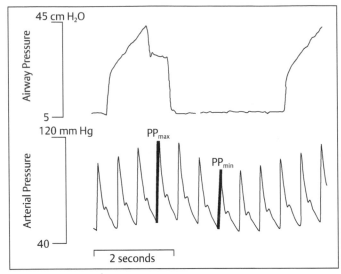

Fig. 12.6 Systolic pressure variation (SPV) during controlled ventilation. Abbreviation: PP, pulse pressure.

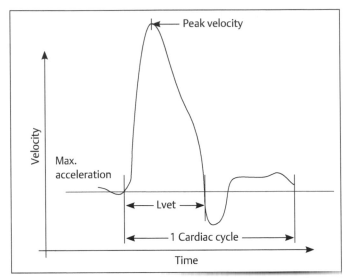

Fig. 12.7 Measuring the peak velocity with the esophageal Doppler.

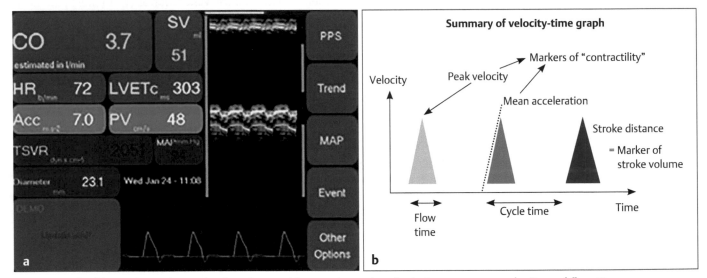

Fig. 12.8 **(a, b)** Esophageal Doppler for advanced haemodynamic calculations measure velocity and flow time.

the presence of mitral E/A >2, deceleration time >160 msec, tissue Doppler e/e' >15 for septal and >12 for lateral mitral annulus. A left atrial size >40 mm also elevates PCWP. Cardiac output can also be measured by measuring the stroke volume by velocity time integral of the Doppler signal obtained from the LV outflow tract multiplied by the cross-sectional area of the LV outflow tract in the absence of significant aortic regurgitation and multiplying it by heart rate (**Figs. 12.8–12.12**). It measures this by the use of ultrasonic cardiac output monitor (USCOM) which is the ultrasonic cardiac monitor (USCCM, USCOM). They accurately measures blood flow, stroke volume and cardiac output using state-of-the-art, high-fidelity ultrasonic (USCOM) users.

Ultrasonic cardiac output monitor (USCOM):
- Uses continuous wave Doppler technology to assess the hemodynamic variables.
- Probe: 2.2 MHz transducer.
- Position: 2 to 4 ICS L-parasternal for the pulmonary artery view and the suprasternal notch for the aortic view.

Other noninvasive cardiac output monitors:
- Four dual sensors with 8 lead wires placed on the neck and chest.
- Thoracic electrical impedance is based on principle of impedance, using special sensor.

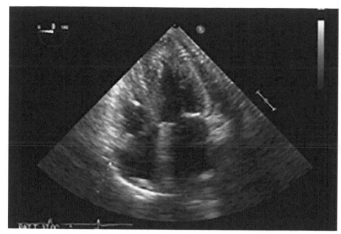

Fig. 12.9 Stroke volume, transgastric midpapillary deep transgastric (DTG) view in transesophageal echocardiography (TEE).

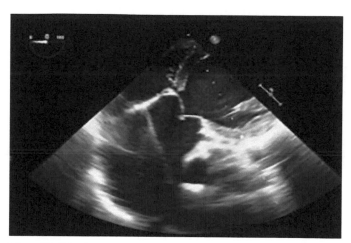

Fig. 12.10 Deep transgastric view on transesophageal echocardiography (TEE) is the best for measuring gradients.

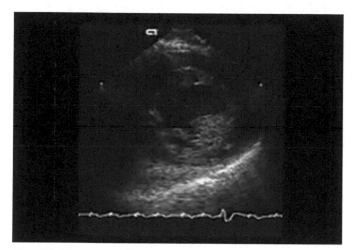

Fig. 12.11 Hypovolemia on transesophageal echocardiography (TEE) in midpapillary short-axis TEE view.

- High-frequency low-amplitude current is transmitted and seeks path of least resistance: blood-filled aorta.
- Baseline impedance (resistance) to signal is measured.
- With each heartbeat, blood volume and velocity in the aorta change.
- Corresponding change in impedance is measured.
- Baseline and changes in impedance are used to measure and calculate hemodynamic parameters (**Fig. 12.13**).

BioZ Machine—all noninvasive monitors on a stand:
- Faster signal processing (**Fig. 12.14**).
- Better signal filtering.
- Improved ECG triggering.
- Improved arrhythmia detection.
- Respiratory filtering.

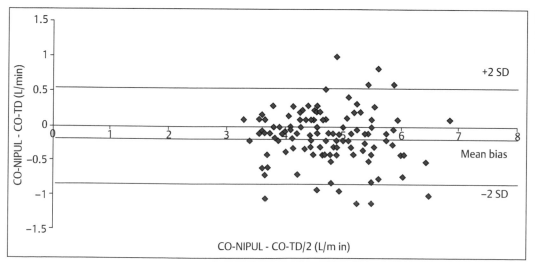

Fig. 12.12 Cardiac output estimation after off-pump coronary artery bypass.

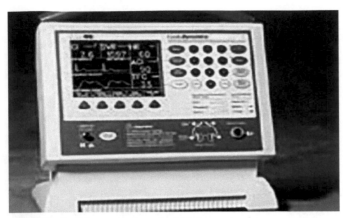

Fig. 12.13 Thoracic electrical bioimpedance.

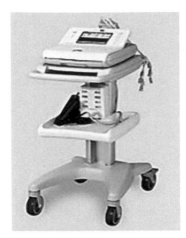

Fig. 12.14 BioZ machine for bioimpedance cardiac output monitoring when all noninvasive monitors come in a potable stand.

Electrodes are placed in specific areas on the neck and thorax. A low-grade electrical current, from 2 to 4 mA, is emitted, and received by the adjacent electrodes. Impedance to the current flow produces a waveform. Through electronic evaluation of these waveforms, the timing of aortic opening and closing can be used to calculate the LV ejection time and stroke volume (**Fig. 12.15**).

The Noninvasive Cardiac Output (NICO) Monitor

- Principle: Differential CO_2 Fick's partial rebreathing method (**Box 12.4**).
- CO = VCO_2/ $CvCO_2$-$CaCO_2$.
- To estimate $CvCO_2$, 150 mL of dead space is added to the ventilator circuit by opening a rebreathing valve (**Boxes 12.5** and **12.6**, **Fig. 12.16**).

Measurements of change in CO_2 elimination and $EtCO_2$ are made first during a period of nonrebreathing and rebreathing.

LiDCO:
- Principle: Indicator dilution.
- A small dose of lithium chloride (0.15–0.30 mmol) is injected via a central or peripheral venous line; the resulting arterial lithium concentration-time curve is recorded by withdrawing blood past a lithium sensor attached to the patient's existing arterial line (**Box 12.6**).

Pulse contour cardiac output (PiCCO):
- Principle: TD + PCA.
- For determination of cardiac output a central venous injection of a saline bolus is required.
- The thermistor on the tip of the arterial PiCCO catheter measures the downstream temperature changes.
- For the PiCCO technology, central venous catheter with a specific arterial PiCCO thermodilution catheter is required.
- The specific PiCCO pressure transducer is validated and optimized for arterial pulse contour analysis (**Fig. 12.17**).

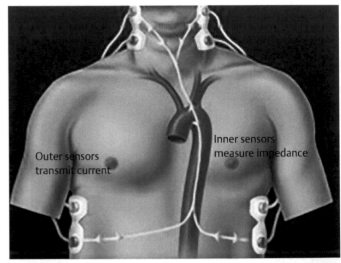

Fig. 12.15 Outer and inner sensors for thoracic bioimpedence cardiac output monitoring.

Box 12.4   Advantages of noninvasive cardiac output (NICO)
- Noninvasive
- No infection risks
- Automated and continuous
- Not technique dependent
- Extremely simple to set up and use
- Can be used in atrial fibrillation

What is the PiCCO technology?

The PiCCO technology is a unique combination of two techniques for advanced hemodynamic and volumetric management without the necessity of a right heart catheter in most patients (**Fig. 12.18**).

Transpulmonary Thermodilution Parameters

Transpulmonary thermodilution measurement only requires central venous injection of a cold (<8°C) saline bolus or a saline bolus at room temperature (<24°C) (**Fig. 12.19**).

Box 12.5 Modified Fick's equation

Applied with and without rebreathing:

$$C.O. = \frac{\dot{V}CO_{2N}}{C_{\bar{v}}CO_{2N} - C_aCO_{2N}} = \frac{\dot{V}CO_{2R}}{C_{\bar{v}}CO_{2R} - C_aCO_{2R}}$$

Combining to form the differential Fick equation (based on the Law of Ratios):

$$C.O. = \frac{\dot{V}CO_{2N} - \dot{V}CO_{2R}}{(C_{\bar{v}}CO_{2N} - C_aCO_{2N}) - (C_{\bar{v}}CO_{2R} - C_aCO_{2R})} = \frac{"\dot{V}CO_2}{"C_aCO_2} = \frac{"\dot{V}CO_2}{S"ETCO_2}$$

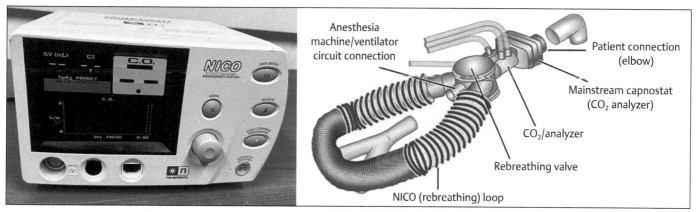

Fig. 12.16 Noninvasive cardiac output (NICO) monitor and connections for re-breathing NICO.

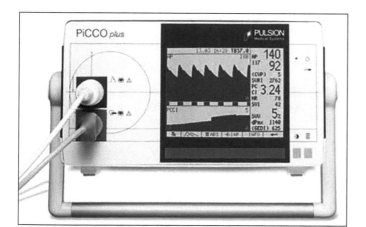

Fig. 12.17 Pulse contour cardiac output (PiCCO) plus monitor used in early 21st century.

The PiCCO technology is a unique combination of 2 techniques for advanced hemodynamic and volumetric management without the necessity of a right heart catheter in most patients:

Transpulmonary thermodilution

CV bolus injection

Pulsiocath

Pulse Contour Analysis

Calibration

Fig. 12.18 Pulse contour analysis using PiCCO technology.

Box 12.6 Advantages of LiDCO

- Provides an absolute cardiac output value via a novel and proven indicator dilution technique
- Requires no additional invasive catheters to insert into the patient
- Is safe—using nontoxic bolus dosages
- Is simple and quick to set up
- Is as accurate as measures triplicate thermodilution
- Is not temperature dependent

Transpulmonary Thermodilution: Cardiac Output

After central venous injection of the indicator, the thermistor at the tip of the arterial catheter measures the downstream temperature changes. Cardiac output is calculated by analysis of the thermodilution curve using a modified Stewart-Hamilton algorithm (**Fig. 12.20**).

Transpulmonary Thermodilution: Volumetric Parameters

The intrathoracic compartments can be considered as a series of "mixing chambers" for the distribution of the injected indicator (intrathoracic thermal volume) (**Flowchart 12.1**).

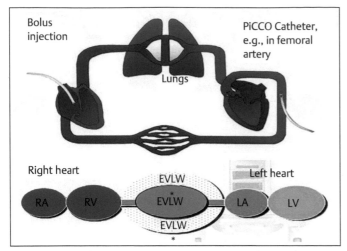

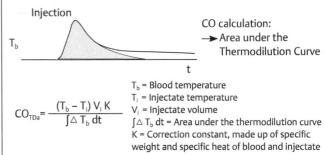

After central venous injection of the indicator, the thermistor at the tip of the arterial catheter measures the downstream temperature changes.
Cardiac output (CO) is calculated by analysis of the thermodilution curve using a modified Stewart-Hamilton algorithm:

$$CO_{TDa} = \frac{(T_b - T_i)\, V_i\, K}{\int \triangle T_b\, dt}$$

T_b = Blood temperature
T_i = Injectate temperature
V_i = Injectate volume
$\int \triangle T_b\, dt$ = Area under the thermodilution curve
K = Correction constant, made up of specific weight and specific heat of blood and injectate

CO calculation:
→ Area under the Thermodilution Curve

Fig. 12.19 Thermodilution parameters with a pulmonary artery catheter. Abbreviations: EVLW, extravascular lung water; LA, left atrium; LV, left ventricle; RA, right atrium; RV, right ventricle.

Fig. 12.20 Transpulmonary thermodilution: cardiac output monitoring measured as area under the curve.

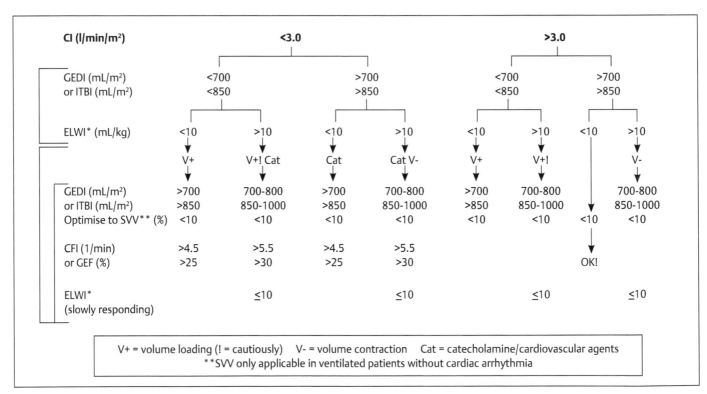

Flowchart 12.1 Decision tree for hemodynamic/volumetric monitoring.

Stroke Volume Variation (SVV): Calculation

SVV represents the variation in stroke volume (SV) over the ventilatory cycle. SVV is measured over the last 30 seconds which is only applicable in controlled mechanically ventilated patients with regular heart rhythm.

Pulse Pressure Variation (PPV): Calculation

PPV represents the variation of the pulse pressure over the ventilatory cycle. PPV is measured over the last 30 seconds

which is only applicable in controlled mechanically ventilated patients with regular beat rhythm (**Fig. 12.21**).

Semi-invasive Cardiac Output Monitoring—The FloTrac Pulse contour analysis—FloTrac:
- Principle—PCA.
- Flow is determined by a pressure gradient along a vessel and the resistance to that flow (F = P/R).
- The FloTrac algorithm uses a similar principle to measure pulsatile flow by incorporating the effects of both

vascular resistance and compliance through a conversion factor known as Khi (**Figs. 12.22** and **12.23**, **Table 12.5**).

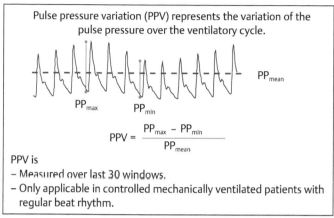

Pulse pressure variation (PPV) represents the variation of the pulse pressure over the ventilatory cycle.

PP_{mean}

PP_{max} PP_{min}

$$PPV = \frac{PP_{max} - PP_{min}}{PP_{mean}}$$

PPV is
– Measured over last 30 windows.
– Only applicable in controlled mechanically ventilated patients with regular beat rhythm.

Fig. 12.21   Pulse pressure variation: calculation.

EV1000 System Overview

The EV1000 monitor, in combination with the EV1000 databox, creates the EV1000 clinical platform. When used with the FloTrac sensor, PreSep and PediaSat oximetry catheters, and VolumeView set (**Figs. 12.24–12.26**), the EV1000 clinical platform transforms into a complete, unified monitoring system—the Edwards Critical Care System. With the use of the advanced EV1000 platform from Edwards Life sciences, the global leader and pioneer in hemodynamic monitoring, the use of FloTrac has decreased.

Central Venous Oxygen Saturation (ScvO$_2$)

It monitors tissue oxygen balance. Addition of fiberoptic bundles to pulmonary artery catheter (PAC) enables continuous monitoring of SvO$_2$. It correlates (rather precedes) with changes in CO and indicates trend and response to therapy in critically ill patients (**Fig. 12.27**).

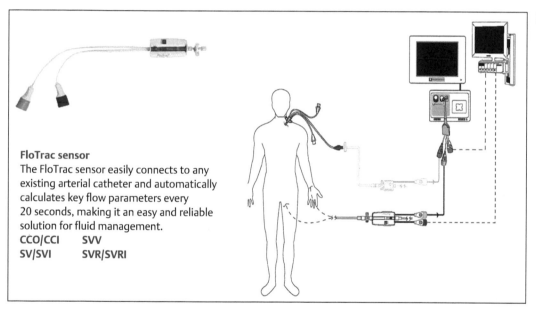

FloTrac sensor
The FloTrac sensor easily connects to any existing arterial catheter and automatically calculates key flow parameters every 20 seconds, making it an easy and reliable solution for fluid management.
CCO/CCI   SVV
SV/SVI   SVR/SVRI

Fig. 12.22   FloTrac sensor.

Table 12.5   Validation studies of the FloTrac/Vigileo device

Authors	Year	Software	Setting	Reference method
Mehta et al	2008	1.07	Cardiac (OP)	PAC (ITD)
Staier et al	2008	1.07	Cardiac (OP)	PAC (ITD)
Compton et al	2008	1.07/1.10	Medical ICU	PiCCO
Chakravarthy et al	2007	NA	Cardiac (OP)	PAC (ITD)
Prasser et al	2007	1.10	Cardiac (ICU)	PAC (ITD)
Mayer et al	2008	1.10	Cardiac (OP/ICU)	PAC (ITD)
Senn et al	2009	1.10	Cardiac (ICU)	PiCCO (ITD)
Mayer et al	2009	1.10	Cardiac (ICU)	PAC (CCO)
Hofer CK et al	2010	1.10	Cardiac (ICU)	PiCCO

Abbreviations: ICU, intensive care unit; ITD, intermittent thermo-dilution; OP, operation theater; PAC, pulmonary artery catheter; PiCCO, pulse contour cardiac output.

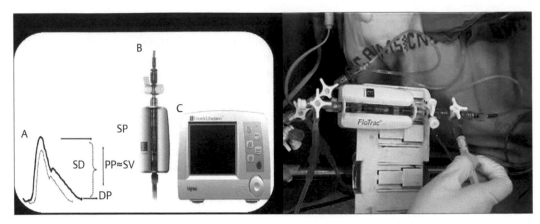

Fig. 12.23 The FloTrac.

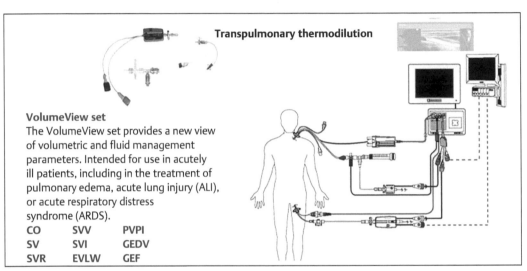

Transpulmonary thermodilution

VolumeView set
The VolumeView set provides a new view of volumetric and fluid management parameters. Intended for use in acutely ill patients, including in the treatment of pulmonary edema, acute lung injury (ALI), or acute respiratory distress syndrome (ARDS).

CO	SVV	PVPI
SV	SVI	GEDV
SVR	EVLW	GEF

Fig. 12.24 VolumeView set.

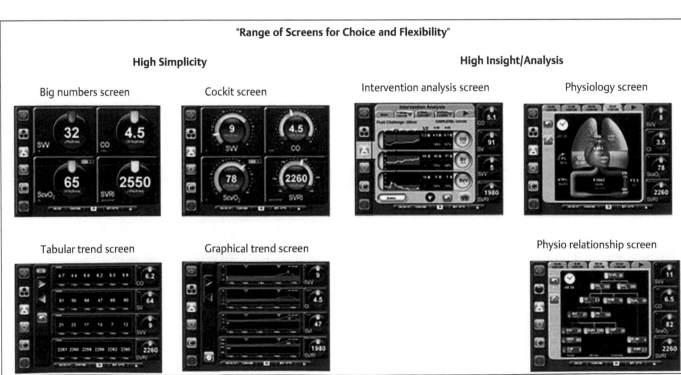

"Range of Screens for Choice and Flexibility"

High Simplicity

High Insight/Analysis

Big numbers screen

Cockit screen

Intervention analysis screen

Physiology screen

Tabular trend screen

Graphical trend screen

Physio relationship screen

Fig. 12.25 EV1000 screens.

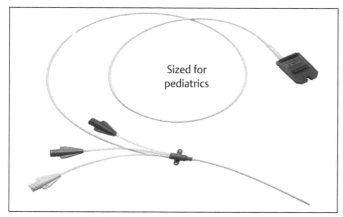

Fig. 12.26 PediaSat continuous $ScvO_2$ oximetry catheter.

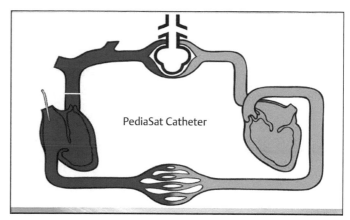

Fig. 12.27 Central venous oxygen saturation.

Fig. 12.28 Reflection spectrophotometry.

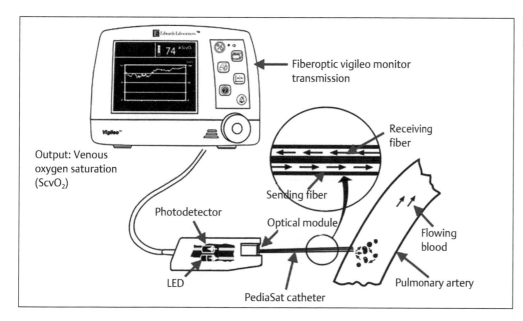

How $ScvO_2$ Is Measured

Reflection spectrophotometry: The amount of light absorbed, refracted, and reflected depends on how much oxygenated and deoxygenated Hb is in the blood (**Fig. 12.28**).

Central (SvO_2) and Mixed Venous Oxygen Saturation (MVO_2)

SvO_2 and $ScvO_2$ are not equivalent. According to an AIIMS study, central venous oxygenation is a reliable surrogate to mixed venous oxygen saturation in cardiac surgical patients.[26]

PediaSat Continuous $ScvO_2$ Oximetry Catheter

Pediaoxymetry Catheter

This catheter is an FDA-approved fiberoptic oximetry catheter fitted with a pediatric multilumen CV catheter. Used in a

size of 5.5 F/8 cm (18 g/23 g/23 g) triple lumen catheter in 10 patients undergoing cyanotic cardiac surgery by the AIIMS team, we found it excellent surrogate of central venous oxygenation, to cardiac output, as no PAV or noninvasive monitor exists for monitoring in cardiac output in neonates and paediatrics population (**Fig. 12.29**).

AIIMS Experience with FloTrac and EV1000 and Hemosphere

- Early goal-directed therapy in moderate high-risk cardiac surgical patients (**Fig. 12.29**).[27]
- Comparative study of myocardial lactate, pyruvate, and lactate pyruvate ratio as markers of myocardial ischemia in adult patients undergoing open heart surgery.[28]
- To study and compare the induction characteristics and hemodynamic effects of induction with etomidate,

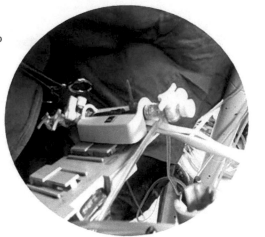

- Cardiac output or similar parameters to guide intravenous fluid and inotropic therapy
- First 6-8 hours– "golden hours"

- Recovery is supposedly early and uneventful

- Very few studies on EGDT in cardiac surgical patients in literature

Fig. 12.29 Early goal-directed therapy (EGDT) in moderate high-risk cardiac surgical patients (EGDT: AIIMS study).

thiopentone, propofol, and midazolam and severe LV dysfunction.[29]
- B-type natriuretic peptide (BNP) and SVV as noninvasive markers of diastolic dysfunction in patients undergoing pericardiectomy.[30]
- The role of blood lactate clearance as a predictor of mortality in children undergoing surgery for tetralogy of Fallot.[31]

Recent Advances in Hemodynamic Monitoring: The Hemosphere

There are many newer devices which can give noninvasive continuous measurement of cardiac output and can eliminate the use of invasive devices like the pulmonary artery catheter (**Fig. 12.30**).

There is a need of pulmonary artery catheterization for cardiac output monitoring. These methods include thoracic electrical bioimpedance device,[24] pulse contour analysis.[25] The aim of hemodynamic management is to optimize the amount of oxygen delivered to tissues. Because direct monitoring of the amount of oxygen delivered remains difficult, hemodynamic variables are monitored instead. Hemodynamic monitoring itself does not improve patient outcomes and needs to be combined with treatment protocols.[32] Detailed discussion is beyond the scope of this chapter.

Acute hemodynamic effects of inhaled nitroglycerine, intravenous nitroglycerine, and their combination with intravenous dobutamine in patients with secondary pulmonary hypertension:[33] When using and studying PVR measurements, then inhalators drugs are of use.

All drugs were of similar efficacy in reducing the pulmonary vascular resistance index (PVRI). Only iNTG produced

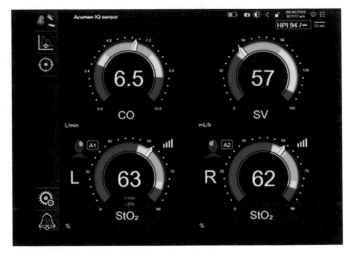

Fig. 12.30 Figure showing hemisphere.

selective pulmonary vasodilatation, while IV NTG. Its combination with IV dobutamine had a significant concomitant systemic vasodilatory effect.

Comparison of BNP and LV dysfunction in patients with constrictive pericarditis undergoing pericardiectomy: BNP released in response to LV wall stress and elevated Kapoor, et al.:[34] BNP in constrictive pericarditis undergoing pericardiectomy filling pressures is a very good comparable and substitutable marker for the E/A ratio, for measuring LV diastolic dysfunction.[34] It is an economical, simple, reliable, reproducible, point-of-care laboratory test, which can be subsequently monitored to evaluate the effect of the therapy provided to the patients in congestive heart failure. However, more studies in a larger number of patients are needed for it to be validated as a "gold standard" noninvasive marker for LV dysfunction.

Renal Resistive Index

Add Text: The renal resistive index is defined as the difference of the peak systolic and end-diastolic blood velocity divided by the peak systolic velocity measured by Doppler ultrasound in kidney arteries. The renal resistive index is used to evaluate vascular and parenchymal renal abnormalities, but growing evidence indicates that it may also reflect systemic vascular properties. Giustiniano et al. investigated whether renal resistive index, alone or combined with other variables, i.e., complexity and time of the surgical procedure, and postoperative serum lactate clearance, can predict postoperative complications in 183 patients undergoing liver resection in a prospective observational study.[35]

Conclusion

Careful interpretation of an optimally performed hemodynamic monitoring guides the management in sick patients. Detailed knowledge of principles of hemodynamic monitoring and troubleshooting of common errors are essential for maximal utilization of data obtained while guiding management in cardiac ICUs. Hemodynamic monitoring enables early detection of change in patient's conditions. New techniques provide reasonably good results and are less invasive.[36] Always correlate the readings/findings with clinical pictures in order to provide the best treatment options. The currently available monitoring technologies vary in cost and diversity of information provided. Critically ill patients may benefit from the more invasive techniques as a result of the greater breadth of information gained.[37] Physicians must thoroughly understand the hemodynamic data obtained and utilize it in a goal-directed fashion if the monitoring technology is to improve patient outcome. Use of PreSep and FloTrac increases the cost. But, a decrease in the duration of ventilation and ICU stay, resulting from its use, may render it cost-effective.

Its future upgradation into hypotension prediction with a Hypotension Prediction Index (HPI) with simulation incorporated technology, launched as hemosphere, is the state-of-the-art technology.[38] Another upcoming parameter is the bioimpedance technology in its advanced format which also measures total fluid content beyond FloTrac and PAC. Hemodynamic monitoring in ICU has a bright future ahead with artificial intelligence based technology like Hemosphere and HPI, predicting intraoperative hypotension on the horizon. The complicated outcome prediction score (COPS), ranging from 5 to 16.5 points, which allows stratifying patients into low (COPS 5–10), medium (COPS 10–12), and high (COPS >12) risk groups of postoperative complication. Additionally, a new scoring system was compared with Surgical Apgar Score and Physiological and Operative Severity Score for the enUmeration of Mortality and Morbidity (POSSUM), but rather scant information was provided, that compared to POSSUM, COPS showed no clinically important difference in the area under the receiver operating characteristics curve, is also an upcoming monitor for perioperative post haemodynamic monitoring.[39]

References

1. Pinsky MR. Hemodynamic evaluation and monitoring in the ICU. Chest 2007;132(6):2020–2029
2. Adler AC, Sharma R, Higgins T, McGee WT. Hemodynamic assessment and monitoring in the intensive care unit: an overview. Enilven: J Anesthesiol Crit Care Med 2014;1:1–13
3. Villegas I, Arias IC, Botero A, Escobar A. Evaluation of the technique used by health-care workers for taking blood pressure. Hypertension 1995;26(6 Pt 2):1204–1206
4. Pickering TG, Hall JE, Appel LJ, et al. Recommendations for blood pressure measurement in humans and experimental animals: part 1: blood pressure measurement in humans: a statement for professionals from the Subcommittee of Professional and Public Education of the American Heart Association Council on High Blood Pressure Research. Circulation 2005;111(5): 697–716
5. Bur A, Hirschl MM, Herkner H, et al. Accuracy of oscillometric blood pressure measurement according to the relation between cuff size and upper-arm circumference in critically ill patients. Crit Care Med 2000;28(2):371–376
6. Severinghaus JW, Honda Y. History of blood gas analysis. VII. Pulse oximetry. J Clin Monit 1987;3(2):135–138
7. Sinex JE. Pulse oximetry: principles and limitations. Am J Emerg Med 1999;17(1):59–67
8. Chan ED, Chan MM, Chan MM. Pulse oximetry: understanding its basic principles facilitates appreciation of its limitations. Respir Med 2013;107(6):789–799
9. Ewer AK, Middleton LJ, Furmston AT, et al; PulseOx Study Group. Pulse oximetry screening for congenital heart defects in newborn infants (PulseOx): a test accuracy study. Lancet 2011;378(9793):785–794
10. Moscucci M, Grossman W, eds. Cardiac catheterization, angiography, and intervention. Lippincott Williams & Wilkins; 2014:223–244
11. Hemodynamic monitoring. 2015. http://www.derangedphysiology.com/main/core-topics-intensive-care/haemodyamic-monitoring
12. Dellinger RP, Levy MM, Rhodes A, et al; Surviving Sepsis Campaign Guidelines Committee including The Pediatric Subgroup. Surviving Sepsis Campaign: international guidelines for management of severe sepsis and septic shock, 2012. Intensive Care Med 2013;39(2):165–228
13. Swan HJ, Ganz W, Forrester J, Marcus H, Diamond G, Chonette D. Catheterization of the heart in man with use of a flow-directed balloon-tipped catheter. N Engl J Med 1970;283(9):447–451
14. Binanay C, Califf RM, Hasselblad V, et al; ESCAPE Investigators and ESCAPE Study Coordinators. Evaluation study of congestive heart failure and pulmonary artery catheterization effectiveness: the ESCAPE trial. JAMA 2005;294(13):1625–1633
15. Sandham JD, Hull RD, Brant RF, et al; Canadian Critical Care Clinical Trials Group. A randomized, controlled trial of the use of pulmonary-artery catheters in high-risk surgical patients. N Engl J Med 2003;348(1):5–14

16. Cohen MG, Kelly RV, Kong DF, et al. Pulmonary artery catheterization in acute coronary syndromes: insights from the GUSTO IIb and GUSTO III trials. Am J Med 2005;118(5):482–488

17. Chatterjee K. The Swan-Ganz catheters: past, present, and future. A viewpoint. Circulation 2009;119(1):147–152

18. Marik PE, Cavallazzi R. Does the central venous pressure predict fluid responsiveness? An updated meta-analysis and a plea for some common sense. Crit Care Med 2013;41(7):1774–1781

19. Saxena A, Garan AR, Kapur NK, et al. Value of hemodynamic monitoring in patients with cardiogenic shock undergoing mechanical circulatory support. Circulation 2020;141(14):1184–1197

20. De Backer D, Heenen S, Piagnerelli M, Koch M, Vincent J-L. Pulse pressure variations to predict fluid responsiveness: influence of tidal volume. Intensive Care Med 2005;31(4):517–523

21. Lakhal K, Ehrmann S, Benzekri-Lefèvre D, et al. Respiratory pulse pressure variation fails to predict fluid responsiveness in acute respiratory distress syndrome. Crit Care 2011;15(2):R85

22. Scheeren TWL, Ramsay MAE. New developments in hemodynamic monitoring. J Cardiothorac Vasc Anesth 2019;33(1):S67–S72

23. Rudski LG, Lai WW, Afilalo J, et al. Guidelines for the echocardiographic assessment of the right heart in adults: a report from the American Society of Echocardiography endorsed by the European Association of Echocardiography, a registered branch of the European Society of Cardiology, and the Canadian Society of Echocardiography. J Am Soc Echocardiogr 2010;23(7):685–713, quiz 786–788

24. Keren H, Burkhoff D, Squara P. Evaluation of a noninvasive continuous cardiac output monitoring system based on thoracic bioreactance. Am J Physiol Heart Circ Physiol 2007;293(1):H583–H589

25. Stok WJ, Stringer RC, Karemaker JM. Noninvasive cardiac output measurement in orthostasis: pulse contour analysis compared with acetylene rebreathing. J Appl Physiol 1999;87(6):2266–2273

26. Agarwal NK, Subramanian A. Central venous oxygenation to be a reliable surrogate to mixed venous oxygen saturation in cardiac surgical patients. J Anaesthesiol Clin Pharmacol 2007;23(1):29–33

27. Kapoor PM, Kakani M, Chowdhury U, Choudhury M, Lakshmy, Kiran U. Early goal-directed therapy in moderate to high-risk cardiac surgery patients. Ann Card Anaesth 2008;11(1):27–34

28. Kapoor P, Mandal B, Chowdhury U, Singh S, Kiran U. Changes in myocardial lactate, pyruvate and lactate-pyruvate ratio during cardiopulmonary bypass for elective adult cardiac surgery: early indicator of morbidity. J Anaesthesiol Clin Pharmacol 2011;27(2):225–232

29. Singh R, Choudhury M, Kapoor PM, Kiran U. A randomized trial of anesthetic induction agents in patients with coronary artery disease and left ventricular dysfunction. Ann Card Anaesth 2010;13(3):217–223

30. Kapoor PM, Aggarwal V, Chowdhury U, Choudhury M, Singh SP, Kiran U. Comparison of B-type natriuretic peptide and left ventricular dysfunction in patients with constrictive pericarditis undergoing pericardiectomy. Ann Card Anaesth 2010;13(2):123–129

31. Ladha S, Kapoor PM, Singh SP, Kiran U, Chowdhury UK. The role of blood lactate clearance as a predictor of mortality in children undergoing surgery for tetralogy of Fallot. Ann Card Anaesth 2016;19(2):217–224

32. de Keijzer IN, Scheeren TWL. Perioperative hemodynamic monitoring: an overview of current methods. Anesthesiol Clin 2021;39(3):441–456

33. Mandal B, Kapoor PM, Chowdhury U, Kiran U, Choudhury M. Acute hemodynamic effects of inhaled nitroglycerine, intravenous nitroglycerine, and their combination with intravenous dobutamine in patients with secondary pulmonary hypertension. Ann Card Anaesth 2010;13(2):138–144

34. Kapoor PM, Aggarwal V, Chowdhury U, Choudhury M, Singh SP, Kiran U. Comparison of B-type natriuretic peptide and left ventricular dysfunction in patients with constrictive pericarditis undergoing pericardiectomy. Ann Card Anaesth 2010;13(2):123–129

35. Giustiniano E, Procopio F, Morenghi E, Gollo Y, Rocchi L, Ruggieri N, Lascari V, Torzilli G, Cecconi M. Renal resistive index as a predictor of postoperative complications in liver resection surgery. Observational study. J Clin Monit Comput. 2021;35(4):731–40

36. Schmidt S, Dieks JK, Quintel M, Moerer O. Hemodynamic profiling by critical care echocardiography could be more accurate than invasive techniques and help identify targets for treatment. Sci Rep 2022;12(1):7187

37. Shang Y, Pan C, Yang X, et al. Management of critically ill patients with COVID-19 in ICU: statement from front-line intensive care experts in Wuhan, China. Ann Intensive Care 2020;10(1):73

38. Koo JM, Choi H, Hwang W, et al. Clinical implication of the acumen hypotension prediction index for reducing intraoperative haemorrhage in patients undergoing lumbar spinal fusion surgery: a prospective randomised controlled single-blinded trial. J Clin Med 2022;11(16):4646

39. Flick M, Bergholz A, Sierzputowski P. et al. What is new in hemodynamic monitoring and management?. J Clin Monit Comput 2022; 36:305–313

13

Recent Advances in Cardiac Pharmacology: Infographics

Ramesh Chand Kashav, Poonam Malhotra Kapoor, Jess Jose, and Rohan Magoon

- ➢ Introduction
- ➢ Novel Antiarrhythmic Drugs
- ➢ Newer Anticoagulants and Its Reversal Agents
- ➢ Novel Antiplatelet Agents
- ➢ Newer Antiheart Failure Drugs
- ➢ Metabolic Modulators and Their Site of Action
- ➢ Gene Therapy in Heart Disease

- ➢ Pathophysiological Pathways Causing Pulmonary Artery Hypertension and Its Pharmacotherapy
- ➢ Free Radicals and Antioxidants
- ➢ Newer Ionotropic Agents
- ➢ Newer Antihypertensive Agents
- ➢ Novel Lipid-Lowering Agents
- ➢ Conclusion

Introduction

The practice of cardiovascular medicine entails the application of a considerably wide range of pharmacological therapies (often, belonging to different classes) for varied indications ranging right from symptomatic relief and preoperative stabilization (such as for those in congestive heart failure or with angina), to heart rate and rhythm control, metabolic modulation, thromboembolic prophylaxis, and favorable modulation of the systemic and pulmonary circuit hemodynamics.

The developments in cardiovascular medicine have been particularly rampant with the impetus primarily driven by the ongoing need for ameliorating the side-effect profile of the existing drug therapies and simultaneously augmenting the inculcation of novel agents with the potential of treating the existing cardiovascular pathologies with the assistance of newer mechanistic pathways.

The anesthesiologists' knowledge needs to be abreast with the pharmacological developments in the cardiovascular medicine for an efficient perioperative and intensive care management. A sound comprehension of these developments can additionally assist in the formulation of pragmatic informed decisions on the preoperative drug continuation-discontinuation, possibility of drug-drug interactions, resultant electrolyte alterations, and the attributable hemodynamic fluctuations.

Cardiovascular pharmacology is a rapidly evolving niche with newer drugs being added to the arsenal every passing year and pragmatic indications being identified for classical agents. With improvements in molecular modeling methods, newer target sites are identified and designer drug structures are manufactured, to selectively target these sites. The onset of SARS-CoV-2 pandemic exposed the underlying limitations of currently available treatment modalities and need for state-of-the-art research and development infrastructure. In this chapter, authors aim to expose the reader to various newer classes of cardiac drugs, currently in clinical practice or in advanced stages of clinical trials, in the form of concise infographics:

- Novel Antiarrhythmic Drugs.
- Newer Anticoagulants and Its Reversal Agents.
- Novel Antiplatelet Agents.
- Newer Antiheart Failure Drugs.
- Metabolic Modulators and Their Site of Action.
- Gene Therapy in Heart Disease.
- Pathophysiological Pathways Causing Pulmonary Artery Hypertension and Its Pharmacotherapy.
- Free Radicals and Antioxidants.
- Newer Ionotropic Agents.
- Newer Antihypertensive Agents.
- Novel Lipid-Lowering Agents.

Novel Antiarrhythmic Drugs

Various newer antiarrhythmic drugs have been introduced in recent years, with improved pharmacokinetic and dynamic properties.[1] With the development of agents with a wide range of mechanisms of action, the classification of antiarrhythmics need to evolve beyond Vaughan Williams Classes, a classification proposed by Lei et al is one such example.[2] Atrial-selective agents offer modality for specific management of atrial fibrillation, with connexins (Cx-40) controlling the electrotonic cell coupling and multiple ionic currents (IKACh, IKur) being the potential targets.[3,4] Upstream therapy is being increasingly used to prevent electrophysiological and/or structural remodeling, especially after ablative therapy.[5] Their mechanism of action is explained in **Fig. 13.1.**

Newer Anticoagulants and Its Reversal Agents

Thrombus formation within the circulatory system regardless of its origin, be it arterial or venous, limits blood flow to target organs. And anticoagulants remain the gold standard therapy for thrombosis prevention and its management. With the arrival of novel anticoagulants, which do not require daily subcutaneous injections, like heparin nor routine monitoring like warfarin, with added advantages like much faster onset of action following first dose and increased ease of use, the patient compliance has improved drastically.[1,6] They are currently approved for venous thromboembolism (VTE) prophylaxis, acute pulmonary embolism (PE), and thromboprophylaxis in atrial fibrillation of nonvalvular origin.[7] Dabigatran etexilate is a prodrug converted to dabigatran by nonspecific esterases, which binds directly to thrombin via ionic interactions, thereby inhibiting thrombin-induced thrombus expansion. The availability of these newer agents facilitates individualized anticoagulant therapy, depending on duration of action required and helps rapidly reverse its effects in emergency situations, like hemorrhage or surgical interventions (**Fig. 13.2**).[8]

Novel Antiplatelet Agents

Antiplatelet drugs have become the mainstay in the prevention of adverse vascular events, such as cerebrovascular accidents and acute coronary syndromes.[1,9] Newer drugs in this class have a wide range of dose duration to offset time like the irreversible inhibitor, Aspirin, which has a duration of action of about 7 to 8 days compared to cangrelor's

Vernakalant

Atrial-selective via IKur blockade. Also Na+ channel and IK-Ach blocking action

Frequency and voltage dependent Na+ channel block of INaL Mx for AF termination

C/I: SBP <100 mmHg, NYHA 3 & 4, Severe AS, QT interval prolongation

Ranolazine

Atrial-selective via blockade of INa, INaL, IKr, and late ICa

Most potent inhibitor of INaL

Increase post repolarization refractoriness Mx for AF termination

C/I: Hepatic cirrhosis

Dronedarone

Amiodarone analogue (Iodine removed methane sulfonyl group added) hence reduced thyroid and pulmonary side effects

Used for persistent AF. Less potent than Amiodarone especially in prevention of reccurent AF

Mx blocks IKs, IKr, IKur, IK-Ach, ICaL, INa+

C/I: Permanent AF, NYHA 4

Selective blockers

Drug	Mx	Comment
Dofetilide	IKr selective blocker	Risk of QT prolongation and polymorphic ventricular tachycardia
Tedisamil	IK-ATP, IKr, IKs blocker	Reducing ventricular tachyarrhythmias with no effect on contractility
Piboserod	5-HT4 blocker	Used for sinus rhythm maintenance in atrial fibrillation
Tecadenoson	Adenosine receptor blocker	Terminates AV node SVT without hypotension and bronchoconstriction
Rotigaptide	Connexin 43 modulator	Normalizes cell-to-cell communication even during acute metabolic stress
Eplerenone	Steroidal Anti-mineralocorticoid	Reduces atrial fibrosis

Azimilide

Class III antiarrhythmics used in SVT and VT

Mx prolongs myocardial repolarization via K+ channel blockade (IKs & IKr)

No survival benefit but reduces rate of AF

C/I: Prolonged QT interval

Upstream Therapy

Drug Class	Mx
ACE inhibitors	Angiotensin II production reduced
ARB	Angiotensin I receptor blocker
Statin	HMG-CoA inhibitor, pleiotropic effects
ω-3 PUFA	Antiarrhythmic, lowers lipids, antioxidant
Spironolactone	Aldosterone blocker
Pirfenidone	Anti-inflammatory
Glucocorticoids	Anti-inflammatory

Fig. 13.1 This infographic represents various newer antiarrhythmic drugs and their mechanism of action. Abbreviations: ω-3 PUFA, Omega-3 polyunsaturated fatty acids; AF, atrial fibrillation; ACE, angiotensin-converting enzyme; ARB, angiotensin receptor blockers; ATP, adenosine triphosphate; AS, aortic stenosis; HMG, high mobility group; NYHA, New York Heart Association; SBP, systolic BP; SVT, supraventricular tachycardia; VT, ventricular tachycardia.

(US FDA 2015) 60 minutes due to degradation in circulation via dephosphorylation [10] Revacept, a GP IV antagonist, has no effect on circulating platelets but exclusively prevents their adhesion at exposed collagen sites, without any additional bleeding tendency,[11] while vorapaxar inhibits thrombin-induced platelet aggregation without effecting impact primary hemostatic functions (**Fig. 13.3**).[12]

Newer Antiheart Failure Drugs

In the pharmacological management of heart failure, in patients with reduced ejection fraction going beyond time-tested beta-blockers, ACE-inhibitors, mineralocorticoid, and aldosterone receptor antagonists, authors specifically

Parenteral Anticoagulants

Idrabiotaparinux and Otamixaban selectively target factor FXa and neutralized by IV **Avidin**
RB006, an anticoagulant RNA aptamer, specifically targets factor FXa and neutralized by **RB007**
These agents have rapid onset of action with a predictable anticoagulant effect

Oral Direct Factor Xa Inhibitors

Rivaroxaban	Apixaban	Edoxaban
$T_{1/2}$ of 7–11 h	$T_{1/2}$ of 8–14 h	$T_{1/2}$ of 9–11 h
Rapid onset of action	The recommended dose is 5 mg BID orally and 2.5 mg orally dose for age >80 years, body weight <60 kg and serum creatinine >1.5 mg/dL	The recommended dose is 60 mg taken OD orally, with reduction to 30 mg OD orally in patients with CrCL < 15–50 mL/min
The recommended initial dose is 10 mg OD orally		

Oral Direct Thrombin Inhibitors

Dabigatran etexilate

Prodrug of dabigatran it reversibly inhibits thrombin

$T_{1/2}$ of 14–17 h

Recommended daily dose is 150 mg BD or 110 mg BD (>75 year)

Significantly decreased the annual rate of stroke or systemic embolus compared to warfarin

Anticoagulant Reversal Agents	
Reversal Agent	Comment
Indarucizumab	Humanized monoclonal antibody fragment (Fab) derived from an IgG1 isotype molecule, against dabigatran
Aripazine	Small molecule (D-arginine compound) which has broad activity against old and new anticoagulants
Andexanet	Recombinant, modified FXa molecule that acts as a direct reversal agent for patients receiving an FXa inhibitor with major bleeding or requiring an emergency surgery

Fig. 13.2 This infographic represents various newer anticoagulants and novel reversal agents highlighting the duration of action and target of these drugs.

focus on two new classes of drugs: hyperpolarization-activated cyclic nucleotide-gated channel blocker (Ivabradine) and angiotensin receptor neprilysin inhibitor (Sacubitril + Valsartan).[13] Ivabradine and Sacubitril + Valsartan both received initial US FDA approval in 2015. Ivabradine is usually started at an initial dose of 5 mg, twice a day titrated to a heart rate of 50 to 60 beats per min to a maximum dose of 7.5 mg, twice a day. Animal models have demonstrated fetal toxicity and therefore concomitant beta-blocker use is not recommended.[1] Sacubitril/Valsartan, on the other hand, is started at an initial dose of 24 mg/26 mg twice per day with routine serum potassium level monitoring (**Fig. 13.4**).[16]

Metabolic Modulators and Their Site of Action

Metabolic modulators are drugs that optimize cardiac metabolism without exerting hemodynamic effects.[1] They are beneficial in patients who are refractory to treatment despite being on optimal conventional therapy.[17] Various agents have been shown to have metabolic modulatory properties in addition to their well-established actions, for example, metformin, ranolazine, and niacin. The core concept is based on the fact that oxygen requirement per molecule of adenosine triphosphate (ATP) produced via fatty

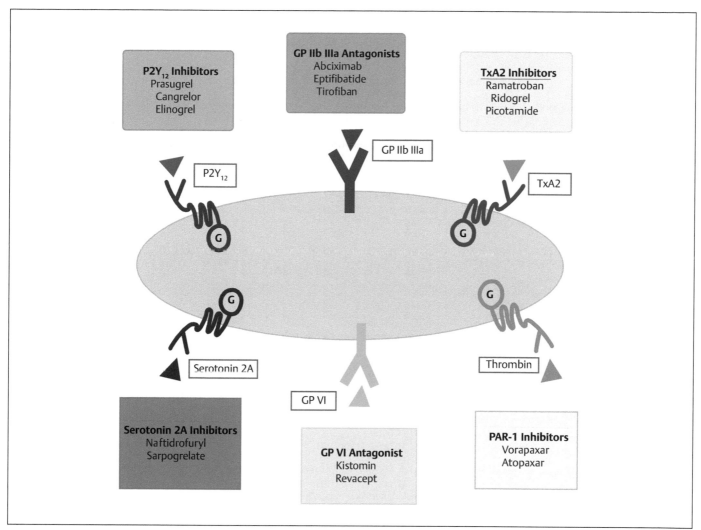

Fig. 13.3 This diagram shows various receptors on a platelet and the drugs which inhibit its normal functioning. Abbreviations: GP, glycoprotein; PAR-1, protease-activated receptor-1.

acid oxidation is more than what is required by glucose oxidation; metabolic modulators shift substrate utilization from fatty acid to glucose through inhibition of free fatty acid oxidation or by stimulation of enzymes in glycolysis (**Fig. 13.5**).[18]

Gene Therapy in Heart Disease

Based on WHO factsheet 2016, an estimated 17.9 million people died of cardiovascular diseases, a vast majority of which are coronary vascular disease and heart failure. Currently available treatment modalities have decreased the mortality and morbidity significantly, but the long-term outcome remains poor. Gene therapy involves transferring genes to target organs using vectors like adenoassociated viral vector and synthetic-modified messenger RNA (modRNA). One particular agent of interest is VEGF-D[dNdC], an angiogenic and lymphangiogenic growth factor under trial for the management of refractory angina. Apart from angiogenic effects it improves lymphatic circulation, thereby reducing myocardial edema, a common side effect of neovascularization.[19] Currently, these techniques are limited by its inability to effectively transfer genes, but with the development of newer gene transfer techniques and vectors it has the potential to be a game changer in the management of cardiac diseases (**Fig. 13.6**).[20,21]

Sinoatrial Node Modulator
Ivabradine

Hyperpolarization-activated cyclic nucleotide-gated channel blocker

Decreases spontaneous activity of the sinus node by inhibiting the if-current (If) Rate reduction with no negative impact on myocardial contractility

Reduces the risk of hospitalization in: Chronic heart failure (HF) with left ventricular ejection fraction (LVEF) ≤35%.
Sinus resting heart rate ≥70 beats/min
Contraindication to beta-blocker therapy

Contraindicated in: Bradycardia, BP <90/50 mmHg, acute decompensated heart failure, sick sinus syndrome
Adverse effects: Bradycardia, hypertensive (HT), atrial fibrillation (AF), and luminous phenomena

Newer Anti-heart Failure Drugs

Angiotensin Receptor Neprilysin Inhibitor (ARNI)

It's a combination of two compound:

Sacubitril (Neprilysin inhibitor) and **Valsartan** (Angiotensin II receptor blocker)

Decreases the risk of cardiovascular death and hospitalization in chronic HF (NYHA Class II–IV) and reduced ejection fraction (EF)

Dose reduction required in patients with severe renal impairment and hepatic impairment

Should not be used in conjunction with Aliskiren; causes renal failure, hyperkalemia, and hypotension

Adverse effects: Hypotension, hyperkalemia, cough, dizziness, and renal failure

Fig. 13.4 This infographic illustrates two new groups of drugs: hyperpolarization-activated cyclic nucleotide-gated channel blocker (ivabradine) and angiotensin receptor neprilysin inhibitor (sacubitril + valsartan) used in the management of heart failure. Abbreviation: NYHA, New York Heart Association.

Pathophysiological Pathways Causing Pulmonary Artery Hypertension and Its Pharmacotherapy

Pulmonary arterial hypertension (PAH) is a progressive disorder characterized by vascular remodeling and endothelial dysfunction of small pulmonary arteries, leading to elevated pulmonary vascular resistance and pulmonary artery pressures, further progressing to reduced cardiac output, right heart failure, and even death. Macitentan, an orally active, dual endothelin (ET) receptor antagonist, exhibits higher antagonistic potency than bosentan and ambrisentan in pulmonary smooth muscles, along with longer duration of action, due to its active metabolite, ACT-132577.[22] Riociguat is a soluble guanylate cyclase (sGC) stimulator that is US FDA approved for the management of PAH, chronic thromboembolic pulmonary hypertension (CTEPH), persisting or recurring postpulmonary endarterectomy, and in inoperable CTEPH.[23] Prior to discovery of these agents, management of PAH relied primarily on intravenous vasodilators which were nonselective and resulted in systemic side effects, with the alternative being inhaled nitric oxide, which has a short duration of action (**Fig. 13.7**).[24]

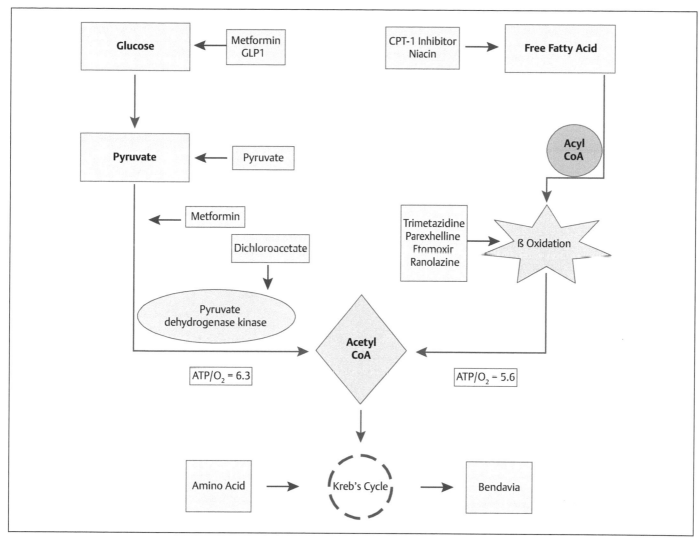

Fig. 13.5 This flowchart depicts various metabolic modulators of cardiac drugs origin and their respective site of action. Abbreviations: ATP, adenosine triphosphate; CPT-1, carnitine palmitoyltransferase 1; GLP-1, glucagon-like peptide 1.

Free Radicals and Antioxidants

Patients undergoing cardiac surgery, especially ones involving cardiopulmonary bypass, are under severe oxidative stress, due to production of free radicals during periods of ischemia and reperfusion.[25] Activated oxygen species, like singlet oxygen, hydrogen peroxide, superoxide, and hydroxyl radical, are highly unstable and extremely reactive.[26] Anesthetic induction agents like thiopental and propofol have direct ROS scavenging property and inhibit lipid peroxidation.[27] Administration of antioxidants may help reduce the free radical-induced cell damage and improve outcome (**Fig. 13.9**)

Newer Ionotropic Agents

Despite the vast strides made in the field of intra-aortic balloon pump and ventricular-assist device technology, inotropes remain an integral part of management of low cardiac output states. Classical agents belong to two broad groups: catecholamines and phosphodiesterase inhibitors (PDE). Catecholamine and PDE-based inotropes have been shown to achieve only short-term hemodynamic goals in heart failure, while novel agents acting via alternative mechanisms help tide over this limitation.[28] Currently, newer agents targeting alternate sites have been gaining momentum, such as ryanodine receptor stabilizers limit leak of calcium from

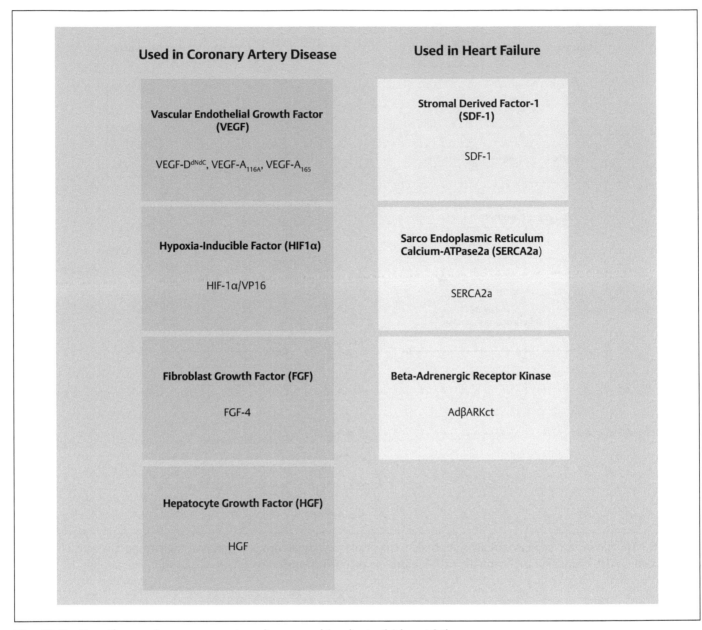

Fig. 13.6 Gene therapy for coronary artery disease and (under trails) heart failure.

the sarcoplasmic reticulum; metabolic energy modulators offer improvement in contractility by optimizing cardiac metabolism; istaroxime is a prototype, dual-action, luso-inotropic agent that enhances myocardial contractility via Na^+/K^+-ATPase inhibition while omecamtiv mecarbil is a cardiac-specific myosin activator (**Fig. 13.9**).[29,30]

Newer Antihypertensive Agents

It is estimated that the global burden of hypertension is around 1.13 billion people out of which two-thirds hail from middle- and low-income countries. Multiple newer

agents have been identified in recent years, with few entering routine clinical practice, such as landiolol and clevidipine. Landiolol is an ultra-short-acting, highly β1-selective, β-adrenergic blocker that is rapidly metabolized by pseudocholinesterase with minimal negative inotropic effects and is currently approved for intraoperative tachyarrhythmias whereas clevidipine is a short-acting IV agent with similar profile as sodium nitroprusside.[31] Firibastat is an orally active, centrally acting renin-angiotensin system blocker via brain aminopeptidase A inhibition, and is currently under investigation for difficult-to-treat hypertension.[32] Various alternate target sites are under investigation, most of which are in phase II trials, including a vaccine against

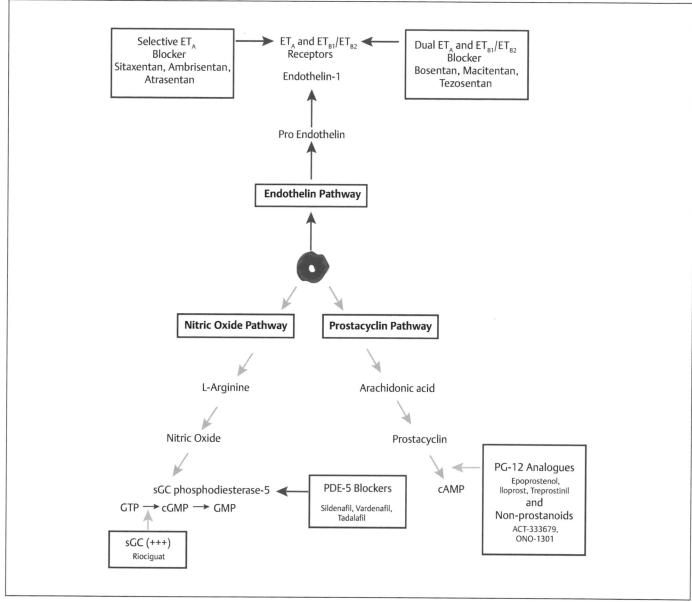

Fig. 13.7 This flowchart illustrates three major pathways involved in regulation of pulmonary artery pressures and the agents which reduces pulmonary artery hypertension (PAH). The green arrows represent the pathways when inhibited decrease PAH. The *red arrows* represent the pathways when stimulated decrease PAH. Abbreviations: cAMP, cyclic adenosine monophosphate; cGMP, cyclic guanosine monophosphate; ET, endothelin; PDE, phosphodiesterases; sGC, soluble guanylate cyclase.

angiotensin II, called CYT006-AngQb for noncompliant high-risk patients (**Fig. 13.10**).[33,34]

Novel Lipid-Lowering Agents

Dyslipidemia has been identified as a major independent risk factor for adverse cardiovascular events, with primary (hereditary) and secondary (acquired) subtypes requiring different management strategies. With the arrival of these newer agents we can target specific lipid component

and go beyond blanket therapy with statins especially in familial genetic disorders.[35] Drugs that were under trial, like CSL-112, intended to raise HDL-C levels failed to show very promising results in reducing atherosclerotic cardiovascular disease while agents like evinacumab are shown to be useful in patients refractory to conventional agents.[36] Various PCSK9 blocking strategies have also been developed to reduce LDL-C including monoclonal antibody mediated (alirocumab, evolocumab, and bococizumab) and nonantibody mediated via inclisiran, a small interfering RNA against PCSK9 with prolonged duration of action (**Table 13.1**).[37]

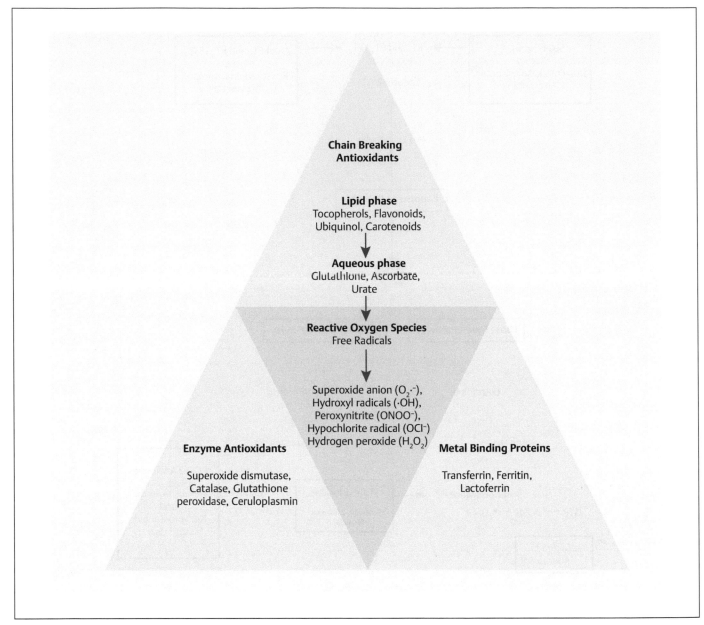

Fig. 13.8 This infographic flowchart depicts common free radicals in the body and the respective antioxidants.

Conclusion

The high incidence of cardiovascular diseases globally, and its debilitating effect on the society at large, highlights the importance of well-funded and ethical research into drug development. With changing environmental conditions and sedentary lifestyle, incidence of cardiac illnesses is expected to increase. Availability of newer agents with different pharmacokinetic and pharmacodynamic properties helps achieve better pharmacoergonomics. The authors hope that the above infographics helps the reader to get an overview of the recent advances in cardiac pharmacology, in a concise and comprehensive format. Few important take-away points are:

- Cardiovascular practice involves the utilization of a gamut of pharmacological therapies wherein the potency, efficacy, drug-drug interaction profile, and

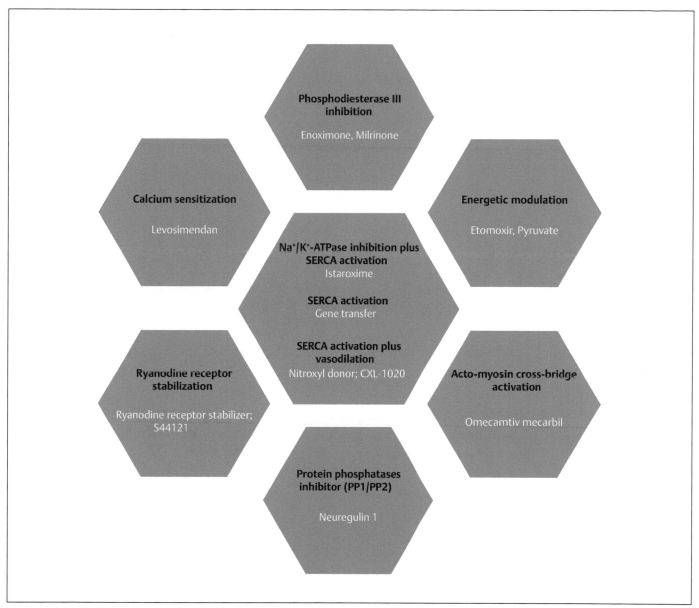

Fig. 13.9 This infographic depicts newer ionotropic agents currently in use and under trial, out of which milrinone and levosimendan are US FDA approved. Abbreviation: SERCA2a, sarco endoplasmic reticulum calcium-ATPase2a.

adverse effects need to be meticulously considered as per the underlying clinical context.

- An anesthesiologist needs to keep pace with the evolving drug developments and the concomitant drug-based recommendations in this ever-dynamic cardiovascular medicine field.

- The aforementioned can assist an anesthesiologist in staging an efficient management of challenging perioperative and intensive care clinical scenarios, which can go a long way in strengthening the formers' role as a true perioperative physician.

Azilsartan medoxomil

It is a prodrug which is hydrolyzed to Azilsartan
A selective AT1 subtype angiotensin II receptor antagonist

Not to be used with Aliskiren

The recommended initial dose in adults is 80 mg taken orally once daily

Clevidipine

Short-acting dihydropyridine calcium channel antagonist

Metabolized by plasma esterase

The initial dose of the drug is 1–2 mg/h until optimal BP reduction. The desired therapeutic response usually occurs at 4–6 mg/h

Aliskiren

Orally active potent renin inhibitor

Not to be combined with angiotensin-converting enzyme inhibitors angiotensin receptor blockers, Azilsartan

The recommended initial dose of the drug is 150 mg once daily increased up to 300 mg

Nebivolol

Third-generation beta-blocker

Has nitric oxide (NO) mediated vasodilation in addition to beta-blocking effects

Contraindicated in severe hepatic impairment

The recommended starting dose is 5 mg OD, up to a maximum dose of 40 mg/day

Under Trial Agents

Site of action	Agent
Mineralocorticoid receptor antagonist	Finerenone
Dual acting endothelin-converting enzyme–neprilysin inhibitor	Daglutril
Nitric oxide donor	Riociguat
Dopamine beta-hydroxylase inhibitor	Etamicastat
Vaccine against Angiotensin II	CYT006-AngQβ

Fig. 13.10 Infographics representing newer antihypertensive drugs with US FDA approved azilsartan (2011), clevidipine (2008), aliskiren (2007), and nebivolol (2007).

Table 13.1 List of novel therapeutics agents for dyslipidemia

Drug	Target	Effects	Indications
RGX-501	LDL receptor	Reduces LDL-C	Homozygous familial hypercholesterolemia
Mipomersen	Apolipoprotein B	Reduces LDL-C	Homozygous familial hypercholesterolemia
Inclisiran	Proprotein convertase subtilisin kexin type 9	Reduces LDL-C	Heterozygous familial hypercholesterolemia
Bempedoic acid	ATP citrate lyase	Reduces LDL-C	Hypercholesterolemia
Alipogene tiparvovec	Lipoprotein lipase	Reduces triglyceride	Familial chylomicronaemia syndrome
Pradigastat	Diacylglycerol acyltransferase 1	Reduces triglyceride	Familial chylomicronaemia syndrome
Volanesorsen	Apolipoprotein C-III	Reduces triglyceride	Familial chylomicronaemia syndrome
Lomitapide	Microsomal triglyceride transfer protein	Reduces LDL-C and triglyceride	Homozygous familial hypercholesterolemia
Gemcabene	Reduced apolipoprotein C-III mRNA expression	Reduces LDL-C and triglyceride	Hypercholesterolemia
Evinacumab	Angiopoietin-like protein 3	Reduces triglyceride, LDL-C and HDL-C	Hypercholesterolemia
Sebelipase	Lysosomal acid lipase	Reduces triglyceride, LDL-C and Liver lipids	Lysosomal acid lipase deficiency
CSL-112	Apolipoprotein A1	Raises HDL-C	Low HDL-C
ACP-501	Lecithin cholesterol acyltransferase	Raises HDL-C	Lecithin cholesterol acyltransferase deficiency
IONIS-APO(A)-Lrx	Apolipoprotein (A)	Reduces lipoprotein (A)	Elevated lipoprotein (A) levels

References

1. Magoon R, Choudhury A, Malik V, Sharma R, Kapoor PM. Pharmacological update: new drugs in cardiac practice: a critical appraisal. Ann Card Anaesth 2017;20(Supplement):S49–S56
2. Lei M, Wu L, Terrar DA, Huang CL. Modernized classification of cardiac antiarrhythmic drugs. Circulation 2018;138(17): 1879–1896
3. Ehrlich JR, Biliczki P, Hohnloser SH, Nattel S. Atrial-selective approaches for the treatment of atrial fibrillation. J Am Coll Cardiol 2008;51(8):787–792
4. Karagueuzian HS, Klein U. Wanted: class VI antiarrhythmic drug action; new start for a rational drug therapy. J Heart Health 2018;5(1): 10.16966/2379-769X.148
5. De Vecchis R, Paccone A, Di Maio M. Upstream therapy for atrial fibrillation prevention: the role of sacubitril/valsartan. Cardiol Res 2020;11(4):213–218
6. Yeh CH, Hogg K, Weitz JI. Overview of the new oral anticoagulants: opportunities and challenges. Arterioscler Thromb Vasc Biol 2015;35(5):1056–1065
7. Priyanka P, Kupec JT, Krafft M, Shah NA, Reynolds GJ. Newer oral anticoagulants in the treatment of acute portal vein thrombosis in patients with and without cirrhosis. Int J Hepatol 2018;2018:8432781
8. Yee J, Kaide CG. Emergency reversal of anticoagulation. West J Emerg Med 2019;20(5):770–783
9. Koenig-Oberhuber V, Filipovic M. New antiplatelet drugs and new oral anticoagulants. Br J Anaesth 2016;117(Suppl 2): ii74–ii84
10. Feng KY, Mahaffey KW. Cangrelor in clinical use. Future Cardiol 2020;16(2):89–102
11. Schüpke S, Hein-Rothweiler R, Mayer K, et al; ISAR-PLASTER-Trial Investigators. Revacept, a novel inhibitor of platelet adhesion, in patients undergoing elective PCI-design and rationale of the randomized ISAR-PLASTER trial. Thromb Haemost 2019;119(9):1539–1545
12. Gryka RJ, Buckley LF, Anderson SM. Vorapaxar: the current role and future directions of a novel protease-activated receptor antagonist for risk reduction in atherosclerotic disease. Drugs R D 2017;17(1):65–72
13. Badu-Boateng C, Jennings R, Hammersley D. The therapeutic role of ivabradine in heart failure. Ther Adv Chronic Dis 2018;9(11):199–207
14. Solomon SD, Vaduganathan M, Claggett B, et al. Sacubitril/Valsartan across the spectrum of ejection fraction in heart failure. Circulation 2020;141(5):352–361
15. Dodd K, Lampert BC. The use and indication of ivabradine in heart failure. Heart Fail Clin 2018;14(4):493–500
16. Fala L. Entresto (Sacubitril/Valsartan): first-in-class angiotensin receptor neprilysin inhibitor FDA approved for patients with heart failure. Am Health Drug Benefits 2015;8(6):330–334
17. Lopaschuk GD. Metabolic modulators in heart disease: past, present, and future. Can J Cardiol 2017;33(7):838–849
18. Palaniswamy C, Mellana WM, Selvaraj DR, Mohan D. Metabolic modulation: a new therapeutic target in treatment of heart failure. Am J Ther 2011;18(6):e197–e201
19. Ylä-Herttuala S, Baker AH. Cardiovascular gene therapy: past, present, and future. Mol Ther 2017;25(5):1095–1106

20. Deng J, Guo M, Li G, Xiao J. Gene therapy for cardiovascular diseases in China: basic research. Gene Ther 2020;27(7-8):360–369

21. Donahue JK. Cardiac gene therapy: a call for basic methods development. Lancet 2016;387(10024):1137–1139

22. Bedan M, Grimm D, Wehland M, Simonsen U, Infanger M, Krüger M. A focus on macitentan in the treatment of pulmonary arterial hypertension. Basic Clin Pharmacol Toxicol 2018;123(2):103–113

23. Khaybullina D, Patel A, Zerilli T. Riociguat (adempas): a novel agent for the treatment of pulmonary arterial hypertension and chronic thromboembolic pulmonary hypertension. P&T 2014;39(11):749–758

24. Sitbon O, Gomberg-Maitland M, Granton J, et al. Clinical trial design and new therapies for pulmonary arterial hypertension. Eur Respir J 2019;53(1):1801908

25. Kurutas EB. The importance of antioxidants which play the role in cellular response against oxidative/nitrosative stress: current state. Nutr J 2016;15(1):71

26. Zakkar M, Guida G, Suleiman MS, Angelini CD. Cardiopulmonary bypass and oxidative stress. Oxid Med Cell Longev 2015;2015:189863

27. Farías JG, Molina VM, Carrasco RA, et al. Antioxidant therapeutic strategies for cardiovascular conditions associated with oxidative stress. Nutrients 2017;9(9):966

28. Long L, Zhao HT, Shen LM, He C, Ren S, Zhao HL. Hemodynamic effects of inotropic drugs in heart failure: a network meta-analysis of clinical trials. Medicine (Baltimore) 2019;98(47):e18144

29. Psotka MA, Gottlieb SS, Francis GS, et al. Cardiac calcitropes, myotropes, and mitotropes: JACC review topic of the week. J Am Coll Cardiol 2019;73(18):2345–2353

30. Bistola V, Arfaras-Melainis A, Polyzogopoulou E, Ikonomidis I, Parissis J. Inotropes in acute heart failure: from guidelines to practical use: therapeutic options and clinical practice. Card Fail Rev 2019;5(3):133–139

31. Alviar CL, Gutierrez A, Cho L, et al. Clevidipine as a therapeutic and cost-effective alternative to sodium nitroprusside in patients with acute aortic syndromes. Eur Heart J Acute Cardiovasc Care 2020;9(3_suppl):S5–S12

32. Ferdinand KC, Balavoine F, Besse B, et al. Efficacy and safety of firibastat, a first-in-class brain aminopeptidase A inhibitor, in hypertensive overweight patients of multiple ethnic origins. Circulation 2019;140(2):138–146

33. Samuelsson O, Herlitz H. Vaccination against high blood pressure: a new strategy. Lancet 2008;371(9615):788–789

34. Wong D, Tsai PNW, Ip KY, Irwin MG. New antihypertensive medications and clinical implications. Best Pract Res Clin Anaesthesiol 2018;32(2):223–235

35. Hegele RA, Tsimikas S. Lipid-lowering agents. Circ Res 2019;124(3):386–404

36. Rosenson RS, Brewer HB Jr, Barter PJ, et al. HDL and atherosclerotic cardiovascular disease: genetic insights into complex biology. Nat Rev Cardiol 2018;15(1):9–19

37. Chaudhary R, Garg J, Shah N, Sumner A. PCSK9 inhibitors: a new era of lipid lowering therapy. World J Cardiol 2017;9(2):76–91

14

Recent Advances in the Pharmacological Management of Pulmonary Hypertension

Ramesh Chand Kashav, Iti Shri, Souvik Dey, and Poonam Malhotra Kapoor

- ➢ Definition
- ➢ Conventional Pharmacological Agents for Treating PH
- ➢ Recent Advances with Selective Pulmonary Vasodilators
- ➢ Conclusion

Definition

Pulmonary hypertension (PH) is defined by a mean pulmonary arterial pressure (PAP) ≥20 mmHg at rest in the presence of pulmonary capillary wedge pressure ≤15 mmHg as measured during right heart catheterization.[1] Comprehensive classification of PH by WHO is provided in **Box 14.1** while **Table 14.1** lists the updated definitions of 6th world symposium on PH. The comparative analysis of precapillary and postcapillary hypertension, keeping in mind, the right atrium and right ventricle size with the pulmonary capillary wedge pressure as well is provided in **Table 14.2**. **Flowchart 14.1** provides a detailed sequence of events constituting the pathophysiology of PH.

Box 14.1 Comprehensive clinical classification of pulmonary hypertension (PH) (WHO)

- Group 1: Pulmonary arterial hypertension
- Group 2: PH due to left-sided heart disease
- Group 3: PH due to lung disease and/or hypoxia
- Group 4: Chronic thromboembolic PH and other pulmonary artery obstructions
- Group 5: PH due to unclear and/or multifactorial etiology

Conventional Pharmacological Agents for Treating PH

- **Calcium channel blockers:** Can be efficacious only in idiopathic pulmonary arterial hypertension (PAH) patients with positive vasoreactivity test (defined by a decrease of at least 10 mmHg or an absolute value of 40 mmHg or less for mean PAP with preserved or increased cardiac output). Longer acting agents like nifedipine, amlodipine, and diltiazem have been used with variable success (<7% chronic responders).[2] Verapamil should not be given due to its negative inotropic effect.
- **Phosphodiesterase inhibitors:** This group of drugs acts by inhibiting phosphodiesterase (PDE) group of enzymes (hence, half-life of cyclic guanosine monophosphate [cGMP] is increased promoting vasodilation). PDE type 5 enzymes are exclusively present in the vascular endothelium of lung. Sildenafil, the prototype PDE5 selective inhibitor, has been used orally and found to improve functional class of the patients with improved 6 minutes walking (6MW) distance in PH. The current FDA recommendation approves 20 mg thrice a day oral dose. An intravenous preparation with a recommended dose of 1.6 mg/kg/d is also

Table 14.1 Sixth World Symposium on PH (Nice, France 2018) updated definitions[1]

Characteristics	Mean PAP	PVR	PAWP
Precapillary PH (primarily pulmonary arterial hypertension)	>20 mmHg	≥3 woods unit	≤15 mmHg
Isolated postcapillary PH (pulmonary venous hypertension, e.g., left heart disease)	>20 mmHg	<3 woods unit	>15 mmHg
Combined pre- and postcapillary PH	>20 mmHg	≥3 woods unit	>15 mmHg

Abbreviations: PAP, pulmonary arterial pressure; PAWP, pulmonary artery wedge pressure; PH, pulmonary hypertension; PVR, pulmonary vascular resistance.

Table 14.2 Comparison between precapillary and postcapillary PH[2]

Parameters	Precapillary hypertension	Postcapillary hypertension
Right ventricle size	Increased	Normal/increased
Right atrium: left atrium size ratio	<1	>1
Interatrial septum	Shifted to left	Shifted to left
RVOT notching	Common	Rare
Lateral E/e'	<8	>10
PCWP	≤15 mmHg	>15 mmHg
DPG = PADP-PCWP	>7 mmHg	<5 mmHg

Abbreviations: DPG, diastolic pressure gradient; PADP, pulmonary arterial diastolic pressure; PCWP, pulmonary capillary wedge pressure; PH, pulmonary hypertension; RVOT, right ventricular outflow tract.

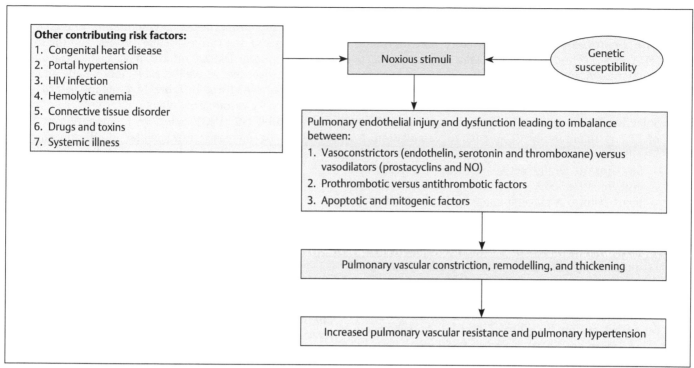

Flowchart 14.1 Pathophysiology of pulmonary hypertension. Abbreviations: HIV, human Immune deficiency virus; NO, nitric oxide.

available.[3] Milrinone, an inodilator, acts by inhibiting PDE type 3 (promoting intracellular cyclic adenosine monophosphate [cAMP]) in cardiac myocytes and vascular smooth muscle cells. Increased cAMP in cardiac myocytes causes positive inotropy, lusitropy, bathmotropy, and chronotropy and causes smooth muscle relaxation in the vascular bed. Milrinone is used in intravenous infusion with loading dose of 50 µg/kg over 10 minutes followed by infusion at the rate of 0.375 to 0.75 µg/kg/min.

- **Inodilators:** For example, dobutamine, a synthetic catecholamine, with partial β-agonist activity. It has both inotropic (mediated by β_1-agonist property) and vasodilation (mediated by β_2-agonist property; pulmonary > systemic = milrinone > dobutamine) properties, and hence the name "inodilator." Dobutamine is given at a continuous infusion rate of 2 to 10 µg/kg/min intravenously.
- **Vasodilators:** Nitroglycerine given at the rate of 0.5 to 20 µg/kg/min intravenously effectively reduces PAP by promoting nitric oxide (NO)-mediated vasodilation.
- **Prostaglandin:** Epoprostenol intravenous infusion at 25 to 40 ng/kg/min rate is also effective. Unstable preparation, relatively short half life (3 6 min) necessitating continuous administration, and uncertainty of the amount of drug delivered to the lung limit the routine use of the drug.[4]
- **Endothelin receptor antagonist:** Bosentan, an orally active endothelin-1 receptor antagonist, has

been widely used in various subgroup of population including congenital systemic-pulmonary shunt and Eisenmenger physiology. An improved hemodynamics, 6MW distance, and functional class were noted without any change in oxygen saturation level.[5] Hepatic derangement is the primary concern and liver function test should be periodically done during the treatment. Other important side effects include headache, anemia, and peripheral edema.

- Other than individual drug side effects, the main disadvantage of the above-mentioned pharmacological agents is the nonspecificity of the drugs with systemic adverse effects including hypotension, drop in oxygen saturation, etc.

Recent Advances with Selective Pulmonary Vasodilators

1. At present three pathways are targeted for pharmacological treatment of the PH as depicted in **endothelin (ET) pathway:** There are two receptors for ET1:
- ET_A receptor which is present on vascular smooth muscle, heart, kidney, and lung and has vasoconstrictor, mitogenic, and fibrogenic effects.
- ET_B receptor which is present on vascular smooth muscle (same as ET_A) and vascular endothelium (causes NO-mediated vasodilation).

- ET$_A$ and ET$_B$ dual receptor antagonists, for example, macitentan. This has been studied in a phase III trial with improved long-term morbidity and mortality (FDA 2013). Three-mg and 10-mg doses have also been studied. Important side effects include anemia, bronchitis, nasopharyngitis, urinary infection, and headache.[6]
- Selective ET$_A$ antagonists block vasoconstrictive effect of ET$_A$ by maintaining ET$_B$-mediated vasodilation. A few examples are:
  - ➤ **Sitaxentan:** Orally active selective ET$_A$ receptor antagonist (6500:1) used in PAH and congestive heart failure. A placebo controlled trial (STRIDE I) with 100- and 300-mg dosage (half-life 6–7 h) demonstrated improved 6MW distance, NYHA class, and hemodynamics. Important side effects include hepatic derangements, headache, peripheral edema, nausea, and nasal congestion. It can interact with warfarin dosing. It was withdrawn from the market due to associated liver toxicity.
  - ➤ **Ambrisentan:** The phase III trial demonstrated an improved 6MW distance and longer time to clinical worsening. FDA (2007) requires no longer periodic monitoring of liver function tests like in case of bosentan once daily dose as the half life of Ambrisentan is 9 to 5 hours (half-life 9–15 h). Other side effects include headache and lower extremity edema (age > 65 y).[7]

2. Prostacyclin pathway:[8] Most therapies for management of PH, using the prostacyclin pathway, have so far only been given by the inhaled route or as subcutaneous infusions. Oral therapy is in vogue today, as it is more convenient and can be started at an early stage of the disease (**Table 14.3**).

3. Nitric oxide (NO) pathway: Nitric oxide has intense anti-inflammatory properties and vasodilating effects on the gastric mucosa, the cardiovascular system, and the musculoskeletal system. Dietary nitrates have a beneficial effect in metabolic disorders as well as have antidiabetic and antilipemic effects. As listed in **Table 14.4**, the inhaled NO (iNO) has pulmonary vasodilatory effects.

- **Inhaled NO (iNO):** Selective pulmonary vasodilator acts by increased intracellular cGMP concentration causing vasodilation. It is used in a closed circuit with continuous patient site concentration monitoring at a dose of 8 to 20 ppm usually. Major indications include persistent pulmonary hypertension (PPHN), acute respiratory distress syndrome (ARDS), post-CPB (cardiopulmonary bypass) PH crisis, etc. **Table 14.4** provides a comparative analysis between iNO and other inhaled pharmacological agents.
- **PDE type 5 inhibitor:** Verdenafil, tadalafil.

A drug that blocks one or more of the five subtypes of the enzyme phosphodiester (PDE), thus preventing the inactivation of the intracellular second messengers, cAMP and cGMP, by the respective PDE subtypes. **Table 14.5** lists a few PDE5 molecules, which help in PH treatment.

- Other investigational approaches:
  - ➤ GENE therapy: COXAGEN—cyclooxygenase gene formulated with cationic lipid encoded in a plasmid vector and delivered to lung via aerosol administration—acts via increasing prostanoids and decreased pulmonary vascular reactivity. Effect lasts for a week after administration. Preclinical stage.
  - ➤ End products of endogenous NO metabolism, nitrate (NO_2^-) and nitrite (NO_3^-) ions can be recycled to reproduce NO in hypoxic state and catalyzed

Table 14.3   Comparison of inhalational, subcutaneous, and oral prostacyclin analogues

Drugs	Iloprost	Treprostinil[9]	Selexipag[10]
MOA	Prostacyclin analogue	Prostacyclin analogue	Prostacyclin receptor agonist
Route	Inhalation	Subcutaneous/intravenous infusion (Remodulin); oral (Orenitram), inhalation (Tyvaso)	Oral selexipag
Dose	2.5–5 µg/dose, 6–9 inhalations/d, 8–10 min each	3 breaths 18 µg/session, 6 hourly	200 µg BD weekly to 1600 µg BD
Half-life	20–30 min	4 h	0.7–2.3 h
Indication	WHO class III & IV patients with PH	PH	PH
Trial		TRIUMPH FREEDOM C	GRIPHON
Side effects	Cough, headache, flushing, and jaw pain	Cough, headache, flushing, throat irritation	Headache, flushing, jaw pain, nausea, diarrhea, myalgia

Abbreviations: MOA, mode of action; PH, pulmonary hypertension.

Table 14.4 Comparison between iNO and other inhaled pharmacological agents

Criteria	iNO	Other inhaled pharmacological agents
Approval status by regulatory bodies	Approved by many	Approval for only iloprost and treprostinil is available
Drug delivery	Continuous inhalation with closed loop feedback system; closed circuit with mechanical ventilation is mandatory	Nebulization with frequent bolus administration or continuous administration
Disadvantages and potential risks	• Rebound PH with abrupt cessation, transiently increases ET1 levels. Therefore, adding sildenafil an hour before discontinuation of iNO prevents rebound PH by sustaining cGMP levels • Risk of NO_2 built up requires high gas flow >6 L/min and lowest possible FiO_2 • Requires closed circuit with continuous monitoring: anesthetic gases may alter the measured NO value • Risk of methemoglobinemia	• Rebound PH possible with short-acting agents • Accidental intravenous administration is harmful • May cause sticking of ventilator valves due to additive agents • Jet nebulizer requires high oxygen flow • Tipping of the nebulization chamber can cause accidental administration of high dose
Cost	Expensive delivery system and cost of the cylinder	Cost of the ultrasonic/jet nebulizer and drugs are comparatively lower than iNO

Abbreviations: cGMP, cyclic guanosine monophosphate; ET, endothelin; iNO, inhaled nitric oxide; PH, pulmonary hypertension.

Table 14.5 Soluble guanylate cyclase (sGC) stimulant: riociguat

Drugs	Tadalafil[11]	Riociguat[12]
MOA	PDE5 inhibitor	sGC stimulator
Route	Oral	Oral
Dose	40 mg/d, single daily dosing	1–2.5 mg thrice daily dosing
Indication	PAH	PAH and CTEPH
Trial	PHIRST	Chest-1 CTEPH Patent-1 PAH
Side effects	Headache, dyspepsia, myalgia, nausea, back pain, nasopharyngitis	Headache, dizziness, dyspepsia/gastritis, nausea, diarrhea, and hypotension
FDA approval	2009	2013

Abbreviations: CTEPH, chronic thromboembolic pulmonary hypertension; MOA, mode of action; PAH, pulmonary arterial hypertension; PDE, phosphodiesterase.

by deoxyhemoglobin, deoxymyoglobin, and xanthine oxidoreductase. Therapeutic use of inorganic anions (mentioned above) is still in investigational stage with promising results in animal models. Apart from inorganic nitrite anions, amyl nitrite, an alkyl nitrite, was historically used as a bedside tool to differentiate between the murmur of mitral stenosis and mitral regurgitation. In an animal study, use of amyl nitrite has demonstrated promising results with significant reduction in mean PAP and pulmonary vascular resistance (PVR). Another small human study involving newborn patients with PH depicted significant improvement in hemodynamics with inhaled ethyl nitrite.

➤ Inhaled PDE3 inhibitor, milrinone, has been demonstrated to be efficacious to reduce mean PAP, PVR, transpulmonary gradient, and PVR/SVR ratio in perioperative settings at a concentration of 1 mg/mL. It also has a synergistic role when coadministered with inhaled prostacyclin analogues.

Conclusion

We cannot ignore the fact that there are still multiple challenges associated with PHTN management. One of the important aspects is PHTN in patients with connective tissue disorders. The diagnosis and treatment for these groups of these patients are challenging most of the time. The reasons are patients may present with multiple systemic involvement and symptoms, patients may develop different classes of PHTN simultaneously, and finding a guideline for treating these patients is often difficult. Managing patients with PHTN is always challenging. But there are already different options available for the treatment of PHTN. Various newer studies are awaiting to show the potential therapeutic benefit of the new drugs/molecules in the management of the PHTN.[13,14]

References

1. Simonneau G, Montani D, Celermajer DS, et al. Haemodynamic definitions and updated clinical classification of pulmonary hypertension. Eur Respir J 2019;53(1):1801913

2. Mclaughlin VV, Humbert M. Pulmonary hypertension. In: Zipes DP, Libby P, Bonow RO, Mann DL, Tomaselli GF, Braunwald E, eds. Braunwald's heart disease: a textbook of cardiovascular medicine. 11th ed. Elsevier Inc.; 2019:1699–1718

3. Buck ML. Sildenafil for the treatment of pulmonary hypertension in children. Pediatr Pharm 2004;10:2

4. Barst RJ, Rubin LJ, Long WA, et al; Primary Pulmonary Hypertension Study Group. A comparison of continuous intravenous epoprostenol (prostacyclin) with conventional therapy for primary pulmonary hypertension. N Engl J Med 1996;334(5):296–301

5. Rubin LJ, Badesch DB, Barst RJ, et al. Bosentan therapy for pulmonary arterial hypertension. N Engl J Med 2002;346(12):896–903

6. Pulido T, Adzerikho I, Channick RN, et al; SERAPHIN Investigators. Macitentan and morbidity and mortality in pulmonary arterial hypertension. N Engl J Med 2013;369(9):809–818

7. Galiè N, Olschewski H, Oudiz RJ, et al; Ambrisentan in Pulmonary Arterial Hypertension, Randomized, Double-Blind, Placebo-Controlled, Multicenter, Efficacy Studies (ARIES) Group. Ambrisentan for the treatment of pulmonary arterial hypertension: results of the ambrisentan in pulmonary arterial hypertension, randomized, double-blind, placebo-controlled, multicenter, efficacy (ARIES) study 1 and 2. Circulation 2008;117(23):3010–3019

8. Magoon R, Choudhury A, Malik V, Sharma R, Kapoor PM. Pharmacological update: new drugs in cardiac practice: a critical appraisal. Ann Card Anaesth 2017;20(Suppl):S49–S56

9. McLaughlin VV, Benza RL, Rubin LJ, et al. Addition of inhaled treprostinil to oral therapy for pulmonary arterial hypertension: a randomized controlled clinical trial. J Am Coll Cardiol 2010;55(18):1915–1922

10. Simonneau G, Torbicki A, Hoeper MM, et al. Selexipag: an oral, selective prostacyclin receptor agonist for the treatment of pulmonary arterial hypertension. Eur Respir J 2012;40(4):874–880

11. Galiè N, Brundage BH, Ghofrani HA, et al; Pulmonary Arterial Hypertension and Response to Tadalafil (PHIRST) Study Group. Tadalafil therapy for pulmonary arterial hypertension. Circulation 2009;119(22):2894–2903

12. Ghofrani HA, Galiè N, Grimminger F, et al; PATENT-1 Study Group. Riociguat for the treatment of pulmonary arterial hypertension. N Engl J Med 2013;369(4):330–340

13. Tudoran C, Tudoran M, Lazureanu VE. Evidence of pulmonary hypertension afterSARS-CoV-2 infection in subjects without previous significant cardiovascular pathology. J Clin Med 2021;10:199

14. Hajraa A, Safiriyua I, Balasubramaniana P, et al. Recent Advances and Future Prospects of Treatment of Pulmonary Hypertension. Curr Probl Cardiol 2022;00:101236

15

Surgical Treatment of Pulmonary Hypertension

Julius Punnen, Devi Prasad Shetty, Varun Shetty, Hema C. Nair, and Bahsa J. Khan

Introduction

Pulmonary hypertension (PH) is not a pleasant condition for surgeons, and in general, PH becomes a contraindication to many operations, or it makes the operation a lot more complex. The increased morbidity and mortality that PH causes and the additional requirement of monitoring using a pulmonary artery catheter makes many people uncomfortable with PH of any cause. However, there are some situations where PH itself is amenable to surgical cure or surgical palliation. Many of the diseases classified under the WHO Group IV at the 6th World Symposium on Pulmonary Hypertension (WSPH) held at Nice in 2018[1] including chronic thromboembolic pulmonary hypertension (CTEPH) and other pulmonary artery obstructions such as malignant or nonmalignant tumors, congenital pulmonary artery stenosis, and parasitosis will require surgical intervention as a diagnostic, therapeutic, or palliative procedure. Besides, these surgical or interventional palliative procedures such as the reversed Potts shunt or atrial septostomy have a beneficial effect on right-ventricular (RV) failure and prevention of sudden death in other WHO PH groups as well. Reversed Pott's shunt has been given an IIb class of recommendation as destination therapy or as bridge to bilateral lung transplantation in children with end-stage pulmonary artery hypertension (PAH).[2] Finally, lung transplantation or combined heart-lung transplantation is also to be mentioned as surgical treatment for PH. For the purpose of this chapter, the discussion will be limited to aspects of CTEPH.

Definitions

CTEPH is a form of precapillary pulmonary hypertension; it is a complication of acute pulmonary embolism that occurs in approximately 3.5% of patients who develop acute pulmonary embolism.[3] The 2015 European Respiratory Society (ERS)/European Society of Cardiology (ESC) guidelines for the diagnosis and treatment of pulmonary hypertension stated, "The diagnosis of CTEPH is based on findings obtained after at least 3 months of effective anticoagulation in order to discriminate this condition from subacute PE. These findings are mean pulmonary artery pressure (mPAP) >/= 25 mm Hg with pulmonary artery wedge pressure (PAWP) </= 15 mm Hg, mismatched perfusion defects on lung scan, and specific diagnostic signs for CTEPH seen by multidetector CT angiography, MR imaging, or conventional pulmonary cine angiography, such as ring-like stenoses, webs/slits, and chronic total occlusions (pouch lesions or tapered lesions)."[4] Some patients may have similar perfusion defects and symptoms but show no PH. This condition was referred to as chronic thromboembolic disease (CTED).[5] Since this definition, the threshold of mPAP for diagnosis of PH has been revised. In 1961, a report by the WHO Expert Committee on chronic cor pulmonale mentioned that the mPAP doesn't normally exceed 15 mm Hg and is not affected by age and never exceeds 20 mm Hg.[6] The first WSPH held in Geneva in 1973, organized by WHO[7] defined PH as mPAP of =/>25 mm Hg measured by right heart catheterization (RHC) at rest, in supine position. This definition was empirical and defined arbitrarily. In 2009,[8] data from 1187 normal subjects were analyzed from 47 studies. The mPAP at rest was found to be 14.0 +/- 3.3 mm Hg. This mPAP of 14 mm Hg and two standard deviations above this as the upper limit of normally raised mPAP above 20 mm Hg were taken as cutoff values to define pulmonary hypertension, and this is no longer arbitrary since there is scientific reasoning to it. For defining precapillary pulmonary hypertension hemodynamically the 6th WSPH also made the requirement of having a PAWP of </= 15 mm Hg and a pulmonary vascular resistance (PVR) of 3 woods units (WU).[1] The PVR threshold was further revised to 2 WU in the 2022 ESC/ERS Guidelines for the diagnosis and treatment of pulmonary hypertension.[9] The European Respiratory Society in its statement on CTEPH in 2021 proposed the term "chronic thromboembolic pulmonary diseases (CTEPD)" to include all symptomatic patients with or without PH having this disease. The term "CTEPH" was maintained for those who have PH at rest. PH in this setting can be from proximal organized thrombotic obstruction, which can also be due to secondary microangiopathy affecting vessels smaller than 500 micrometres.[10]

Diagnosis

Among the various etiologies of pulmonary hypertension, CTEPH is the only condition that has a curative treatment option, though it may be debatable if one is entirely cured of this disease with treatment. Therefore, it is important to establish the correct diagnosis in this group of patients who have pulmonary hypertension. Patients may present with exercise intolerance, shortness of breath, signs and symptoms of right heart failure. The diagnosis of pulmonary hypertension is usually first made on echocardiography showing raised systolic pulmonary artery pressure (sPAP). In the evaluation and categorization of PH, usually the first diagnostic test aimed at excluding or confirming CTEPH would be a ventilation-perfusion scan (V/Q). A negative V/Q scan effectively rules out a diagnosis of CTEPH; therefore, as a screening tool, it remains the most effective method of imaging. A high-quality computed tomography (CT) pulmonary angiogram (CTPA) is also quite good at diagnosing CTEPH; however, it should be kept in mind that a negative CTPA does not completely exclude CTEPH as very distal disease can be missed by conventional CTPA. Though dual-energy CT and magnetic resonance imaging (MRI) can also be useful screening tools with some advantages, they do not replace V/Q scan in today's clinical practice.[10]

Echocardiography

Besides being the usual modality for the first diagnosis of PH, it can also look for the structure and function of the heart that is relevant to PH. The commoner cause of PH is left heart disease, and echocardiography can diagnose this with good specificity. Echo also helps to determine the function of the right heart and the degree of tricuspid regurgitation (TR). Though the fibrous clots in the pulmonary arteries are rarely seen on echo, clots in the right-sided cardiac chambers can be demonstrated.

Computed Tomography Pulmonary Angiogram

It is the go-to imaging modality in most centers and might replace angiogram to assess operability and define the disease anatomically to provide a roadmap for pulmonary thromboendarterectomy (PTE). Besides the anatomical definition, CT also demonstrates the condition of the lung parenchyma and the presence or absence of systemic–pulmonary collaterals. These collaterals are an important determinant of operability and can help to distinguish from WHO Group 1 PH with in situ thrombosis. The collateral flow can be up to 30% of the systemic blood flow in CTEPH but rarely exceeds 1% of systemic blood flow in WHO Group I PH.[11,12] CT is also helpful to differentiate CTEPH from other conditions that may mimic it, such as pulmonary artery sarcoma, vasculitis, fibrosing mediastinitis, and as mentioned earlier in situ thrombosis.

Magnetic Resonance Angiography

Magnetic resonance angiography (MRA) when used with maximum intensity projection (MIP) can demonstrate the pulmonary arteries well. In addition, MR has the advantage of being able to assess the function of the right ventricle and perfusion in the lungs. It is also useful as a follow-up tool following surgical or interventional therapy.

Cardiac Catheterization and Catheter-Based Angiography

In most CTEPH centers all the patients undergo cardiac catheterization before undergoing treatment for the disease. Right heart catheterization (RHC) is done and all the hemodynamic measurements are obtained. The mPAP and PVR are determined only on RHC. Echo estimates of sPAP can be inaccurate in this setting; mPAP and PVR and PAWP which are required for defining and categorizing PH are available only through RHC. It should be remembered that measurement of PAWP may not always be accurate in CTEPH due

to obstruction of the pulmonary arteries. In order to rule out left heart disease, left ventricular end-diastolic pressure may need to be measured. Historically, catheter-based angiography was used as the roadmap for surgical PTE, though currently, some centers use CTPA for that purpose; digital subtraction angiography is also a good alternative, and some consider it to be the gold standard in CTEPH imaging. Additional dye injections are done in the coronary arteries, bilateral internal mammary arteries, and the descending thoracic aorta to look for and demonstrate systemic–pulmonary collaterals and to rule out coronary artery disease. During the capillary phase of the pulmonary angiogram, poor subpleural perfusion may indicate small vessel disease and therefore increased mortality.[13] In the setting of balloon pulmonary angioplasty (BPA), the lesions in CTEPH were classified by the lesion morphology as type A through E, ring-like lesion was called type A, web lesions type B, subtotal and total occlusions types C and D, respectively, and a tortuous lesion was described as type E.[14] Advanced imaging combined with high computing power has led to the application of artificial intelligence in image analysis using machine learning. A model has been developed to better predict patient outcomes in various PH groups including CTEPH.[15,16] This will be a space to watch for in the next decade, particularly if quantum computing becomes more accessible and is used more widely in healthcare analytics. At the moment, it is difficult to predict accurately which patients have significant microvascular disease in addition to surgically accessible obstructive disease (**Fig. 15.1**).

A multidisciplinary team consisting of cardiologists preferably those who have the ability to perform BPA, PH specialist pulmonologists, cardiac imaging specialists, and an experienced PEA surgeon should review the patient data and imaging in detail and make an individualized plan for each patient which may include surgical, interventional, medical, or a combination of various modalities whichever is appropriate for the given patient.

Patients with no history of deep vein thrombosis (DVT), having signs of right heart failure, in functional class IV, having no disease appreciable in the lower lobes, and showing inconsistencies on various imaging modalities, particularly if PVR is >15 WU and out of proportion to the amount of obstruction seen on imaging and having high PA diastolic pressure, are thought to be a high-risk group.[5]

The University of California San Diego (UCSD) group has proposed a surgical classification based on the level where the disease starts with level 1 starting in the main pulmonary arteries, level 2 at the level of the lobar, level 3 (**Fig. 15.2**) at segmental level, and level 4 at subsegmental level. Level 1C refers to complete obstruction of one of the branch of pulmonary arteries (**Fig. 15.3**) and level 0 refers to having no thromboembolic disease in either lung.

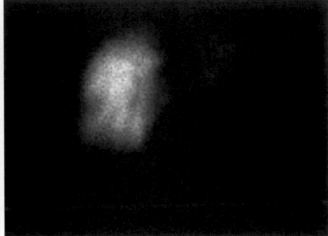

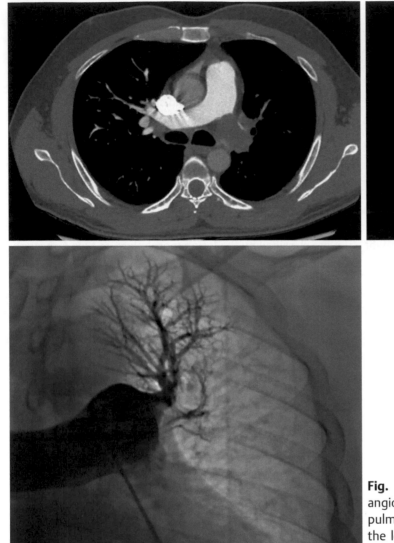

Fig. 15.1 Computed tomography (CT) pulmonary angiogram, ventilation perfusion scan, and catheter pulmonary angiogram showing complete occlusion of the left pulmonary artery showing correlation between all imaging modalities.

Treatment

General Treatment

All patients who have been diagnosed to have CTEPH should be on lifelong anticoagulation. This has been traditionally done with Vitamin K antagonists (VKA); however, novel oral anticoagulants (NOACs) are increasingly replacing VKA, though most CTEPH centers continue to use VKA. NOACs are not recommended for use in patients who have antiphospholipid antibody.[17] If the patient is hypoxic, oxygen supplementation may be required and those with right heart failure may need diuretics.

Pulmonary Thromboendarterectomy/ Pulmonary Endarterectomy

The treatment of choice for CTEPH is pulmonary endarterectomy (PEA), also called pulmonary thromboendarterectomy

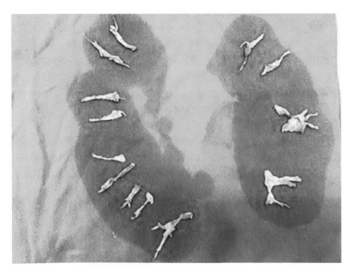

Fig. 15.2 Pulmonary thromboendarterectomy (PTE) specimen showing level 3 disease commencing at segmental level extending distally.

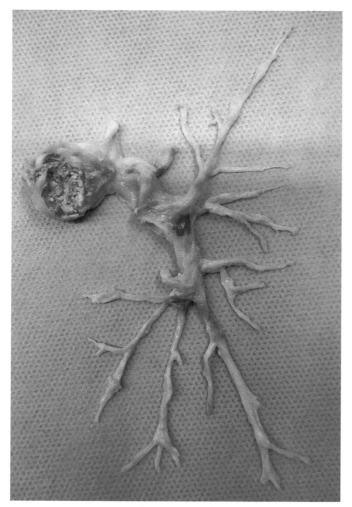

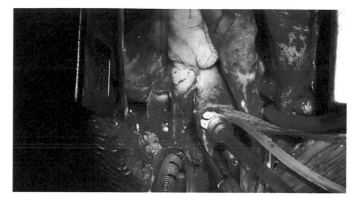

Fig. 15.4 Bubbles seen in the open pulmonary artery on ventilating, indicating a breach of the blood–air barrier during endarterectomy.

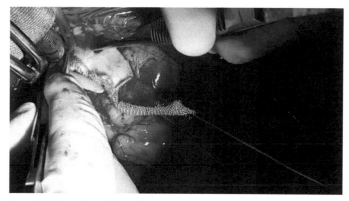

Fig. 15.5 After identifying the subsegmental artery from where air bubbles are coming, a long strip of Surgicel is used to plug the injured vessel.

Fig. 15.3 Pulmonary thromboendarterectomy (PTE) specimen showing complete obstruction of the left pulmonary artery with calcification. The fibrous clots extend distally into the subsegmental level but since the disease commences at the level of the left pulmonary artery it is level 1 and as it causes complete obstruction it is level 1C.

(PTE). Other treatment modalities are only offered to those who cannot be offered PTE. Data published by an international registry showed a survival advantage for operated patients, with 90% 3-year survival in operated patients compared to 70% in nonoperated patients.[18] The importance of the assessment of operability, preferably by a multidisciplinary team, cannot be overemphasized.

Patients who have severe parenchymal lung diseases such as emphysema or destroyed lungs from previous infections, do not benefit from PTE and that would represent a contraindication. Caution is also advised in patients who have severe left ventricular dysfunction, since the increase in the return to the left artery following PTE may put additional strain on an already dysfunctional left ventricle. Contrary to popular belief, there is no upper limit to the PVR of patients who may be accepted for surgery, but patients with PVR exceeding

12.5 WU may have a higher surgical risk, although the gain from surgery is also high in patients with high PVR.[19] If the patient requires any concomitant cardiac surgery, live coronary artery bypass grafts, or heart valve surgery, they can be combined without much additional risk. Most patients who undergo PTE have severe TR; this need not be addressed in the absence of organic tricuspid valve disease, since the TR will improve once the PAP normalizes.

The operation is usually done through a median sternotomy, though a minimally invasive approach is done in highly selected cases in some very experienced centers, particularly when one is absolutely certain that the disease is entirely unilateral. Cardiopulmonary bypass is established with superior and inferior vena cava cannulas for drainage and ascending aortic cannula for arterial return. The patient is cooled to 18°C in preparation for deep hypothermic total circulatory arrest. The left heart is vented adequately to prevent distention of the left ventricle; authors use vents in the left superior pulmonary vein, pulmonary arteries, and the left ventricular apex. Aortic cross-clamp may be applied, and myocardial protection achieved by a combination of hypothermia and intermittent cardioplegia delivery as appropriate; alternatively aortic cross-clamp may be avoided with diligent de-airing at the commencement of circulation each time. During this period any concomitant procedures that may be required can be performed. The PEA is performed through incisions in the intrapericardial portions of the left and right branch pulmonary arteries sequentially. This being a bilateral disease, bilateral endarterectomy will be required generally. A critical step in the operation is to identify and raise the correct plane of dissection carefully, the site of which depends on the level of the disease as described earlier. Once the plane is identified, the fibrous clots are held, and the pulmonary artery wall is gently dissected away from the fibrous clot circumferentially. This part of the dissection is done on total circulatory arrest; if the requirement of the arrest period exceeds 20 minutes a period of reperfusion of 10 minutes is done.

The most important step in the operation is to trace all the distal tail ends and remove them completely to remove the obstruction in the pulmonary arteries. Usually, a period of 20 minutes for each side would suffice; sometimes more than one 20-minute period is needed, particularly when the disease is very distal. Once the fibrous clots are removed, the pulmonary artery is filled with saline and the lung is inflated fully, and the artery is inspected for bubbles of air indicating a breach of the blood–air barrier by damage to the pulmonary artery (**Fig. 15.4**). In case such a breach is detected, the injured segmental/sub-segmental branch is identified and plugged[20] with Surgicel (**Fig. 15.5**) or occluded with glue. Several other techniques and algorithms are reported to prevent/manage catastrophic bleeding following PEA. The endarterectomy is always done bilaterally in a sequential manner. After completion of the endarterectomy, the pulmonary artery is closed, and the patient is fully rewarmed and separated from cardiopulmonary bypass.

A continuous cardiac output catheter, pulmonary artery catheter, is floated into the pulmonary artery either in the beginning of the operation or later on. This will give good guidance for the appropriate use of vasoactive medications. The usual drips to start with would be dopamine and noradrenaline, though milrinone has a beneficial effect on the right ventricle and pulmonary vasculature, due to its inodilator effect. If the cardiac index goes up very high, one aims to keep the cardiac index at around 2.5 L/min/m². A higher cardiac index may result in reperfusion pulmonary edema. In a hypertrophied right ventricle like the one in CTEPH patients, the coronary blood flow is predominant during diastole, unlike a normal right ventricle where the coronary flow occurs during systole and diastole. Therefore, it is important to maintain adequate diastolic pressure by maintaining adequate systemic vascular resistance (SVR). A low SVR also results in a "steal" from the right coronary artery among other undesirable effects.

Complications

There are some specific complications that may occur following this operation. RV failure following surgery manifests as low PAP and a high central venous pressure and RV contractility can be seen to be low on direct inspection and on transesophageal echocardiography. Appropriate inotropic therapy including use of milrinone may help if the dysfunction is not severe; in severe dysfunction early institution of extracorporeal life support is indicated. Early reperfusion edema may manifest as hypoxia with a low pulmonary flow (PF) ratio. Early initiation of extracorporeal membrane oxygenation (ECMO) would be indicated in this situation as well. Airway bleeding is a very important and life-threatening complication of this operation. This may occur either from a breach in the blood–air barrier from surgical injury to a pulmonary artery branch during endarterectomy or from the systemic to pulmonary collaterals bleeding into the parenchyma. The first thing to be attended to in this situation is to prevent soiling of the contralateral lung. Detection and prevention of airway hemorrhage from surgical injury were described earlier, Kanchi et al[11] have published details of managing airway bleeds of various kinds. Bleeding from collaterals may resolve once the antegrade flow through native pulmonary arteries are re-established. One may need to use ECMO for oxygenation, neutralize the heparin completely, and at times perform embolization of the bleeding collateral with the help of interventional radiologists. The most difficult complication to deal with is persistent pulmonary hypertension. This may be from a mistaken diagnosis of CTEPH; if the pulmonary hypertension was not the result of fibrous clots in the pulmonary arteries, the pressure will not come down by doing endarterectomy, and there may be small vessel disease that is responsible for the high PVR leading to persistent pulmonary hypertension. Inability to obtain adequate surgical clearance may be a rare cause of persistent pulmonary hypertension, particularly in subsegmental disease. ECMO may help to tide over the immediate crisis; further imaging can show if any lesions can be addressed further by interventions and targeted pulmonary vasodilators can also help sometimes. The mortality in this situation is high and transplantation of lungs or heart and lungs with ECMO as bridge to transplant can be done if unable to wean off ECMO. For reperfusion edema venovenous ECMO is used, and for hemorrhage, RV failure, and persistent pulmonary hypertension venoarterial ECMO is used. While on venoarterial ECMO it is important to maintain some antegrade flow in the pulmonary arteries which are now devoid of intima and in the absence of adequate blood flow would form a fresh intraluminal thrombus.

Balloon Pulmonary Angioplasty (BPA)

Though the golden standard for the treatment of this disease is PTE, some patients who are technically inoperable due to very distal disease may benefit from BPA. This has re-emerged with expertise and specific hardware being developed in Japan. In the earlier era the complication rate was unacceptably high but with increasing expertise and better technology, the complication rates are much lower and might one day replace PTE as the treatment of choice in subsegmental and further distal disease. Currently, the number of centers performing this procedure is low, and it should be restricted to expert CTEPH centers where multimodality treatment facilities are available. A clear correlation is demonstrable between BPA experience and outcomes; also non-BPA interventional experience has not been shown to improve BPA outcomes.[22]

Medical Treatment

All patients following PTE should be on lifelong anticoagulation. Use of targeted pulmonary vasodilators is recommended only in inoperable CTEPH or in those with persistent pulmonary hypertension or recurrent pulmonary hypertension after successful PTE. Some patients with recurrent PH may be eligible for redo-PTE. The approved drug in these situation is Riociguat. Other classes of pulmonary vasodilators have been used off-label for treating CTEPH. In patients who have severe PH and who await surgery or BPA are sometimes treated with pulmonary vasodilators; it may be useful to do so in patients awaiting BPA but the utility of this approach has not been shown to be beneficial in patients undergoing PTE.

Outcomes of Pulmonary Thromboendarterectomy

Successful PEA provides excellent short-term outcomes by improving hemodynamics, exercise capacity, and functional capacity. The in-hospital mortality reported from an experienced center in the most recent 500-patient cohort is 2.2%.[23] A complete follow-up study reported from the UK national series of 880 consecutive patients reported an overall survival of 86% at 1 year, 84% at 3 years, 79% at 5 years, and 72% at 10 years. A mPAP of >30 mm Hg correlated with the need for pulmonary vasodilator therapy postoperatively and a mPAP of >38 mm Hg and PVR of >425 dynes.s^{-1}.cm^{-5} predicted worse long-term survival.[24]

Conclusion

Patients who have had acute pulmonary embolism should be followed up routinely for the development of CTEPH. Though international guidelines do not recommend this, Indian data show a higher number of acute PE patients developing CTEPH than reported elsewhere.[25] A multidisciplinary team should review all the patient data and make the therapeutic choices; the team should determine whether there is pulmonary hypertension, whether the organized, fibrous clots in the pulmonary arteries are the cause for the PH, and what is the best modality of treatment. All operable patients should be offered PTE, and if deemed inoperable, getting a second opinion from an expert CTEPH center would be recommended.

Acknowledgment
We would like to express our heartfelt thanks to Dr. Vimal Raj for providing **Fig. 15.1**.

References

1. Simonneau G, Montani D, Celermajer DS, et al. Haemodynamic definitions and updated clinical classification of pulmonary hypertension. Eur Respir J 2018; In press [https://doi.org/10.1183/13993003.01913-2018]
2. Hansmann G, Koestenberger M, Alastalo TP, et al. 2019 updated consensus statement on the diagnosis and treatment of pediatric pulmonary hypertension: the European Pediatric Pulmonary Vascular Disease Network (EPPVDN), endorsed by AEPC, ESPR and ISHLT. J Heart Lung Transplant 2019;38(9):879–901
3. Pepke-Zaba J, Delcroix M, Lang I, et al. Chronic thromboembolic pulmonary hypertension (CTEPH): results from an international prospective registry. Circulation 2011;124(18):1973–1981
4. Galiè N, Humbert M, Vachiéry J-L, et al. 2015 ESC/ERS Guidelines for the diagnosis and treatment of pulmonary hypertension: The Joint Task Force for the Diagnosis and Treatment of Pulmonary Hypertension of the European Society of Cardiology (ESC) and the European Respiratory Society (ERS): Endorsed by: Association for European Paediatric and Congenital Cardiology (AEPC), International Society for Heart and Lung Transplantation (ISHLT). Eur Respir J 2015;46(4):903–975
5. Kim NH, Delcroix M, Jais X, et al. Chronic thromboembolic pulmonary hypertension. Eur Respir J 2019;53(1):1801915
6. Chronic cor pulmonale. Report of an expert committee. World Health Organ Tech Rep Ser 1961;213:35
7. Hatano S, Strasser T, eds. Primary pulmonary hypertension. Report on a WHO Meeting. Geneva, World Health Organization, 1975
8. Kovacs G, Berghold A, Scheidl S, Olschewski H. Pulmonary arterial pressure during rest and exercise in healthy subjects: a systematic review. Eur Respir J 2009;34(4):888–894
9. Humbert M, Kovacs G, Hoeper MM, et al; ESC/ERS Scientific Document Group. 2022 ESC/ERS Guidelines for the diagnosis and treatment of pulmonary hypertension. Eur Heart J 2022; 43(38):3618–3731
10. Delcroix M, Torbicki A, Gopalan D, et al. ERS statement on chronic thromboembolic pulmonary hypertension. Eur Respir J 2021;57(6):2002828
11. Endrys J, Hayat N, Cherian G. Comparison of bronchopulmonary collaterals and collateral blood flow in patients with chronic thromboembolic and primary pulmonary hypertension. Heart 1997;78(2):171–176
12. Gopalan D, Blanchard D, Auger WR. Diagnostic evaluation of chronic thromboembolic pulmonary hypertension. Ann Am Thorac Soc 2016;13(Suppl 3):S222–S239
13. Tanabe N, Sugiura T, Jujo T, et al. Subpleural perfusion as a predictor for a poor surgical outcome in chronic thromboembolic pulmonary hypertension. Chest 2012;141(4):929–934
14. Kawakami T, Ogawa A, Miyaji K, et al. Novel angiographic classification of each vascular lesion in chronic thromboembolic pulmonary hypertension based on selective angiogram and results of balloon pulmonary angioplasty. Circ Cardiovasc Interv 2016;9(10):e003318

15. Dawes TJW, de Marvao A, Shi W, et al. Machine learning of three-dimensional right ventricular motion enables outcome prediction in pulmonary hypertension: a cardiac MR imaging study. Radiology 2017;283(2):381–390

16. Madani M, Mayer E, Fadel E, Jenkins DP. Pulmonary endarterectomy. Patient selection, technical challenges, and outcomes. Ann Am Thorac Soc 2016;13(Suppl 3):S240–S247

17. Pengo V, Denas G, Zoppellaro G, et al. Rivaroxaban vs warfarin in high-risk patients with antiphospholipid syndrome. Blood 2018;132(13):1365–1371

18. Delcroix M, Lang I, Pepke-Zaba J, et al. Long-term outcome of patients with chronic thromboembolic pulmonary hypertension: results from an International Prospective Registry. Circulation 2016;133(9):859–871

19. de Perrot M, Gopalan D, Jenkins D, et al. Evaluation and management of patients with chronic thromboembolic pulmonary hypertension - consensus statement from the ISHLT. J Heart Lung Transplant 2021;40(11):1301–1326

20. Shetty DP, Nair HC, Shetty V, Punnen J. A novel treatment for pulmonary hemorrhage during thromboendarterectomy surgery. Ann Thorac Surg 2015;99(3):e77–e78

21. Kanchi M, Nair HC, Natarajan P, et al. Management of intrapulmonary hemorrhage in patients undergoing pulmonary thrombo-endarterectomy. Ann Card Anaesth 2021;24(3):384–388

22. Shimura N, Kataoka M, Inami T, et al. Additional percutaneous transluminal pulmonary angioplasty for residual or recurrent pulmonary hypertension after pulmonary endarterectomy. Int J Cardiol 2015;183:138–142

23. Madani MM, Auger WR, Pretorius V, et al. Pulmonary endarterectomy: recent changes in a single institution's experience of more than 2,700 patients. Ann Thorac Surg 2012;94(1):97–103, discussion 103 [Discussion, p. 103.]

24. Cannon JE, Su L, Kiely DG, et al. Dynamic risk stratification of patient long-term outcome after pulmonary endarterectomy: results from the United Kingdom National Cohort. Circulation 2016;133(18):1761–1771

25. Sen Dutt T, Murali Mohan BV, Tousheed SZ, Ramanjenaya R, Shetty DP. Incidence of chronic thrombo-embolic pulmonary hypertension following acute pulmonary thrombo-embolism: an Indian perspective. Indian J Chest Allied Sci 2013;55:205–207

16

Conduction Defects in ICU

K. K. Kapur, Rohan Kapur, Pranav Kapoor, and Poonam Malhotra Kapoor

Introduction

Conduction defects are a common clinical finding in the ICU. Disturbance in both sinoatrial (SA) and atrioventricular (AV) conduction exist as conduction defects, which are commonly observed in ICU patients. The atrial and ventricular contraction of the heart reflects as bradyarrhythmias and tachyarrhythmias, which are the synchronous contractility of the atria and ventricles, that is, conduction across the SA node and the AV or the Aschoff-Tawara node (**Fig. 16.1a, b**) and also the bundle of His and the Purkinje fibers showing or fastened controllability.

Bradyarrhythmias

Bradycardia is an abnormally slow heart rate of less than 60 beats per minute. All slow heart rhythms are referred to as bradyarrhythmias. The bradyarrhythmic disorder as shown in **Flowchart 16.1** could be either extrinsic or intrinsic.

Sinus Node Dysfunction (SND)

There are broadly two types of bradyarrhythmias: (1) the sick sinus syndrome when the sinus node fails (SND), and (2) heart block or AV block, which is a complete or partial interruption of electrical impulses on their way to the ventricles, resulting in a slow, unreliable heartbeat (**Box 16.1**).

Atrioventricular Blocks

The three types of AV block are referred to as first degree, second degree, and third degree AV block. The AV node

provides a short delay in conduction which helps the atrial blood to completely empty into the ventricle before the ventricles begin to contract as well. Thus, the conduction is slow. **Table 16.1** highlights various electrocardiogram (ECG) leads and their corresponding chambers. **Table 16.2** enumerates the various AV conduction defects.

Box 16.1 Sinus node dysfunction

- Persistent sinus bradycardia
- Sinus pauses or arrest
- Sinoatrial exit block
- Chronotropic incompetence
- Atrial tachycardia (including atrial fibrillation or atrial flutter)
- Bradycardia-tachycardia syndrome

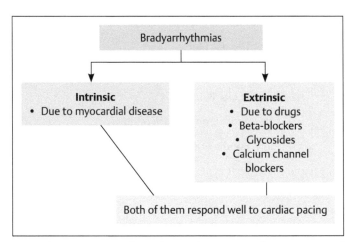

Flowchart 16.1 Algorithm depicting the origin of bradyarrhythmia.

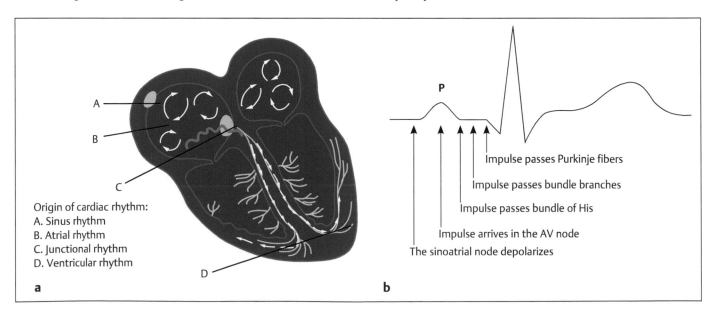

Fig. 16.1 (a) Level of etiopathogenesis of conduction defect in the intensive care unit (ICU) for different conduction rhythms at the sinoatrial (SA) and atrioventricular (AV) node levels. (b) Mode of conduct of the impulse in the conduction system and the impulse transmission and its correlation to electrocardiogram (ECG) waves.

Bifascicular Block

When there is a conduction delay below the level of the AV node and both fascicles of the right bundle branch and one of the two on the left side it is called bifascicular block (**Fig. 16.2** and **Flowchart 16.2**). The PR interval incorporate the time from the depolarization of the sinus node to the onset of ventricular depolarization. The measurement is from the beginning of P wave to the first part of QRS complex. North PR interval is 0.12 to 0.20 seconds. The QRS on ECG signifies time for ventricular depolarization. Its duration is normally 0.06 to 0.10 seconds. Important features are:

1. Normal PR interval.
2. A left-axis deviation (QRS rate 55) and a right bundle branch block (RBBB).

The ECG shows the QRS axis as 81 which suggests that it is a left-axis deviation along with a RBBB and a PR interval, making it a first-degree AV block (**Fig. 16.3**).

Table 16.1 ECG leads and cardiac chambers

Leads	Corresponding cardiac chamber
V1 and V2	Form the RV on ECG
V3 and V5	Correspond to the septum
V5 and V6	Left side of the heart
Lead I	Left side of the heart
Lead II	Inferior territory

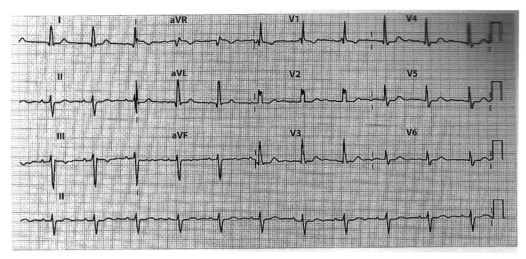

Fig. 16.2 Electrocardiogram (ECG) strip depicting bifascicular block.

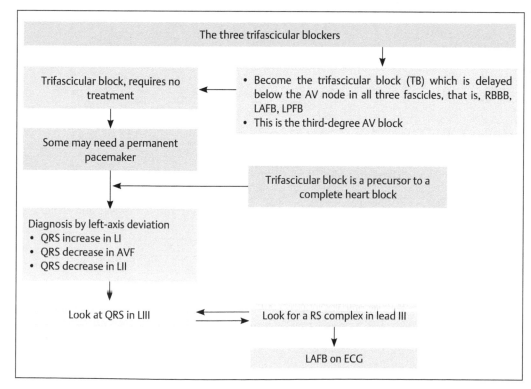

Flowchart 16.2 Algorithm depicting the management of three bifascicular blockers. Abbreviations: AV, atrioventricular; LAFB, left anterior fascicular block.

Table 16.2   ECG of the atrioventricular (AV) blocks

AV block type	Diagnostic points	Treatment	ECG strip
First-degree AV blocks	• PR interval greater than 0.2 s; no variation in PR interval and P followed by QRS interval	• No specific therapy needed • Beta-blocker or calcium channel blockers, sotalol, verapamil • Pacemaker may be considered in specific situations	 Sinus rhythm with first-degree AV block. Note prolonged PR interval
Second-degree AV block (Mobitz type 1)	• There are at least two regular atrial impulses which are consecutive and conducted with a PT interval, which remains same with each beat	• Asymptomatic: observation and monitoring with holding drugs that can slow AV node conduction • Symptomatic atropine and/or temporary pacing only	 Second-degree AV blocks Mobitz type 1. Note PR interval gradually increased until P-wave is blocked (Wenckebach periodicity). Note after the blocked P-wave PR interval is short. PR interval containing blocked P-wave is smaller than the two consecutive PP intervals
Second-degree AV block (type 2) Mobitz	• **New MI:** seen more commonly with acute anterior MI • Either seen postoperative in cardiac ICU or in Cath Lab	As above	 • It is an "infranodal conduction disease of the His-Purkinje system" • Occurs after an anterior MI
Third-degree AV block	• **Complete AV or third-degree block.** The atrial impulses do not empty into the ventricles, which keeps contracting on its own • This is known as AV dissociation when atria and ventricles have no relationship to each other	As above and additionally administer dopamine infusion if hypotensive	 "These strips show a normal QRS; absence of P-waves and earlier than expected junctional premature beats." • Idioventricular AV escape rhythm is 30 bpm • When there is AV dissociation, always the ventricle rate is greater than the atrial rate (VR > AR) • In above AV dissociation is different in that it shows AR > VR • An RBBB morphology as well

Abbreviations: AR, atrial regurgitation; AV, atrioventricular; MI, myocardial ischemia; RBBB, right bundle branch block; VR, ventricular regurgitation.

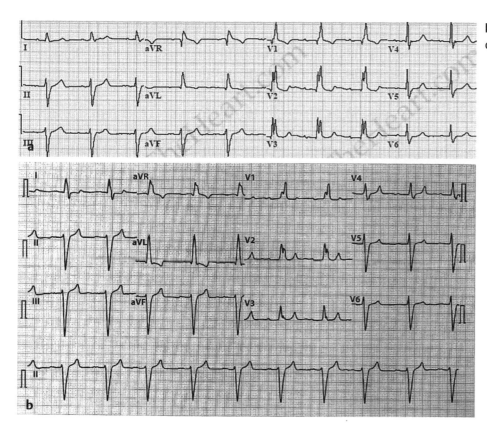

Fig. 16.3   (a, b) Trifascicular block as depicted in electrocardiogram (ECG).

Trifascicular Block

A trifascicular block is the combination of a RBBB, a left anterior or posterior fascicular block, and a first-degree AV block (prolonged PR intervals). This term is a misnomer, as AV node is not a fascicle (**Box 16.2**).

Left Bundle Branch Block (LBBB)

In India, there are more than one million cases of LBBB per year. LBBB is a delay or blockage of electrical impulses on the left side of the heart, making it harder for the heart to pump blood into circulation. It is seen in patients of hypertension, delayed and/or hypertrophic cardiomyopathy aortic valve disease, coronary artery disease, etc. It is rarely caused by stress tests like myocardial perfusion imaging when vasodilatory agents such as regadenoson are used (0.51% in incidence).[1] A simple way to diagnose LBBB in an ECG with a widened QRS complex (>120 ms) would be to look at V1. If the QRS complex is widened then look for other features of LBBB in lead I, lead V5, and lead V6 (**Fig. 16.4** and **Box 16.3**).

Right Bundle Branch Block

RBBB is a bundle block on the right side of the bundle of His of the conduction system. In an RBBB, the right ventricle (RV), which is not activated by the impulse travelling through the bundle branch on the right side, is involved. The ECG of an RBBB is shown in **Fig. 16.5**. RBBB characteristics are listed in **Box 16.4**. Today, RBBB is associated with cardiac-related morbidity and mortality.[2,3]

Box 16.2   The trifascicular block (TFB)

- Due to ischemic heart disease (IHD), congenital heart disease (CHD), hyperkalemia, digoxin toxicity
- It may be complete or incomplete trifascicular block (TFB)
- Right bundle branch block (RBBB) and Left bundle branch block (LBBB) may alternate in a TFB
- Bizarre QRS
- Complete or incomplete AV block with a slow ventricular escape rhythm
- Fixed RBBB with alternative left anterior fascicular (LAF) and left posterior fascicular block (LPFB)

Box 16.3   The features of LBBB

- QRS duration is more than 120 million seconds (>120 ms)
- Absence of Q-waves in leads I, V5, and V6
- Presence of a monomorphic R-wave in lead I, V5, and V6
- LBBB is also characterized by a typical ST- and T-wave displacement opposite to the major deflection of QRS complex

---

Around 4.5% of the general population may also have an RBBB pattern in their ECG.[2] RBBB is associated with more cases of hypertension, decreased aerobic capacity, slower heart rate, and more dyspnea when tested on exercise. RBBB seen in heart failure has a negative predictive valve.[4] Many

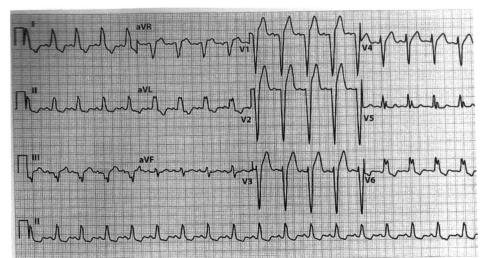

Fig. 16.4   Left bundle branch block.

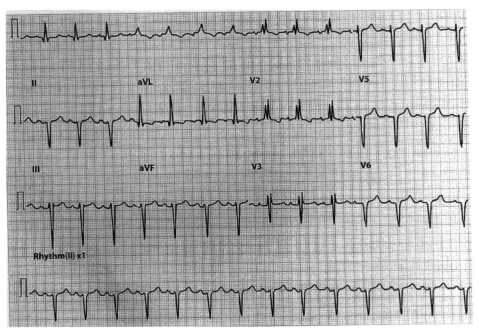

Fig. 16.5   Electrocardiogram (ECG) of a right bundle branch block (RBBB). An RBBB is a heart block in the right bundle branch of the electrical conduction system. During an RBBB, the right ventricle is not directly activated by impulses travelling through the right bundle branch.

Box 16.4   RBBB characteristics on ECG

ECG shows the following in an RBBB:
- QRS complex duration more than 120 million seconds
- Anterior chest leads (V1–V2) show a typical "RSR" bunny ear pattern; a secondary R-wave in V1 and V2
- As shown in **Fig. 16.5**, a slurred S-wave in LI, VL, and V5 and V6 occasionally are seen
- MI and RBBB are generally seen together (**Fig. 16.6**)

Abbreviation: MI, myocardial infarction; RBBB, right bundle branch block.

studies have shown RBBB to be an independent predictor of in-hospital mortality[5] when associated with acute coronary syndromes such as unstable angina and ST-elevation myocardial infarction (MI). Outcomes of RBBB are worst with presence of a decreased ejection fraction of RV in patients with ischemic cardiomyopathy.[6] On its own, RBBB may be transient, requiring no treatment. Acute treatment of RBBB alone or RBBB with a hemiblock consists of observing and treating the clinical condition that causes the conduction disturbances or removing the drug that causes the disease.

Myocardial Infarction and Ischemic Heart Disease

A vasospastic chest pain or angina may occur and show (**Fig. 16.6**) an anterior ST-segment elevation in the anterior chest leads, which resolves with rest and treatment. This is the basis of an myocardial infarction (MI) with an ischemic

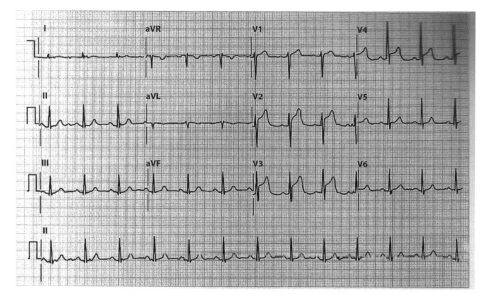

Fig. 16.6 Prinzmetal (vasospastic) angina.

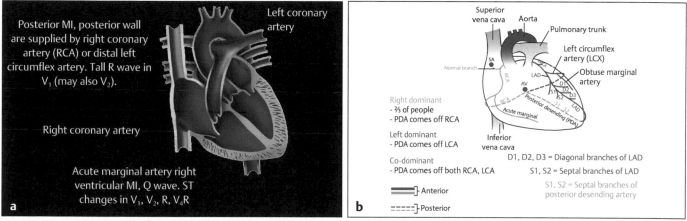

Fig. 16.7 **(a)** Schematic diagram showing coronary arteries areas infarcted and lead changes. **(b)** The left anterior descending (LAD) artery gives off the septal and diagonal arteries. The diagonal arteries (D1, D2, D3) supply the lateral wall of the left ventricle.

heart disease (IHD). In case of MI, changes in coronary arteries with simultaneous involvement in the ECG is shown in **Fig. 16.7** and listed in **Table 16.3**. It is important to know this and treat accordingly.

All the coronary blood supply into the myocardium ultimately drains into the great cardiac vein or the left marginal vein, the small cardiac and middle cardiac vein, or the left posterior ventricular vein. **Figs. 16.8** and **16.9** give good examples of ECG changes and recognition in anterolateral MI in anterolateral leads of ECG (**V1** to **V6** in **Fig. 16.8**).

ST segment is seen to be elevated in the interpolated leads, V3 to V6, and lead I and VL suggesting the inferior territory is involved.

Inferior wall ST-segment elevation (MI), there is injury or thrombosis of the right coronary artery, giving rise to myocardial tissue. When an inferior wall MI extends to the infarcted posterior regions as well, it is known as a posterior wall MI.

ECG for Electrolyte Disturbances: Hypokalemia

A majority of the cardiovascular drugs cause changes that lead to either bradyarrhythmias or tachyarrhythmias. Drugs especially the antiarrhythmic diuretics, digoxin, etc., generally cause these electrolyte disturbances. Commonest electrolyte imbalances seen on an ECG involve potassium, calcium, and magnesium. Just like increased potassium levels, the low potassium levels too can cause conduction defects such as arrhythmias and ectopy. ECG changes are shown in **Figs. 16.10** and **16.11** and are listed in **Box 16.5**.

Hyperkalemia occurs when potassium levels rise above 5.5 mL. Early changes of ECG show peaked T-waves with increase in PR interval in interspatial leads.

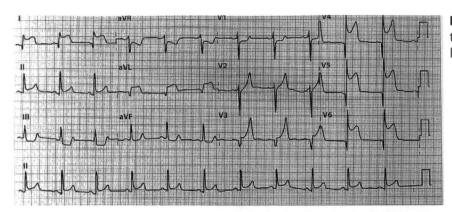

Fig. 16.8 An anterolateral myocardial infarction produces changes in the anterolateral leads.

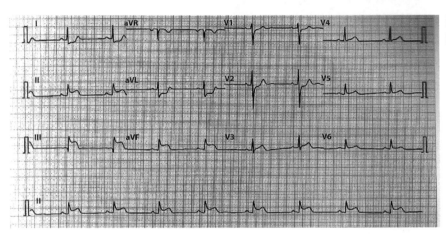

Fig. 16.9 An inferior myocardial infarction produces changes in the inferior leads.

Table 16.3 The coronary artery and the cardiac region it supplies

Coronary branch	Cardiac chamber supplied
The right coronary artery	• Right atrium • SA and AV nodes • Posterior part of IVS
The right marginal artery	• Right ventricle • Apex
The posterior interventricular artery	• Right ventricle • Left ventricle • Posterior 1/3 of IVS
The left coronary artery	• Left atrium • Left ventricle • IVS • AV bundles
The left anterior descending artery	• Right ventricle • Left ventricle • Anterior 2/3 IVS
The left marginal artery	• Left ventricle
The circumflex artery	• Left atrium • Left ventricle

Abbreviations: AV, atrioventricular; IVS, interventricular septum; SA, sinoatrial.

Box 16.5 ECG changes in hypokalemia (Fig. 16.9)

- T-waves become flattened
- ST elevation in the inferior leads, leads II, III, and a VF
- Reciprocal T-segment depression in the lateral and/or high lateral leads (leads I, aVL, V5, and V6)
- Hypokalemia is slowed conduction delayed ventricular repolarization

Abbreviation: VF, ventricular fibrillation.

Severe hyperkalemia with potassium more than 7 mmol/L leads to heart block, a systole, and ventricular tachycardia/ventricular fibrillation (VT/VF) cardiac arrest (**Box 16.6**).

Digitalis Effect on ECG

Digitalis produces an increase in blood flow, a decrease in vascular resistance, vasodilation, a decrease in heart rate, and central venous pressure. Normal changes on ECG with therapeutic levels of digitalis include the first change that occurs in T-Wave (flattening to inversion to peaking of T-wave). Later, it is QT-interval shortening with secondary repolarization abnormalities (**Fig. 16.12** and **Box 16.7**).

To conclude, on ECG tall QT and shortening inverted T-wave need to be differentiated. **Box 16.8** sums up various

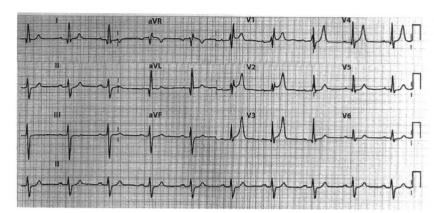

Fig. 16.10 Electrocardiogram (ECG) changes in hyperkalemia.

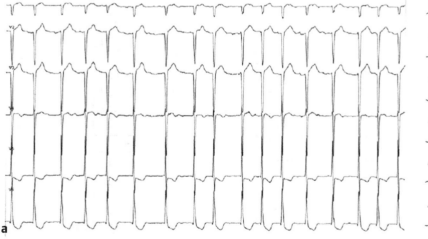

Fig. 16.11 Electrocardiogram (ECG) changes in severe hyperkalemia.

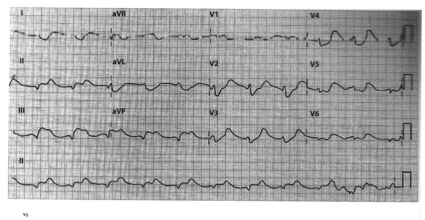
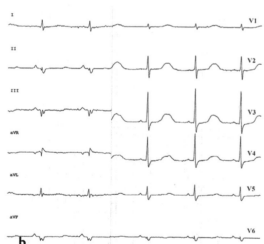

Fig. 16.12 **(a)** Electrocardiogram (ECG) of the digital is effect. Typical ST depression in lead V6 with atrial fibrillation and prolonged PR interval. **(b)** Due to the vagus effect of digitalis, the QT interval also gets shortened.

Box 16.6 ECG changes in hyperkalemia
• Tall T-waves as T-wave interval increases
• Absent P-waves or diminished P-wave
• Widened complex prolongation of the PR and QRS intervals
• ST segment depression
• Heart rate begins to slow as potassium levels increase

Box 16.7 ECG and digitalis
• Downsloping ST depression with a characteristic "Salvador Dali sagging" appearance
• Flattened inverted or biphasic T-waves
• Shortened QT interval
• Decreased heart rate as it slows AV conduction heart block
• Prolonged PR interval
• Toxicity: second and third degree

Box 16.8 Differential diagnosis of tall and inverted T-waves

- Peaked T-waves = hyperkalemia
- Hyperacute T-waves = STEMI; Prinzmetal angina
- Upright tall T-wave (New) NTTV1 in V1 = suggests a high likelihood of coronary artery disease
- Dynamic T-wave inversions = acute MI
- Fixed T-wave inversions = following MI with pathological Q-wave

Abbreviations: MI, myocardial infarction; STEMI, ST-elevation myocardial infarction.

Box 16.9 ECG for torsades de pointes

- Undulating QRS axis with shifting of complexes from the baseline
- Presence of ventricular tachycardia
- Rapid irregular QRS complexes
- Long QTc interval
- P-wave shows AV dissociation
- Heart rate 150–300 bpm

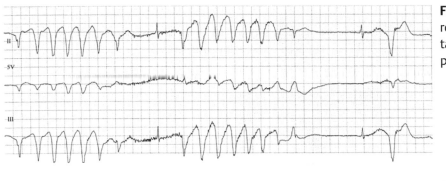

Fig. 16.13 Electrocardiogram (ECG) shows recurrent torsades de pointes with ventricular tachycardia and prolonged QT interval due to possible ingestion of antibiotics.

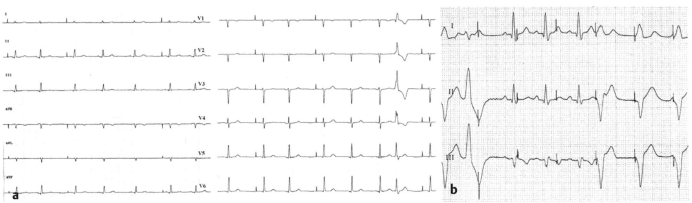

Fig. 16.14 **(a)** Schematic diagram of ECG showing atrial pacing (AAI) pacing. **(b)** If we exclude the sensing circuit then the electrocardiogram (ECG) in a patient with a pacemaker on whom a magnet is put would read as shown in this figure.

differential diagnosis of the same. High lateral STEMI: High lateral STEMI can present as ST elevation involving lead I and aVL. Subtle ST elevation in V5, V6 and reciprocal changes in lead III and avF may be present. This is usually caused by occlusion of the first diagonal branch of LAD and is sometimes referred to as the South African flag sign.[7]

Torsades De Pointes

In long QT syndrome, the ventricles take too long to contract and release, which could be due to some drugs, antibiotics, or antidepressants (**Fig. 16.13** and **Box 16.9**). Beta-blockers,

implantable cardioverter defibrillator (ICD), and pacemakers are the treatment of choice.

Torsades de pointes is a polymorphic ventricular tachycardia, with oscillatory changes in the QRS complex and a prolonged QTc interval due to drugs such as quinidine, procainamide, calcium, and disopyramide.

Pacing and Conduction Defect in ICU

Pacemakers help achieve the sinus rhythm in a patient who has an irregular heart rate. The electrical stimulus must be adequate in both amplitude and duration. The ECG on a pacemaker shows pacemaker spikes, which are vertical signals that show the electrical activity of the pacemaker. In **Fig. 16.14**, these changes are seen as a stimulation artifact. Two artifacts are seen if both chambers are paced. The P-waves conduct normally to the ventricle in this ECG and in this pacing ECG the sensed sinus rhythm is seen to alternate in a regular fashion with the pacing spikes with P-wave following it.

Here the pacing spikes are seen independent of patient's spontaneous rhythm once ventricular pacing (VOO) is added with the application of a magnet.[8,9]

Pericardial Disease and Conduction Defect

In an ECG of conduction defects in patients with pericardial disease, especially acute pericarditis, it is seen that there are inflammatory changes from the subepicardium to the myocardium. These appear on an ECG as diffuse ST-segment and T-wave changes, as shown in **Fig. 16.15** and listed in **Box 16.10**.

The key feature of pericardial disease on ECG is a significant decrease in the QRS voltage in all leads. Treatment for bradycardia and conduction defects depends on the type of

electrical conduction problem, the severity of symptoms, and the cause of the slow heart rate (**Flowchart 16.3**).[10,11]

On bradyarrhythmias whether it is a drug therapy in the ICU, such as digoxin, magnesium, or corduroyed or an electrolyte imbalance or ischemia, an algorithm with ECG changes does wonders to the patient's outcomes. With a increase in the heart failure it is of utmost importance in patients with conduction bocks, to consider alternative options, for cardiac resynchronization therapy (CRT), wherein bundle branch pacing (LBB/PCRT) biventricular pacing (BiVP - CRT). this increases ejection fraction, there BiVP - CRT alone.[12] Patients with idiopathic pulmonary hypertension (IPAH) have a higher prevalence of conduction disease than patients without IPAH, according to recent study results published in the *Journal of Heart and Lung Transplantation.* The study confirmed that IPAH patients with conduction disorder have reduced physical functioning and a poor prognosis, typically resulting in right ventricular (RV) failure and death. This could be due to raised pulmonary vascular resistance seen in PAH patients.[13]

Conclusion

In case of conduction defects in the ICU, it is important to assess patients for adverse signs including heart rate less than 40 bpm, chest pain, heart failure, or hypotension (systolic BP [SBP] <90 mmHg). If no adverse signs, then observe and monitor the patient in the ICU. Consider use of glycopyrrolate, or administer intravenous atropine. Consider whether the patient has an indication for elective pacing to avert the risk of a systole. Detailed knowledge of

Box 16.10   ECG changes in acute pericardial disease
• The ST segment is concave upwards with ST elevation • ST segment may be depressed in aVR • PR segment depression in leads II and V3 • No reciprocal ST segment changes are seen (vis-à-vis MI ECG)

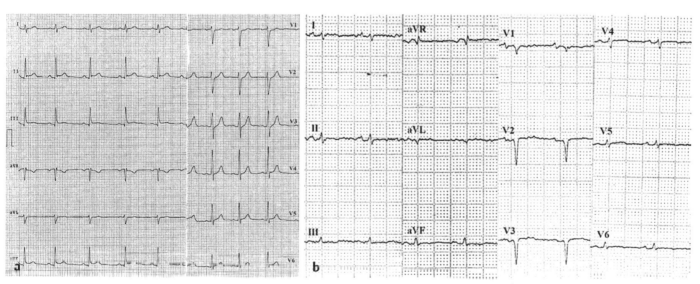

Fig. 16.15 **(a)** Diffuse ST-segment elevation with ST-segment depression in V1 and augmented ECG lead (aVR). **(b)** Electrocardiogram (ECG) in a patient with massive pericardial effusion causing pericardial tamponade.

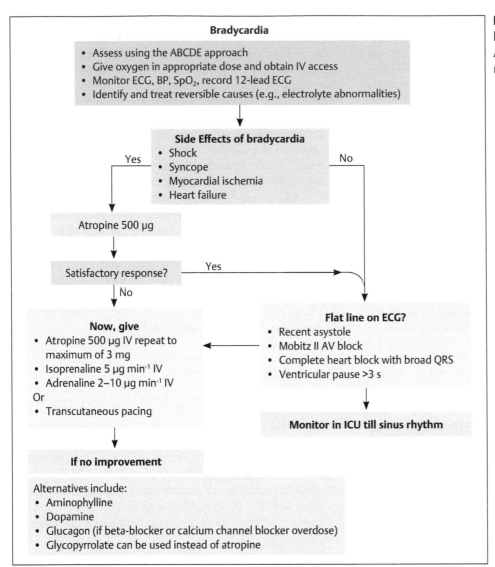

Flowchart 16.3 Management of bradycardia in ICU. (A flowchart from AIIMS protocol in ICU on "Bradycardia management.")

ECG of these conduction defects helps solve the treatment dilemma, in these very sick patients. Incident arrhythmias in patients hospitalized with COVID-19 are associated with an increased risk of mortality, likely reflective of underlying COVID-19 disease severity more than intrinsic cardiac dysfunction.[14] Odds for conduction abnormalities increased with age; and the odds of cardiologist involvement increased with age and cardiovascular disease.[15]

References

1. Assaad M, Berry A, Palanisamy J, Fenner J, Zughaib M. Differential effect of regadenoson versus dipyridamole on heart rate in patients with left bundle branch block: How does it affect the results of pharmacological nuclear stress testing? JRSM Cardiovasc Dis 2019;8:2048004019828257

2. Gholampour-Dehaki M, Zareh A, Babaki S, Javadikasgari H. Conduction disorders in continuous versus interrupted suturing technique in ventricular septal defect surgical repair. Res Cardiovasc Med 2016;5(1):e28735

3. Fazelifar S, Bigdelian H. Effect of esmolol on myocardial protection in pediatrics congenital heart defects. Adv Biomed Res 2015;4:246

4. Chan WK, Goodman SG, Brieger D, et al; ACS I and GRACE Investigators. Clinical characteristics, management, and outcomes of acute coronary syndrome in patients with right bundle branch block on presentation. Am J Cardiol 2016;1 17(5):754–759

5. Widimsky P, Roháč F, Stásek J, et al. Primary angioplasty in acute myocardial infarction with right bundle branch block: should new onset right bundle branch block be added to future guidelines as an indication for reperfusion therapy? Eur Heart J 2012;33(1):86–95

6. Sabe MA, Sabe SA, Kusunose K, Flamm SD, Griffin BP, Kwon DH. Predictors and prognostic significance of right ventricular ejection fraction in patients with ischemic cardiomyopathy. Circulation 2016;134(9):656–665

7. Ludhwani D, Chhabra L, Goyal A, et al. Lateral Wall Myocardial Infarction. [Updated 2022 Sep 12]. In: StatPearls [Internet]. Treasure Island (FL): StatPearls Publishing; 2022

8. Smerup M, Hjertholm T, Johnsen SP, et al. Pacemaker implantation after congenital heart surgery: risk and prognosis in a population-based follow-up study. Eur J Cardiothorac Surg 2005;28(1):61–68

9. Shepard SM, Tejman-Yarden S, Khanna S, Davis CK, Batra AS. Dexmedetomidine-related atrial standstill and loss of capture in a pediatric patient after congenital heart surgery. Crit Care Med 2011;39(1):187–189

10. Monsieursa KG, Nolanc JP, Bossaerte LL, et al. European Resuscitation Council Guidelines for Resuscitation 2015: Section 1. Executive summary. Resuscitation 2015;95:1–80

11. Khan UA, Sharma D, McGlinchey P, Peace A. Percutaneous coronary intervention to left anterior descending artery/right coronary artery bifurcation: this is not a typo! A case report. Eur Heart J Case Rep 2019;3(3):ytz137

12. Heart Rhythm 2022 Reveals Latest Advances in Conduction System Pacing. Heart Rhythm Society. April 30, 2022; https://www.hrsonline.org/news/press-releases/hr22-latest-advances-conduction-system-pacing

13. Brick P, Reddy SA, et al. Is Conduction Disease More Prevalent in Idiopathic Pulmonary Hypertension? J Heart Lung Transplant. published on June 10, 2022

14. Patel NH, Rutland J, Tecson KM. Arrhythmias and Intraventricular Conduction Disturbances in Patients Hospitalized With Coronavirus Disease 2019. Am J Cardiol. 2022; 162:111-115

15. Gerges L, D'Angelo K, Bass D, Haghshenas A, Kersten DJ, Ahluwalia M, Zelster R, Makaryus AN. Cardiac conduction disturbances in rheumatologic disease: a cross-sectional study. Am J Cardiovasc Dis. 2022 ;12(1):31–37

17

Management of Cardiac Implantable Electronic Devices in Cardiac Surgery and Intensive Care

Iti Shri

Introduction

Cardiac implantable electronic devices (CIEDs) are designed to either monitor or treat irregular heart beat in people with rhythm disorder or heart failure. The term encompasses implantable loop recorders (ILMs) for monitoring rhythm disorders, pacemakers (PPMs) for bradyarrhythmia treatment, implantable cardioverter defibrillators (ICDs) for tachyarrhythmia management, and cardiac resynchronization therapy (CRT) devices for systolic dysfunction in heart failure with conduction delays.

More than 10,000 ICDs and 18,000 PPMs are implanted each month in the United States alone.[1]

In a survey conducted in 2016, Shenthar et al reported that about 37,000 cardiac device implantations take place annually in India. Pacemaker (PPM) for bradyarrhythmic indication constituted 80% of the devices implanted with ICDs and CRT forming approximately 10% each.[2]

Pacemakers

As the indication for device placement expands with advances in understanding of pathophysiology and management of arrythmias and heart failure, so do significant advances which have been witnessed in pacing technology. These multichamber and multisite pacing with cardiac resynchronization, preservation of atrioventricular (AV) synchronization as in dual-chamber PPMs, rate responsiveness that adjusts to metabolic demands, battery longevity and remote internet-based monitoring, and magnetic resonance are safe for a paradigm shift to even leadless and batteryless devices. The future may be belonging to gene- or cell-based biological PPMs.[3,4]

Cardiac pacing is based on the principle that myocardial cells can be depolarized repeatedly by electrical stimulation.

The battery and electronics are contained in a pulse generator or can, and are implanted subcutaneously infraclavicularly, sometimes in abdomen. The leads travel from the can to contract the myocardium, to deliver a depolarizing pulse, and to sense intrinsic cardiac activity. Pacing occurs when a potential difference (voltage) is applied between the two electrodes.

The minimum amount of energy required to depolarize myocardium is called the stimulation threshold. The acceptable stimulation threshold is under 1.5 V with a pulse width of 0.5 ms, and high resistance at lead tips so as to minimize current flow and preserve battery.[5] PPM leads are built with steroid-eluting collars to prevent tissue-lead fibrosis in case of passive fixation of leads,[6] and hence mitigate the threshold rise over time. Active fixation is when leads are screwed into the myocardium.[6]

Present PPMs can have sensing ability apart from pacing. In such PPMs near-field depolarization signals are sensed while near-field repolarization signals (T-waves) and far-field signals are rejected so as to begin cardiac depolarization.[5] Atrial channels are optimized to sense in the frequency range of 80 to 100 Hz and ventricular channels in the 10 to 30 Hz range. Typical amplitude ranges for signals recorded from atrial and ventricular leads are 1.5 to 5 mV and 5 to 25 mV, respectively.[5]

The pacing mode is described with a 4- or 5-letter code and in response to a sensed intracardiac signal. A PPM may inhibit output, trigger output, or pace in a different chamber after a timed delay. The first position identifies the chamber paced, second position is for the chamber sensed, the third position tells what device responds for the sensed events, while the fourth position indicates whether rate response is on, and the fifth position (when used) indicates whether multisite pacing is employed as in case of CRT (**Table 17.1**).[7]

Few Pacemaker Modes

VVI or VVIR: VVI(R) is ventricular demand pacing. The ventricle is paced, sensed, and inhibited in response to a sensed ventricular event. This mode of pacing prevents ventricular bradycardia and is primarily indicated in patients with atrial fibrillation with a slow ventricular response.

AAI or AAI(R): AAI(R) is atrial demand pacing. The atrium is paced, sensed, and the pulse generator inhibits pacing output in response to a sensed atrial event. This mode is used for patients purely with sinus node dysfunction, yet maintain AV nodal function.

DDD or DDD(R): DDD or DDD(R) is a dual-chamber system. It possesses pacing and sensing capabilities in both the atrium and the ventricle, and it is the most commonly used pacing

Table 17.1 Generic pacemaker code (North American Society of Pacing and Electrophysiology [NASPE]/British Pacing and Electrophysiology Group [BPEG] generic [NBG] code)

First position	Second position	Third position	Fourth position	Fifth position
Chamber paced	Chamber sensed	Response	Rate modulation	Multisite pacing
None (O)	None (O)	Inhibited (I)	None (O)	None (O)
Atrium (A)	Atrium (A)	Triggered (T)	Rate responsive (R)	Atrium (A)
Ventricle (V)	Ventricle (V)	Dual (D)		Ventricle (V)
Dual (D)	Dual (D)			Dual (D)

mode. This mode is most appropriate for patients with combined sinus node dysfunction and AV nodal dysfunction.

Rate responsive sensors are incorporated to overcome chronotropic incompetence of the sinus node to exercise and nonexercise requirements. Sensors can be classified by the method they detect a physiological change: vibration or acceleration of movement, impedance sensing to minute ventilation or pulmonary fluid status, evoked QT interval, and response to physical or chemical parameters such as central venous temperature or blood pH.[8,9] The role of sensors has been expanded to include functions other than rate augmentation—such as detection of atrial and ventricular capture, and monitoring of heart failure, sleep apnea, and hemodynamic status.[10]

So with the dual mode (e.g., dual chamber pacemaker rate modulate [DDDR]) both triggering and inhibition are used. In the dual chamber pacemaker (DDD) mode, inhibition occurs in the atrium if the intrinsic atrial rate exceeds the programmed lower rate. An AV clock is then started. In the absence of an intrinsic ventricular event, a ventricular pacing spike is triggered; a sensed intrinsic ventricular event inhibits pacing.

Following conditions are included in the ACC/AHA/HRS guidelines for the PPM insertion:[11]
1. Sinus node dysfunction.
2. Acquired AV block.
3. Chronic bifascicular block.
4. After acute phase of myocardial infarction (MI).
5. Neurocardiogenic syncope and hypersensitive carotid sinus syndrome.
6. Postcardiac transplantation.
7. Hypertrophic cardiomyopathy.
8. Pacing to detect and terminate tachycardia.
9. CRT in patients with severe systolic heart failure.
10. Patients with congenital heart disease.

Some terminologies associated with PPMs:[12,13]
1. Oversensing: Interpreting external stimuli as cardiac depolarization and failure to pace.
2. Undersensing: Failure to detect cardiac depolarization and so inappropriate delivery of pacing pulses.
3. AV delay: Time that a dual-chamber system waits after detecting or initiating an atrial event before pacing ventricle.
4. Hysteresis: A programmable feature that allows the PPM to begin ventricular pacing only if the spontaneous rate falls below a set rate.
5. Programmed or automatic rate: Lowest sustained regular rate during which the generator will pace.
6. Upper-rate behavior: Pacing in dual-chambered PPMs programmed such that as the atrial rate increases and reaches a set threshold, it limits the rate at which the ventricle can pace.
7. Ventricular fusion: The electrical summation of a heart's intrinsic beat and depolarization from a pacing stimulus.

8. Pseudomalfunctions: Unusual and unexpected ECG findings that appear to be malfunctions but actually are normal PPM behavior.
9. Runaway PPM: Malfunction of the generator resulting in life-threatening tachycardia, mostly due to battery failure or external damage.
10. Crosstalk: Failure of DDD pacing; atrial pacing spike is mistaken for a QRS by the ventricular lead. The QRS complex on an ECG strip is the most central and most visually obvious part of the ECG tracing.
11. PPM syndrome: Most commonly seen in the setting of a single-chamber device with ventricular sensing and pacing lead. In the absence of atrial lead, the ventricle contracts at the programmed rate, and reverse ventriculoatrial contraction may occur. This causes loss of AV synchrony, resulting in heart failure and loss of cardiac output. PPM syndrome may also be induced by preferential right ventricular (RV) pacing. Therefore, features that avoid RV pacing result in very long AV delays (>400 ms) that cause atrial contraction during early diastole, resulting in cannon a-waves and adverse hemodynamics, referred to as "pseudopacemaker syndrome." The reported incidence of PPM syndrome has ranged from 2 to 83%. Because of the high incidence of PPM syndrome in VVIR-paced patients, atrial-based pacing is preferred.

Acute complications occur in approximately 2 to 4% of PPM implantations (e.g., lead dislodgement, perforation, pneumothorax, pocket hematoma, or infection).

Perforation of a vein, atrium or ventricle may also occur.[14,15]

Implantable Cardioverter Defibrillator

An ICD is a specialized device to treat many dysrhythmias, specifically ventricular tachyarrhythmias. All modern ICDs also function as PPMs.[14] A meta-analysis of the Antiarrhythmic versus Implantable Defibrillator (AVID), Canadian Implantable Defibrillator Study (CIDS), and Cardiac Arrest Study of Hamburg (CASH) trials clearly demonstrate benefit of ICD over medical therapy in secondary prevention of sudden cardiac death (SCD) in survivors of ventricular fibrillation (VF) and tachycardia.[16] Multicenter Automatic Defibrillator Implantation Trial (MADIT), MADIT II, Multicenter Unsustained Tachycardia Trial (MUSTT), and Coronary Artery Bypass Graft Patch (CABG-Patch) evaluated ICD for primary prevention of SCD in patients with coronary artery disease and showed that use of ICD is associated with a substantial reduction in both absolute and relative risk reduction in mortality rates as compared to conventional antiarrhythmic therapy.[17] However, based on Defibrillator in Acute Myocardial Infarction Trial (DINAMIT) results, it is recommended that ICD placement be delayed for at least 40 days in patients with acute myocardial infarction.[17]

ICDs also find an indication for implantation in nonischemic cardiomyopathy such as hypertrophic cardiomyopathy, and various infiltrative and inherited conditions such as long QT syndrome and Brugada syndrome type I.[17-19]

The ICD consists of a generator, which has a battery with 4–7 years of longevity and a circuitry that contains the capacitor that determines how and when both bradycardia pacing and antitachycardia therapies are delivered. The ventricular defibrillator leads function similar to PPM lead except for shock coils. The ventricular ICD lead is essentially a bipolar lead.

The ICD system needs to be sensitive enough to detect the VF wavelength that occurs in a tenth of millivolts, and also not to oversense the T-wave, far fields, or myopotential. Most ICDs now offer three-tiered therapy to terminate the tachycardia:[20]

- Antitachycardia pacing (ATP).
- Cardioversion or low-energy shocks.
- Defibrillation or high-energy shocks.

Rhythm detection is also crucial in therapy delivering so as to differentiate supraventricular tachycardia (SVT) from ventricular tachycardia (VT) and prevent inappropriate shock therapy.

There is also a code used to identify ICDs. The NBD Code (*North American Society of Pacing and Electrophysiology/ British Pacing and Electrophysiology Group Defibrillator Code*) has four letters as given in **Table 17.2**.[17]

Leads within the central venous circulation and cardiac chambers can cause vascular obstruction, thrombosis, infection, and cardiac perforation. Moreover, lead failure has been estimated at 0.58%/y and up to 20% at 10 years. This led to the development of subcutaneous ICDs.[21]

Indications of ICD

ICDs are broadly indicated either in secondary prophylaxis against SCD or in its primary prophylaxis.[22]

Class I indications (i.e., the benefit greatly outweighs the risk):

- Survivors of cardiac arrest due to VF or sustained VT after excluding reversible causes.
- Patients with structural heart disease and spontaneous, sustained VT, whether hemodynamically stable or unstable.

- Patients with syncope of undetermined origin with clinically relevant sustained VT or VF induced at electrophysiology study.
- Patients with a left ventricular ejection fraction (LVEF) ≤35% due to prior MI occurring at least 40 days earlier and who have NYHA functional Class II or Class III disease.
- Patients with nonischemic-dilated cardiomyopathy who have an LVEF ≤35% and NYHA functional Class II or III disease.
- Patients with left-ventricular (LV) dysfunction due to prior MI occurring at least 40 days earlier with an LVEF ≥ 30% and who have NYHA Class I disease.
- Patients with nonsustained VT due to prior MI with an LVEF ≤ 40% with inducible VF or sustained VT at electrophysiology study.

Contraindications to ICD Implantation[22]

- Estimated life expectancy of less than 1 year and/or poor functional capacity.
- Incessant ventricular tachyarrhythmias.
- NYHA Class IV patients who fail to respond to GDMT and are not deemed suitable for cardiac transplantation or CRT.
- Ventricular tachyarrhythmias that are amenable to surgical/catheter ablation or secondary to reversible causes.

Indications for ICD Deactivation[14]

- End-of-life care.
- Inappropriate shocks.
- During resuscitation.
- With external pacing that can cause an ICD to fire.
- During procedures such as central lines or surgery with electrocautery.

Cardiac Resynchronization Device

CRT provides a mechanical advantage to symptomatic systolic heart failure patients with abnormal QRS duration by targeting AV and inter- and intraventricular

Table 17.2 The NBD code to identify implantable cardioverter defibrillators (ICDs)

	First position	**Second position**	**Third position**	**Fourth position**
Category	Shock chamber	Antitachycardia pacing chamber	Tachycardia detection	Antibradycardia pacing chamber
	O (None)	O (None)	E (Electrocardiogram)	O (None)
	A (Atrium)	A (Atrium)	H (Hemodynamic)	A (Atrium)
	V (Ventricle)	V (Ventricle)		V (Ventricle)
	D (Dual)	D (Dual)		D (Dual)

dyssynchrony.[22,23] As a consequence, isovolumic contraction and isovolumic relaxation are prolonged with decreased cardiac output, and a dilated left ventricle can result in mitral regurgitation (MR) as well.[23]

CRT is typically accomplished by adding an LV pacing lead (placed through coronary sinus) to a standard PPM (CRT-P) or defibrillator system (CRT-D). When the two leads are activated, coordinated pacing of the left ventricle and right ventricle results.

At present patients eligible for CRT are those with mild heart failure symptoms or even asymptomatic ones with QRS duration >120 ms, LVEF ≤35%. In fact the EchoCRT (Echocardiography-Guided Cardiac Resynchronization Therapy) study even showed an increase in mortality with CRT implantation in cohort with relatively narrow QRS duration.[23,24] CRT leads to further improvement in the structure and function of the heart (reverse-remodeling), but the benefit disappears with the removal of CRT.[25]

Perioperative Management of Patients with CIEDs

With the rise in the number of patients with CIEDs and an elevation in their life expectancy, it is undoubtful that anesthesiologists will encounter CIEDs more and more in their practice. Current CIEDs are sophisticated and better shielded in insulated titanium or stainless steel case.[26] Use of Zener diode[27] and use of bipolar leads[28] mitigate the effects of electromagnetic interference (EMI), which is defined as interference of CIED function by the signals generated by external sources. EMI occurs in two forms: (1) conducted (e.g., electrocautery and defibrillation), and (2) radiated (e.g., magnetic resonance imaging [MRI]), positron emission tomography (PET), and radiation therapy. CIED systems are capable of filtering out some noncardiac signals by using bandpass filters.[27,28] However, if the energy level of a nearby electromagnetic field is very high, or has a frequency component close to that generated by the heart, it may lead to inappropriate inhibition or triggering of CIED, induction of fixed rate pacing, software reset, inappropriate patient movement, ventricular or atrial fibrillation, and even loss of battery output or damage to the generator.[26]

The role of electrocautery in the presence of CIED is of interest to an anesthesiologist. It (monopolar or bipolar) involves passing a high-voltage, high-frequency (10,000 Hz) current through tissue to cut or coagulate. Normally, it poses no risks but if activated before contacting the surgical instrument, its frequency might fluctuate and fall into the frequency range that PPMs and ICDs sense, interpreting them as cardiac output and generating inappropriate responses.[29]

Now since the CIED properties vary in structure and function from manufacturer to manufacturer, their indications vary from patient to patient. According to British Heart Rhythm Society (BHRS)[30] and practice advisory by American Society of Anaesthesiologist (ASA),[31] a single recommendation for all CIED patients is not appropriate and there should be individualized care of each patient through clear bilevel communication among the anesthesia professionals, surgeon, and CIED team.

Approach to Perioperative Management of Patients with a CIED

1. Determine whether a patient has a CIED.
2. Determine the CIED type, manufacturer, and primary indication for placement: obtain medical record form or chest X-ray if needed.
   Chest X-ray helps in identifying the type of CIED, lead location, integrity of device implantation, and even the manufacturer in emergency, in the absence of records.[29,32]
   ICD can be recognized by thicker white bands (shock coils) along the course of leads, while in CRT device a third lead can be identified in the coronary sinus.[33]
3. The CIED team should know the type of procedure, the patient position, the type of EMI that will be used, anticipated cardioversion, and postoperative disposition in order to make recommendations.
4. To know if the patient is pacing dependent based on history or no detectable ventricular activity if put on nontracking mode.[7]
   Tracking mode: Atrial events are tracked by the ventricle and so in DDD mode, during atrial tachyarrhythmias, ventricle is paced at inappropriate rates.
   Nontracking mode: VVI, DVI, or DDI.
   Automatic mode switching is defined as the ability of a PPM to reprogram itself from tracking to nontracking mode in response to atrial tachyarrhythmias.[34] Determine the current settings, obtain recent interrogation report, and reinterrogate if situation demands so. The ASA practice advisory suggests timely reinterrogation in the absence of surety of proper functioning before elective surgery. However, HRS suggests that interrogation should be done at proper intervals and that the CIED personnel should provide prescription for intraoperative care.
5. Consider replacing any CIED near its elective replacement period in a patient scheduled to undergo either a major operation or surgery within 15 cm of the generator. Three months of battery duration is reasonable in the perioperative period[35] because there is an increase in physiologic demands due to decreased systemic vascular resistance and hypovolemia during anesthesia.
6. Ideally, devices should be interrogated at specified intervals and this varies with the time of implantation of the device. As such PPMs should be interrogated every 12 months and ICDs and CRT devices should be evaluated every 6 months considering patients with these have significant comorbidities.

7. Determine the electromagnetic interference potential of the procedure. As far as the cardiac surgery is concerned it is a high-risk procedure occurring in the vicinity of the CIED and involves use of electrocautery. Therefore, the CIED should be interrogated before the procedure.
8. Put the PPM in asynchronous mode in pacing-dependent patient.
   What is asynchronous mode of pacing? No sensing of events occur and pulse generator delivers pacing stimulus at a fixed rate (e.g., VOO, DOO). Here pacing may occur in the vulnerable period (R on T phenomenon) resulting in lethal ventricular arrhythmias. Reprogramming to asynchronous pacing will prevent bradycardia or asystole during electrocautery use by not oversensing the signals; however, this will not protect it from internal damage or reset caused by EMI.[29]
9. Disable the rate modulating feature (e.g., minute ventilation which might otherwise erroneously sense extra cardiac signals) (e.g., positive pressure ventilation, or use of depolarizing muscle relaxant).
10. Suspend antitachycardia function of the ICD. Remember this will not abolish its pacing function. Always do this in a monitored environment and ensure there is at hand availability of temporary pacing and defibrillation equipment all through and after the procedure.
11. The ASA advisory recommends against the use of magnet while the HRS suggests for a magnet use.

Role of magnet: The response of a CIED to magnet depends on the type and manufacturer of the device. A magnet refers to a specifically designed ring or block magnet, which should be available in all hospitals.

It should be realized that magnet-activated switches were incorporated to produce a pacing behavior. Each PPM type has a unique asynchronous rate for beginning of life (BOL), elective replacement indicator (ERI), and end of life (EOL),[36] and therefore pacing thresholds and battery life can be predicted. Any device with inadequate battery life may actually be harmed by the application of magnet. One can even identify the manufacturer by the magnet response.[36]

The majority of manufacturers of the ICDs advise positioning the magnet directly over the device. However, St. Jude Medical and LivaNovs recommend that the magnet is offset from the device.[30]

Most PPMs respond with fixed rate (asynchronous) pacing while a magnet is held over the generator. However, the Medtronic "Micra" leadless IC-PM has no magnet sensor, whereas magnet mode is permanently disabled in Biotronik (Boston Scientific, St. Jude Medical) or temporarily suspended (e.g., Medtronic).[17] Thus, magnet response of the device is unstandardized and complicated. Although most PPMs provide asynchronous pacing at a rate of 85 to 100 with magnet application, it may be even lesser (i.e., 10 to 80 beats). Hence, response to magnet becomes inadequate in cases of increased oxygen requirements.[17]

For ICDs, placing a magnet over the device will inhibit delivery of ATP and shock therapy but will have no effect on bradycardia pacing. Some devices from Boston Scientific, Pacesetter, and St. Jude Medical can be programmed to ignore magnet placement. If the magnet mode is off, then intraoperative EMI is likely to produce repeated shocks. Antitachycardia therapy in some Guidant and CPI devices can be permanently disabled by magnet placement for 30 seconds.[17] Caution should be exercised when using magnetic drapes to hold surgical equipment. Placement of magnetic drapes on the patient thorax should be avoided.[30]

12. Intraoperatively monitor continuously patient's electrocardiography (ECG) while filtering out high-frequency components and disabling artifact filters, pulse oximetry (SpO$_2$) for oxygen saturation, and peripheral arterial pulse monitoring for observing mechanical systoles because EMI and some devices such as nerve stimulator may interfere with QRS or pacing spikes on ECG. Also pacing artifacts may be misinterpreted as heartrate for an asystolic patient. This should continue in the postoperative recovery room till the device is reprogrammed. In case of CRT while inserting central line one should be careful of spontaneous coronary sinus lead dislodgement or guidewire may dislodge sensing electrodes of ICD.
13. If unanticipated CIED interactions occur, suspend the procedure until the source of interference is identified and managed.
14. Use of electrocautery: Open heart surgery cannot be performed without electrocautery and the field of surgery too is near the PPM generator and leads. Hence require a cautious approach. Also patients with a rate-dependent permanent PPM present the potential problem of persistent cardiac electrical and mechanical activity intraoperatively that increases the potential for myocardial injury. A technique is described that makes use of chest wall stimulation through external pacing electrodes and thereby inhibiting the PPM.[37]
    a. Position the electrosurgical instrument and dispersive electrode so the current pathway does not pass through or near the CIED generator or leads.
    b. Avoid proximity of the electrosurgery electrical field to the generator and leads.
    c. Use short, intermittent, and irregular bursts of electrosurgery at the lowest feasible energy levels (limit ESU bursts to <4 s separated by at least 2 s).[38]
    d. Use bipolar electrosurgery or an ultrasonic (harmonic) scalpel, if possible.

Considerations during cardiac surgery:[39,40]
- Device reprogramming (in the asynchronous mode) should occur in the immediate preoperative period since placement of magnet is impractical due to surgical incision.
- Temporary epicardial pacing wires should be routinely inserted because ischemia reperfusion injury

and direct myocardial damage may result in loss of capture.

- Repeated attempts at defibrillation during a cardiac surgery if required may exhaust shielding function of PPM and cause permanent device dysfunction. It may also cause burn at lead–tissue interface, again to result in loss of capture.
- PPMs may have to be inactivated to sensing mode during cardioplegia to guide in assessing return of intrinsic electrical activity.
- Symptoms that led to PPM insertion and heart failure need to be optimized before surgery.
- ODO mode needs a temporary backup. According to Sathyanarayana et al, VVI pacing mode is optimal, as it provides electrical quiescence during the period of arrest.[39]

Studies have shown poor perioperative outcome in PPM patients, mainly related to the underlying cardiac disease, and confirmed the necessity to check the cardiac device in both the preoperative and postoperative period.[41]

15. In the circumstance when an external defibrillator or cardioversion has to be used, initially try re-enabling ICD antitachycardia therapy. There is no significant risk to someone performing CPR or touching the patient even if a shock is delivered through the patient's ICD. If this measure fails, try minimizing flow of current across the generator or leads by careful positioning of pads away (at least 8 cm) from the device and in anteroposterior position. Resuscitate as if the device was not present and use energy for defibrillation in clinically appropriate doses. Reinterrogate the device immediately after external defibrillation.

16. Intraoperatively, none of the anesthetic techniques claim advantage over one another. Literature reviews showed that isoflurane or sevoflurane prolong QT interval, whereas halothane shortens this interval. High-dose opiates and dexmedetomidine suppress underlying rhythms, rendering a patient pacing dependent. Etomidate, ketamine, and succinylcholine should be avoided as these may cause myoclonus or fasciculations.[17]

17. Postoperative management:
    a. Primarily, interrogate and restore CIED function.
    b. Continuously monitor rate and rhythm of the patient.
    c. Ensure availability of backup pacing and external defibrillation.

18. If on interrogation postsurgery it is determined that CIED has been reprogrammed to inappropriate settings, program it to the appropriate setting as soon as possible.

Perform a postoperative interrogation if emergency surgery occurred without appropriate preoperative evaluation, antitachycardia therapy is disabled or malfunctions, and significant EMI occurred in close proximity to the CIED.

HRS suggests that if the CIED is not reprogrammed or if the EMI procedure was infraumbilical, one can interrogate the device within 30 days after the procedure.

ASA, however, recommends interrogation of device after every procedure.

Emergency Protocol

1. Obtain information from the patient's CIED wallet card, medical records, or CIED team note, or from the chest X-ray.
2. Establish if the patient is PPM dependent.
3. Establish the risk of EMI.
4. Consider the use of magnet and use short bursts of cautery.
5. Monitor pulse oximetry, invasive arterial line if required, and transcutaneous external pacing and external defibrillator should be available.
6. For patients with ICDs, defibrillator pads should be placed.
7. Interrogation of the device as soon as possible.

PPM Implantation after Cardiac Surgery

Conduction disturbances necessitating permanent PPM implantation after cardiac surgery occur in 1 to 5% of patients.[42]

Early PPM implantation may reduce morbidity and postoperative hospital stay. However, Bis et al recommend implanting a PPM on postoperative day 7 to prevent unnecessary implantations and avoid prolonged hospitalization.[42] But patients undergoing redo double-valve surgery who continue to be asystolic or undergoing aortic root replacement and having persistent complete heart block postoperatively may need an earlier PPM implantation.[43]

Elective valve surgery: Associated bradycardia leads to the highest number of PPM implantations at a rate of 3.3%, while CABG and congenital heart surgery have a PPM rate of 0.8 and 2.4%, respectively.[44] Postoperative pacing need arises if either operative procedure injures the conduction system or there is a compromised myocardial protection and ischemic injury due to extensive coronary artery disease. Patients at high risk for PPM implantation after cardiac surgery include those with pulmonary hypertension, reoperation, and pre-existing left bundle branch block (LBBB).

Age, female sex, history of prior myocardial infarction, and impaired left ventricular function are risk factors for postoperative PPM insertion after open heart surgery. Similarly bypass time, cross clamp time, intra-aortic balloon pump, and type of surgery have a bearing on the rate of PPM implantation while electrolyte imbalance, AV block, and redo-operation are postoperative factors that may influence PPM implantation.[44]

Care of Patients with CIED or Temporary Pacemakers in Intensive Care

Apart from having knowledge of the types and indication of CIED, the treating intensivist as well as the nurse should have a sound knowledge of programmed modes, parameter settings, underlying rhythm, and cardiac function, and should be able to recognize complications such as failure to pace, capture (myocardial changes that result in noncapture include myocardial ischemia or infarction, acid-base disturbances, electrolyte abnormalities, or abnormal levels of antiarrhythmic drug[17]), or sense. They should understand the level of device dependency, and should be able to troubleshoot in case of device failure and provide timely external support.[45] In the critical care setting temporary pacing is applied to treat bradycardia in hemodynamically unstable patients, as a bridge to permanent PPM and for overdrive pacing.

Other problems that may be encountered in critical care is infection and even infective endocarditis due to the CIED, venous thromboembolism, and PPM malfunction. Some of the PPM malfunctions include failure of output (if no sensing on magnet application, with the main reason being either battery discharge or generator defect), failure to capture (evidence of pacing artifacts without resultant paced P-waves or QRS complexes results from lead failure, lead dislodgement, lead–tissue interface problem, or lead insulation break increasing stimulation threshold), oversensing that might result in prolonged asystole managed by reprogramming, and finally undersensing.[46] In case of infection, apart from systemic antibiotics, the whole device is explanted, measures are taken for temporary pacing on the contralateral side, and a new device is implanted. The common organisms that cause infection are *Staphylococcus aureus* and *Staphylococcus epidermidis*. Antibiotics are usually continued for 3 to 6 weeks. In case of venous thromboembolism anticoagulation is instituted at least for 3 months.[46]

Temporary Cardiac Pacing

Cardiac anesthesiologists may perform temporary pacing more often considering more frequent rhythm disorders in cardiac subset of patients. This serves as an emergency measure for managing bradycardia in hemodynamically unstable patients, and a bridge to permanent therapy in case of brady-tachy arrhythmias. The various forms of temporary pacing include transvenous catheter systems, transcutaneous pads, transthoracic wires, and epicardial and esophageal pacing techniques. It is imperative to reprogram the permanent device if present because if it senses the energy transvenous device it could result in inappropriate shock delivery by ICD, pacing inhibition (if sensed by ventricular lead), or rapid ventricular rate (if sensed by atrial lead) in case of PPM.[17]

Leadless and Subcutaneous Pacemakers

Leadless pacemakers and subcutaneous ICDs (s-ICDs) have emerged as novel alternatives to traditional CIEDs.

Respectively, these devices have minimal or no intravascular components, hence they should be less prone to infection. However, haematogenous seeding of leadless pacemakers from a distant site of infection is possible, and no definitive randomised controlled trial data currently exist to support a reduced risk of infection.

Currently, two types of leadless pacemakers have been developed for use in patients: the Micra Transcatheter Pacing System (Medtronic) and the Nanostim Leadless Cardiac Pacemaker (Abbott Cardiovascular, Plymouth, MN, USA). Avoiding a transvenous system may be preferential in patients at high risk of infection, particularly in those patients for whom central venous access is also challenging. Preliminary studies show that in selected high-risk patients—namely those with valve prosthesis or indwelling central venous catheters for haemodialysis—undergoing Micra implantation, no infections were reported after a year's follow-up. Leadless pacemakers may also confer a reduced risk of infection in those patients undergoing extraction of transvenous devices. Subcutaneous ICDs are an option for patients who only require protection from sudden ventricular arrhythmias and have no indication for pacing.[47]

Conclusion

Despite advances in technology as well as medical care, perioperative care of patients with CIED still remains a challenge for anesthesiologists. With more and more patient population already with underlying complex disease presenting for surgery, knowing the various CIEDs, understanding the targeted perioperative care they demand, and troubleshooting complications is an absolute necessity. Despite concerted efforts to mitigate the risk of CIED infections, the incidence has doubled in the last two decades.[1] CIED infections continue to be a significant cause of morbidity and mortality among device patients, with substantial associated health care costs associated with intensive care unit stays, complex diagnostics, prolonged antibiotic therapy, and additional invasive procedures.[48]

References

1. Naraparaju V, Almnajam M, Joseph L, et al. A survey on patient preferences towards CIED implantation. Indian Pacing Electrophysiol J 2021;21(4):227–231
2. Shenthar J, Bohra S, Jetley V, et al. A survey of cardiac implantable electronic device implantation in India: by Indian Society of Electrocardiology and Indian Heart Rhythm Society. Indian Heart J 2016;68(1):68–71
3. Verma N, Knight BP. Update in cardiac pacing. Arrhythm Electrophysiol Rev 2019;8(3):228–233
4. Cingolani E, Goldhaber JI, Marbán E. Next-generation pacemakers: from small devices to biological pacemakers. Nat Rev Cardiol 2018;15(3):139–150
5. Mulpuru SK, Madhavan M, McLeod CJ, Cha YM, Friedman PA. Cardiac pacemakers: function, troubleshooting, and

management: Part 1 of a 2-Part series. J Am Coll Cardiol 2017;69(2):189–210

6. Liu L, Tang J, Peng H, et al. A long-term, prospective, cohort study on the performance of right ventricular pacing leads: comparison of active-fixation with passive-fixation leads. Sci Rep 2015;5:7662

7. Lak HM, Goyal A. Pacemaker types and selection. [Updated 2020 Dec 1]. In: StatPearls [Internet]. Treasure Island, FL: StatPearls Publishing; 2021. https://www.ncbi.nlm.nih.gov/books/NBK556011/

8. Dell'Orto S, Valli P, Greco EM. Sensors for rate responsive pacing. Indian Pacing Electrophysiol J 2004;4(3):137–145

9. Kaszala K, Ellenbogen KA. Device sensing: sensors and algorithms for pacemakers and implantable cardioverter defibrillators. Circulation 2010;122(13):1328–1340

10. Lau C-P, Tse H-F, Camm AJ, Barold SS. Evolution of pacing for bradycardias: sensors. Eur Heart J Suppl 2007;9:I11–I22

11. Puette JA, Malek R, Ellison MB. Pacemaker. [Updated 2021 Sep 18]. In: StatPearls [Internet]. Treasure Island, FL: StatPearls Publishing; 2021. https://www.ncbi.nlm.nih.gov/books/NBK526001/

12. Farmer DM, Estes NA III, Link MS. New concepts in pacemaker syndrome. Indian Pacing Electrophysiol J 2004;4(4):195–200

13. Safavi-Naeini P, Saeed M. Pacemaker troubleshooting: common clinical scenarios. Tex Heart Inst J 2016;43(5):415–418

14. Beyerback DM. Pacemakers and implantable cardioverter defibrillators.[Updated 2019 Oct 11]. In: The heart.org Medscape [Internet]: Medscape Publishing. https://emedicine.medscape.com/article/162245-overview#a1

15. Townsend T. Five common permanent cardiac pacemaker complications. Nurs Crit Care 2018;13:46–48

16. Kedia R, Saeed M. Implantable cardioverter-defibrillators: indications and unresolved issues. Tex Heart Inst J 2012;39(3):335–341

17. Rozner MA. Cardiac implantable electronic device. In: Kaplan JA, ed. Kaplans cardiac anaesthesia. 7th ed. Philadelphia, PA: Elsevier; 2017:118–139

18. Trivedi A, Knight BP. ICD therapy for primary prevention in hypertrophic cardiomyopathy. Arrhythm Electrophysiol Rev 2016;5(3):188–196

19. El-Battrawy I, Roterberg G, Liebe V, et al. Implantable cardioverter-defibrillator in Brugada syndrome: Long-term follow-up. Clin Cardiol 2019;42(10):958–965

20. Ghzally Y, Mahajan K. Implantable defibrillator. [Updated 2021 Oct 9]. In: StatPearls [Internet]. Treasure Island, FL: StatPearls Publishing; 2021. https://www.ncbi.nlm.nih.gov/books/NBK459196/

21. Cappelli S, Olaru A, Maria ED. The subcutaneous defibrillator: who stands to benefit. ESC Council Cardiol J. 2014;12:17. https://www.escardio.org/Journals/E-Journal-of-Cardiology-Practice/Volume-12/The-subcutaneous-defibrillator-who-stands-to-benefit

22. Chia PL, Foo D. Overview of implantable cardioverter defibrillator and cardiac resynchronisation therapy in heart failure management. Singapore Med J 2016;57(7):354–359

23. Jaffe LM, Morin DP. Cardiac resynchronization therapy: history, present status, and future directions. Ochsner J 2014;14(4):596–607

24. Marek J, Gandalovicova J, Kejrova E, et al. Echocardiography and cardiac resynchronization therapy. Cor Vasa 2016;58:e340–e351

25. Sutton MS, Keane MG. Reverse remodelling in heart failure with cardiac resynchronisation therapy. Heart 2007;93(2):167–171

26. Erdogan O. Electromagnetic interference on pacemakers. Indian Pacing Electrophysiol J 2002;2(3):74–78

27. Waller C, Callies F, Langenfeld H. Adverse effects of direct current cardioversion on cardiac pacemakers and electrodes: is external cardioversion contraindicated in patients with permanent pacing systems? Europace 2004;6(2):165–168

28. Beinart R, Nazarian S; From Engineering Principles to Clinical Practice. Effects of external electrical and magnetic fields on pacemakers and defibrillators: from engineering principles to clinical practice. Circulation 2013;128(25):2799–2809

29. Madigan JD, Choudhri AF, Chen J, Spotnitz HM, Oz MC, Edwards N. Surgical management of the patient with an implanted cardiac device: implications of electromagnetic interference. Ann Surg 1999;230(5):639–647

30. Thomas H, Turley A, Plummer C. British Heart Rhythm Society guidelines for the management of patients with cardiac implantable electronic devices (CIEDs) around the time of surgery. [Updated February 2019]. https://bhrs.com/wp-content/uploads/2019/05/Revised-guideline-CIED-and-surgery-Feb-19.pdf

31. Practice Advisory for the Perioperative Management of Patients with Cardiac Implantable Electronic Devices: Pacemakers and Implantable Cardioverter-Defibrillators 2020: an updated report by the American Society of Anesthesiologists Task Force on perioperative management of patients with cardiac implantable electronic devices: erratum. Anesthesiology 2020;132(4):938

32. Torres-Ayala SC, Santacana-Laffitte G, Maldonado J. Radiography of cardiac conduction devices: a pictorial review of pacemakers and implantable cardioverter defibrillators. J Clin Imaging Sci 2014;4:74

33. Mathew RP, Alexander T, Patel V, Low G. Chest radiographs of cardiac devices (Part 1): Cardiovascular implantable electronic devices, cardiac valve prostheses and Amplatzer occluder devices. SA J Radiol 2019;23(1):1730

34. Israel CW. Mode-Switch-Algorithmen: Programmierbarkeit und Nutzen. [Mode-switching algorithms: programming and usefulness] Herz 2001;26(1):2–17

35. Mahajan A, Neelankavil JP. Implantable cardiac pulse generators: pacemakers and cardioverters-defibrillators. In: Gropper M, ed. Miller's anaesthesia. 9th ed. Philadelphia, PA: Elsevier; 2019:1231–1242e1

36. Jacob S, Panaich SS, Maheshwari R, Haddad JW, Padanilam BJ, John SK. Clinical applications of magnets on cardiac rhythm management devices. Europace 2011;13(9):1222–1230

37. Hakki HI, Goel IP, Mundth ED. Pacemaker inhibition in cardiac surgery. Ann Thorac Surg 1982;33(3):295–296

38. Cardiac Electrophysiology. Diagnosis and treatment. In: Anesthesia key fastest anesthesia & intensive care & emergency medicine insight engine. https://aneskey.com/cardiac-electrophysiology-diagnosis-and-treatment-2/

39. Sathyanarayana LA. Open heart surgery in a patient with dual chamber pacemaker. Res Inno in Anesth 2018;3:66–69

40. Barbeito A. Preanaesthesia evaluation for cardiac surgery. [Updated 2021 October 07]. https://www.uptodate.com/contents/preanesthesia-evaluation-for-cardiac-surgery?csi=9c69dc00-93da-4ee4-a8a1-6b28128e89fd&source=contentShare

41. Pili-Floury S, Farah F, Samain E, Schauvliege F, Marty J. Perioperative outcome of pacemaker patients undergoing non-cardiac surgery. Eur J Anaesthesiol 2008;25(6):514–516

42. Bis J, Gościńska-Bis K, Gołba KS, Gocoł R, Zębalski M, Deja MA. Permanent pacemaker implantation after cardiac surgery:

Optimization of the decision making process. J Thorac Cardiovasc Surg 2021;162(3):816–824.e3

43. Sultan I. Commentary: permanent pacemakers after cardiac surgery: are we jumping the gun? J Thorac Cardiovasc Surg 2021;162(3):826–827

44. Harky A, Gatta F, Noshirwani A, et al. Permanent pacemaker post cardiac surgery: where do we stand? Rev Bras Cir Cardiovasc 2021;36:94–105

45. Chui-Man C, MacGill-Lane S, Murphy C. Care of the patient with temporary pacemaker in the neonatal and pediatric cardiac patient what the nurse caring for a patient with congenital heart disease needs to know. https://pcics.org/wp-content/uploads/nursing/Temporary_Pacemaker_-_Final_2016.pdf

46. Hongo RH, Goldschlager NF. Cardiac pacing in the critical care setting. In: Kusumoto FM, Goldschlager NF, eds. Cardiac pacing for the clinician. Boston, MA: Springer; 2008

47. Uslan DZ, Dowsley TF, Sohail MR, Hayes DL, Friedman PA, Wilson WR, Steckelberg JM, Baddour LM. Cardiovascular implantable electronic device infection in patients with Staphylococcus aureus bacteremia. Pacing Clin Electrophysiol. 2010;33(4):407–13

48. Mahtani K, Maclean E, Schilling RJ. Prevention and Management of Cardiac Implantable Electronic Device Infections: State-of-the-Art and Future Directions. Heart, Lung and Circulation. 2022; 31(11):1482–1492

18

Antibiotics in Cardiac Surgery

Poonam Malhotra Kapoor, Rohan Magoon, Iti Shri, and Jess Jose

Introduction

Cardiac surgery is a unique surgery that employs cardiopulmonary bypass (CPB) pump, implants, grafts especially in coronary artery disease, in-dwelling catheters, and prolonged intubation, making the patients prone to inflammation and infection. The CPB in itself is associated with systemic inflammation, impaired humoral immunity, reduced phagocytosis and activation of white blood cells and bleeding, and hypothermia, which together predispose to the perils of infection.[1] The saphenous vein graft-harvesting sites and various in-dwelling devices such as chest drain, pacemaker wires, central venous line serve as potential routes of bacterial access into the body.[2] Also, a longer duration of surgery increases their propensity to infection.[3]

The most common noncardiac complication after cardiac surgery is nosocomial infection (NI), which includes surgical site infection (SSI), respiratory and urinary tract infection, central venous catheter-related infection, approximately in 5 to 21% of cases.[4]

These not only just increase cost of care but also prolong recovery (more than 14 days), reduce patient satisfaction, and are associated with considerable morbidity and mortality (attributable mortality fraction, 17.1%).[5,6] The most common sites of infection are the respiratory tract (45.7–57.8%), the surgical site (27.7%), and catheters or devices (20.5–25.2%).[4]

In a prospective study by Jiang et al, NI rates following surgery for congenital malformation, valve replacement, and coronary artery bypass graft (CABG) were 2.6, 5.5, and 13.6%, respectively.[5] The NI rate was highest with aortic aneurysms and dissection repair (16.8%) presumably owing to emergency nature of the intervention.[5] Superficial sternal wound infection (SSWI), which involves the skin, subcutaneous tissue, and the pectoralis fascia, has an incidence of 0.5 to 8%, with an associated morbidity and mortality rate ranging from 0.5 to 9%[7] while the incidence of deep sternal wound infection (DSWI) or mediastinitis is 0.25 to 6.8% with in-hospital mortality rates between 7 and 47%.[8]

Such patients incur approximately 2.8 times the expenditure as compared to those with uncomplicated course. In the United States, they contribute to patients spending more than 400,000 extra days in hospital at a cost of an additional US$ 10 billion per year.

Fowler et al identified subset of patients that are at high risk of major infection following cardiac surgery:[9]
- Age (more than 65 years).
- BMI ($18.5 \leq$ BMI <25 Kg/m^2).
- Female gender.
- Diabetes.
- Renal failure.
- Congestive heart failure, cardiogenic shock, myocardial infarction.
- Peripheral vascular disease.
- Chronic lung disease.
- Concomitant surgery.
- Perfusion time 100 to 300 minutes.
- Intra-aortic balloon pump.

CABG surgery with pedicled harvesting of the internal mammary artery is associated with the maximum rate of sternal wound infection.[10] Postoperative bleeding, reoperations, sternal rewiring, excessive electrocautery, razors, administration of prophylactic antibiotics >60 minutes prior to incision, inadequate antibiotic doses, and the use of bone wax are other commonly implicated factors.[7,11,12]

Here comes the role of antibiotic prophylaxis, although it's just one of the measures to prevent SSI, other measures, such as meticulous aseptic surgical technique, care bundles, preoperative screening for carriage of resistant organisms together with decolonization, preoperative showering and hair removal, perioperative skin preparation, temperature and blood glucose control, maintenance of adequate hemoglobin saturation, and postoperative wound management, together form a comprehensive approach in preventing SSI.[13]

Antibiotic Prophylaxis

Surgical antibiotic prophylaxis (SAP) is defined as the use of antibiotics to prevent infections at the surgical site. A single antibiotic dose, given immediately before the start of surgery, may be just as effective in preventing infection, while reducing the risk of drug side effects. Primary prophylaxis refers to the prevention of an initial infection. Secondary prophylaxis refers to the prevention of recurrence or reactivation of a preexisting infection. Eradication refers to the elimination of a colonized organism to prevent the development of an infection.

American Society of Healthcare Pharmacy (ASHP), Society for Healthcare Epidemiology of America (SHEA), National Health Service (NHS), American College of Cardiology Foundation/American Heart Association (ACC/AHA), European Society of Cardiology (ESC) and Centers for Disease Control and Prevention (CDC), Society of Thoracic Surgeons (STS), and World Health Organization (WHO) have all come up with various guidelines on SAP during cardiac surgery and broadly follow the same general principles. A major limitation of the available literature on antimicrobial prophylaxis is the difficulty in establishing significant differences in efficacy between prophylactic antimicrobial agents and controls (including placebo, no treatment, or other antimicrobial agents) due to study design and low SSI rates for most procedures.

The mean frequency of SSIs in cardiac procedures (CABG) ranges from 0.23 to 5.67 per 100 operations.[14] Almost two-thirds of organisms isolated in both adult and pediatric patients undergoing cardiac procedures are gram-positive, including *Staphylococcus aureus* (in three-quarters of patients and when combined with other gram-positive organisms account for approximately 80% of DSWI), coagulase-negative staphylococcus (CoNS), and, rarely, *Propionibacterium acnes*.[2,15]

Gram-negative organisms are less commonly isolated in these patients and include *Enterobacter* species, *Pseudomonas aeruginosa*, *Escherichia coli*, *Klebsiella pneumoniae*, *Proteus mirabilis*, and *Acinetobacter* species.[2,16] The SSI rate in cardiac procedures is low, but there are potential consequences if infection occurs. Multiple studies have found that antimicrobial prophylaxis in cardiac procedures lowers the occurrence of postoperative SSI up to fivefold.[17]

But three cardinal questions to be answered here are:

1. Which antibiotic and dose?
2. When to administer?
3. Duration of administration?

Ideally, an antimicrobial agent for surgical prophylaxis should:

- Prevent SSI by acting on the pathogen causing it.
- Attains adequate serum and tissue concentration during the period of potential infectivity.
- Prevent SSI-related morbidity and mortality.
- Be cost-effective.
- Produce no adverse effects.
- No adverse consequences for the normal microbial flora.

Suitable antibiotic choices require gram-positive activity because these organisms account for 80% of SSIs. Since predominant organism for cardiac surgical infections is a *Staphylococcus* spp., the earlier generation cephalosporins are likely to be preferred for prophylaxis, and the cephalosporin of choice, which is recommended by the Society of Thoracic Surgeons, is cefazolin (cheap and has better gram-positive activity than later generations of cephalosporins). Although there's no cephalosporin that conclusively has been shown to be superior in affecting a lower infection rate, a recent meta-analysis concluded that second- or third-generation cephalosporins should be used based on lower postoperative ventilator-associated pneumonia (VAP) rates and all-cause mortality.[18]

But the choice of a prophylactic antibiotic has become increasingly controversial with the emergence of methicillin-resistant *Staphylococcus aureus* (MRSA) and methicillin-resistant coagulase-negative *Staphylococcus* (MRCNS). In a study by Mekontso-Dessap et al, overall mortality was 53.3% for MRSA poststernotomy infections as compared to 19.2% for MSSA infections, with corresponding 3-year survival rates of 26% versus 79%.[19] In such cases prophylaxis by vancomycin is considered to be more effective. In 2008, it was reported that when the hospital MRSA infection rate reached 60%, changing to vancomycin decreased the monthly SSI rate (2.1 cases per 100 surgical procedures).[20]

Also in patients with a history of an immunoglobulin-E (IgE)–mediated reaction to penicillin or cephalosporin (anaphylaxis, angioedema), if reaction persists after a skin test, vancomycin should be given preoperatively and for no more than 48 hours (Class I, Level of Evidence A). If its non-IgE-mediated reaction, then either vancomycin or a cephalosporin is recommended for prophylaxis (Class I, Level of Evidence B).[21]

However, overall, vancomycin has a narrower antimicrobial spectrum, inferior tissue and bone penetration, poor performance on CPB, and poor and slow bactericidal properties;[9] and high incidence of SSI due to methicillin-sensitive organisms, emergence of enterococcus organisms as well, has been higher when only vancomycin has been employed for prophylaxis.[22]

According to a Class IIB recommendation by STS society, in the setting of either a presumed or known staphylococcal colonization, the institutional presence of a "high incidence" of MRSA, patients susceptible to colonization (hospitalized longer than 3 days, transfer from other inpatient facility, already receiving antibiotics), or an operation for a patient having prosthetic valve or vascular graft insertion, it would be reasonable to combine the β-lactam (cefazolin) with a glycopeptide (vancomycin) for prophylaxis, with the restriction to limit vancomycin to only one or two doses (Level of Evidence C).[23]

Appropriate perioperative dosing of antibiotics during cardiac surgery presents unique challenges, not only because of altered pharmacokinetics on CPB but also because of tissue levels, specifically in bone and sternal fat, that may be more relevant than the serum concentrations. The standard cefazolin antibiotic prophylaxis regimen of 1 g was not reliable in patients with normal renal function undergoing elective cardiac surgery with CPB.[24] In fact, even with 2-g cefazolin, therapeutic tissue levels may not be achieved in the morbidly obese patients. Readministration of a prophylactic antibiotic during surgery should be within two half-lives of the antibiotic, exclusive of any influence of the effects of CPB.[25] Therefore, cefazolin, which has a half-life of approximately 1.8 hours, an additional dosing during surgery every 3 to 4 hours is recommended with an open wound beyond that period. If CPB is to be discontinued within 4 hours, then it is appropriate to delay redosing until perfusion is complete to maximize effective blood levels (Class I, Level of Evidence B).[23]

A dose of 1 to 1.5 g or 15 mg/kg of vancomycin administered intravenously slowly over 1 hour is considered appropriate.[23] Gentamicin, an aminoglycoside may be added, in a dose of 4 mg/kg to vancomycin if gram-negative prophylaxis is necessary.

Redosing an aminoglycoside during CPB is not indicated and may be harmful (Class III, Level of Evidence C) because of associated nephrotoxicity and ototoxicity, and excretion is delayed after CPB.[23]

CPB over the years have evolved into a keystone component of most major cardiac surgical procedures, but they impart various physiological alterations to circulatory system and pharmacokinetic changes. These changes are primarily due to hemodilution, sequestration of antibiotics within the CPB circuit, hypothermia and lung isolation leading to trapping of drugs administered prior to initiation of CPB.[26] Various studies have been conducted to better understand and standardize antibiotic prophylaxis in adult patients undergoing CPB:[27]

- Cefuroxime: 3.0 g at induction of anesthesia followed by 1.5 g at initiation of CPB plus 1.5 g 8 hours after surgery or 1.5 g at induction of anesthesia followed by 750 mg every 6 h for 24 hours have been shown to achieve adequate minimum inhibitory concentrations (MIC) for most common pathogens.
- Ceftriaxone: 1 g given approximately 2 hours prior to CPB achieved adequate tissue concentration.
- Daptomycin: At 8 mg/kg around 30 to 60 minutes prior to surgery have been shown to produce consistently high tissue concentrations.
- Teicoplanin: 12 mg/kg at induction of anesthesia followed by 6 mg/kg after 12 hours attained adequate tissue concentrations for common pathogens.
- Vancomycin: 15 mg/kg prior to anesthesia over 60 minutes or 1 g within 1 to 2 hours prior to surgery.
- Levofloxacin: 500 to 1,000 mg once daily achieved required tissue concentration.
- Linezolid: 600 mg every 12 hours had same tissue concentrations as patients who were not on CPB and was found to be adequate for methicillin-resistant *Staphylococcus aureus* (MRSA) infections with MIC < 1 mg/L.
- Meropenem: 1 g every 8 hours for susceptible organisms (MIC < 2) and 2 g every 8 hours for resistant organisms (MIC < 2–8) was found to be adequate.
- Piperacillin/tazobactam: 3.375 g every 6 hours or 4.5 g every 6 to 8 hours achieved necessary tissue concentrations similar to non-CPB patients.
- Tigecycline: 100 mg once followed by 50 mg every 12 hours achieved required tissue levels.

The findings from a prospective cohort study of more than 5,000 patients found that pneumonia, bloodstream infections, and *Clostridium difficile* colitis accounted for 79% of all major postoperative infections following surgery with a major burden of readmissions, morbidity, and mortality. In this scenario, second-generation cephalosporins (± vancomycin) were more commonly used than first-generation antibiotics and were strongly associated with reduced infection risk.[28]

When to Administer?

It is imperative that the antibiotic used for prophylaxis attains bactericidal concentrations at the most critical time and at the most critical site as to prevent the bacterial contamination of the surgical site, and provide adequate duration of coverage both before and throughout the procedure.

According to WHO summary of systematic review over the optimal timing of administration of antibiotic for prophylaxis, the retrieved evidence can be summarized as follows:[29]

- Low-quality evidence of a significant harm if SAP is withheld prior to incision.
- Moderate-quality evidence of significant harm if SAP is administered before 120 minutes prior to incision than within 120 minutes.
- It is not possible to establish more precisely the optimal timing within the 120-minute interval as no significant difference was found between the different time intervals within this period.

Exceptions include vancomycin and levofloxacin, which require administration within 120 minutes of the procedural incision due to longer administration times.

If a patient is already receiving an antibiotic for another infection before surgery, and it is appropriate for surgical prophylaxis, an extra dose of the antibiotic can be administered within 60 minutes of the incision.

Duration of Prophylaxis

In cardiac surgery, a low-quality evidence exists that continuation of antibiotic prophylaxis for up to 24 hours postoperatively has a benefit in reducing the SSI rate when compared to a single dose of antibiotic prophylaxis, with no benefits if extended beyond 24 hours (very low-quality evidence). A prolonged (24–48 hours) prophylactic regimen is considered beneficial in cardiac surgery in view of use of CPB, systemic cooling for myocardial protection, invasive devices remaining after surgery, high risk of bleeding requiring blood transfusion and re-exploration, and delayed extubation after surgery.[30]

It has also been found that reducing the duration of antibiotic prophylaxis (AP) from 56 to 32 hours in adult cardiac surgery contributes to reduced antibiotic resistance and healthcare costs.[31]

But the optimal duration of antibiotic prophylaxis in cardiac surgery is still controversial. Lador et al found from 23 randomized controlled trials (RCTs) that prophylaxis of ≤24 hours postoperation led to higher rates of DSWI, as compared to longer duration prophylaxis. However, there was no advantage of regimens lasting >48 hours postoperation, rather only grow and emergence of *C. difficile* infection (CDI).[32]

Prophylactic Nasal Mupirocin Ointment

Nasal carriage of *S. aureus* is now considered a well-defined risk factor for subsequent infection in various groups of patients. Mupirocin nasal ointment (applied two times daily for 5 days) is an effective, safe, and relatively low-cost treatment for the eradication of carriage. Overall, a moderate quality of evidence shows that the use of mupirocin 2% ointment in combination with or without chlorhexidine gluconate (CHG) body wash in cardiothoracic surgical patients with nasal *S. aureus* carriage has significant benefit when compared to placebo/no treatment.[33-35]

However, there is evidence that the increased short-term use of mupirocin leads to an increase in resistance to mupirocin and other antibiotics.[35]

Good quality RCTs are needed to test other options than mupirocin.

Deep Sternal Wound Infection

DSWI, if happens,[36] is associated with:
- An organism isolated from culture of mediastinal tissue or fluid.
- Evidence of mediastinitis seen during operation.
- Presence of chest pain, sternal instability, or fever (>38.8°C).
- Purulent drainage from the mediastinum, isolation of an organism present in a blood culture, or culture of the mediastinal area.

These patients require a much more aggressive treatment regimen.

Gardlund et al stratified DSWI into three forms:[37]
1. Coagulase negative *Staphylococcus* is the dominant species in which dehiscence is associated with obesity and chronic obstructive pulmonary disease (COPD).
2. In the second form, *S. aureus* is predominant and is associated with perioperative or nasopharyngeal contamination and often presents with bacteremia.
3. The third form involves gram-negative DSWI, most commonly *E. coli*, *Klebsiella*, or *Enterobacter* and is associated with bacterial spread from other sites.

Here the empiric antibiotic therapy is initiated to include broad coverage against methicillin-resistant gram-positive, gram-negative, and anaerobic organisms. Culture-directed therapy should be initiated as soon as microbiological analysis is available. Blood, urine, and sputum cultures should also be obtained. Systemic antibiotics are typically given for 6 weeks. Antifungal therapy is often administered in the absence of clinical improvement on antibiotics.

There is a multitude of current treatment options available for sternal wound closure including closed suction antibiotic catheter irrigation systems, vacuum-assisted closure, the omental transposition, flap and major muscle rotation, etc. Treatment of any DSWI consists of early wound exploration.[7,37]

Pediatric Cardiac Procedures

SSI rates after pediatric cardiac surgery range from 2.3 to 9.9%.[38] Significant risk factors are presence of other infections, young age, small body size, the duration of the procedure, the need for an intraoperative blood transfusion, an open sternum postoperatively, re-exploration, and the length of stay in the intensive care unit. The organisms of concern in pediatric patients are the same as those in adult patients. No well-controlled studies have evaluated the efficacy of antimicrobial prophylaxis in pediatric patients undergoing cardiac procedures and for infectious endocarditis (IE).[39]

Antibiotic Prophylaxis for Infective Endocarditis

Infective endocarditis (IE) is an infection of the endocardium (particularly the valve leaflets) with a yearly incidence of 3 to 10 per 100,000 and is characterized by the development of infected heart valve vegetations. It has a poor prognosis with high morbidity and an in-hospital mortality of 15 to 20%, rising to approximately 30% at 1 year. Therefore, prevention strategies are considered mainstay in avoiding the burden.[40]

Major revisions in guidelines focus on the treatment and prevention of IE; the AHA guidelines 2007 is focused on those at greatest risk of adverse outcomes from IE rather than only a life-time risk of developing IE. The major factors contributing to this change in recommendation are lack of RCT data demonstrating benefit from AP, lack of data demonstrating consistent associations between procedures and development of IE, lack of cost-effectiveness of AP, and an increasing antibiotic resistance. Finally, the cumulative lifetime risk of developing IE from tooth brushing and mastication was estimated to be higher than from a single tooth extraction.

The European Society of Cardiology (ESC) followed in 2009 with similar recommendations to the American Heart Association (AHA), whereas in the United Kingdom the National Institute for Health and Care Excellence (NICE) endorsed complete restriction of AP regardless of risk in 2008. However there was an increase in the rate of hospitalization because of IE and this increase occurred in both high- and moderate-risk groups and the relative proportion of streptococcal IE versus staphylococcal IE decreased, especially in the younger adult population, over time. But as noted patients with bicuspid aortic valves and mitral valve prolapse have a higher rate of viridans group streptococci and IE of suspected odontological origin, AP should be reconsidered in such patients.[41] Therefore, prevention of IE remains an empirical practice. Antibiotic regimens for endocarditis prophylaxis are directed toward *S. viridans*, and the recommended standard prophylactic regimen is a single dose of oral amoxicillin. Amoxicillin, ampicillin, and penicillin V are equally effective in vitro against alpha-hemolytic streptococci; however, amoxicillin is preferred because of superior gastrointestinal absorption.[42]

All doses shown below are administered once as a single dose 30 to 60 minutes before the procedure:

- Standard general prophylaxis: Amoxicillin 2 g PO.
- Unable to take oral medication: Ampicillin 2 g IV/IM or cefazolin/ceftriaxone 1 g IM or IV.
- Allergic to penicillin: Clindamycin 600 mg PO.
- Allergic to penicillin: Cephalexin 2 g PO or other first- or second-generation oral cephalosporin in equivalent dose (do not use cephalosporins in patients with a history of immediate-type hypersensitivity penicillin allergy, such as urticaria, angioedema, anaphylaxis).
- Allergic to penicillin: Azithromycin or clarithromycin: 500 mg PO.
- Allergic to penicillin and unable to take oral medication: Clindamycin 600 mg IV.
- Allergic to penicillin and unable to take oral medication: Cefazolin or ceftriaxone (do not use cephalosporins in patients with a history of immediate-type hypersensitivity penicillin allergy, such as urticaria, angioedema, anaphylaxis): 1 g IV/IM.

Conclusion

Unfortunately, there are no data concerning the risk of inducing antibiotic resistance associated with AP. However, most concern relates to the use of lower dose therapeutic antibiotic regimens over several days and not to use a single high dose of a bactericidal antibiotic, such as amoxicillin.

A major limitation of the available literature on antimicrobial prophylaxis is the difficulty in establishing significant differences in efficacy between prophylactic antimicrobial agents and controls (including placebo, no treatment, or other antimicrobial agents) due to study design. A small sample size increases the likelihood of a Type II error; therefore, there may be no apparent difference between the antimicrobial agent and placebo.

Prophylactic antibiotic protocols in cardiac surgery remain far from standardized and in this era of antibiotic stewardship, enhanced recovery after surgery pathway protocols, early postoperative discharge and preventable readmissions, finance and healthcare infrastructure, which are all heavily influenced by infections, we need to dynamically revise and re-evaluate our guidelines, and monitor our incidence of infection and effectiveness and adequacy of management practices.

There is an over prescription of broad spectrum antibiotic and high frequency of antibiotic combination for all causes of admission to CCUs in primary and secondary hospitals in India. It is crucial to implement the surveillance of antibiotic use in CCUs and establish a protocol the empirical antibiotic treatment to improve overall patients' outcome.[43]

References

1. Laffey JG, Boylan JF, Cheng DC. The systemic inflammatory response to cardiac surgery: implications for the anesthesiologist. Anesthesiology 2002;97(1):215–252
2. Cove ME, Spelman DW, MacLaren G. Infectious complications of cardiac surgery: a clinical review. J Cardiothorac Vasc Anesth 2012;26(6):1094–1100
3. Sulzgruber P, Schnaubelt S, Koller L, et al. An extended duration of the pre-operative hospitalization is associated with an increased risk of healthcare-associated infections after cardiac surgery. Sci Rep 2020;10(1):8006
4. Michalopoulos A, Geroulanos S, Rosmarakis ES, Falagas ME. Frequency, characteristics, and predictors of microbiologically documented nosocomial infections after cardiac surgery. Eur J Cardiothorac Surg 2006;29(4):456–460
5. Jiang WL, Hu XP, Hu ZP, et al. Morbidity and mortality of nosocomial infection after cardiovascular surgery: a report of 1606 cases. Curr Med Sci 2018;38(2):329–335
6. Massart N, Mansour A, Ross JT, et al. Mortality due to hospital-acquired infection after cardiac surgery. J Thorac Cardiovasc Surg 2020;2: S0022–5223(20)32486–7
7. Singh K, Anderson E, Harper JG. Overview and management of sternal wound infection. Semin Plast Surg 2011;25(1):25–33
8. Cotogni P, Barbero C, Rinaldi M. Deep sternal wound infection after cardiac surgery: evidences and controversies. World J Crit Care Med 2015;4(4):265–273
9. Fowler VG Jr, O'Brien SM, Muhlbaier LH, Corey GR, Ferguson TB, Peterson ED. Clinical predictors of major infections after cardiac surgery. Circulation 2005;112(9, Suppl):I358–I365
10. Sá MP, Ferraz PE, Escobar RR, et al. Skeletonized versus pedicled internal thoracic artery and risk of sternal wound infection after coronary bypass surgery: meta-analysis and meta-regression of 4817 patients. Interact Cardiovasc Thorac Surg 2013;16(6):849–857
11. Tang GH, Maganti M, Weisel RD, Borger MA. Prevention and management of deep sternal wound infection. Semin Thorac Cardiovasc Surg 2004;16(1):62–69
12. Bryan CS, Yarbrough WM. Preventing deep wound infection after coronary artery bypass grafting: a review. Tex Heart Inst J 2013;40(2):125–139
13. Rogers L, Vaja R, Bleetman D, Ali JM, Rochon M, Sanders J, et al. Interventions to prevent surgical site infection in adults undergoing cardiac surgery. Cochrane Database Syst Rev 2019;2019(5):CD013332
14. Basicmedical Key. Practice guidelines for antimicrobial prophylaxis in surgery[Internet].[cited on 20 December 2020]. https://basicmedicalkey.com/practice-guidelines-for-antimicrobial-prophylaxis-in-surgery/
15. Sommerstein R, Kohler P, Wilhelm MJ, Kuster SP, Sax H. Factors associated with methicillin-resistant coagulase-negative staphylococci as causing organisms in deep sternal wound infections after cardiac surgery. New Microbes New Infect 2015;6:15–21
16. Garey KW, Kumar N, Dao T, Tam VH, Gentry LO. Risk factors for postoperative chest wound infections due to gram-negative bacteria in cardiac surgery patients. J Chemother 2006;18(4): 402–408

17. Bratzler DW, Dellinger EP, Olsen KM, et al; Surgical Infection Society Guidelines. Clinical practice guidelines for antimicrobial prophylaxis in surgery. Surg Infect (Larchmt) 2013;14

18. He S, Chen B, Li W, et al. Ventilator-associated pneumonia after cardiac surgery: a meta-analysis and systematic review. J Thorac Cardiovasc Surg 2014;148(6):3148–55.e1, 5

19. Mekontso-Dessap A, Kirsch M, Brun-Buisson C, Loisance D. Poststernotomy mediastinitis due to Staphylococcus aureus: comparison of methicillin-resistant and methicillin-susceptible cases. Clin Infect Dis 2001;32(6):877–883

20. Carrier M, Marchand R, Auger P, et al. Methicillin-resistant Staphylococcus aureus infection in a cardiac surgical unit. J Thorac Cardiovasc Surg 2002;123(1):40–44

21. WHO Department of Service Delivery and Safety (SDS). EML GUIDANCE ON SAP, FINAL VERSION 1 Application for the 21st Model List of Essential Medicines Antibiotics of choice for surgical antibiotic prophylaxis.[Internet][cited on 20 December 2020] https://www.who.int/selection medicines/committees/expert/22/applications/s6.2_surgical-antibiotic-prophylaxis.pdf

22. Garey KW, Dao T, Chen H, et al. Timing of vancomycin prophylaxis for cardiac surgery patients and the risk of surgical site infections. J Antimicrob Chemother 2006;58(3):645–650

23. Engelman R, Shahian D, Shemin R, et al; Workforce on Evidence-Based Medicine, Society of Thoracic Surgeons. The Society of Thoracic Surgeons practice guideline series: antibiotic prophylaxis in cardiac surgery, part II: antibiotic choice. Ann Thorac Surg 2007;83(4):1569–1576

24. Calic D, Ariano RE, Arora RC, et al. Evaluation of cefazolin antimicrobial prophylaxis during cardiac surgery with cardio-pulmonary bypass. J Antimicrob Chemother 2018;73(3):768–771

25. Woods RK, Dellinger EP. Current guidelines for antibiotic prophylaxis of surgical wounds. Am Fam Physician 1998;57(11):2731–2740

26. Hall RI, Blaine Kent B. Changes in the pharmacokinetics and pharmacodynamics of drugs administered during cardio-pulmonary bypass. In: Gravlee GP, ed. Cardiopulmonary bypass: principles and practice. 3rd ed. Philadelphia, USA: Lippincott Williams & Wilkins; 2007:190–260

27. Paruk F, Sime FB, Lipman J, Roberts JA. Dosing antibiotic prophylaxis during cardiopulmonary bypass-a higher level of complexity? A structured review. Int J Antimicrob Agents 2017;49(4):395–402

28. Gelijns AC, Moskowitz AJ, Acker MA, et al; Cardiothoracic Surgical Trials Network (CTSN). Management practices and major infections after cardiac surgery. J Am Coll Cardiol 2014;64(4):372–381

29. Global WHO. Guidelines for the Prevention of Surgical Site Infection Web Appendix 5. Summary of a systematic review on optimal timing for preoperative surgical antibiotic prophylaxis. [Internet][cited on 14 December 2020]. https://www.who.int/gpsc/Appendix5.pdf

30. Kappeler R, Gillham M, Brown NM. Antibiotic prophylaxis for cardiac surgery. J Antimicrob Chemother 2012;67(3):521–522

31. Hamouda K, Oezkur M, Sinha B, et al. Different duration strategies of perioperative antibiotic prophylaxis in adult patients undergoing cardiac surgery: an observational study. J Cardiothorac Surg 2015;10:25

32. Lador A, Nasir H, Mansur N, et al. Antibiotic prophylaxis in cardiac surgery: systematic review and meta-analysis. J Antimicrob Chemother 2012;67(3):541–550

33. Bode LG, Kluytmans JA, Wertheim HF, et al. Preventing surgical-site infections in nasal carriers of Staphylococcus aureus. N Engl J Med 2010;362(1):9–17

34. Kluytmans J, van Belkum A, Verbrugh H. Nasal carriage of Staphylococcus aureus: epidemiology, underlying mechanisms, and associated risks. Clin Microbiol Rev 1997;10(3):505–520

35. Global Guidelines for the Prevention of Surgical Site Infection. Summary of a systematic review on decolonization with mupirocin ointment with or without chlorhexidine gluconate body wash for the prevention of Staphylococcus aureus infection in nasal carriers undergoing surgery. Web Appendix 3. [Internet][cited on 15 December 2020]. https://www.ncbi.nlm.nih.gov/books/NBK536421/

36. De Feo M, Gregorio R, Della Corte A, et al. Deep sternal wound infection: the role of early debridement surgery. Eur J Cardiothorac Surg 2001;19(6):811–816

37. Gårdlund B, Bitkover CY, Vaage J. Postoperative mediastinitis in cardiac surgery: microbiology and pathogenesis. Eur J Cardiothorac Surg 2002;21(5):825–830

38. Murray MT, Corda R, Turcotte R, Bacha E, Saiman L, Krishnamurthy G. Implementing a standardized perioperative antibiotic prophylaxis protocol for neonates undergoing cardiac surgery. Ann Thorac Surg 2014;98(3):927–933

39. Woodward CS, Son M, Taylor R, Husain SA. Prevention of sternal wound infection in pediatric cardiac surgery: a proto-colized approach. World J Pediatr Congenit Heart Surg 2012;3(4):463–469

40. McDonald JR. Acute infective endocarditis. Infect Dis Clin North Am 2009;23(3):643–664

41. Zegri-Reiriz I, de Alarcón A, Muñoz P, et al; Spanish Collabo-ration on Endocarditis—Grupo de Apoyo al Manejo de la Endocarditis infecciosa en España (GAMES). Infective endocarditis in patients with bicuspid aortic valve or mitral valve prolapse. J Am Coll Cardiol 2018;71(24):2731–2740

42. Nguyen VQ. Endocarditis prophylaxis. Medscape. [Internet] [cited on 14 December 2020]. https://www.medscape.com/answers/2172262-200355/what-are-the-recommended-antibiotic-regimens-for-infective-endocarditis-ie-prophylaxis

43. Dat VQ, Dat TT, Hieu VQ, et al. Antibiotic use for empirical therapy in the critical care units in primary and secondary hospitals in Vietnam: a multicenter cross-sectional study. The Lancet Regional Health - Western Pacific 2022;18: 100306

19

Challenges in ALCAPA Repair

Poonam Malhotra Kapoor, Shivani Aggarwal, Amita Sharma, and Sandeep Sharan

Introduction

In the human heart the left coronary artery (LCA), which provides oxygenated blood to the left ventricle, arises from the aorta (above the left cusp of the aortic valve). When the LCA arises abnormally from the pulmonary artery, it is referred to as anomalous left coronary artery. This chapter briefly outlines ALCAPA (anomalous left coronary artery from the pulmonary artery) repair and its challenges to the anesthesiologists.

ALCAPA is also known as Bland-White-Garland syndrome or White-Garland syndrome, instead of arising from the aortic sinus, the LCA branches off from the pulmonary artery instead of the aortic sinus.[1] The incidence of anomaly is rare and so are its complications, but the challenges remain in the perioperative and postoperative period.[2]

A Left-to-Right Shunt is Created after Birth

In ALCAPA patients, the creation of a left-to-right coronary artery increases the pressure in the LCA. This causes the blood to flow from the right coronary artery (RCA) into the LCA (**Fig. 19.1** and **Flowchart 19.1**), thus creating a left-to-right shunt.

History of ALCAPA

Anomalous arteries arising from anterior part of pulmonary artery were first described by Krause in 1865[3] and Brooks in 1885.[4] These arteries have vein-like morphology and joined vessels arising from mediastinum, thorax, and aorta. Adult ALCAPA was first described by Maude Abbott

in 1908 following autopsy in a 60-year-old woman who had died accidently and was asymptomatic.[5] It was in 1993, that Bland and his colleagues first described this syndrome, in a 3-month-old infant.[6] They described an infant having pallor, irritability, diaphoresis, and dyspnea attributed to cardiac ischemia which came to be known as Bland-White-Garland syndrome. In a review by Kaunitz et al, it was demonstrated that the onset of symptoms often parallel the closure of ductus arteriosus after 2 months of birth.[7] Jurishica et al reported a high incidence of sudden early death in 11 adult ALCAPA patients.[8] Only 18% were symptomatic prior to death. Thus early surgical intervention was advocated though with limited success. Earliest procedures to be attempted were pulmonary artery banding or ligation in an

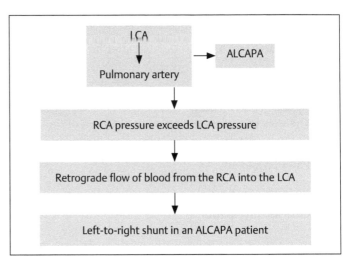

Flowchart 19.1 In ALCAPA patients, the creation of a left to right coronary artery increase pressure in the LCA causing the blood to flow from the RCA into LCA. Abbreviations: ALCAPA, anomalous left coronary artery from the pulmonary artery; LCA, left coronary artery; RCA, right coronary artery.

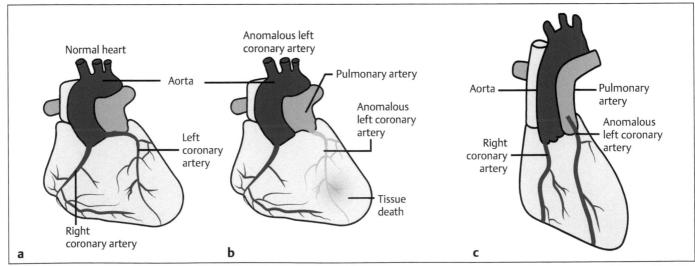

Fig. 19.1 The normal heart **(a)** and the ALCAPA (anomalous left coronary artery from the pulmonary artery) heart **(b, c)** in which a left-to-right shunt is created.

attempt to increase coronary perfusion pressure in the LCA.[9] With the development of cardiopulmonary bypass in 1953, varied surgical procedures were attempted including left common carotid artery bypass, creation of aorta-pulmonary window, pericardial poundage with talcum powder, and de-epicardialization for promoting collateral circulation, and internal mammary artery bypass.[10] ALCAPA today has good postsurgical prognosis due to improvements in (i) diagnosis of ALCAPA as a disease entity early using echocardiography with color flow mapping, (ii) adequate myocardial protection during cardiopulmonary bypass, and (iii) improved surgical techniques. All the above three favor a better outcome in the operative room.

Types of ALCAPA

ALCAPA is a rare but serious congenital cardiac anomaly, observed in up to 0.25 to 0.50% of all congenital heart diseases.[11] ALCAPA is of two types based on the survival pattern: the adult and the infantile type. In the infantile type, the collateral circulation is poorly developed and therefore, if left untreated, the mortality rate in the first year of life is 90% secondary to myocardial infarction and mitral valve insufficiency leading to congestive heart failure. In the adult type, delayed presentation is due to development of good collateral circulation.[12,13] The incidence of sudden death remains as high as 80 to 90% after the age of 35 years. The mortality in ALCAPA is sudden death in nearly 90% of patients and mortality occurs around 35 years of age.

Theories to Explain the Anomalous Origin of the Coronary Artery from the Pulmonary Artery

Over the years, many theories exist about the genesis of this syndrome. The best one states that there is a defective embryological division of the truncus arteriosus[14] (**Table 19.1**). The coronary artery originates from the embryological pulmonary artery origin instead of from the aorta. According to this theory, there is abnormal division by the developing truncal septum which results in incorporation of one of both coronary artery buds into the pulmonary artery.

Due to this replacement of the coronaries (either one or both) from the pulmonary artery the term is named "ALCAPA."

Pathophysiology

The perfusion of the left ventricle is from the collaterals of the LCA. Death ensues if collaterals are poorly developed and immediate surgery is not performed.

The physiology of ALCAPA is described under three phases:

- **In the newborn period:** A phase of high pulmonary vascular resistance (PVR) and pulmonary artery pressure (PAP). There are no symptoms or signs of ischemia because of adequate myocardial perfusion. There is no shunt or coronary steal as PVR is high.

Table 19.1 Theories to explain embryological origin of ALCAPA

Theory	Embryological origin of ALCAPA
Theory 1	Definitive embryological division of the truncus arteriosus (TA)
Normal embryology of TA	Truncus arteriosus: LCA RCA } From coronary endothelial buds truncal septum ↓ Development of septum ↙ ↘ LCA RCA ↓ Definitive aorta
Theory 2 Harkenseller theory	The aortic bud of the truncus arteriosus involutes and the pulmonary bud of the truncus arteriosus persists
Abrikososoff theory	Abnormal division by the developing truncal septum, wherein both the coronary arteries develop from the pulmonary artery

Abbreviations: ALCAPA, anomalous left coronary artery from the pulmonary artery; LCA, left coronal artery; RCA, right coronal artery.

- **After birth:** Immediately after birth, a transition phase is seen when PVR and PAP falls. There is retrograde flow in the LCA from the pulmonary artery (**Fig. 19.2**). If collaterals from the RCA do not develop, ischemia occurs, resulting in typical sign and symptoms of angina, congestive heart failure, and even sudden death (**Fig. 19.3**). Survival beyond infancy is usually uncommon because of myocardial necrosis and left heart failure. Eighty-five percent die while remaining 15% may enter the next stage.

- **Adulthood:** Patients who develop collaterals remain asymptomatic and enter adulthood without any obvious signs and symptoms. This is called adult ALCAPA. Patients with ALCAPA surviving through childhood have varying symptoms of myocardial ischemia and heart failure, 90% dying by 35 years of age with very few older than 50 years surviving without surgical correction.[13] Overtime papillary muscle dysfunction may result in overt mitral regurgitation.

Diagnosis of ALCAPA

Diagnosis of ALCAPA mandates, due to its varied etiologies, a detailed diagnostic work-up. The various investigations which can be done are as follows:

- **Electrocardiogram (ECG):** In infancy, abnormal Q-waves in lead I, avL, V5, V6 with transient ST-segment changes in chest leads may be seen. Q-waves may not be seen in 20 to 45% of cases; therefore, it is suggested to suspect ALCAPA whenever abnormal R-wave progression is found on chest leads.[16] ECG typically shows signs of anterolateral myocardial infarction (55–80%) and left ventricular (LV) hypertrophy in adults.

- **Chest X-ray:** In infants and adults cardiomegaly with LV apex may be seen.

- **Echocardiography:** Echocardiography, due to its advanced probes and machinery, is a reliable tool today for diagnosing ALCAPA. All types of Echo, chiefly transthoracic and transesophageal in 2D and 3D modes, can be used, even in pediatric patients today. The color-flow Doppler mode on Echo remains the chief diagnostic mode of reliability. Echo, today, has replaced angiography as a diagnostic tool, chiefly because of its noninvasive nature. The criteria are a dilated right coronary system with flow reversal in at least two of the three left coronary segments. There is a flow reversal into the pulmonary trunk with the turbulence along the medial wall as against the lateral wall in a patent ductus. The location of left coronary segments and demonstration of flow reversal are however difficult. Transesophageal echocardiography (TEE), midesophageal aortic-valve long-axis view, can demonstrate the large orifice of the RCA with laminar diastolic antegrade flow by color Doppler mapping. 3D echo can clearly delineate the coronary system than the conventional 2D echocardiography and make the diagnosis of ALCAPA simpler.

The findings in infants and children include severe dilatation of left ventricle with dysfunction. The RCA is prominent, dilated with origin from aorta, and collateral flow into the anomalous LCA may also be seen. LCA may be seen originating from the pulmonary artery (lateral part just distal to main pulmonary artery). It can be seen in parasternal short-axis view in transthoracic echocardiography (**Fig. 19.4**) or midesophageal aortic long-axis and short-axis view in transesophageal echocardiography (**Figs. 19.4–19.8**). Mild-to-moderate mitral regurgitation may be present due

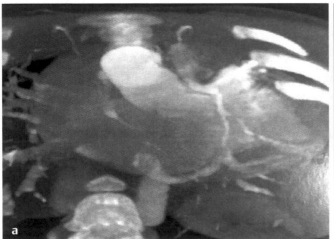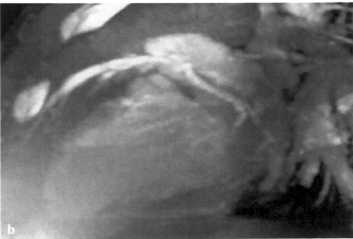

Fig. 19.2 **(a)** Computed tomography (CT) angiogram showing how the left coronary artery (LCA) originates from the pulmonary artery. **(b)** CT angiogram showing the dilated LCA arising from the pulmonary artery.

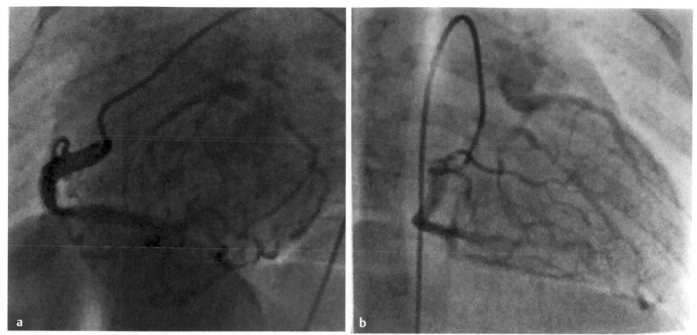

Fig. 19.3 **(a, b)** Coronary angiogram in left anterior oblique (LAO) and right anterior oblique (RAO) projection showing the origin of right coronary artery (RCA) from the right coronary sinus and filling of the left coronary artery (LCA) from the RCA during the levo phase.

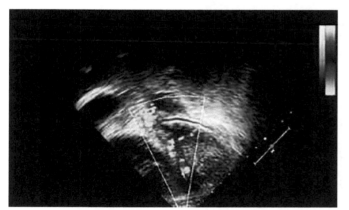

Fig. 19.4 2D apical four-chamber view with color-flow Doppler displaying septal perforator coronary arteries which are seen in diastole as abnormal septal color flows.

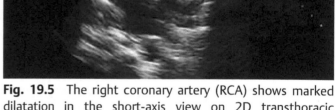

Fig. 19.5 The right coronary artery (RCA) shows marked dilatation in the short-axis view on 2D transthoracic echocardiography.

to ischemia. The LV papillary muscles are usually more echogenic. The pulsed-wave spectral Doppler at the right coronary origin shows presence of systolic coronary flow predominance.[17]

- **Angiography:** This is the gold standard for the diagnosis of ALCAPA and is mandatory before surgery. An aortic root angiogram shows a dilated RCA arising from aorta with collateral flow in the LCA which finally drains into the pulmonary artery (**Fig. 19.9**). Limitations include invasive procedure, overlapping of vascular structures, and difficulty in identifying an interarterial course.[18]

- **Other valuable noninvasive technique is coronary CT angiogram:** We can demonstrate the origin of RCA alone from the right coronary sinus whereas the left coronary sinus is devoid of any coronary origin. It arises from the aorta above the aortic left cusp of the aortic valve, and feeds blood to the left side of the heart muscle.

- **Cardiac catheterization:** It also reveals the absence of the left main coronary artery (LMCA) in the left sinus of Valsalva. Contrast dye injected into the RCA fills the main branches of the LMCA with anomalous drainage through the LMCA into the pulmonary

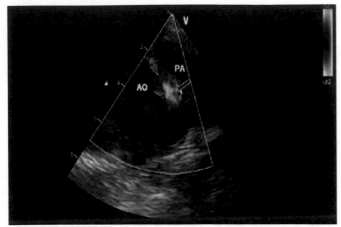

Fig. 19.6 The figure shows on the transthoracic Echo the pulmonary artery and aorta close to each other and the right coronary artery (RCA) arises from the pulmonary artery.

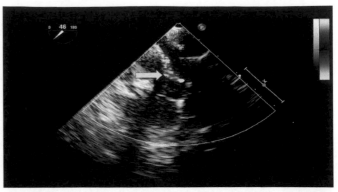

Fig. 19.7 The 46-degree midesophageal (ME) ascending aortic short-axis view, with a prominent *yellow-colored* Doppler flow arising from the left coronary artery (LCA) into the pulmonary artery.

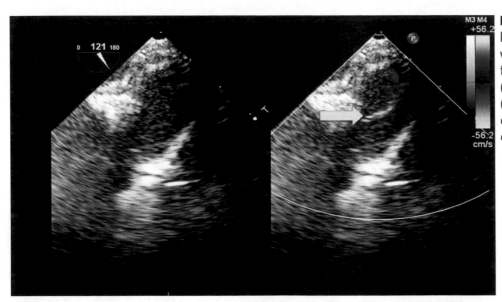

Fig. 19.8 A midesophageal aortic long-axis view at 121 degrees which displays with *yellow arrow* flow from the left coronary artery (LCA) into the left pulmonary artery (LPA). Multiple transesophageal echocardiography (TEE) views clinch the diagnosis.

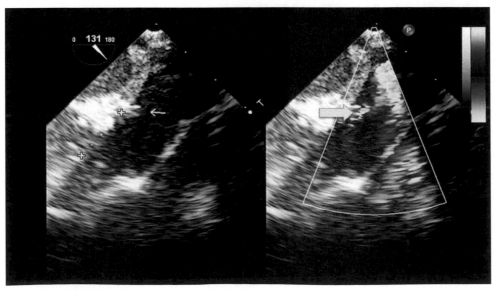

Fig. 19.9 Midesophageal aortic long-axis view at 131 degrees showing with a *yellow arrow* flow from the left coronary artery (LCA) to pulmonary artery, that is, it has coronary stenosis pattern.

artery (**Figs. 19.10** and **19.11**). Management of ALCAPA has evolved dramatically over the years. Management is surgical. Initial days saw bypass grafting procedures using the subclavian artery. Now, most preferred treatment is the reimplantation of the LCA into the aortic sinus. Rarely, aortopulmonary window with a tunnel to divert the blood into the LCA is used.

- **CT and MRI:** Development of cardiac CT and MRI has revolutionized the way congenital heart diseases are diagnosed. The LCA can be seen originating posteriorly from pulmonary artery with a dilated and tortuous RCA originating from the aorta (**Fig. 19.12**). The intercoronary collaterals both external and within the interventricular septum can be seen. Both modalities may be used to assess LV systolic function. Multidetector computed tomography (MDCT) can be used as a confirmatory test when in doubt about the diagnosis. MRI offers several additional advantages. These include visualization of origin as well as flow of LCA into the pulmonary artery, assessment of mitral valve function, and determination of viability of myocardium with delayed gadolinium enhancement. Magnetic resonance angiography (MRCA) is helpful in cases of equivocal coronary angiography.[19–21]

Clinical Presentation

Patients become symptomatic early in life, usually within the first year after birth. The signs and symptoms are usually due to chronic ischemia resulting from anomalous take off of LCA from PA which may lead to congestion in heart and lungs and cause sudden cardiac death. Infants may have vague complaints like irritability, difficulty in breastfeeding, diaphoresis, tachycardia, and tachypnea. The chest pain occurring as a result of myocardial ischemia may mimic infantile colic. The symptoms resemble that of dilated cardiomyopathy so ALCAPA should be excluded by appropriate investigations described later. If collaterals develop between the RCA and LCA, these patients may remain asymptomatic till adulthood. Physical examination may reveal cardiomegaly, S3 gallop, hepatomegaly, and pansystolic murmur of mitral regurgitation.

Most adults surviving with ALCAPA are generally women. There is a common history of associated metabolic disorders like hypertension and diabetes with occasional episodes of exertional dyspnea and angina. They manifest typical chest pain from myocardial ischemia at rest or exercise, dyspnea, exercise intolerance, and even sudden death resulting from

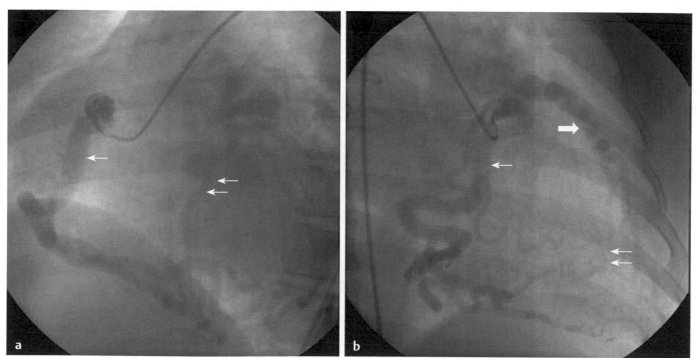

Fig. 19.10   (a, b) Angiographic left anterior oblique (LAO) and right anterior oblique (RAO) views portraying right coronary artery (RCA) as dilated and tortuous (*single arrow*) and left coronary artery (LCA [*wide arrow*]) filling through intercoronary collaterals (*double arrow*)

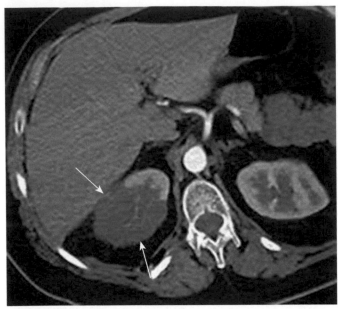

Fig. 19.11 In this view the left coronary artery is not seen. This computed tomography (CT) is at the level of the right coronary artery (RCA), which is originating at its normal position.

acute myocardial ischemia during exercise/intense activity or ventricular dysrhythmias (due to scarred myocardium).

Physical examination may reveal a gallop rhythm or murmur of ischemic mitral regurgitation or a continuous murmur due to collateral flow from the aorta into the pulmonary circulation. A study by Conde et al[22] has found high incidence of atherosclerosis in adults with coronary artery abnormalities, with significant stenosis (>50%) in 40% of patients. This might explain why ALCAPA mimics acute coronary syndrome in adults.

Mortality

Mortality remains high in ALCAPA patients. Inadequate collateral shunt circulation between the right and left coronary arteries (L→R shunt already exists and presence of collaterals worsens it!) may lead to sudden death; fulminant arrhythmias, mitral insufficiency, and myocardial ischemia or infarction may all cause mortality up to 90% in the first year of life in an ALCAPA patient.

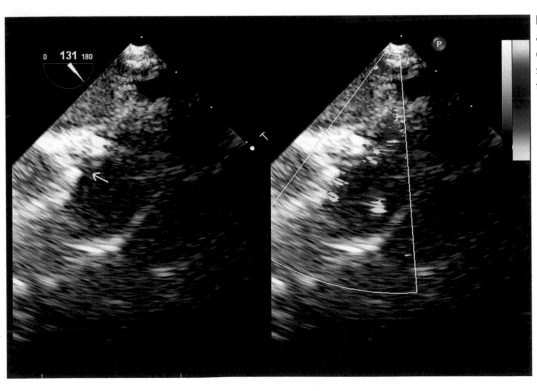

Fig. 19.12 Midesophageal aortic long-axis view at 131 degrees on color Doppler showing left coronary artery to pulmonary artery.

Treatment of ALCAPA

Mortality remains high in the first year of life after birth in both symptomatic and asymptomatic patients. In asymptomatic ALCAPA patients the mortality is sudden death in and around the fourth decade of the patient's life.

Surgical correction of the ALCAPA anomaly is the only definitive treatment modality. The four major surgical interventions for treatment have been described by Zheng et al and are enumerated in **Box 19.1**. They include (i) LCA ligation; (ii) LCA ligation with coronary artery bypass grafting; (iii) the Takeuchi procedure; and (iv) LCA reimplantation.[23]

Postsurgery, mortality may remain high—as observed in six patients in this study by Zheng et al.[23] The survivors' ejection fraction, LV size, and abnormal Q-wave, all returned to near normal, once the mitral regurgitation was corrected.

Yau et al in a study showed that a 21% of ALCAPA patients underwent an LCA ligation and nearly 79% had dual coronary perfusion.[24] Surgical mortality in these patients according to Yau et al was between 1 and 4% only in both adults and children in most studies.

Prognosis of ALCAPA

In a famous study of seven ALCAPA patients who remained on medical management, five remained stable for up to 5 years postdiagnosis. In adults an interposition graft is generally required. This mandates creating a dual coronary system with coronary button transfer.[25]

Coronary artery ligation had a high morbidity and mortality as compared to dual coronary system. Complications include presence of a residual shunt, severe mitral regurgitation, and reoccurrence of anginal pain.[25] The methods for establishing dual coronary system include:

- **Takeuchi procedure:** This involves creation of a tunnel between LCA and aorta by means of a pulmonary artery baffle. Complications of this procedure were aortic regurgitation, supravalvular pulmonary stenosis, and obstruction of the baffle.[25]
- **Implantation of LCA into the ascending aorta:** Direct implantation of the LCA in the ascending aorta is the preferred method nowadays in children.[26] The pulmonary trunk is transected above the level of commissures and the anomalous LCA. The LCA ostium is excised and anastomosed with ascending aorta. The pulmonary sinus of Valsalva is reconstructed with autologous pericardium and end-to-end anastomosis of divided pulmonary trunk is done. In case mitral valve is incompetent, mitral annuloplasty is also performed.

Anesthetic Management

The anesthetic goals for ALCAPA repair are to strike a balance between preload and afterload while maintaining cardiac contractility and prevention of tachycardia (**Box 19.2**). The anesthetic management is briefly summarized in **Box 19.3**.

Anesthetic management in ALCAPA patients focuses on striking a balance between preload and after-load systemic oxygen saturation while maintaining myocardial contractility and preventing untoward increases in myocardial oxygen demand. As there is severe ventricular dysfunction it is important to avoid too many anesthetic agents. A bispectral Index (BIS) or near infrared spectroscopy (NIRS) guides

---

Box 19.1   Surgical treatment of the ALCAPA anomaly

- LCA ligation
- LCA ligations with coronary artery bypass grafting
- Takeuchi procedure
- LCA reimplantation

Abbreviations: ALCAPA, anomalous left coronary artery from the pulmonary artery; LCA, left coronary artery.

Box 19.2   Anesthetic goals for ALCAPA repair

The anesthetic goals are to:
- Maintain optimum preload
- Prevent a decrease in pulmonary vascular resistance (PVR)
- Maintain myocardial contractility
- Maintain low or normal systemic vascular resistance (SVR)
- Prevent tachycardia

Abbreviation: ALCAPA, anomalous left coronary artery from the pulmonary artery.

Box 19.3   Anesthetic considerations for ALCAPA

For favorable outcomes in perioperative period, follow:
- No swings in blood pressure, preoperative and perioperative period
- Smooth induction and laryngoscopy
- Keep PVR on higher side to obtund coronary steal
- Judicious inotropic use
- Postoperative vasodilators such as NTG and SNP
- Decreased afterload
- Postoperative intubation for sometime
- Normal coronary circulation restoration takes up to 2 y
- Functional postoperative recovery is good if preoperative and perioperative period are meticulous

Abbreviations: ALCAPA, anomalous left coronary artery from the pulmonary artery; NTG, nitroglycerin; PVR, pulmonary vascular resistance; SNP, sodium nitroprusside.

well, when to give the maintenance fentanyl and midazolam during the surgical repair on cardiopulmonary bypass.

Factors which cause coronaries steal such as fluctuations in PVR, $PaCO_2$, and high FiO_2 should all be circumvented. FiO_2 should be avoided. Intraoperative goals are as listed in **Box 19.4**. To arrest the heart, anterograde and retrograde cardioplegia is given while the surgeons snare the right and left pulmonary arteries. Surgical correction is usually accomplished by explanting origin of the LCA from the main by reimplantation in a normal anatomic position on the ascending aorta.

Inotropic Drug Administration

To overcome increase in myocardial oxygen consumption and risk of arrhythmias, the use of inotropes should be judiciously weighed and the right inotrope started. Use of a mechanical circulatory support (MCS) device such as integrated extracorporeal membrane oxygenation (ECMO)[27,28]

Box 19.4 Intraoperative goals in ALCAPA repair

- Decreased heart rate <75 bpm
- Normal or slightly increased PVR
- Optimized cardiac output
- Low FiO_2 of 21%
- $PaCO_2$: 45–55 mmHg
- MAP within 10% of the baseline
- Optimal preload to maintain the cardiac output

Abbreviations: ALCAPA, anomalous left coronary artery from the pulmonary artery; FiO_2, fraction of inspired oxygen; MAP, mean arterial pressure; $PaCO_2$, partial pressure of carbon dioxide; PVR, pulmonary vascular resistance.

---

or a ventricular-assist device may be the best option. The MCS devices are especially useful when separation from cardiopulmonary bypass is arduous. In cases of low cardiac output sternal closure may be delayed. This secondary sternal closure is particularly helpful in cases of hemodynamic instability which becomes worst when primary sternal closure is done at the same setting. Chances of infection do not increase with a delayed sternal closure. In case of a patient with associated mitral regurgitation, polytetrafluoroethylene surgical membrane may be utilized in place of a pericardial patch.

Complications of ALCAPA Repair

Following ALCAPA repair, complications are not many if done by an expert. There may be following ALCAPA repair surgery permanent damage of the mitral valve apparatus, leading to hemodynamic instability.

Late complications associated with coronary revascularization are seen more with the following:

- Surgical ligation.
- Bypass grafts which get occluded.
- Supraventricular pulmonary stenosis due to intrapulmonary tunnel technique.
- Least common, aneurysms at the surgically created aortopulmonary window (**Fig. 19.13**).

Inadequate growth of the coronary anastomosis is possible, although unlikely, if surgical reimplantation of the LCA was performed. This occurrence is similar to the rare reports of late coronary artery problems following the arterial switch procedure for transposition of the great vessels that also requires direct coronary transfer and reimplantation.

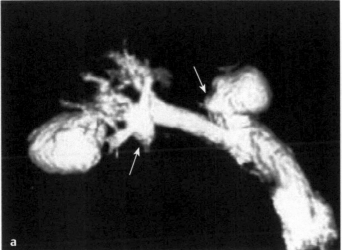 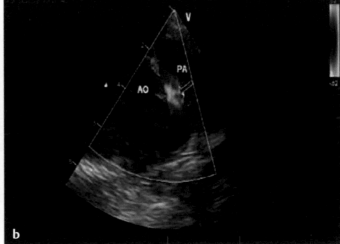

Fig. 19.13 **(a, b)** Anomalous pulmonary artery aneurysms (*arrows*) where the right coronary artery (RCA) is arising from the pulmonary artery post-ALCAPA (anomalous left coronary artery from the pulmonary artery) repair.

Postoperative Function

The patients undergoing ALCAPA repair show improvement in LV function, reduction in mitral regurgitation with improvement in quality on long-term follow-up, provided the dual coronary system is well established following surgical repair.

Mechanical Support for ALCAPA

Mechanical circulatory support in the form of ECMO and LVAD can be used post-ALCAPA repair as a bridge to recovery. Authors at AIIMS have used integrated ECMO in ALCAPA for better survival.[28] The risk factors for perioperative death of patients suffering from ALCAPA are low output syndrome and acute myocardial infarction. In only 33% ECMO support is initiated in postoperative period post cardiopulmonary bypass for supporting a failing heart survival. Authors have found integrated ECMO to be a safer strategy aiding recovery of cardiac function in critically compromised cardiosurgical patients and enhancing survival of the patient when ECMO is initiated as bypass circuitry, preemptively saving time for set-up and also being cost-effective and preventing sepsis.[28]

Conclusion

The total duration of perioperative ischemia and the LV dysfunction that occurs during the ALCAPA repair determines the need for an MCS device postoperatively. The determinants for an MCS arise, when there is inability to wean from cardiopulmonary bypass due to a prolonged aortic cross-clamp time (exceeding 56 min or more) or there is severe LV dysfunction with a fractional shortening of less than 20%.[29,30]

Anesthetic management should revolve around preventing further decrease in myocardial contractility, maintaining adequate diastolic blood pressure and preventing tachycardia as the myocardium is already ischemic with poor contractility.

Although many congenital coronary abnormalities have a benign outcome, natural history of ALCAPA shows a poor outcome in untreated patients. ALCAPA is a rare coronary anomaly that usually manifests in the first month of life. Multimodality imaging is crucial for the initial diagnosis, therapeutic management and follow up. Surgical repair provides symptomatic and prognostic benefit, and it is recommended in all cases of ALCAPA, regardless of age, symptomatic status or presence of inducible myocardial ischemia. Assessment of the risk of recurrent ventricular arrhythmias despite full revascularization should be performed in all adults with ALCAPA.[31]

References

1. Chang RR, Allada V. Electrocardiographic and echocardiographic features that distinguish anomalous origin of the left coronary artery from pulmonary artery from idiopathic dilated cardiomyopathy. Pediatr Cardiol 2001;22(1):3–10
2. Crawford M, DiMarco J, Paulus W. Cardiology. 3rd ed. St. Louis, MO: Mosby; 2009:229. ISBN: 0723434859
3. Krause W. Cber den Ursprung einer akzessorischen A. coronaria aus der A. pulmonalis. Ztschr rat Med. 1865;24:225–227
4. Brooks HS. Two cases of an abnormal coronary artery of the heart arising from the pulmonary artery: with some remarks upon the effect of this anomaly in producing cricoid dilatation of the vessels. J Anat Physiol 1885;20(Pt 1):26–29
5. Abbott ME. Congenital heart disease. In: Osler W, ed. Modern medicine: its theory and practice. Philadelphia, PA: Lea & Febiger; 1908:420–421
6. Bland EF, White PD, Garland J. Congenital anomalies of the coronary arteries: report of an unusual case associated with cardiac hypertrophy. Am Heart J 1933;8:787–801
7. Kaunitz PE. Origin of left coronary artery from pulmonary artery: review of the literature and report of two cases. Am Heart J 1947;33(2):182–206
8. Jurishica AJ. Anomalous left coronary artery: adult type. Am Heart J 1957;54(3):429–436
9. Case RB, Morrow AG, Stainsby W, Nestor JO. Anomalous origin of the left coronary artery: the physiologic defect and suggested surgical treatment. Circulation 1958;17(6):1062–1068
10. Dodge-Khatami A, Mavroudis C, Backer CL. Anomalous origin of the left coronary artery from the pulmonary artery: collective review of surgical therapy. Ann Thorac Surg 2002;74(3):946–955
11. Al Umairi RS, Al Kindi F, Al Busaidi F. Anomalous origin of the left coronary artery from the pulmonary artery: the role of multislice computed tomography (MSCT). Oman Med J 2016;31(5):387–389
12. Wesselhoeft H, Fawcett JS, Johnson AL. Anomalous origin of the left coronary artery from the pulmonary trunk. Its clinical spectrum, pathology, and pathophysiology, based on a review of 140 cases with seven further cases. Circulation 1968;38(2):403–425
13. Alexi-Meskishvili V, Berger F, Weng Y, Lange PE, Hetzer R. Anomalous origin of the left coronary artery from the pulmonary artery in adults. J Card Surg 1995;10(4 Pt 1):309–315
14. Satpathy M, Mishra BR. Clinical Diagnosis of Congenital Heart Disease. 1st ed. India: Jaypee Brothers Medical Publishers; 2008: 185
16. Hoffman JI. Electrocardiogram of anomalous left coronary artery from the pulmonary artery in infants. Pediatr Cardiol 2013;34(3):489–491
17. Ghaderi F, Gholoobi A, Moeinipour A. Unique echocardiographic markers of anomalous origin of the left coronary artery from the pulmonary artery (ALCAPA) in the adult. Echocardiography 2014;31(1):E13–E15
18. Tariq R, Kureshi SB, Siddiqui UT, Ahmed R. Congenital anomalies of coronary arteries: diagnosis with 64 slice multidetector CT. Eur J Radiol 2012;81(8):1790–1797
19. Hejmadi A, Sahn DJ. What is the most effective method of detecting anomalous coronary origin in symptomatic patients? J Am Coll Cardiol 2003;42(1):155–157

20. Post JC, van Rossum AC, Bronzwaer JG, et al. Magnetic resonance angiography of anomalous coronary arteries. A new gold standard for delineating the proximal course? Circulation 1995;92(11):3163–3171

21. Taylor AM, Thorne SA, Rubens MB, et al. Coronary artery imaging in grown up congenital heart disease: complementary role of magnetic resonance and X-ray coronary angiography. Circulation 2000;101(14):1670–1678

22. Conde D. Anomalous origins of coronary arteries: frequency and association with coronary disease. Am J Emerg Med 2013;31(10):1528

23. Zheng JY, Han L, Ding WH, et al. Clinical features and long-term prognosis of patients with anomalous origin of the left coronary artery from the pulmonary artery. Chin Med J (Engl) 2010;123(20):2888–2894

24. Yau JM, Singh R, Halpern EJ, Fischman D. Anomalous origin of the left coronary artery from the pulmonary artery in adults: a comprehensive review of 151 adult cases and a new diagnosis in a 53-year-old woman. Clin Cardiol 2011;34(4):204–210

25. Bunton R, Jonas RA, Lang P, Rein AJ, Castaneda AR. Anomalous origin of left coronary artery from pulmonary artery. Ligation versus establishment of a two coronary artery system. J Thorac Cardiovasc Surg 1987;93(1):103–108

26. Alexi-Meskishvili V, Hetzer R, Weng Y, et al. Anomalous origin of the left coronary artery from the pulmonary artery. Early results with direct aortic reimplantation. J Thorac Cardiovasc Surg 1994;108(2):354–362

27. del Nido PJ, Duncan BW, Mayer JE Jr, Wessel DL, LaPierre RA, Jonas RA. Left ventricular assist device improves survival in children with left ventricular dysfunction after repair of anomalous origin of the left coronary artery from the pulmonary artery. Ann Thorac Surg 1999;67(1):169–172

28. Singh P, Kapoor PM, Devagourou V, Bhuvana V, Kiran U. Use of integrated extracorporeal membrane oxygenator in anomalous left coronary artery to pulmonary artery: better survival benefit. Ann Card Anaesth 2011;14(3):240–242

29. Edwin F, Kinsley RH, Quarshie A, Colsen PR. Prediction of left ventricular assist device implantation after repair of anomalous left coronary artery from the pulmonary artery. J Thorac Cardiovasc Surg 2012;144(1):160–165

30. Biçer M, Korun O, Yurdakök O, et al. Anomalous left coronary artery from the pulmonary artery repair outcomes: preoperative mitral regurgitation persists in the follow-up. J Card Surg 2021;36(2):530–535

31. Prandi FR, Zaidi AN, LaRocca G, Hadley M, Riasat M, Anastasius MO, Moreno PR, Sharma S, Kini A, Murthy R, Boateng P, Lerakis S. Sudden Cardiac Arrest in an Adult with Anomalous Origin of the Left Coronary Artery from the Pulmonary Artery (ALCAPA): Case Report. Int J Environ Res Public Health. 2022 Jan 29;19(3):1554

20

Future of Pediatric Cardiac Intensive Care

Devarakonda Bhargava Venkata, G. Srinivas, Rupa Sreedhar, and Sukesan Subin

Evolution of a Pediatric Cardiac Intensive Care Unit: Team and Its Organization

Setting up dedicated pediatric cardiac intensive care units (PCICU) has been adequately justified after the demonstration of tangible outcomes.[1,2] However, the variety of unique skill sets required in this complex environment dealing with a dynamic clinical situation in an ever-challenging patient population can be overwhelming for a conventional organizational setup of the PCICU. Also, the facets of conflict management, the need for continuous learning, adaptability, outcome-oriented practice, and shared accountability pose additional challenges to building resonant teams that are congruent, coherent, and concordant.[3,4] Besides, the advances in catheter-based approaches to complex congenital cardiac problems, the capability to perform a successful hybrid procedure, and encouraging advances in the field of pediatric electrophysiology and arrhythmia management[5,6] are likely to broaden the spectrum of clinical challenges faced in PCICU by introducing additional factors for a successful outcome. A review of experience in fetal cardiac interventions[7-9] points toward altering disease course and changing dynamics of emergent perinatal interventions in specific conditions like pulmonary atresia with an intact ventricular septum and fetal aortic stenosis with hypoplastic left heart syndrome. Further, encouraging outcomes of duct stenting compared to Blalock-Taussig shunt in congenital cardiac defects with duct-dependent pulmonary circulation[10] are likely to pave the way for the widespread acceptance of these techniques. Complete repair of tetralogy of Fallot in the neonatal period is rapidly emerging as a gold standard in symptomatic neonates[11,12] and is therefore likely to pose novel clinical challenges to the PCICU team. Hence, the leadership in PCICU is evolving from a hierarchical individual leadership, usually by a surgeon with obligatory acknowledgment of team members, to the present day PCICU team with all members of the team, including bedside intensive care unit nurse, perfusionist, physiotherapist, pediatric cardiac surgeon, and the pediatric cardiac intensive care specialist, displaying distinct leadership skills, coping ability to evolving challenges, management capabilities, communication skills, and emotional intelligence. This evolved team would be poised to accommodate a multidisciplinary approach to handle complex clinical problems in PCICU by integrating as team players in progressive work culture. The wisdom gained from various established centers is being increasingly put to test during medical missions providing pediatric cardiac surgery in low- to middle-income countries.[13,14] Also, various other independent initiatives like HeartLink®[15] are likely to make an increasing impact through enhanced training opportunities by developing centers of excellence in various parts of the world. These far-reaching economic benefits, availability of specialty training within local resources, and audit of clinically measurable outcomes are likely to provide real-world solutions which may result in a diverse spectrum of self-governed and self-financed pediatric cardiac programs in all parts of the globe.[16]

Empowered Nursing Care

Nursing considerations in pediatric cardiac intensive care are unique,[17] especially in resource-poor settings.[18] The evolution of nursing leadership and empowered nursing staff, whose opinion is valued in the shared decision-making process,[19] would continue to improve successful patient outcomes. The inputs provided by the bedside PCICU nurse in a multidisciplinary round can be reckoned far beyond the tangible gains of a clinical outcome. Quality improvement initiatives including implementation of effective care bundles to prevent surgical site infections[20] are difficult to succeed without adequate training and involvement of PCICU nursing care personnel. Repetitive emphasis on the implementation of care bundles by nurse educators and middle-level nurse managers at various staff meetings will find mention in all modern-day protocols. The perception of empowerment by middle management nurses and training to enhance problem-solving ability is increasingly shown to improve patient outcomes.[21,22] A significant evolution in the application of extracorporeal life support that improves survival to discharge poses a new challenge to the orthodox nursing training curriculum. Also, the additional resource utilization required for the application of extracorporeal membrane oxygenation (ECMO) therapy in PCICU puts strain on the number of nursing personnel required per patient. Presently, this number is arbitrarily set at 2 nursing personnel per patient undergoing ECMO therapy in most established centers. Simulation-based training of nursing personnel with scenarios specific to pediatric cardiac critical care[23] has been reported. Adoption of these training methods as part of the prescribed nursing curriculum should be considered a natural progression. Assessment of nutritional adequacy after implementation of a nurse-led protocol for feeding has been reported.[24] The involvement of the parent, under the guidance of nursing personnel, in nutritional rehabilitation during the acute phase of stay in PCICU is an area that would warrant attention in the future. This will possibly reduce the need for patient sedation as well as improve satisfaction levels of parents due to their involvement in care processes. Changing demographic distribution, with a shortage of nursing personnel for the care of the elderly, has envisaged the increasing role of robotic nurses that are programmed to perform certain repetitive tasks to help in nursing care.[25] Some of the repetitive tasks proposed for robotic nurses use triage process, transfer patients, schedule appointments, provide patient education, turn patients in bed, and provide reminders for care and medications. These robots can be tailored to the specific needs of PCICU care.

Transfer of Care Information: Shift Change and Adaptive Learning

Various strategies for the safe transfer of patient information ranging from simple standardized protocols for handover[26] to the adoption of models from formula-1 pitstop and present-day aviation industry[27] have been practiced and reported in the literature. The essence of these interventions lies in the implementation of a locally suitable format to facilitate the transfer of patient information without any loss. Hence, success depends on team dynamics at the time of handover. The traditional "swarming-in" on the arrival of a new patient needs constant review and refinement to remain efficient. These can be improved by the incorporation of prompts at each stage (in a standard format) of handover to minimize missing information. Robots have a potential role to play in supervising the daily transfer of care by providing cues for each stage of handover, patient monitoring during the transfer of care, and preventing interruptions during handover between health care personnel. Inbuilt audit of such handing-over processes would then be a consistent offshoot. Besides, siting of PCICU in proximity, not necessarily in geographical terms, to the operating rooms and cardiac intervention labs needs early planning.

Immediate Extubation after Cardiac Surgery and Airway Interventions in PCICU

Cardiac arrest rate of 7% and peri-intubation mortality rate of 1.6%, along with various risk factors for adverse events during intubation, have been reported in a patient cohort in PCICU.[28] Identification of unique patient subgroups in PCICU with a higher risk of nonrevivable cardiac arrest that occurs during airway events (systemic ventricle with systolic dysfunction,[28] single ventricle physiology with borderline obligatory mixing lesions, preintubation hypotension, elevated lactate levels, aortic stenosis, etc.) will pave way for additional specific preparations for handling these unique situations in the form of inotropic support, prostaglandin infusions, and rarely extracorporeal support. Similarly, PCICU-specific risk factors (pulmonary hypertension, single ventricle physiology, cardiac outflow obstructive lesions, etc.) and preparations (ketamine, adrenaline, etc.) need to be included and highlighted in various intubation checklists used during airway management. A meta-analysis of seven trials has demonstrated that ketamine, when used in children with congenital heart disease, has minimal effects on systemic vascular resistance, pulmonary vascular resistance, as well as blood gas parameters.[29] Evidence for alterations in a hemodynamic profile specific to each anesthetic agent, in the context of pulmonary hypertension, is still emerging to guide safe practice during intubation in PCICU. Supraglottic

airway devices have found their way into the PCICU as conventional guideline-directed rescue devices in life-threatening difficult airway situations. In addition, the scope for using supraglottic airway devices to facilitate early recovery after cardiac surgery among selected patient subgroups has been explored, albeit with clear limitations.[30] Also, traditional indications for bronchoscopy in certain challenging cases of bronchomalacia and vocal cord palsy associated with certain cardiac surgical interventions have not changed. The technological improvements in flexible bronchoscopy, such as smaller scopes, do not necessarily reduce the risks associated with the procedure. But, the modalities for evaluation now increasingly involve the use of virtual bronchoscopy in the form of computerized tomographic 3D reconstruction. Ultrasonography (USG) has been used as an alternative to fluoroscopy for diagnosing diaphragmatic palsy after cardiac surgery by evaluating diaphragmatic movements. The normal values for diaphragmatic thickness during various phases of respiration have been reported recently.[31] The increased use of USG in intensive care has led to the use of various specific measurements of diaphragm, such as diaphragmatic thickness, diaphragmatic excursion, and diaphragmatic thickening fraction, for predicting successful weaning from mechanical ventilation.[32] The widespread application of this knowledge in PCICU is likely to improve patient outcomes in the future. The use of artificial intelligence (AI) to predict prolonged mechanical ventilation (>7 d) and the need for tracheostomy in critically ill patients have been explored using large databases.[33] However, these prediction models for prolonged ventilation need to be modified by incorporating specific cardiac risk factors that suit the unique characteristics of patients in PCICU. Benefits and risks of tracheostomy in pediatric cardiac patients need to be reviewed and studied in a fashion similar to popular large-scale studies conducted in adult population.

Pharmacology of PCICU: Newer Agents and Routes Challenge the Age-Old Practices

Nanomedicine is a rapidly evolving technological offshoot of nanotechnology with advantages like better bioavailability, transport across tissue barriers, prolonged availability in circulation, reduced toxicity, and immunogenicity.[34] Nanoparticles that are biodegradable as well as biocompatible, administered by inhalation, are being developed to specifically tackle adult patients with heart failure. In a rodent model of diabetic cardiomyopathy, it was demonstrated that an inhalation therapy with calcium phosphate nanoparticles loaded with therapeutic mimotic peptide improves cardiac function.[35] The argument in support of a reduction in opioids for postoperative sedation is fueled by the rapid advent of multimodal analgesia techniques, nonopioid analgesics, and regional anesthetic techniques applicable for cardiac surgery.[36] Further, inhalational anesthetics such as sevoflurane, using the AnaConDa device, have been used for postoperative sedation in critically ill children. However, 30% of the children suffered hypotension while 26% suffered withdrawal after cessation of sevoflurane sedation.[37] Nevertheless, sedation using inhalational anesthetic agents can be considered another viable option in selected patients. Closed-loop delivery of anesthesia and sedation is a well-validated practice. However, the routine adoption of such algorithm-based closed-loop delivery of medications (such as insulin for glycemic control and inotropic/vasopressor support specific to each cardiac condition) is still to emerge. After the acceptance of milrinone or levosimendan infusions as the most sought-after supports along with epinephrine in most critical situations, basal vasopressin infusion continued for the first 24 hours after weaning from cardiopulmonary bypass remains an interesting regimen to counteract postoperative vasoplegia. Advantages of alpha-2 adrenergic agonists such as dexmedetomidine for postoperative sedation and further continuation with oral clonidine for reducing central sympathetic drive are evolving. The benefits do not remain limited to sedation but extend to a reduction in the incidence of acute kidney injury and postoperative delirium. Monitoring of anticoagulation during ECMO therapy by activating clotting time is being rapidly replaced by anti-Xa factor assays in various centers.[38] The pharmacologic armamentarium for PCICU care is transforming into one that is opioid-free, patient-specific, and accommodating newer routes and modes of drug administration.

Regional Anesthetic Techniques for Postoperative Care: The Challenger in the Ring

Regional anesthetic techniques such as caudal block, thoracic epidural analgesia,[39] and various chest wall blocks are rapidly emerging as the thrust for an opioid-free and multimodal analgesic regimen for pediatric cardiac surgery. The safety of thoracic epidural analgesia infusion in adult cardiac surgery has been demonstrated in a large audit of 2113 cases.[40] In addition, combinations of chest wall blocks like transverse thoracic muscle plane block and abdominal wall blocks like rectus sheath block,[41] to reduce epigastric pain due to sternotomy, are soon finding a place in the anesthetic regimen for pediatric cardiac surgery. However, the thoracic epidural block can be seen just as a casual mention in some recent fast-tracking targeted anesthetic protocols for pediatric cardiac surgery.[42] The safety of thoracic epidural in pediatric cardiac surgery is still debated in spite of evidence that suggests reliable safety of one-hour gap between insertion of epidural catheter and heparin administration during surgery.[43] The numerous advantages ranging from reduction in opioid requirements to reduction in pulmonary

hypertensive crises and stress response are likely to be supported by robust evidence in the future, leading to wider acceptance of regional anesthetic techniques for pediatric cardiac surgery.

Ultrasound IN and X-ray OUT!

Guidelines for point-of-care ultrasound (POCUS) in critically ill neonates and children are available.[44] The use of POCUS is beneficial for almost every imaging need, like atelectasis, pneumothorax, pulmonary edema, for vascular access fluid responsiveness, evaluation of hypotension, lung ultrasound to assess diaphragmatic function, and during cardiac arrest resuscitation. Lung ultrasound also has been utilized in assessing pulmonary blood flow in children with congenital heart disease,[45] lung recruitment after cardiac surgery, extravascular lung water,[46] and retrosternal clots after Fontan surgery.[47] **Fig. 20.1** depicts the various applications of POCUS in PCICU. However, the role of a conventional chest radiograph for determination of the correct position of endotracheal tube tip in the trachea safely above the carina can still be considered as the "*last man standing*" in its battle against USG.

It has been demonstrated that lung ultrasound provides a new diagnosis, thereby changing therapeutic management after pediatric cardiac surgery.[48] Various scoring systems have been validated to facilitate reporting, decision-making, and outcomes. It has also been reported that lung USG scoring system can be used to predict PCICU stay after pediatric cardiac surgery.[49] Ultrasound has been used as an alternative to fluoroscopy for the evaluation of diaphragm after cardiac surgery. The normal values for diaphragmatic thickness during various phases of respiration in children have been reported recently.[31] USG can be used to predict successful weaning from mechanical ventilation in intensive care based on the assessment of diaphragmatic thickness, diaphragmatic excursion, and diaphragmatic thickening fraction.[32] The diagnostic accuracy of these parameters is likely to be determined. Finally, it has been demonstrated that selective use of lung ultrasound reduces the number of radiographic examinations after pediatric cardiac surgery, thereby reducing costs without any adverse patient outcomes. Measurement of optic nerve sheath diameter (ONSD) by USG is potentially useful in detecting cerebrovascular accidents (intracranial hemorrhage) by the detection of elevated intracranial pressure. Renal ultrasound has been validated to determine renal resistive index in critically ill pediatric patients. Bowel ultrasound (BUS) for early diagnosis of necrotizing enterocolitis instead of abdominal radiograph has been evaluated.[50] Cardiac, cerebral, renal, optic nerve, and lung ultrasound study (CCROSS) protocol[51] was proposed for evaluating critically ill cardiac patients. Also, a POCUS protocol for evaluating pediatric shock was proposed.[52] These protocols are likely to be validated in pediatric cardiac surgical patients. Besides, VExUS

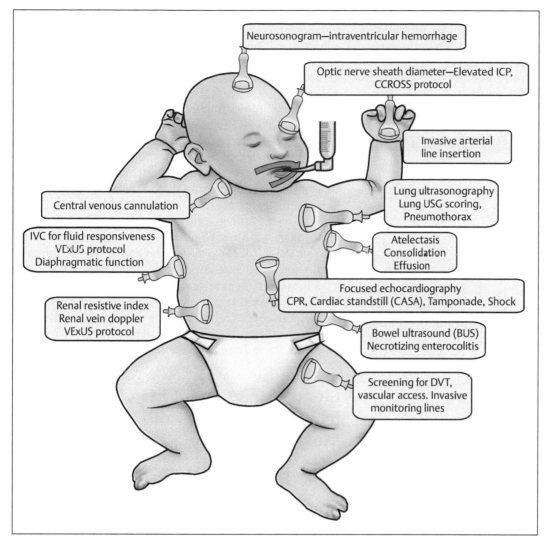

Fig. 20.1 Applications of point-of-care ultrasound (POCUS) in pediatric cardiac intensive care unit (PCICU). Abbreviations: CASA, cardiac arrest sonographic assessment; CPR, cardiopulmonary resuscitation; CROSS, chemoradiotherapy for oesophageal cancer followed by surgery study; USG, ultrasonography; VExUS, venous excess ultrasonography score.

protocol[53] for systemic congestion, combining portal vein, hepatic vein, and renal vein Doppler, has been evaluated in pediatric patients after cardiac surgery.

Ultrasound during cardiac arrest is evolving as an important adjunct to the diagnosis and management of cardiac arrest. Evaluating cardiac standstill using USG is an important area of emerging research.[54] Cardiac arrest sonographic assessment (CASA) is a protocol for assessment by USG during cardiac arrest.[55] ONSD is very useful for prognostication after the return of spontaneous circulation.[56] In addition to transthoracic echocardiography, a protocol for evaluation by transesophageal echocardiography during cardiac arrest[57] has been proposed. Hence, AI and machine learning are the tools that are most appropriate in this situation when disease management involves complex scoring systems involving multiple variables. The future cardiac arrest scenario would involve active goal-directed therapy based on the early application of ultrasound-based protocols for determining etiology, assessing the effectiveness of the resuscitation, and meaningful prognostication.

Mechanical Ventilation: Return to Non-invasive Ventilation

Mechanical ventilatory support for critically ill pediatric cardiac patients involves balancing multiple competing interests arising from various unique cardiopulmonary interactions experienced in PCICU patient population. After the rise of oxygenation index, hybrid modes of ventilation, and high-frequency oscillatory ventilation in critically ill patients with lung hemorrhages, the noninvasive ventilatory support with the use of high-flow nasal cannula is gaining popularity due to scientific evidence in favor of improved outcomes in the neonatal population. Simultaneously, the popularity of early (within 6 h)/immediate extubation (in operation theater) has paved the way for the widespread adoption of noninvasive ventilation. This is likely to progress to intravenous oxygenation using lipidic oxygen-filled microparticles, as demonstrated in rabbits.[58] This therapy holds promise for the rescue of profoundly hypoxemic patients with accurate titration of oxygen levels, once human trials are reported. However, the present-day limitations of this technology still include the removal of carbon dioxide from the body. Decision support in mechanical ventilation using AI tools is rapidly emerging[33,59] and is likely to improve the success rates of weaning from mechanical ventilation.

Acute Kidney Injury: There Is Light at the End of the Tunnel

Acute kidney injury (AKI) in PCICU was dominated by the rapid emergence of various biomarkers for early detection of cardiac surgery–associated AKI. However, a better understanding of the dynamics of intrarenal oxygenation, renal autoregulation, pressure differences between renal cortex and medulla, and the inevitable but transient effects of the cardiopulmonary bypass has led to the widespread application of renal oximetry using near-infrared spectroscopy (NIRS) in the critically ill pediatric population. The present trend toward determining the effect of the renal resistive index, time-weighted expression of renal oxygenation deficits,[60] and trends in cerebral-somatic NIRS gradient[61] in predicting AKI is gaining importance. Prediction models for AKI after pediatric cardiac surgery are likely to include these evolving parameters in addition to age, the complexity of the surgery, and cardiopulmonary bypass parameters. However, the use of renal replacement therapy (peritoneal dialysis or after cardiac surgery) has evolved from an empirical therapy to an elective procedure in selected patient subgroups like smaller and younger children. Prospective data is still awaited while retrospective data[62] provides limited insights into this subgroup of patients with high mortality.

Monitoring: Conventional Bedside Nurse Employs the Latest Gadgets

The monitoring and treatment of a critically ill neonate after cardiac surgery using cardiopulmonary bypass remains one of the most challenging employment for a healthcare professional, which requires distinct skill sets and technical knowledge in an ever-challenging environment. The advent of logical evaluation of trends in markers of oxygenation at tissue level (lactate, an arterial-venous difference of carbon dioxide) as well as point-of-care USG has rather added more pieces to the puzzle. The identification of the central role of the endothelial glycocalyx in the pathogenesis of microcirculatory alterations and monitoring of microcirculation by videomicroscopy has led to the identification of four different patterns of microcirculation.[63,64] Trends in microcirculation after cardiac surgery have been demonstrated to be different for cyanotic and acyanotic patients.[65] The accurate determination of variations in vessel density,[66] diffusive capacity, heterogeneity, and convective flow capacity along

with actionable therapeutic target values is likely to provide insights for a tailored management of each microcirculatory abnormality. The role of cerebral, somatic, and renal oximetry[60,67] and trends in cerebral-somatic NIRS gradient[61] will be coupled with electroencephalography-based monitors to provide better insights into the perfusion and functional paradigms of cerebral monitoring. Second-generation NIRS monitors (FORESITE Elite®) utilizing reference oxygen saturation based on arterial and jugular bulb oxygen saturations have been validated in pediatric cardiac patients undergoing cardiac catheterization.[68] Apart from the conventional clinical methods of determining low cardiac output states (peripheral temperature, urine output, tachycardia), transthoracic echocardiography and thermodilution techniques still remain reliable methods. Electric velocimetry (ICON®) was not found to be a reliable technique for determining cardiac output.[69] The analysis of continuous oximetry curves from the respiratory gas analysis is likely to find importance. Amid all the latest technological advancements, the age-old "*red-flag*" of a well-trained bedside nurse caring for the critically ill child, despite being subjective at times, will continue to remain the most indispensable monitor.

Blood Management in PCICU: Synthetic Products and Viscoelastic Measures

Blood management guidelines[70] for neonates and children undergoing cardiac surgery advocate antifibrinolytics, miniaturized cardiopulmonary bypass circuits, cell salvage, and viscoelastic test-based transfusion therapy. The trend toward reducing allogeneic transfusions by the use of synthetic products is palpable. Platelet dysfunction encountered after cardiopulmonary bypass is not completely reversed by platelet transfusion in spite of rising platelet count. Hence, the use of platelet-like particles[71] has been reported to be effective in forming a fibrin network.[71] The clot structure of neonates is different from that of adults. Hence, adult fibrinogen may not necessarily integrate well. However, rFVIIa resembles and suits neonatal clot structure.[72] Further, the use of fibrinogen concentrates toward the treatment of hypofibrinogenemia due to the hemodilution of cardiopulmonary bypass can be comparable to cryoprecipitate administration, thereby reducing allogeneic transfusions. Also, the increased thrombosis after cardiac surgery among infants is attributed to an imbalance between von Willebrand factor and ADAMTS-13.[73] Transfusion based on point-of-care viscoelastic coagulation parameters (ROTEM)[74] has been adopted in regular patient blood management algorithms in various centers across the world. This is likely to gain wider acceptance. In the future, the variations in results of point-of-care test parameters due to the sampling site (arterial vs. venous) could be minimized by the use of the Quantra system.[75]

Chronic Pain: Anticipation and Preparation

The development of persistent postsurgical pain (PPSP) is multifactorial, resulting due to the interplay of behavioral, acute pain characteristics and familial, psychological, and genetic mechanisms. The incidence of chronic pain in 121 children, described as pain near the surgical scar in last week, was 21% after a median of 3.8 years after sternotomy.[76] The intensity of pain on a numeric rating scale was >4 in 46% of the studied children. The risk factors proposed for children, some derived from adult studies, include older age, the extent of preoperative pain, postoperative pain after 2 weeks, and psychosocial factors.[77] Multidisciplinary assessment and management of PPSP in children by medical, physical, and psychological strategies have been proposed.[78] Management of acute pain by multimodal pre-emptive analgesia regimen, including regional anesthetic techniques and nonopioid analgesics, remains the cornerstone for the prevention of PPSP. The evidence for use of pharmacologic methods directly useful to prevent PPSP in children is still emerging. Since mechanisms for PPSP in children also include a neuropathic component, the efficacy of perioperative gabapentinoids and tricyclic antidepressants needs rigorous evaluation in the setting of pediatric cardiac surgery. Pain education of patients and families before surgery makes them understand the scientific basis of any pain likely to be experienced. This will be helpful in better coping mechanisms and compliance with management strategies. Genetic polymorphisms associated with chronic pain,[79] although emerging, still remain to be accurately established to offer tailormade solutions in the future. Age-appropriate assessment of physiological and psychological functions alongside the daily assessment of pain severity needs attention. The sensitization of the PCICU staff for identifying patients predisposed for developing PPSP, based on existing evidence, will be the first major step toward minimizing a complication that has a major effect on the quality of life and experience later in the child's life.

Sepsis in PCICU

The immunoparalysis after pediatric cardiac surgery using cardiopulmonary bypass is likely to predispose these children to sepsis. Postoperative sepsis occurs in 3% of children undergoing cardiac surgery.[80] The therapeutic principles for sepsis management in PCICU still aim to recognize the condition early, control the source early, early administration of antibiotic therapy, and reversal of shock state.[81] Biomarkers for sepsis in children have not been encouraging enough for routine use. Sepsis associated with necrotizing enterocolitis is usually fatal. A recent retrospective study, with 458 infants born at term undergoing cardiac surgery, showed that enteral feeding (fully fed or at least 45 mL/kg daily before

cardiac surgery) is associated with reduced incidence of necrotizing enterocolitis.[82] Enteral probiotic supplementation has a protective role against necrotizing enterocolitis.[83] The use of bedside bowel ultrasound to monitor a premature baby for necrotizing enterocolitis was demonstrated to be a feasible alternative to abdominal radiograph.[50] A POCUS protocol has been proposed for the evaluation of pediatric shock.[52] However, fluid bolus for hypotension has to be administered with the existing cardiac condition in mind. The appropriate use of POCUS for guiding fluid bolus in PCICU needs attention. Further, the effect of underlying heart disease and chronic hypoxemia on outcomes from sepsis in this patient population remains to be determined to guide the best clinical practices. The emerging role of POCUS in evaluating shock, guiding fluid therapy, and monitoring for necrotizing enterocolitis is likely to dominate the future landscape of PCICU.

Pulmonary Hypertension: Always a Difficult Case

Pediatric patients with pulmonary hypertension due to any etiology, admitted to PCICU, constitute a high-risk subset. The Paediatric Index of Pulmonary Hypertension Intensive Care Mortality model was developed after analysis of data from 14,268 patients under 21 years of age with pulmonary hypertension admitted to ICU and found to be better than Paediatric Risk of Mortality 3 and Paediatric Index of Mortality 2.[84] Multiple factors such as accepting patients with borderline pulmonary vascular resistance for corrective cardiac surgery and the advent of total intracardiac repair at a younger age for congenital cardiac defects might put patients with pulmonary hypertension at higher risk of perioperative morbidity. The wider availability as well as the adoption of intravenous Sildenafil as the first-line agent, initiated soon after weaning from cardiopulmonary bypass, in such high-risk patients, coupled with close monitoring using bedside echocardiography is likely to reduce the incidence of adverse events in these patients. The guidelines for preoperative pulmonary vasoreactivity testing for children are likely to incorporate children with improvements after the administration of pulmonary vasodilators as suitable candidates for surgery. The future is likely to see the advent of a wider spectrum of patients with pulmonary hypertension, earlier considered unsuitable for intervention, admitted to PCICU after surgery.

Scoring Systems and Prognostication

Databases for pediatric cardiac intensive care patients have been widely encouraged and accepted.[85,86] The clinical decision support systems,[87] however, were not tailored for use in PCICU. Recently, the Paediatric Index of Cardiac Surgical Intensive Care Mortality model (PICSIM)[88] was derived from

16,574 patients and proposed for use in PCICU. International databases with collaborations from various continents have been envisaged to understand the longitudinal outcomes from various parts of the world, standardization of nomenclature, protocols, and data collection.[89] Prediction of outcomes at admission by various prognostication models is available.[49,84,88] Further, disease-specific prognostication models are likely to be proposed and validated.

Nutrition: Prehabilitation to Catch Them Early

The role of "prehabilitation" in improving outcomes after cardiac surgery in children is rapidly gaining acceptability. Anthropometric measurements suggestive of wasting and stunting are associated with adverse outcomes after cardiac surgery in children. Hence, in children undergoing nonurgent cardiac surgery, nutritional rehabilitation before surgery may improve the surgical outcome. The PREQUEL study protocol[90] for adult frail patients planned for elective coronary artery bypass graft surgery has been proposed. Similar studies in children with cardiac ailments may guide goal-directed nutritional rehabilitation techniques. The role of bedside nurse-led nutritional protocol[24] is being explored. The involvement of parents in daily feeding in the acute phase of the PCICU stay is likely to gain wider acceptance in the future.

ECMO: Where Death Is an Option

We live in an era of "Code ECMO" where Code Blue is augmented with a call to a specialized ECMO team with preheparinized circuits, connections, and other equipment ready to connect. This availability of extracorporeal life support (ECLS) in a Code Blue situation has added ECMO to the latest list of "all things that can be done" for saving a cardiac arrest patient.[91] There is no evidence for the period after which ECLS is considered futile. In the future, the success of extracorporeal cardiopulmonary resuscitation (ECPR) for specific patient groups is likely to be accurately determined. The existing data suggest certain high-risk groups for the application of ECMO. Anticoagulation monitoring during ECMO is transforming into a wider application of anti-Xa factor assays (65%) and thromboelastography (43%), although activating clotting time (97%) is still employed by the majority of the centers.[38]

Communication, Counseling, and Consent in Future

Communication with parents and loved ones of a critically ill child is a vital part of professional commitment.

Counselors specifically trained in dealing with psychological issues specific to the PCICU patient disease spectrum are now employed in advanced centers that augment the communication provided by the intensive care physicians and other caregivers. They provide the necessary psychological support to the parents in dealing with this stressful situation. In times to come, addressing the father/mother's stress[92-94] is likely to gain attention in order to provide a holistic approach to the problem. Transparency between caregivers and parents is likely to reap dividends beyond the conventional dimension of trust and legal problems. The present era of end-stage heart failure, heart transplantation, ventricular-assist devices, and ECMO demands that this communication link be strong enough, right from the time of PCICU admission to the time when parents have to take difficult (end-of-life/terminal care) decisions without any predicament. The era of AI and fog computing has brought about the novel ethical dilemma and legal issues related to data sharing and patient privacy.[95,96] These aspects would also be addressed in the future as the adoption of advanced healthcare technology becomes extensive.

The Big Data, Internet of Things (IoT), and Artificial Intelligence (AI)

Cybercare 2.0 has been proposed as the next destination of health care for meeting the challenges of global burden of disease by employing existing technological advancements.[97,98] It envisages the concept of a paradigm shift to predominantly home-based care with a network of distributed health care while hospital-based care existing for specialized services. Health care in cyberspace is likely to evolve into care based on a network with consultation using smartphones or wearable devices or at minute clinics in the neighborhood. The augmented reality using wearable smart devices will facilitate a better chance of patient evaluation for the physician and a pleasant experience for the patient. The vital components of this structure of care are genomics, telemedicine, robotics, simulation, AI, electronic medical records, and smartphones.[97] Various innovative examples of the Internet of things (IoT)[99-102] have been employed in other fields of medicine. These principles are likely to be applied to individual patient care in PCICU where remote monitoring by an international physician with a link for decision-making after clinical evaluation using augmented reality is likely to gain popularity.[103-105] This may reduce the need for a physician at the bedside for each patient but is likely to require more staff at the bedside including nurses, respiratory therapists, ECMO teams, and other support staff for care as well as maintaining this technology. Clinical engineers and biomedical engineers are likely to positively impact global outcomes of disease by affecting the optimum application of health technology.[106] Further, the increased interface between the health care system and mobile communication technologies is likely to increase the reach of health technology.[107] This may facilitate easy data collection and real-time prediction of trends to appropriately caution the clinician. Hence, the PCICU physician must stay up to date with the existing technological advancements affecting the delivery of health care. The real-time availability of innumerable data points in a health technology–embedded patient care environment would augment AI and machine learning–based decision-making in the future.[108–112] Similarly, augmented reality has the potential to be utilized for simulation and training of multidisciplinary PCICU team.[113–115]

Conclusion

Despite advances in the management of pediatric acute respiratory distress syndrome (PARDS) and shock, once refractory to conventional treatment these patients have very high risk of death. Extracorporeal therapies have shown promise in such cases with increased survival rates in refractory shock and PARDS. Survival with ECMO in neonates has improved over the decades. However, many of these survivors develop chronic lung disease. In a retrospective series of 91% neonates by Ortiz et al. from a neonatal ECMO centre, the authors report 76% of survivors developing CLD and factors such as prolonged ECMO, early initiation of ECMO (<24 h of life) and Congenital diaphragmatic hernia as risk factors for the same. Pediatric cardiac critical care one of the most challenging disciplines in medicine has come a long way but not limited to education, personalised medicine, newer surgical techniques, nanomedicine, machine learning and quality and safety that will expand the horizon of Pediatric cardiac critical care.[115,116]

Acknowledgment
We would like to express our heartfelt thanks Dr Abhishek Rathore for providing **Fig. 20.1**.

References

1. Balachandran R, Nair SG, Gopalraj SS, Vaidyanathan B, Kumar RK. Dedicated pediatric cardiac intensive care unit in a developing country: does it improve the outcome? Ann Pediatr Cardiol 2011;4(2):122–126
2. Varma A. Pediatric cardiac intensive care units: the way forward. Ann Pediatr Cardiol 2011;4(2):127–128
3. da Cruz EM, Ivy D, Jaggers J. Pediatric and congenital cardiology, cardiac surgery and intensive care. London: Springer; 2014: 1–3572
4. Ungerleider RM, Ungerleider JD. Whole brain leadership for creating resonant multidisciplinary health care teams. Vol. 108, Annals of Thoracic Surgery. The Society of Thoracic Surgeons; 2019:978–986
5. Chubb H, Rosenthal DN, Almond CS, et al. Impact of cardiac resynchronization therapy on heart transplant-free survival in pediatric and congenital heart disease patients. Circ Arrhythmia Electrophysiol 2020;291–301
6. Ceresnak SR, Perera JL, Motonaga KS, et al. Ventricular lead redundancy to prevent cardiovascular events and sudden death from lead fracture in pacemaker-dependent children. Heart Rhythm 2015;12(1):111–116
7. Friedman KG, Tworetzky W. Fetal cardiac interventions: where do we stand? Arch Cardiovasc Dis 2020;113(2):121–128
8. Strainic J, Armstrong A. Fetal cardiac intervention: a review of the current literature. Curr Pediatr Rep 2020;8(1):1–9
9. Tulzer A, Arzt W, Prandstetter C, Tulzer G. Atrial septum stenting in a foetus with hypoplastic left heart syndrome and restrictive foramen ovale: an alternative to emergency atrioseptectomy in the newborn-a case report. Eur Heart J Case Rep 2020;4(1):1–4
10. Alsagheir A, Koziarz A, Makhdoum A, et al. Duct stenting versus modified Blalock–Taussig shunt in neonates and infants with duct-dependent pulmonary blood flow: a systematic review and meta-analysis. J Thorac Cardiovasc Surg 2021;161(2):379–390.e8
11. Bailey J, Elci OU, Mascio CE, Mercer-Rosa L, Goldmuntz E. Staged versus complete repair in the symptomatic neonate with tetralogy of fallot. Ann Thorac Surg 2020;109(3):802–808
12. Menaissy Y, Omar I, Mofreh B, Alassal M. Total correction of tetralogy of fallot in the first 60 days of life in symptomatic infants: is it the gold standard? Thorac Cardiovasc Surg 2020;68(1):45–50
13. Molloy FJ, Nguyen N, Mize M, et al. Medical missions for the provision of paediatric cardiac surgery in low- and middle-income countries. Cardiol Young 2017;27(S6):S47–S54
14. Nguyen N, Pezzella AT. Pediatric cardiac surgery in low- and middle-income countries or emerging economies: a continuing challenge. World J Pediatr Congenit Heart Surg 2015;6(2):274–283
15. Children's Heartlink: Healing hearts worldwide [Internet]. 2019 [cited 2020 Aug 10]. http://childrensheartlink.org/wp-content/uploads/2020/05/CHL.Overview-Fact-Sheet.2020.pdf
16. El Rassi I, Assy J, Arabi M, et al. Establishing a high-quality congenital cardiac surgery program in a developing country: lessons learned. Front Pediatr 2020;8(July):357
17. Jones MB, Tucker D. Nursing considerations in pediatric cardiac critical care. Pediatr Crit Care Med 2016;17(8, Suppl 1):S383–S387
18. Murni IK, Musa NL. The need for specialized pediatric cardiac critical care training program in limited resource settings. Front Pediatr 2018;6(March):59
19. Boydston J. Use of a standardized care communication checklist during multidisciplinary rounds in pediatric cardiac intensive care: a best practice implementation project. JBI Database Syst Rev Implement Reports 2018;16(2):548–564
20. Caruso TJ, Wang EY, Schwenk H, et al. A postoperative care bundle reduces surgical site infections in pediatric patients undergoing cardiac surgeries. Jt Comm J Qual Patient Saf 2019;45(3):156–163
21. Raines K, Sevilla Berrios RA, Guttendorf J. Sepsis education initiative targeting qSOFA screening for non-ICU patients to improve sepsis recognition and time to treatment. J Nurs Care Qual 2019;34(4):318–324
22. Regan LC, Rodriguez L. Nurse empowerment from a middle-management perspective: nurse managers' and assistant nurse managers' workplace empowerment views. Perm J 2011;15(1):e101–e107
23. Brown KM, Mudd SS, Hunt EA, et al. A multi-institutional simulation boot camp for pediatric cardiac critical care nurse practitioners. Pediatr Crit Care Med 2018;19(6):564–571

24. Ang B, Han WM, Wong JJM, Lee AN, Chan YH, Lee JH. Impact of a nurse-led feeding protocol in a pediatric intensive care unit. Proc Singapore Healthc. 2016;25(1):35–42

25. Hamstra B. Will these nurse robots take your job? Don't freak out just yet. [Internet]. 2018 [cited 2020 Aug 10]. https://nurse.org/articles/nurse-robots-friend-or-foe/

26. Joy BF, Elliott E, Hardy C, Sullivan C, Backer CL, Kane JM. Standardized multidisciplinary protocol improves handover of cardiac surgery patients to the intensive care unit. Pediatr Crit Care Med 2011;12(3):304–308

27. Catchpole KR, de Leval MR, McEwan A, et al. Patient handover from surgery to intensive care: using Formula 1 pit-stop and aviation models to improve safety and quality. Paediatr Anaesth 2007;17(5):470–478

28. Esangbedo ID, Byrnes J, Brandewie K, et al. Risk factors for peri-intubation cardiac arrest in pediatric cardiac intensive care patients: a multicenter study. Pediatr Crit Care Med 2020;21(12):e1126–e1133

29. Bernier ML, Jacob AI, Collaco JM, McGrath-Morrow SA, Romer LH, Unegbu CC. Perioperative events in children with pulmonary hypertension undergoing non-cardiac procedures. Pulm Circ 2018;8(1):2045893217738143

30. Elgebaly AS, Eldabaa AA. Is I-gel airway a better option to endotracheal tube airway for sevoflurane-fentanyl anesthesia during cardiac surgery? Anesth Essays Res 2014;8(2):216–222

31. El-Halaby H, Abdel-Hady H, Alsawah G, Abdelrahman A, El-Tahan H. Sonographic evaluation of diaphragmatic excursion and thickness in healthy infants and children. J Ultrasound Med 2016;35(1):167–175

32. Xue Y, Zhang Z, Sheng CQ, Li YM, Jia FY. The predictive value of diaphragm ultrasound for weaning outcomes in critically ill children. BMC Pulm Med 2019;19(1):270

33. Parreco J, Hidalgo A, Parks JJ, Kozol R, Rattan R. Using artificial intelligence to predict prolonged mechanical ventilation and tracheostomy placement. J Surg Res 2018;228:179–187

34. Pasut G. Grand challenges in nano-based drug delivery. Front Med Technol 2019;1(December):1

35. Miragoli M, Ceriotti P, Iafisco M, et al. Inhalation of peptide-loaded nanoparticles improves heart failure. Sci Transl Med 2018;10(424):1–12

36. Chakravarthy M. Opioid free cardiac anesthesia: a flash in the pan? Ann Card Anaesth 2020;23(2):113–115

37. Mencía S, Palacios A, García M, et al. An exploratory study of sevoflurane as an alternative for difficult sedation in critically ill children. Pediatr Crit Care Med 2018;19(7):e335–e341

38. Bembea MM, Annich G, Rycus P, Oldenburg G, Berkowitz I, Pronovost P. Variability in anticoagulation management of patients on extracorporeal membrane oxygenation: an international survey. Pediatr Crit Care Med 2013;14(2):e77–e84

39. Vakamudi M, Kodali RKV, Karthekeyan RB, Thangavel P, Sambandham KG. A comparative study on safety and efficacy of caudal, thoracic epidural and intra venous analgesia in paediatric cardiac surgery: a double blind randomised trial. World J Cardiovasc Surg 2020;10:101–114

40. Chakravarthy M, Thimmangowda P, Krishnamurthy J, Nadiminti S, Jawali V. Thoracic epidural anesthesia in cardiac surgical patients: a prospective audit of 2,113 cases. J Cardiothorac Vasc Anesth 2005;19(1):44–48

41. Yamamoto T, Seino Y, Matsuda K, et al. Preoperative implementation of transverse thoracic muscle plane block and rectus sheath block combination for pediatric cardiac surgery. J Cardiothorac Vasc Anesth 2020;34(12):3367–3372

42. Sharma VK, Kumar G, Joshi S, Tiwari N, Kumar V, Ramamurthy HR. An evolving anesthetic protocol fosters fast tracking in pediatric cardiac surgery: a comparison of two anesthetic techniques. Ann Pediatr Cardiol 2020;13(1):31–37

43. Weiner MM, Rosenblatt MA, Mittnacht AJC. Neuraxial anesthesia and timing of heparin administration in patients undergoing surgery for congenital heart disease using cardiopulmonary bypass. J Cardiothorac Vasc Anesth 2012;26(4):581–584

44. Singh Y, Tissot C, Fraga MV, et al. International evidence-based guidelines on Point of Care Ultrasound (POCUS) for critically ill neonates and children issued by the POCUS Working Group of the European Society of Paediatric and Neonatal Intensive Care (ESPNIC). Crit Care 2020;24(1):65

45. Steppan D, DiGiusto M, Steppan J. Perioperative lung ultrasound in the pediatric intensive care unit-beyond the vasculature and parenchyma. J Cardiothorac Vasc Anesth 2020;34(4):956–958

46. Kaskinen AK, Martelius L, Kirjavainen T, Rautiainen P, Andersson S, Pitkänen OM. Assessment of extravascular lung water by ultrasound after congenital cardiac surgery. Pediatr Pulmonol 2017;52(3):345–352

47. Cantinotti M, Giordano R, Marchese P, et al. Retrosternal clots after Fontan surgery by systematic evaluation with transthoracic ultrasound. J Cardiothorac Vasc Anesth 2020;34(4):951–955

48. Cantinotti M, Ait Ali L, Scalese M, et al. Lung ultrasound reclassification of chest X-ray data after pediatric cardiac surgery. Paediatr Anaesth 2018;28(5):421–427

49. Cantinotti M, Giordano R, Scalese M, et al. Prognostic value of a new lung ultrasound score to predict intensive care unit stay in pediatric cardiac surgery. Ann Thorac Surg 2020;109(1):178–184

50. Alexander KM, Chan SS, Opfer E, et al. Implementation of bowel ultrasound practice for the diagnosis and management of necrotising enterocolitis. Arch Dis Child Fetal Neonatal Ed 2021;106(1):96–103

51. Garduño-López J, García-Cruz E, Baranda-Tovar FM. Cardiac, cerebral, renal, optic nerve, and lung ultrasound study (CCROSS) protocol. Arch Cardiol Mex 2019;89(1):126–137

52. Hardwick JA, Griksaitis MJ. Fifteen-minute consultation: point of care ultrasound in the management of paediatric shock. Arch Dis Child Educ Pract Ed 2021; 106(3):136–141

53. Beaubien-Souligny W, Rola P, Haycock K, et al. Quantifying systemic congestion with Point-Of-Care ultrasound: development of the venous excess ultrasound grading system. Ultrasound J 2020;12(1):16

54. Hussein L, Rehman MA, Sajid R, Annajjar F, Al-Janabi T. Bedside ultrasound in cardiac standstill: a clinical review. Ultrasound J 2019;11(1):35

55. Clattenburg EJ, Wroe PC, Gardner K, et al. Implementation of the Cardiac Arrest Sonographic Assessment (CASA) protocol for patients with cardiac arrest is associated with shorter CPR pulse checks. Resuscitation 2018;131:69–73

56. Lee SH, Jong Yun S. Diagnostic performance of optic nerve sheath diameter for predicting neurologic outcome in post-cardiac arrest patients: a systematic review and meta-analysis. Resuscitation 2019;138(138):59–67

57. Nazerian P, De Stefano G, Albano G, et al. Transesophageal echocardiography (TEE) in cardiac arrest: results of a hands-on training for a simplified TEE protocol. Ultrasound J 2020; 12(1):41

58. Kheir JN, Scharp LA, Borden MA, et al. Oxygen gas-filled microparticles provide intravenous oxygen delivery. Sci Transl Med 2012;4(140):140ra88

59. Prasad N, Cheng LF, Chivers C, Draugelis M, Engelhardt BE. A reinforcement learning approach to weaning of mechanical

ventilation in intensive care units. Uncertain Artif Intell - Proc 33rd Conf UAI 2017

60. Ruf B, Bonelli V, Balling G, et al. Intraoperative renal near-infrared spectroscopy indicates developing acute kidney injury in infants undergoing cardiac surgery with cardiopulmonary bypass: a case-control study. Crit Care 2015;19(1):27

61. Bernal NP, Hoffman GM, Ghanayem NS, Arca MJ. Cerebral and somatic near-infrared spectroscopy in normal newborns. J Pediatr Surg 2010;45(6):1306–1310

62. Hames DL, Ferguson MA, Kaza AK, et al. Renal replacement therapy in the pediatric cardiac intensive care unit. J Thorac Cardiovasc Surg 2019;158(5):1446–1455

63. Ince C. Hemodynamic coherence and the rationale for monitoring the microcirculation. Crit Care 2015;19(Suppl 3):S8

64. Erdem Ö, Kuiper JW, Tibboel D. Hemodynamic coherence in critically ill pediatric patients. Best Pract Res Clin Anaesthesiol 2016;30(4):499–510

65. Scolletta S, Marianello D, Isgrò G, et al. Microcirculatory changes in children undergoing cardiac surgery: a prospective observational study. Br J Anaesth 2016;117(2):206–213

66. González R, Urbano J, Solana MJ, et al. Microcirculatory differences in children with congenital heart disease according to cyanosis and age. Front Pediatr 2019;7(July):264

67. Flechet M, Güiza F, Scharlaeken I, et al. Near-infrared-based cerebral oximetry for prediction of severe acute kidney injury in critically ill children after cardiac surgery. Crit Care Explor 2019;1(12):e0063

68. Nasr VG, Bergersen LT, Lin HM, et al. Validation of a second-generation near-infrared spectroscopy monitor in children with congenital heart disease. Anesth Analg 2019;128(4):661–668

69. Sanders M, Servaas S, Slagt C. Accuracy and precision of non-invasive cardiac output monitoring by electrical cardiometry: a systematic review and meta-analysis. J Clin Monit Comput 2020;34(3):433–460

70. Faraoni D, Meier J, New HV, Van der Linden PJ, Hunt BJ. Patient blood management for neonates and children undergoing cardiac surgery: 2019 NATA guidelines. J Cardiothorac Vasc Anesth 2019;33(12):3249–3263

71. Nandi S, Sommerville L, Nellenbach K, et al. Platelet-like particles improve fibrin network properties in a hemophilic model of provisional matrix structural defects. J Colloid Interface Sci 2020;577:406–418

72. Nellenbach K, Guzzetta NA, Brown AC. Analysis of the structural and mechanical effects of procoagulant agents on neonatal fibrin networks following cardiopulmonary bypass. J Thromb Haemost 2018;16(11):2159–2167

73. Hunt R, Hoffman CM, Emani S, et al. Elevated preoperative von Willebrand factor is associated with perioperative thrombosis in infants and neonates with congenital heart disease. J Thromb Haemost 2017;15(12):2306–2316

74. Bolliger D, Tanaka KA. Transfusion makeovers by thrombo-elastometry: does it work for everyone? J Cardiothorac Vasc Anesth 2019;33(2):318–320

75. Groves DS, Winegar DA, Fernandez LG, Huffmyer JL, Viola F. Comparison of coagulation parameters in arterial and venous blood in cardiac surgery measured using the Quantra system. J Cardiothorac Vasc Anesth 2019;33(4):976–984

76. Lauridsen MH, Kristensen AD, Hjortdal VE, Jensen IS, Nikolajsen L. Chronic pain in children after cardiac surgery via sternotomy. Cardiol Young 2014;24(5):893–899

77. Nikolajsen L, Brix LD. Chronic pain after surgery in children. Curr Opin Anaesthesiol 2014;27(5):507–512

78. Williams G, Howard RF, Liossi C. Persistent postsurgical pain in children and young people: prediction, prevention, and management. Pain Rep 2017;2(5):e616

79. Buskila D. Genetics of chronic pain states. Best Pract Res Clin Rheumatol 2007;21(3):535–547

80. Wheeler DS, Jeffries HE, Zimmerman JJ, Wong HR, Carcillo JA. Sepsis in the pediatric cardiac intensive care unit. World J Pediatr Congenit Heart Surg 2011;2(3):393–399

81. Wheeler DS, Wong HR. Sepsis in pediatric cardiac intensive care. Pediatr Crit Care Med 2016;17(8, Suppl 1):S266–S271

82. Nordenström K, Lannering K, Mellander M, Elfvin A. Low risk of necrotising enterocolitis in enterally fed neonates with critical heart disease: an observational study. Arch Dis Child Fetal Neonatal Ed 2020;105(6):609–614

83. Pierro A, Zani A. Necrotizing enterocolitis: controversies and challenges. F1000 Res 2015;4:F1000

84. Balkin EM, Zinter MS, Rajagopal SK, Keller RL, Fineman JR, Steurer MA. Intensive care mortality prognostic model for pediatric pulmonary hypertension. Pediatr Crit Care Med 2018;19(8):733–740

85. LaRovere JM, Jeffries HE, Sachdeva RC, et al. Databases for assessing the outcomes of the treatment of patients with congenital and paediatric cardiac disease: the perspective of critical care. Cardiol Young 2008;18(Suppl 2):130–136

86. Jacobs ML, Jacobs JP, Franklin RC, et al. Databases for assessing the outcomes of the treatment of patients with congenital and paediatric cardiac disease: the perspective of cardiac surgery. Cardiol Young 2008;18(Suppl 2):101–115

87. Mack EH, Wheeler DS, Embi PJ. Clinical decision support systems in the pediatric intensive care unit. Pediatr Crit Care Med 2009;10(1):23–28

88. Jeffries HE, Soto-Campos G, Katch A, Gall C, Rice TB, Wetzel R. Pediatric index of cardiac surgical intensive care mortality risk score for pediatric cardiac critical care. Pediatr Crit Care Med 2015;16(9):846–852

89. Jacobs JP, Maruszewski B, Kurosawa H, et al. Congenital heart surgery databases around the world: do we need a global database? Semin Thorac Cardiovasc Surg Pediatr Card Surg Annu 2010;13(1):3–19

90. Yau DKW, Wong MKH, Wong WT, et al. PREhabilitation for improving QUality of recovery after ELective cardiac surgery (PREQUEL) study: protocol of a randomised controlled trial. BMJ Open 2019;9(5):e027974

91. Brauner DJ, Zimmermann CJ. Will we code for default ECMO? AMA J Ethics 2019;21(5):E443–E449

92. Prouhet PM, Gregory MR, Russell CL, Yaeger LH. Fathers' stress in the neonatal intensive care unit: a systematic review. Adv Neonatal Care 2018;18(2):105–120

93. Govindaswamy P, Laing SM, Waters D, Walker K, Spence K, Badawi N. Fathers' needs in a surgical neonatal intensive care unit: assuring the other parent. PLoS One 2020;15(5):e0232190

94. Neubauer K, Williams EP, Donohue PK, Boss RD. Communication and decision-making regarding children with critical cardiac disease: a systematic review of family preferences. Cardiol Young 2018;28(10):1088–1092

95. Gerke S, Minssen T, Cohen G. Ethical and legal challenges of artificial intelligence-driven healthcare. Artificial Intelligence in Healthcare 2020;295–336

96. King DK, Toobert DJ, Portz JD, et al. What patients want: relevant health information technology for diabetes self-management. Health Technol (Berl) 2012;2(3):147–157

97. Rosen JM, Kun L, Mosher RE, et al. Cybercare 2.0: meeting the challenge of the global burden of disease in 2030. Health Technol (Berl) 2016;6(1):35–51

98. Hammami R, Hatem B, Hadj Kacem A. Interoperability for medical information systems: An overview. Health Technol (Berl) 2014;4(3):261–272

99. Gharehbaghi A, Lindén M. An internet-based tool for pediatric cardiac disease diagnosis using intelligent phonocardiography. LNICST 2016;169:443–447

100. de Moura Costa HJ, da Costa CA, da Rosa Righi R, Antunes RS. Fog computing in health: a systematic literature review. Health Technol (Berl) 2020;10:1025–1044

101. Li C, Hu X, Zhang L. The IoT-based heart disease monitoring system for pervasive healthcare service. Procedia Comput Sci 2017;112:2328–2334

102. Hayek A, Telawi S, Börcsök J, Abi Zeid Daou R, Halabi N. Smart wearable system for safety-related medical IoT application: case of epileptic patient working in industrial environment. Health Technol (Berl) 2020;10(1):363–372

103. Lopez-Magallon AJ, Otero AV, Welchering N, et al. Patient outcomes of an international telepediatric cardiac critical care program. Telemed J E Health 2015;21(8):601–610

104. Ramnath VR, Ho L, Maggio LA, Khazeni N. Centralized monitoring and virtual consultant models of tele-ICU care: a systematic review. Telemed J E Health 2014;20(10):936–961

105. Young K, Gupta A, Palacios R. Impact of telemedicine in pediatric postoperative care. Telemed J E Health 2019;25(11):1083–1089

106. David Y, Judd T. Evidence-based impact by clinical engineers on global patients outcomes. Health Technol (Berl) 2020;10(2):517–535

107. Nair P, Bhaskaran H. The emerging interface of healthcare system and mobile communication technologies. Health Technol (Berl) 2015;4(4):337–343

108. Gutierrez G. Artificial intelligence in the intensive care unit. Crit Care 2020;24(1):101

109. Gearhart A, Gaffar S, Chang AC. A primer on artificial intelligence for the paediatric cardiologist. Cardiol Young 2020;30(7): 934–945

110. Bærøe K, Miyata-Sturm A, Henden E. How to achieve trustworthy artificial intelligence for health. Bull World Health Organ 2020;98(4):257–262

111. Ishii E, Ebner DK, Kimura S, Agha-Mir-Salim L, Uchimido R, Celi LA. The advent of medical artificial intelligence: lessons from the Japanese approach. J Intensive Care 2020;8(1):35

112. Mlodzinski E, Stone DJ, Celi LA. Machine learning for pulmonary and critical care medicine: a narrative review. Pulm Ther 2020;6(1):67–77

113. Merkle F, Kurtovic D, Matschke A, Haupt B, Falk V, Starck C. Simulation-based training of critical events during cardiopulmonary bypass: importance of a critical events checklist. Perfus (United Kingdom); 2020

114. Lal A, Pinevich Y, Gajic O, Herasevich V, Pickering B. Artificial intelligence and computer simulation models in critical illness. World J Crit Care Med 2020;9(2):13–19

115. Aneman A, Brechot N, Brodie D, et al. Advances in critical care management of patients undergoing cardiac surgery. Vol. 44, Intensive Care Medicine. Berlin, Heidelberg: Springer; 2018:799–810

115. Alibrahim OS, Heard CMB. Extracorporeal life support: four decades and counting. Curr Anesthesiol Rep. (2017) 7:168–82

116. Sankar J and Kissoon N (2022) Editorial: Insights and advances in pediatric critical care. Front. Pediatr. 10:1057991

21

Acyanotic Congenital Heart Disease and Transesophageal Echocardiography

Rupa Sreedhar

Introduction

Transesophageal echocardiography (TEE) is an essential diagnostic and monitoring device in pediatric cardiac surgery for confirming preoperative diagnoses, demonstrating previously unappreciated anatomic details, formulating surgical plans, evaluating immediate surgical results, detecting residual lesions which are significant, and guiding surgical revisions.[1,2]

Atrial Septal Defect (ASD)

1. **Secundum ASD:** Defect is seen in the foramen ovale area in midesophageal four-chamber view (ME 4C V), midesophageal bicaval view (ME bicaval V), midesophageal aortic valve short-axis view (ME AV SAX V), midesophageal right ventricular inflow-outflow view (ME RV inflow-outflow V), and transgastric (TG) bicaval equivalent views (**Fig. 21.1a, b**).

   TEE guidance is used for transcatheter closure. Mitral and tricuspid valves as well as total septal length is assessed in ME 4C view. Mitral valve must be examined for prolapse. When a large device is deployed, atrioventricular valve (AVV) closure may be affected.[3] Diameter of atrial septal defect, septal rims, and total septal length are measured using TEE.

Baseline view of valve function prior to device deployment must be acquired to enable comparison with post deployment image. Catheter course from inferior vena cava (IVC) to right atrium (RA) and then to left atrium (LA) via defect is seen in ME AV SAX view. The superior and inferior septal rims are seen in the bicaval view.[4]

2. **Primum ASD:** Defect is seen using ME 4 C view in the posterior and inferior part of interatrial septum, above the AVVs. Both these valves originate at the same level. Primum ASD is frequently associated with partial or complete atrioventricular septal defect. It is also commonly associated with cleft mitral valve. Using color-flow Doppler (CFD) and spectral Doppler, mitral regurgitation if present must be diagnosed and graded (**Fig. 21.1c**).

   It is necessary to look for left ventricular outflow tract (LVOT) obstruction using two-dimensional (2D) TEE, CFD, and spectral Doppler in modified midesophageal five-chamber view (ME 5C V), midesophageal aortic valve long-axis view (ME AV LAX V), midesophageal long-axis view (ME LAX V), and deep transgastric long-axis view (Deep TG LAX V). LVOT obstruction may be present due to:
   - Aberrant chords inserting into interventricular septum.
   - Discrete membrane in LVOT.

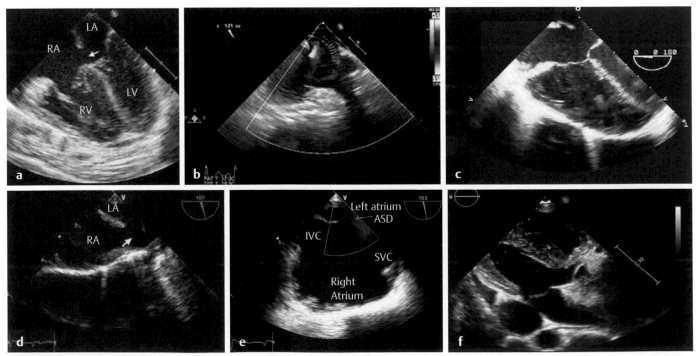

Fig. 21.1 **(a)** Secundum atrial septal defect (ASD) in midesophageal four-chamber view; **(b)** secundum ASD in midesophageal bicaval view; **(c)** primum ASD in midesophageal four-chamber view; **(d)** superior vena cava-type sinus venosus ASD in midesophageal bicaval view; **(e)** inferior vena cava-type sinus venosus ASD in midesophageal bicaval view; **(f)** coronary sinus ASD with dilated coronary sinus in deep midesophageal four-chamber view. Abbreviations: LA, left atrium; LV, left ventricle; RA, right atrium; RV, right ventricle.

- Goose neck deformity or long-tunnel-type obstruction of LVOT.

3. **Sinus venosus ASD:** The defect is to be looked for in ME 4 Chamber, ME bicaval, and deep TG bicaval equivalent views. Superior defect (more common) is located near superior vena cava (SVC) above foramen ovale (**Fig. 21.1d**). The inferior defect (rare) is situated below foramen ovale, in inferior part of interatrial septum, near IVC (**Fig. 21.1e**). These ASDs are associated with partial anomalous pulmonary venous drainage. CFD and pulse-wave Doppler (PWD) are used to assess drainage of all pulmonary veins. ME 4C and ME bicaval views with rightward rotation is used to look for right pulmonary veins. ME 4C and ME 2C views are used to look for left pulmonary veins. By advancing and withdrawing the probe, the SVC and IVC needs to be searched for high-normal-velocity flow or aliasing, suggestive of anomalous pulmonary venous drainage of upper and lower pulmonary veins.

4. **Coronary sinus ASD:** The defect may be anywhere along the course of the coronary sinus. It is looked for using ME 4C (in area of coronary sinus in AV groove), modified ME bicaval view near entrance of IVC, and midesophageal two-chamber view (ME 2 CV) (**Fig. 21.1e**).

Contrast saline solution should be injected into left hand to determine whether left SVC (LSVC) is present. Immediate opacification of LA occurs prior to RA if LSVC and coronary sinus ASD are present. Bubbles first enter RA (via innominate and right SVC) when there is coronary sinus ASD without LSVC.[5]

In all types of ASD:

- The interatrial septum must be examined for multiple defects and the size of ASD must be measured in multiple planes. CFD and PWD are used to identify the size and direction of flow.
- The pulmonary veins must be examined to find out where they drain. Using PWD, velocity of flow in pulmonary veins can be assessed. Although the velocity of flow in pulmonary veins may be high due to high pulmonary blood flow, peak and mean velocities are not significantly elevated.
- It is necessary to look for RA and right ventricular (RV) enlargement, and to assess biventricular function.
- Mitral valve (MV) and tricuspid valve (TV) annulus must be measured. Prolapse or cleft in MV needs to be looked for. CFD and spectral Doppler is used to grade any mitral or/and TR. LSVC is searched for between left upper pulmonary vein (LUPV) and left atrial appendage (LAA) in ME 2C and ME 4C views.
- The pulmonary valve must be examined (ME ascending aortic SAX and TG RV basal view[6]) for leaflets doming, commissural fusion, and restricted motion. From TG basal SAX view, turn the probe clockwise to see transgastric (TG) RV basal view.[6] CFD and continuous-wave Doppler (CWD) are used to look for

pulmonary stenosis. Velocities of up to 2.5 m/s at the pulmonary valve may occur due to ASD flow.[7,8]

TEE assessment after surgery/device closure:

- ASD closure is confirmed preferably with bubble contrast study.
- Mitral valve needs to be assessed and any MR quantified.
- Following sinus venosus ASD repair, proper drainage of pulmonary veins into LA and absence of narrowing of pulmonary veins, SVC, SVC baffle, and SVC-RA appendage anastomosis (post-Warden repair) must be confirmed. If SVC-RA appendage anastomosis is narrow, increased PWD gradients are observed at this site in TG RV inflow view and TG RV inflow-outflow view. Usually, SVC-RAA gradient of more than 5 mm Hg is unacceptable. Tacy et al have mentioned that loss of biphasic pattern in SVC is more indicative of obstruction rather than absolute value of gradient as it varies with the loading conditions.[6]
- Absence of pulmonary vein obstruction must be confirmed after device closure of ASD. If the PWD gradient is less than 2 mm Hg, pulmonary venous obstruction is ruled out.

Ventricular Septal Defect (VSD)

1. **Perimembranous VSD:** This VSD is seen in ME RV inflow-outflow (**Fig. 21.2a**), ME AV SAX, and modified ME 5C views (obtained by withdrawing and flexing the probe from the ME 4C view). The defect is adjacent to septal leaflet of TV. The leaflet tissue may completely or partially close the defect. In the ME AV LAX view, the defect is seen adjacent to right coronary cusp of aortic valve which may be prolapsed into the defect due to venturi effect from VSD flow (**Fig. 21.2c**).

2. **Inlet VSD:** Inlet VSD is located inferiorly in the ventricular septum close to AVVs. It is seen in ME 4C and in TG basal SAX views. It is often associated with atrioventricular canal defect. The AVV must be examined for override. More than 50% of the TV may open into LV. It may also be associated with LVOT obstruction. The LVOT must be examined for membranes, chords, and tunnel-like obstruction (use ME LAX, TG LAX, and Deep TG LAX views). CFD and CWD is used to look for stenosis/regurgitation of AVVs (**Fig. 21.2b**).

3. **Outlet VSD:** It is observed adjacent to pulmonary valve in ME RV inflow-outflow view. In the ME AV LAX view with outward rotation, it is seen adjacent to the right coronary cusp. This view is used to look for aortic regurgitation (CFD) and prolapse of right coronary cusp (**Fig. 21.2c**).

4. **Muscular VSD:** Muscular VSDs are looked for using 2D and CFD in ME 4C, ME LAX, ME AV LAX, TG mid-SAX, and Deep TG LAX views. The entire interventricular septum must be searched for multiple defects.

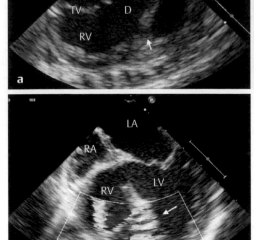
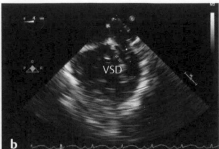
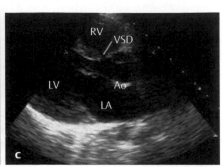
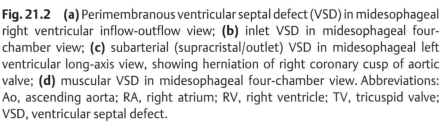

Fig. 21.2 **(a)** Perimembranous ventricular septal defect (VSD) in midesophageal right ventricular inflow-outflow view; **(b)** inlet VSD in midesophageal four-chamber view; **(c)** subarterial (supracristal/outlet) VSD in midesophageal left ventricular long-axis view, showing herniation of right coronary cusp of aortic valve; **(d)** muscular VSD in midesophageal four-chamber view. Abbreviations: Ao, ascending aorta; RA, right atrium; RV, right ventricle; TV, tricuspid valve; VSD, ventricular septal defect.

Muscular VSD may be anterior, midventricular, posterior, and apical, depending on their location in the muscular septum. It has a rim totally made up of muscle (**Fig. 21.2d**).

In all types of VSD:
- Search for multiple VSDs should be done and the size of each VSD assessed (small 1–2 mm; moderate 3–5 mm; large >5 mm).
- It is necessary to look for left atrial enlargement (LAE), left ventricular enlargement (LVE), right atrial enlargement (RAE).
- Measure annulus of TV if dilated and assess biventricular function.
- Direction of blood flow must be assessed using CFD. Flow is left to right in uncomplicated VSD. However, in early part of diastole, a short reversal of flow is usual.
- CWD is used to measure RV pressure which is = PAP = Systolic BP minus four multiplied by square of velocity across VSD.
- Presence of any AR is assessed using CFD, CWD/PWD.

TEE assessment after surgical repair:
- Closure of VSD (and any coexisting ASD) must be confirmed and diligent search must be done to look for residual or additional VSDs.
- Residual defects <3 mm are detected by TEE but are hemodynamically insignificant and usually do not require immediate reoperation.
- RV pressure or PA pressure is measured using VSD flow or TR jet velocity if present.

- Search is done for AR, aortic cusp perforation or prolapse, TR.
- Biventricular function needs to be assessed (can be affected by injury to coronary artery, ventriculotomy).

In ASD and VSD:
- Pulmonary hypertension, RV hypertrophy, right-to-left shunt, and systolic flattening of interventricular septum points toward the possibility of Eisenmenger syndrome.
- TR is searched for (using CFD) and if it is present, CW is used to measure RVP = PAP = systolic BP = $4V^2$ + RAP.
- QP: QS (ratio measured [before and after surgery]) using VTI at LVOT and RVOT as well as diameter of LVOT and RVOT.

Atrioventricular Canal Defect (AVCD)

Interatrial septum is examined for primum ASD (ME 4C) and interventricular septum for inlet VSD (ME 4C, TG mid-SAX). Partial AVCD consists of primum ASD and cleft MV (**Fig. 21.3a**). Complete AVCD consists of primum ASD, inlet VSD, and common AVV (**Fig. 21.3b**). Size of defect and direction of flow are assessed using CFD and PWD.

- AVVs are examined for MV cleft, leaflet prolapse, and straddling using ME 4C, ME LAX, TG Basal SAX, TG LAX views. ME 4C and TG mid-SAX views are used to assess whether the defect is balanced. If the LV is small (unbalanced AVCD), single-ventricle repair

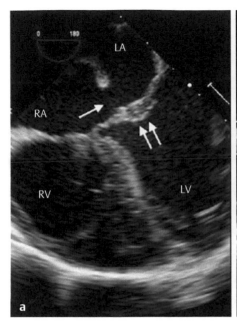
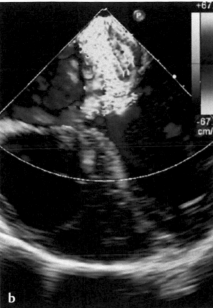

Fig. 21.3 (a) Partial atrioventricular canal defect (AVCD): primum atrial septal defect (ASD), cleft left atrioventricular valve, no ventricular septal defect (VSD). **(b)** Complete AVCD consisting of primum ASD, common atrioventricular valve (AVV) and inlet VSD. Abbreviations: RA, right atrium; RV, right ventricle; LV, left ventricle.

may be required. Size and function of ventricles are assessed. When insertions of straddling cords are into the opposite ventricle, it may not be possible to obtain two competent AVVs (necessitating single-ventricle repair).[10]

- Any stenosis or regurgitation of AVVs should be graded. Any LVOT should be identified using CFD (ME LAX) and the gradient measured (TG LAX, deep TG LAX views).
- It is necessary to look for LSVC. If LSVC draining into coronary sinus is present, the atrial patch should not be placed in such a way that the coronary sinus drains into LA.
- RV pressure or PA pressure is measured using TR or VSD jet.

Postoperative TEE:

- Closure of ASD and VSD is confirmed and AVVs are examined for any residual stenosis/regurgitation/prolapse/flail.
- Biventricular function is assessed and PA pressure is measured if there is TR.

Persistent Ductus Arteriosus (PDA)

ME ascending aorta SAX view is used to image PDA. Although it is difficult to visualize PDA by 2D TEE, ductal flow can be seen in this view (using CFD) as continuous high-velocity turbulent aliased flow in the MPA. CWD at this site shows flow throughout the cardiac cycle and it may be possible to delineate the PDA and its attachment to PA using CFD. The same views obtained after surgery should show absence of turbulence in the MPA (**Fig. 21.4a**).

In postsurgical period: Any persistent shunt is looked for and biventricular function is assessed.

Aortopulmonary Window

In this anomaly, both aortic and pulmonary valve apparatus are well defined and there is a communication between the ascending aorta and the pulmonary trunk and/or the right pulmonary artery. The defect can be imaged in midesophageal ascending aorta short-axis view (**Fig. 21.4b**).

Coarctation of Aorta

The narrow coarctation segment (including posterior shelf inside aortic lumen) and poststenotic dilation of descending thoracic aorta distal to the coarctation site can be seen in UE Ao Arch SAX and descending thoracic aortic LAX view (**Fig. 21.5a–c**). Color-flow Doppler shows aliased flow. CW Doppler measures gradient of >2.5 m/s. In descending aortic SAX view, collateral vessels which bring blood flow to descending aorta may be visualized (using CFD). PWD interrogation of these collateral vessels show flow signals in systole and diastole.

Using ME 4-CH, ME 2-CH, AV LAX, and TG SAX, mitral and aortic valvular morphology and function are assessed, any subvalvular and supravalvular aortic obstruction is searched for, and LV mass and function are assessed (**Fig. 21.5d**).

Residual gradient, re-coarctation, and aortic aneurysm formation is searched for during postsurgical TEE examination.

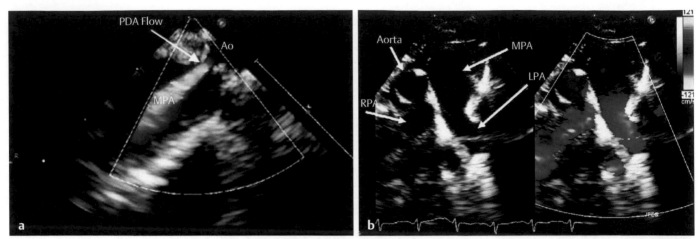

Fig. 21.4 **(a)** Turbulent flow signals from aorta to pulmonary artery (PA) through persistent ductus arteriosus (PDA) shown in color-flow Doppler at midesophageal (ME) ascending aorta short-axis (SAX) view. Continuous flow can be demonstrated at the area of PDA using pulsed Doppler. **(b)** Division of main pulmonary artery into right (RPA) and left (LPA) pulmonary artery is seen in this ME short-axis view showing the A-P window. Abbreviations: Ao, ascending aorta; PDA, posterior descending artery; LPA, left pulmonary arteries; MPA, main pulmonary arteries; RPA, right pulmonary arteries.

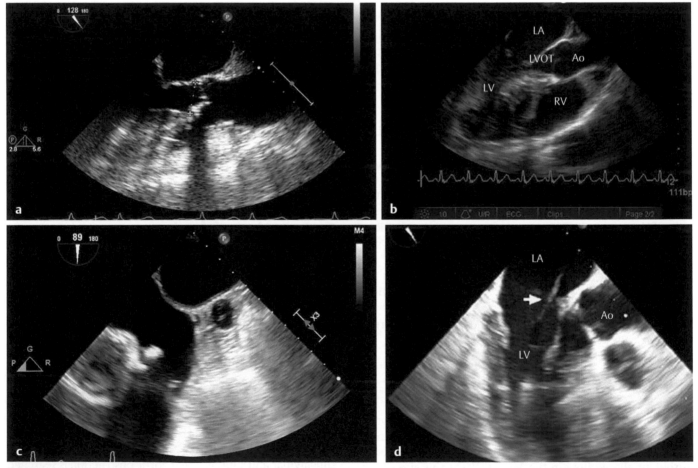

Fig. 21.5 **(a)** Descending aortic long-axis (LAX) view showing the narrow coarctation segment; **(b)** supravalvular aortic stenosis seen in midesophageal aortic valve long-axis view; **(c)** upper esophageal aortic arch SAX view showing thickening and doming of pulmonary valve leaflets in pulmonary stenosis; **(d)** midesophageal commissural view showing a membrane between atrial septum and junction of left atrial appendage and left upper pulmonary vein (cor triatriatum). Abbreviations: Ao, ascending aorta; LA, left atrium; LV, left ventricle; LVOT, left ventricular outflow tract; RV, right ventricle.

Aortic Stenosis

Pre-CPB TEE: ME AV SAX view is used to see morphology of AV. Deep TG LAX view is used to assess aortic stenosis (measure peak gradient across obstruction), any associated aortic regurgitation, and to measure the aortic root size. Location and severity of obstruction (subvalvar, valvar, supravalvar) must be evaluated. To look for LV hypertrophy and to assess LV function, ME 4C view is used.

Post-CPB TEE: After surgery, TEE is used to look for any residual outflow obstruction or aortic insufficiency, any new ventricular septal defect, or mitral regurgitation. Ventricular function (segmental and global) is also assessed. Function of right ventricular homograft is assessed after Ross procedure.[6,11]

Pulmonic Stenosis

For valuation of RV outflow tract and PV, ME RV inflow-outflow view is used. ME ascending aortic SAX view is used to evaluate the main pulmonary artery and right pulmonary artery. For measurement of gradients across the pulmonary valve, TG RV basal view, TG RV inflow-outflow view, and upper esophageal aortic arch SAX views can be used. Anatomy of pulmonary valve, the location and severity of obstruction (subvalvar, valvar, supravalvar), and size of pulmonary arteries must be determined. It is also necessary to evaluate for intracardiac shunts, to evaluate for ventricular hypertrophy, and to assess ventricular function.

Postsurgical evaluation includes assessment of RV size and function as well as any residual pulmonary outflow tract obstruction or pulmonary regurgitation.

Cor Triatriatum

Midesophageal four-chamber, midesophageal commissural, and ME two-chamber views enable visualization of a fibromuscular membrane which courses between the atrial septum and the junction of the left upper pulmonary vein (LUPV) and the LAA. The atrial accessory chamber (AC) receives the LUPV. 2D TEE shows the opening in the membrane. Using PWD, the degree of narrowing can be assessed.

Conclusion

Congenital cardiac defects are the most common developmental anomaly, with an incidence of 4 to 10 per 1000 live births. They are the most common noninfectious causes of mortality in pediatrics. Patients suffering from cardiac

diseases are frequently reported with anemia, which is highly prevalent without vitamin or mineral insufficiency or other definable reasons. ACHD patients, especially patients with VSD, should be considered a group with a potential risk of neutropenia and be evaluated to avoid remaining misdiagnosed as well as to reduce the risk of infection and its consequences. Using TEE preoperative, peri-operative and postoperative helps discern concomitant lesions.[12]

References

1. Joffe D. Intraoperative transesophageal echocardiography. In: Lewin MB, Stout K, eds. Echocardiography in congenital heart disease. Elsevier Saunders; 2012:31–57
2. Ayres NA, Miller-Hance W, Fyfe DA, et al; Pediatric Council of the American Society of the Echocardiography. Indications and guidelines for performance of transesophageal echocardiography in the patient with pediatric acquired or congenital heart disease: report from the task force of the Pediatric Council of the American Society of Echocardiography. J Am Soc Echocardiogr 2005;18(1):91–98
3. Click RL, Oh JK. Intraoperative echocardiography (Chapter 21). In: Oh JK, Seward JB, Jamil Tajik A, eds. The echo manual, 3rd ed. Lippincott Williams & Wilkins; 2006:368–382
4. Miller-Hance Wanda C, Russel Isobel A. Intraoperative and postoperative transesophageal echocardiography in congenital heart disease. In: Wong PC, Miller-Hance WC, eds. Transesophageal echocardiography for congenital heart disease. Springer; 2014:383–395
5. Russell I, Foster E, Rouine-Rapp K. Assessment of congenital heart disease in the adult patient. In: Savage RM, Aronsen S, Shermane SK, eds. Comprehensive textbook of perioperative transesophageal echocardiography, 2nd ed. Lippincott Williams and Wilkins; 2011: 390–405
6. Tacy TA. Systemic and pulmonary venous anomalies. In: Wong PC, Miller-Hance WC, eds. Transesophageal echocardiography for congenital heart disease. Los Angeles, CA: Springer-Verlag; 2014:145–168
7. Perrino Albert C, Reeves Scott T, eds. Practical approach to transesophageal echocardiography, A. 3rd ed. Lippincott Williams & Wilkins; 2013
8. Lewin Mark B, Stout Karen, eds. Echocardiography in congenital heart disease. Elsevier Saunders; 2012
9. Nanda NC, Domanski MJ. Atlas of transesophageal echocardiography. 2nd ed. Lippincott Williams & Wilkins; 2007
10. Denault AY, Couture P, Buithieu J, Tardif J-C. Transesophageal echocardiography multimedia manual: a perioperative transdisciplinary approach. Taylor & Francis Group; 2005
11. Hahn RT, Abraham T, Adams MS, et al. Guidelines for performing a comprehensive transesophageal echocardiographic examination: recommendations from the American Society of Echocardiography and the Society of Cardiovascular Anesthesiologists. J Am Soc Echocardiogr 2013;26(9):921–964
12. Mohammadi H, Mohammadpour Ahranjani B, Aghaei Moghadam E, Kompani F, Mirbeyk M, Rezaei N. Hematological indices in pediatric patients with acyanotic congenital heart disease: a cross-sectional study of 248 patients. Egypt J Med Hum Genet. 2022;23(1):47

22

Pediatric Fluid Status

Tanveer Singh Kundra

Introduction

Appropriate fluid management is essential for maintaining adequate tissue perfusion and maintaining homeostasis, especially in perioperative settings. The pediatric population is very heterogeneous,[1] with ages ranging from neonates to 16 years. So, one formula may not suffice for all age groups.

This chapter covers the physiological principles on which pediatric fluid management is based, along with the assessment of fluid status in pediatric patients and the clinical management of the patient based on the assessment done.

Physiological Considerations

The composition of fluid compartments, especially extracellular fluid (ECF) and intracellular fluid (ICF) compartments varies with age (**Table 22.1** and **Fig. 22.1**). The plasma compartment, however, remains constant at 5% of body weight.

Fluid Compartments

ICF accounts for two-thirds of body water. ECF accounts for one-third of body water (**Fig. 22.2**). ECF compartment in

premature babies and infants is much larger than in adults (**Table 22.1**). The *functional ECF compartment* consists of intravascular blood or plasma volume and interstitial fluid. They have the same electrolyte composition, but are separated from each other by the vascular endothelium.

The hemodynamic changes in heart rate (HR), blood pressure (BP), and central venous pressure (CVP) help us to monitor the "size" of the intravascular compartment, which is actually an extension of the large ECF and helps maintain intravascular volume.[2] When the large "buffer compartment" of ECF is depleted and cannot replenish the contracted vascular volume, symptoms of hypovolemia become obvious.

Fluid Assessment in Pediatric Patients

The fluid assessment in any pediatric patient can be done clinically as listed in **Table 22.2**.[3] In the preoperative setting, more specific questions need to be assessed as listed in **Table 22.3**. The importance of assessment of dehydration is in knowing the preoperative estimated fluid deficit (**Table 22.4**).

The serum osmolarity and serum sodium indicate the type of dehydration[2]:

- Hyponatremic (serum osmolarity <270 mOsm/L, serum Na <130 mEq/L), usually seen in children on low-sodium-containing fluids such as Isolyte P or 5% dextrose.
- Isonatremic (serum osmolarity 270–300 mOsm/L, serum Na 130–150 mEq/L).
- Hypernatremic (serum osmolarity >310 mOsm/L, serum Na >150 mEq/L).

Table 22.1 Fluid compartment (% of body weight) and body water changes in premature, neonates, infant, and child

Component	Premature	Neonates	Infant	Child
Extracellular fluid	50	35	30	20
Intracellular fluid	30	40	40	40
Total	80	75	70	60

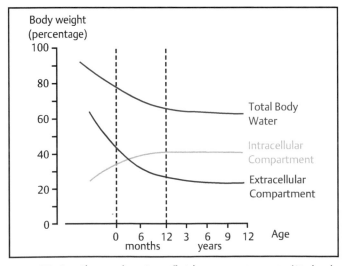

Fig. 22.1 Chart showing fluid compartment (% body weight) and body water changes with age.

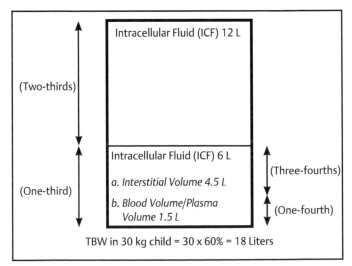

Fig. 22.2 Total body water (TBW) and fluid compartments in a 30-kg child.

Table 22.2   The clinical assessment for degree of dehydration

Severity of dehydration	% Dehydration infant	% Dehydration child	Symptoms
Mild	5	3–4	Thirst, mucous membranes moist, EJV visible in supine, CRT normal, urine sp. gr. >1.020
Moderate	10	6–8	Dry mucous membranes, ↑HR, ↓tears, Sunken fontanelle, decreased skin turgor, CRT 2–4 s, ↓urine output
Severe	15	10	Eye sunken, cool peripheries, apathy, somnolence, orthostatic shock
Shock	>15	>10	Decompensation, poor O$_2$ delivery, ↓BP

Abbreviations: BP, blood pressure; CRT, capillary refill time; EJV, external jugular vein; HR, heart rate.

Table 22.3   Preoperative assessment and preparation for surgery

Symptoms and signs	Mild	Moderate	Severe
Weight loss	3–5%	6–9%	>10%
General condition	Alert, restless, thirsty	Thirsty, lethargic	Cold, sweaty
Pulse	Normal rate, volume	Rapid, weak	Rapid, feeble
Respiration	Normal	Deep, rapid	Deep, rapid
Systolic pressure	Normal	Normal/low	Low, unrecordable
Anterior fontanelle	Normal	Sunken	Very sunken
Skin turgor	Normal	Decreased	Markedly decreased
Eyes	Normal	Sunken, dry	Grossly sunken
Mucous membrane	Moist	Dry	Very dry
Urine output	Adequate	Less, dark colored	Oliguria, anuria
Capillary refill	Normal	>2 s	>4 s

Table 22.4   Estimated fluid deficit based on preoperative clinical assessment of dehydration

Degree of dehydration	Estimated fluid deficit
Mild	30–50 mL/kg
Moderate	60–90 mL/kg
Severe	~100 mL/kg

Management of Dehydration

Management of dehydration is considered under the following headings:
- Initial resuscitation.
- Physiological compensatory responses by body to dehydration.
- Responses in sick child.
- Definitive management of dehydration.

Initial Resuscitation

Initial resuscitation is done with a bolus of normal saline over 10 to 20 minutes. This is done to restore circulation and renal perfusion even before the results of investigations are available.

Physiological Compensatory Mechanisms

Physiological compensatory mechanisms can be temporary or definitive.

Temporary compensatory mechanisms include the production of endogenous vasopressors (such as antidiuretic hormone [ADH], angiotensin II, and catecholamines) and transcapillary refill with fluids shifting from interstitial compartment to vascular compartment. The release of ADH causes water reabsorption from the distal tubule of the kidney.[2]

Definitive compensatory mechanisms are through the renal system. Low blood volume, low blood pressure, or low sodium (Na) in the distal renal tubule causes activation of renin-angiotensin-aldosterone system, which leads to reabsorption of Na and water, and restores euvolemic state and normal serum Na.

Stress Response in Sick Child

The stress response to illness includes secretion of ADH, which causes water retention by the kidney. Children have less space in their cranial vaults for retained water and become symptomatic earlier, with Na levels much higher than the levels at which adults experience signs and symptoms. For this reason, overhydration of sick children with hypotonic fluids such as 4% dextrose and 0.18% sodium chloride (NaCl) should be avoided. The "extra" water in these fluids adds to the volume retained by the kidney. Due to this reason, these fluids have been removed from many pediatric units. Alternative fluids that can be used include 5% dextrose and 0.45% saline, 0.9% saline, and Ringer lactate (RL).

It may be noted that RL contains calcium. This may cause harmful precipitation if administered with drugs like ceftriaxone or blood products.[2]

Definitive Management of Dehydration[2]

Oral Rehydration for Mild Dehydration

For mild dehydration, rehydration is done orally. The WHO-UNICEF formula contains glucose (20 g/L water) and three basic salts: NaCl (3.5 g/L water), KCl (1.5 g/L water), and either trisodium citrate (2.9 g/L water) or sodium bicarbonate (2.5 g/L water).

Correction of Fluid Deficits in Moderate-to-Severe Dehydration

In moderate-to-severe dehydration, correction is done intravenously in three phases:
- **Emergency phase:** Initial resuscitation is done with a fluid bolus of 20–30 mL/kg isotonic crystalloid given over 10–20 minutes. This restores circulation and renal perfusion even before the laboratory tests are available.
- **Repletion phase I:** 25–50 mL/kg of isotonic crystalloid (or half the fluid deficit) is given over 6 to 8 hours.
- **Repletion phase II:** Remainder of deficit is given over 24 hours.

It is important to know the electrolyte composition of various body fluids (**Table 22.5**), so that different IV fluids can be transfused as per their constituents (**Table 22.6**) in different losses.

Based on **Tables 22.4** and **22.5**, RL and Plasmalyte A are isotonic, with osmolarity similar to plasma osmolarity. NS (0.9% NaCl) contains only sodium and chloride and was initially the fluid choice for replacement fluid; however, we must watch for hyperchloremic acidosis. RL is now the fluid choice for replacement; however, it contains lactates and

Table 22.5 Electrolyte composition of body fluids

Electrolytes (mEq/L)	Gastric	Diarrhea	Pancreatic	Bile	Ileostomy
Na⁺	70	50	140	120	130
K⁺	5–15	35	5	5	15–20
Cl⁻	120	40	50–100	100	120
HCO₃⁻	0	50	35	40	25–30

Table 22.6 Composition of commonly used IV fluids in children

Electrolytes (mEq/L)	NS (0.9% NaCl)	RL	Isolyte P in D 5%	Plasmalyte A	Dext. 5%	Albumin 5%	Hexa 6%	Gelofusine
pH	5.5	6.5	5	7.4	4.5			
Na⁺	154	130	26	140	–	145 ± 15	154	154
K⁺	–	4	21	5	–	<2.5	–	–
Cl⁻	154	109	21	98	–	100	154	120
Ca²⁺	–	3	–	–	–	–	–	–
Mg²⁺	–	–	3	3	–	–	–	–
Acetate	–	–	24	27	–	–	–	–
Lactate	–	28	–	–	–	–	–	–
Glucose (g%)	–	–	5	–	5	–	–	–
Phosphate (g%)	–	–	3	–	–	–	–	–
Osmolarity (mOsm/L)	308	274	–	295	252	330	310	274

Abbreviations: Dext., dextrose; IV, intravenous; NS, normal saline; RL, Ringer lactate.

should be avoided in diabetic patients. Further it contains calcium and can cause precipitation when transfused along with blood products. Hence, RL cannot be used in these situations. Dextrose 5% (D5%) and Isolyte P are hypotonic fluids. Plasmalyte A is isotonic and is currently the choice for perioperative fluid replacement.

Determining Fluid Requirements

It measures the energy consumption in children. It was concluded that children <1 year (3–10 kg) consume around 100 kcal/d, while older children consume around 75 kcal/d. Adults consume around 35 kcal/d.

In 1957, Holliday and Segar et al[6] reviewed data which correlated calorie requirements with basal metabolism and active energy needs. They suggested that the caloric requirement is:

- 0–10 kg = 100 kcal/kg/d.
- 10–20 kg = 1000 kcal + 50 kcal for each kg over 10 kg but less than 20 kg.
- 20 kg and up = 1500 kcal + 25 kcal for each kg over 20 kg.
- Metabolism of 1 calorie produces 0.2 mL of water and consumes 1.2 mL of water, so calorie and water consumption are considered equal. For example, a 1-year-old child weighing 10 kg requires 100 kcal/kg/d of energy and 100 mL/kg/d of water.

Holliday and Segar's 4/2/1 formula (**Table 22.7**) is commonly used to guide preoperative fluid therapy.[3] Fever increases the caloric requirement by 10 to 12% for every degree centigrade rise in temperature above normal. Hence, the fluid requirements should be increased accordingly.

Fluid management can be broadly covered in three main parts:

- Resuscitation fluid.
- Maintenance fluid.
- Replacement for losses.

Maintenance fluid is the fluid required for maintaining body functions at a basal rate in the pediatric patient and is required for the following:

- Evaporation from the skin, which is an essential part of thermoregulation in the pediatric patient.

- Excretion of waste products from the kidneys and stool.
- Water loss from the respiratory tract.
- Growth.

Resuscitation/replacement fluid is the fluid which replaces abnormal losses of fluids such as blood, sweat, gastrointestinal fluid, or urine.

Preoperative Management

NPO (Nil Per Oral) Guidelines

In the recent past, NPO guidelines have been modified by European Society of Anaesthesiology and Intensive Care (ESAIC), especially for intake of clear fluids (**Table 22.8**).[4] Children can be given clear fluids up to 1 hour before induction of anesthesia. This has been reduced from the previous recommendations of fasting requirements of 2 hours for clear fluids.[3] It has been suggested that patients fasted for 1 hour have decreased thirst, gastric volume, and hunger compared to children fasted overnight.

Children can be allowed to drink clear fluids safely until 1 hour before surgery. The shortened fasting times for clear fluids have shown to improve perioperative experience for children and parents, without increasing the incidence of pulmonary aspiration. Better experience leads to increased compliance for the fasting guidelines and leads to better outcomes.

Fluid Required to Compensate for Fasting Deficits

It is important to have a realistic estimate of fluid required to "cover" the fasting time. For example, a 25 kg, 8-year-old child scheduled for surgery at 9 am may have his last meal at 7 pm. If one calculates his fluid requirements on the basis of Holliday and Segar (4/2/1) formula for his time of fasting, he would need approximately 1000-mL fluid. This is clearly nonrealistic. It would mean that every child on waking up in the morning is dehydrated and requires a lot of fluid for rehydration.

Table 22.7 Hourly 4/2/1 rule and daily maintenance fluids according to child's weight[5]

Weight	Fluid requirement per h	Daily fluid requirement
<10 kg	4 mL/kg	100 mL/kg
10–20 kg	40 mL + 2 mL/kg for each kg above 10 kg, but <20 kg	1000 mL + 50 mL/kg for each kg above 10 kg, but <20 kg
>20 kg	60 mL + 1 mL/kg for each kg above 20 kg	1500 mL + 25 mL/kg for each kg above 20 kg

Table 22.8 Fasting guidelines for elective surgery (ESAIC)

Type of food	Hours of fasting
Heavy solids	8 h
Light meals (solids)/Formula milk/juice with pulp	6 h
Breast milk	4 h
Clear fluids (water, fruit juices without pulp, carbonated beverages, clear tea, and black coffee excluding alcohol)	1 h

There are specific indications for giving more fluid to "cover" the fasting time:

- Prolonged fasting which occurred inadvertently or out of necessity.
- In hot summer months when evaporation is more, especially in tropical regions.
- In a child with polycythemia, when there is a real danger of dehydration predisposing to thrombosis.

Thus the fluid required to "cover fasting" should be decided on a case-to-case basis.

Encouraging intake of 10 mL/kg of clear fluid up to 1 hour before anesthesia will further decrease intravenous (IV) compensation required.

The main aim of perioperative fluid therapy is to maintain "homeostasis" by re-establishing the normal physiology through central euvolemia and providing adequate electrolytes based on the child's need due to various deficits like preoperative fasting, losses due to renal, cutaneous, gastrointestinal, and third space losses. It should be remembered that children have a higher metabolic rate, a larger surface area to weight ratio, and faster respiration, which results in extensive fluid losses in comparison to adults.

Box 22.1 Guidelines for fluid administration of balanced salt solution in children according to the age and the severity of tissue trauma[6]

1. **First hour (plus item 3 below)**
   25 mL/kg in children aged 3 y and below
   15 mL/kg in children aged 4 y and over
2. **All other hours (plus item 3 below)**
   Maintenance + trauma = basic hourly fluid
   Maintenance volume = 4 mL/kg/h
   Maintenance + mild trauma = 4 + 2 mL/kg/h = 6 mL/kg/h
   Maintenance + moderate trauma = 4 + 4 = 8 mL/kg/h
   Maintenance + severe trauma = 4 + 6 = 10 mL/kg/h
3. **Blood replacement 1:1 with blood or colloid or 3:1 with crystalloids**

Table 22.9 Suggested rates of fluid replacement for common surgeries

Surgical trauma	Type of surgery	Fluid replacement
Minimal/mild trauma	For example, inguinal hernia repair	1–2 mL/kg/h
Moderate trauma	For example, ureteric reimplantation	4 mL/kg/h
Severe trauma	For example, scoliosis, major bowel surgery, burns surgery	>6–8 mL/kg/h

Intraoperative Fluid Management

Intraoperative fluid therapy (**Table 22.9** and **Box 22.1**) is aimed at:

- Providing basal metabolic requirements (maintenance fluids).
- Compensating for preoperative deficits.
- Replacing losses from the surgical field.

Replacement of Fluid Losses

Replacement fluid: This covers losses caused by trauma (including surgery), burns, peritonitis, and bleeding, and losses from gastrointestinal tract. These losses are essentially of ECF and should be replaced by fluid with approximately the same Na^+ concentration. Balanced salt solution such as RL, with Na^+ of 130, and an electrolyte mix similar to ECF, is ideal for this purpose.

Monitoring Fluid Loss and Replacement

In general, routine monitoring (noninvasive blood pressure monitoring, pulse oximetry, electrocardiogram [ECG], and precordial stethoscope) is sufficient for blood losses up to 15 to 20%. If blood loss is anticipated to equal or exceed 20% of blood volume or if blood loss is potentially uncontrollable, then consider using an intra-arterial line and a CVP line for monitoring of blood pressure, hematocrit (Hct), electrolytes, and arterial blood gases.

Should We Give Glucose Containing Fluids for Maintenance?

Presently it is well accepted that to balance between hypoglycemia and hyperglycemia, we should use isotonic fluids with lower glucose concentration (1–2.5%) for children less than 2 years.

Glucose supplementation is required in all children with high risk of developing hypoglycemia as in preterm neonates, patients with liver failure, children receiving hyperalimentation, those with mitochondrial diseases, and children with endocrinopathies.

Which Isotonic Fluid Is Most Preferred?

In children undergoing major pediatric and neurosurgeries, better acid-base status is observed with balanced crystalloids like Plasmalyte A and RL.

Plasmalyte contains acetate instead of lactate. Acetate is metabolized significantly faster and is more independent of hepatic function and causes a lower increase in oxygen consumption. Most of the anesthetic drugs are compatible with acetate, except phenytoin and diazepam.

Colloids and Their Use in Pediatric Population

Administration of colloid solution (albumin or synthetic colloid) is indicated to maintain intravascular osmotic pressure after administration of a total of 30–50 mL/kg of crystalloid solution. Literature published has not shown any alteration of renal parameters, blood transfusion, or blood loss with infusion of low molecular weight 6% hydroxyethyl starch (HES).[1]

There is no role of nonemergency volume replacement with colloids and no advantage of one colloid over other in preventing the shift of fluids to interstitial space. Also, the volume of albumin administered is more important than its concentration (20% vs. 5%) to maintain or restore cardiovascular stability. Hence, 5% albumin remains the preferred colloid in children as it is iso-oncotic to plasma and very effective to maintain blood pressure and plasma colloid perfusion pressure. Also, it is cheaper as compared to 20% albumin.

Table 22.10 Blood volume in children

Age of the child	Blood volume (mL/kg)
Neonates	85–90
Infants	75–80
Children	70–75
Adults	65–70

Table 22.11 Normal hemoglobin values for full-term and premature infants

	Full term (g/dL of blood)	Premature (g/dL of blood)
Birth	19.3	Slightly less than full term
0.5 mo	16.6	15.4
1 mo	13.9	11.6
4 mo	12.2	11.7
6 mo	12.5	12.4

Table 22.12 Normal and acceptable hematocrits in pediatric patients

Age	Normal	Acceptable
Premature	40–45	35
Newborn	45–65	30–35
3 mo	30–42	25
1 y	34–42	20–25
6 y	35–43	20–25

Blood Transfusion in Pediatric Population

The normal blood volume in different age groups is listed in **Table 22.10**.[1]

More important than the hemoglobin value is the hematocrit value as this is used to calculate the maximum allowable blood loss (MABL), after which transfusion is needed. Normal hemoglobin and hematocrit values are listed in **Tables 22.11** and **22.12**.

Normal Hct is defined as Hct within 2 standard deviations for age. If Hct is below 2 standard deviations for age, the child may still be accepted for minor surgery but this does not make him normal. The reason for his anemia should be investigated.

Acceptable Hct is that Hct which is tolerated by the patient without the need for blood transfusion. It must be understood that if the patient has an underlying medical condition, which involves either the respiratory system or the cardiovascular system, which limits either the ability to saturate hemoglobin or the ability to increase cardiac output, then higher values of hemoglobin may be needed.

Before bleeding has crossed 20% of blood volume, preferred ratio of crystalloid to colloid is 2:1 or 3:1 as per institutional guidelines. After 20% of blood volume, the preferred ratio of crystalloid to colloid changes to 1:1.

The decision on when to transfuse blood to children depends on MABL calculated as: MABL = EBV × (H0 – H1)/H0 (EBV = estimated blood volume; H0 = starting Hct; H1 = lowest acceptable Hct).

Intraoperative Targets for Fluid Management

Till date, urine output monitoring is used as intraoperative target for fluid management in pediatric patients.

Literature regarding perioperative use of esophageal Doppler, pulse contour analysis, or mixed venous oxygen saturation is lacking, and this is an area that requires further randomized control trials.

Postoperative Fluid Management

Children should be encouraged to restart oral fluids as early as possible in the absence of surgical contraindication; however, fluid intake need not be insisted before discharge from an ambulatory facility.

Postoperative IV infusions, if required, should be with isotonic fluids, instead of hypotonic fluids, as incidence of hyponatremia is lower. Appropriate potassium chloride and dextrose may be added to the pediatric maintenance IV fluids postoperatively.

Conclusion

Perioperative fluid prescription is very crucial in the management of pediatric patients and should be guided by the physiology and pathology of the child. The main aim of fluid infusion is establishing euvolemia, adequate tissue perfusion, and tissue oxygenation. Recent guidelines have advocated minimal preoperative as well as postoperative fasting times, which significantly impacts the hydration status of the child. Holliday and Segar formula is a decent guide to pediatric fluid management, but the actual fluid therapy should be decided on a case-to-case basis, keeping the surgical catabolic state and stress in mind.

The negative effects of fluid overload make patients more susceptible to an elevated risk of morbidity and death even if fluid overload itself is not a direct indicator of mortality. Further research can in aid in developing preventive and management strategies for the fluid balance in pediatrics settings.[7]

References

1. Mathew A, Rai E. Pediatric perioperative fluid management. Saudi J Anaesth 2021;15(4):435–440
2. Chandrasekaran K, McDougall R, Jacob R, George SP. Fluid management in the pediatric patient. In: Jacob R, Thirlwell J, eds. Understanding pediatric anaesthesia. 3rd ed. New Delhi: Wolters Kluwer Pvt Ltd; 2015:72–79
3. Arya VK. Basics of fluid and blood transfusion therapy in paediatric surgical patients. Indian J Anaesth 2012;56(5):454–462
4. Sümpelmann R, Becke K, Brenner S, et al. Perioperative intravenous fluid therapy in children: guidelines from the Association of the Scientific Medical Societies in Germany. Paediatr Anaesth 2017;27(1):10–18
5. Holliday MA, Segar WE. The maintenance need for water in parenteral fluid therapy. Pediatrics. 1957 May;19(5):823-32.
6. Murat I, Dubois MC. Perioperative fluid therapy in pediatrics. Paediatr Anaesth 2008;18(5):363–370
7. Althagafi TH, Qartali AA, Alasmari NH, et al. Adverse effects of fluid overload in different paediatric age groups International Journal of Community Medicine And Public Health. 2022; 9(10):3960–3964

23

Preoperative Considerations in Lung Transplantation

*Iti Shri, Rohan Magoon, Poonam Malhotra Kapoor, Vijay Hadda,
Saurabh Mittal, and Randeep Guleria*

Introduction

An enhanced quality of life, survival benefits, and improved perioperative techniques make lung transplantation an acceptable treatment option for people with end-stage lung disease.

Apart from these broadened donor selection criteria, induction immunosuppressive regimes and strategies to prevent chronic graft dysfunction have added an incremental value to lung transplant procedure.

According to the International Society for Heart and Lung Transplantation (ISHLT)[1] the indications and contraindications to lung transplant can be summarized as given in **Box 23.1** and **Table 23.1**.

Preoperative Factors Affecting Outcomes After Transplant[2]

These can briefly be summarized as donor, recipient, and surgical aspects as follows:

1. **Donor factors:**
   - Cytomegalovirus infection.
   - Diabetes mellitus.
   - Donor weight 70% of recipient weight.
   - Female donor to male recipient.
   - Smoking.
   - Increased age.
   - High blood pressure however has a protective role in lung transplant sometimes, but SVR should not remain too high.

2. **Recipient factors:**
   - Age more than 70 years.
   - Body mass index <18.5 kg/m² or >30 kg/m².
   - Low cardiac index.
   - Renal dysfunction, increased bilirubin levels.
   - Underlying etiology.
   - Hospitalization.
   - Need for oxygen therapy.
   - Need for extracorporeal membrane oxygenation (ECMO).
   - Retransplantation.
   - Steroid therapy.

3. **Surgical factors:**
   Approach:
   - Use of cardiopulmonary bypass (CPB).
   - Pleurodesis.
   - Use of ECMO, ex vivo lung perfusion (EVLP), and multiorgan transplant are considered to increment long-term survival.

Bridge to transplantation is a strategy that helps in managing acutely decompensating patient or patients in respiratory failure survive until suitable organ is available for the transplant. Two commonly employed strategies for bridge to transplantation are the mechanical ventilation and/or ECLS. Patients breathing spontaneously on ECLS have better survival as compared to those mechanically ventilated. Patients eligible for ECLS are of younger age, with no multiple organ dysfunction syndrome (MODS), and have a good potential for rehabilitation. ECLS is not recommended if the patient is in septic shock for a long time or is in MODS or has severe hemodynamic compromise, is on prolonged mechanical ventilation, is obese, or has heparin-induced thrombocytopenia.[3,4]

Preoperative indications of ECLS are prior ECMO support, pulmonary vascular diseases especially idiopathic pulmonary hypertension, other indications with severe pulmonary arterial hypertension (PAH), refractory hypoxemia, and hypercapnia.[5]

Box 23.1 Indications for lung transplant

- Whenever in risk of mortality within 2 years is more than 50%.
- Chances of 90 days survival are high (>80%)
- Persistence of adequate graft function after optimal medical therapy
- Chances of survival are >80% for 3 months post-transplant.

Table 23.1 Contraindications for lung transplant

Absolute contraindication	Relative contraindications
• Nontreatable coronary artery disease	• Advanced age > 65 years
• Moribund patient with multiple organ dysfunction	• BMI (body mass index) is between 30 and 35
• Bleeding coagulopathy infection resistant	• Malnutrition
• Active tuberculosis	• Osteoporosis
• Chest wall deformity	• Severe lung resection
• BMI > 35.0 kg/m²	• Patient on ECLS and/or mechanical ventilation
• Resistant medical therapy	• Infections like hepatitis A, B or C; HIV; myocobacleiue abcessus
• Drug abuse	
• Inadequate family social support	• Atherosclerosis
• Psychosis and poor chances of rehabilitees	• Diabetes with organ damage

Abbreviations: BMI, body mass index; ECLS, extracorporeal life support; HIV, human immunodeficiency virus.

Disease-Specific Candidate Selection

It is prudent to refer a patient before any acute decompensation, and the patient is able to undergo standard evaluation and treatment.[6] This would not only determine the candidacy or transplantation but also influence the postoperative outcomes. ISHLT has laid down criteria for timing of referral and timing of listing with United Network for Organ Sharing (UNOS) based on the stage of the underlying disease process (**Table 23.2**).[1,6]

The Lung Allocation Score (LAS)

Patients are categorized into four main groups: Group A (COPD, emphysema, alpha-one antitrypsin deficiency), Group B (primary PAH, Eisenmenger syndrome), Group C (cystic fibrosis and immunodeficiency syndromes), Group D (idiopathic pulmonary fibrosis, sarcoidosis, bronchiolitis obliterans following transplant).

LAS ranges from 0 to 100 and is derived from calculation of transplant benefit which is the difference between posttransplant survival in days and waitlist survival in days. Higher score (>60) is given a priority in the organ allocation; however, it also signifies worsened survival. Use of LAS has resulted in an improved 1-year survival rate (**Table 23.3**).[6,7]

ATP11B, FGFR2, EGLN1, and MCPH1 are the genes found to be associated with development of primary graft dysfunction (PGD). Identification of such genetic factors and gene therapy may be used in the evaluations procedure as to predict postoperative complications and help guide therapy as well.[8]

Organ Procurement and Preservation[5]

Donor lung preservation help preserves donor lung function from the time of procurement until reperfusion, minimizing any injury and optimizing posttransplant function as well. This is an integral component especially with the expansion

Table 23.2 Modified ISHLT criteria for disease-specific referral and listing time

Disease	Referral time	Listing time
Restrictive Airway Disease (Interstitial Lung Disease)	• Interstitial pneumonitis on radiograph • FVC <80% predicted • DLCO <40% predicted • Any dyspnoea or functional limitation • Oxygen requirement	• Decline in FVC ≥10% during 6 months of follow-up • Decline in DLCO ≥15% during 6 months of follow-up • Desaturation to <88% or distance of >50 m decline in 6-minute-walk distance over a 6-month period • Pulmonary hypertension • Hospitalization due to respiratory failure
Suppurative disease (cystic fibrosis)	• FEV_1 < 30% or rapidly declining FEV_1 despite therapy • 6-min walk distance <400 m • SPAP > 35 mmHg or mPAP > 25 mmHg • Increased frequency of exacerbation	• Chronic respiratory failure • Pulmonary hypertension • WHO functional class IV • Long-term NIV therapy • Decreasing lung function
Obstructive disease (COPD)	• Progressive disease despite optimal therapy • Not a candidate for LVRS • BODE index of 5 to 6 • $PaCO_2$ > 50 mmHg and/or PaO2 < 60 mmHg • FEV_1 < 25% predicted	• BODE index ≥ 7 • FEV_1 < 15–20% predicted • Three or more severe exacerbations during the preceding year • One severe exacerbation with acute hypercapnic respiratory failure • Moderate to severe pulmonary hypertension
Pulmonary vascular disease	• NYHA Class III or IV • Rapidly progressive disease • Use of parenteral targeted pulmonary arterial hypertension (PAH) therapy • Pulmonary veno-occlusive disease (PVOD) or pulmonary capillary hemangiomatosis	• NYHA Class III or IV • Cardiac index <2 L/min/m² • Mean right atrial pressure of >15 mmHg • 6-min walk test of <350 m • Development of significant hemoptysis, pericardial effusion, or progressive right heart failure

Abbreviations: BODE index, body-mass index (B), degree of obstruction (O), dyspnea (D), and exercise capacity (E); DLCO, diffusing capacity of the lung for carbon monoxide; FEV, forced expiratory volume; FVC, forced vital capacity; mPAP, mean pulmonary arterial pressure; NYHA, New York Heart Association; SPAP, systolic pulmonary arterial pressure.

Table 23.3   Factors affecting posttransplant and waitlist survival

Factors affecting posttransplant survival	Factors affecting waitlist survival measure
Forced vital capacity (FVC)	Forced vital capacity (FVC)
Pulmonary capillary wedge pressure (PCWP)	Pulmonary systolic, mean, and wedge pressures
Requirement of continuous mechanical ventilation	Body Mass Index (BMI)
Age of the patient	Functional status and 6-min walk distance
Functional status	Underlying etiology
Serum creatinine levels	Continuous mechanical ventilation
Underlying etiology	Presence of diabetes
	Requirement of supplemental oxygen
	Partial pressure of carbon dioxide in blood

Table 23.4   Donor selection ensures both ideal and extended donor criteria[9]

Ideal donor criteria	Extended donor criteria
ABO identical matches	ABO compatible
Age <55 y	Age >55 y
Chest X-ray without evidence of infection, trauma, or infiltration	Abnormal chest radiograph, bronchoscopy recommended
Smoking or tobacco chewing history less than 20 packs/y	Tobacco history >20 pack/y
Clear sputum without purulent secretions or gastric aspirate	Presence of cytomegalovirus antibodies
Arterial oxygen tension/inspired oxygen ratio <300 at positive end expiratory pressure of 5 cm H_2O	Low partial pressure of oxygen, intubation >2 d
Donor and recipient size matching	Primary central nervous system tumor unlikely to spread through blood–brain barrier

in the donor lung criteria (**Table 23.4**). Organs for transplant can be procured either after the brain death (DBD) or after the determination of circulatory death (DCD). Graft survival after the donation of either DCD or DBD has been comparable; however, there is a higher incidence of primary graft dysfunction grade 3 (PGD-3) as well as bronchiolitis obliterans syndrome (BOS) following donation after DCD. Strategies to preserve the function of the allograft and reducing ischemia time are the key element of success following transplant.

During DBD, cold flush preferably low potassium dextran is administered antegrade into both the pleural cavities to topically cool the lungs. The cold flush is then retrogradely administered into each pulmonary vein and finally placed in sterile bag with 2 liters of cold flush.

DCD procurement happens using modified ECMO or by following ex vivo machine perfusion.

Various preservative solutions used are Perfadex, Celsior, Papworth. Various pharmacological additives like prostaglandins and glucocorticoids have been also employed in view of their anti-inflammatory properties. Although optimal temperature for preservation is debatable but 4 to 8°C is acceptable with cold ischemia time of 8 to 12 hours, which has been associated with good outcomes. Low perfusion

pressure is applied (10-15 mmHg) while infusion to prevent damage to the pulmonary artery, and lungs are kept in a slightly inflated state.

Normothermic ex vivo lung perfusion (EVLP) and ventilation is a promising preservation technique that can maintain donor lung function with minimal injury.

Apart from preservation, a donor-recipient lung size matching is performed either based on predicted total lung capacity (TLC) or by CT scanning.

Preoperative Anesthetic Evaluation

Aim is to evaluate fitness for surgery, case appropriate investigations and optimization of clinical status, and anesthetic and postoperative analgesic plan.

It is vital to know about the penultimate cause for transplant and the specific prognostic factors (e.g., patients with pulmonary fibrosis who develop PAH have a poorer prognosis). Similarly in cases of cystic fibrosis one should evaluate for antibiotic-resistant organisms like *Burkholderia cepacia* complex. Diabetes, gastroesophageal reflux, and cases of PAH may require an extracorporeal life support (ECLS) if there is a pre-existing severe right ventricular dysfunction.

Recipient Selection[10]

The various indications and contraindications and the disease stage have already been described in **Box 23.1** and **Table 23.1**.

Few factors substantially increase the risk of transplant and impact the outcome. They are age >70 years, concomitant severe coronary artery disease (CAD) or cerebrovascular disease, extremes of Body Mass Index (BMI), concomitant infections, previous cardiothoracic or chest wall surgery, esophageal dysmotility, poor functional or psychiatric status, frailty, poor nutritional status, and retransplant (**Table 23.5**).

If appropriate criteria are applied, few patients with CAD and left ventricular dysfunction may be considered for heart-lung transplantation. If the ventricular function is satisfactory, revascularization may be attempted either prior to or concomitant with the transplant. For cases who become COVID-19-positive, ISHLT advises to temporarily wait for resolution of the disease and two successive negative polymerase chain reaction (PCR) tests at least 24 to 48 hours apart.[11]

Preoperative Evaluation of Lung Transplant Patients

Prior to transplantation, hepatitis A and B vaccination if not immune, pneumococcal pneumonia, and seasonal influenza vaccine should be administered. During preanesthetic evaluation of history of diabetes, hypertension, CAD, PAH, renal and hepatic dysfunction, old age, and high BMI predicate a high-risk transplant. History and site of any chronic pain, allergy should be documented (**Flowchart 23.1**).[4]

Improving Nutritional, Physical, Pulmonary, and Psychological Status

An evaluation of exercise capacity, activities of daily living, and pulmonary function is essential preoperatively. It is imperative to train the inspiratory muscles to improve the outcomes after the transplant. Malnutrition also affects the outcomes and the newly developed muscle index may be a prognostic factor in lung transplantation. Tailored nutrition should be a priority to facilitate early recovery after transplant.

The mental and psychological status of the patients as well as their social support system determine their suitability for transplantation to a great extent. An assessment of patients' compliance, their mental as well as their social well-being has a bearing on the ultimate success of the transplant and their quality of life post-transplant.

Treatment of any concomitant infection too is an integral part of preoperative rehabilitation and sites such as sinuses,

Table 23.5   Evaluation of potential lung transplant patients[6]

Organ system	Investigations
Hematologic	• Complete blood count • PT, APTT, INR
Immunologic	• ABO cross match • HLA I and HLA II antibodies • ANA, DNA antibody, rheumatoid factor, ANCA
Pulmonary	• Pulmonary function test • 6-min walk test • Arterial blood gas analysis • Chest radiograph • High-resolution computerized tomography scan • Ventilation perfusion scan
Cardiac	• Electrocardiogram • 2D echocardiography • Cardiac catheterization
Renal	• Urine analysis • Blood urea • Serum creatinine/creatinine clearance
Gastrointestinal	• Liver function test • Esophagoduodenoscopy (assessment of gastroesophageal reflux) • Gastric emptying by barium swallow • pH probe monitoring • Abdominal ultrasound • Colonoscopy • Serum amylase, serum lipase • Hemoccult stools
Endocrine	• Blood glucose, HbA1C • Thyroid profile • Serum cortisol • Testosterone levels in men • Brain natriuretic peptide
Infection	• Gram stain and culture • Tuberculin test, skin test for coccidiomycosis, histoplasmosis • IgM/IgG antibodies for cytomegalovirus, Epstein-Barr virus, hepatitis B and C, HIV, varicella zoster and herpes simplex, toxoplasma, strongyloides
Other tests	• Vitamin D level • Iron profile • Bone density scan • Mammogram, pregnancy test • Prostate-specific antigen • Dental examination • Sinus CT scan and surgery for cystic fibrosis patients • Toxicology profile in case of substance abuse

Abbreviations: PT, prothrombin time; APTT, aprotinin partial thromboplastin time; INR, international normalized ratio.

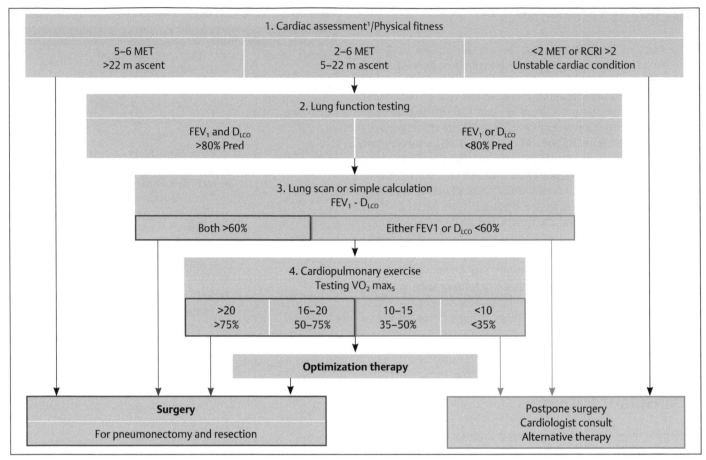

Flowchart 23.1   Algorithm depicting the preoperative assessment of lung transplant patient. Abbreviations: MET, medical emergency team; RCRI, revised cardiac risk index.

indwelling catheters should be investigated and treated appropriately.

Apart from above, airway assessment, vascular access assessment, and a planning for postoperative analgesia form integral component for preanesthetic evaluation. The intensity of perioperative pain is influenced by the patient's psychological status, duration of surgery, extent of incision, and intercostal nerve damage. Various analgesic modes include thoracic epidural, thoracic paravertebral block, systemic opioids, and gabapentin-like drugs.[4]

Preoperative Medications

These patients are on multiple medications (e.g., opioids, steroids, anticoagulants, and drugs) for underlying disease and comorbidities that should be tailored according to the necessity.

Opioid tolerance may be difficult to manage while steroids in low doses (prednisone 0.2–0.3 mg/kg/d) may be safely tolerated without affecting outcomes after surgery. Preoperative medications for PAH should be continued, only to be tapered following reperfusion of the graft.

Conclusion

Good preoperative preparation and evaluation is essential for bilateral lung transplantation in patients with destroyed lung and asymmetric chest deformity[12,13] as discussed by Yue et al in six patients, recently.[12] Adequate blood preparation in the preoperative period, and releasing adhesions with a clamshell incision, can prevent lobectomy or pneumonectomy in a patient with marked collapse/consolidation, thus preserving maximal donor lung function. Improvement in 30-day survival is seen with a PGD incidence of 34%. With the above protocol, the use of statins preoperatively, immensely improves the postoperatives, due to the antioxidant action of statins.[14] Also, monitoring pulmonary artery systolic pressure, with preoperative echocardiography, but performing right heart catheterization is a must, despite echocardiography for best lung transplant outcomes.[15]

Lung transplant is a complex procedure that involves careful donor and recipient selection, appropriate timing of referral and listing, prehabilitation, and a proper understanding and knowledge of natural course of the underlying disease as well as psychosocial implications. However owing to evolving multidisciplinary techniques and teamwork, identification of factors influencing the perioperative outcomes, emergence of bridging techniques, and immunosuppression, and application of rigorous rehabilitation processes make it a viable option for patients with end-stage lung disease. Decide the physical fitness accordingly to a number of meters, walked by the patient. Categorize the patient accordingly. Perform lung function tests on the patient.

Weder et al in 2022 have post COVID-19 with their clinical experience called for a global registry. They reiterate that capturing the experience of lung transplant programs of different sizes from different countries offers important perspectives and will help guide clinical practice for this patient population in the future and encourage transplant centers to share their expertise in transplanting patients with this challenging condition.[16]

References

1. Weill D, Benden C, Corris PA, et al. A consensus document for the selection of lung transplant candidates: 2014—an update from the Pulmonary Transplantation Council of the International Society for Heart and Lung Transplantation. J Heart Lung Transplant 2015;34(1):1–15
2. Martin AK, Yalamuri SM, Wilkey BJ, et al. The impact of anesthetic management on perioperative outcomes in lung transplantation. J Cardiothorac Vasc Anesth 2020;34(6):1669–1680
3. Garijo JM, Cypel M, McRae K, Machuca T, Cunningham CCP, Slinger P. The evolving role of extracorporeal membrane oxygenation in lung transplantation: implications for anesthetic management. J Cardiothorac Vasc Anesth 2019;33:1995–2006
4. Prabhu M, Valchanov K. Pre-anaesthetic evaluation of the patient with end-stage lung disease. Best Pract Res Clin Anaesthesiol 2017;31(2):249–260
5. Hartwig MG, Klapper JA. Lung transplantation: procedure and postoperative management. UpToDate [Internet] Wolters Kluwer. [updated on December 10, 2021; cited on March 22, 2022]. https://www.uptodate.com/contents/lung-transplantation-procedure-and-postoperative-management https://www.uptodate.com/contents/lung-transplantation-procedure-and-postoperative-management
6. Smith CM. Patient selection, evaluation, and preoperative management for lung transplant candidates. Clin Chest Med 1997;18(2):183–197
7. Hachem RR. Lung Transplantation: An Overview. UpToDate [Internet]. Wolters Kluwer. [Updated on November 30, 2021; cited on March 22; 2022]. https://www.uptodate.com/contents/lung-transplantation-an-overview
8. Bag R. Lung transplantation: deceased donor evaluation. UpToDate [Internet]. Wolters Kluwer. [updated on October 07, 2021; cited on March 22, 2022]. https://www.uptodate.com/contents/lung-transplantation-deceased-donor-evaluation
9. Rodrigues ES, Ramakrishna H, Pajaro OE. Lung transplantation: perioperative pharmacology and anesthetic considerations. Curr Clin Pharmacol 2015;10(1):22–34
10. Hachem RR. Lung transplantation: general guidelines for recipient selection. UpToDate [Internet].Wolters Kluwer. [updated on November 24, 2021; cited on March 22, 2022]. https://www.uptodate.com/contents/lung-transplantation-general-guidelines-for-recipient-selection
11. Gerlach RM. Lung transplant: preanaesthetic consultation and preparation. UpToDate [Internet].Wolters Kluwer. [updated on July 09, 2021; cited on March 22, 2022]. https://www.uptodate.com/contents/lung-transplantation-preanesthetic-consultation-and-preparation
12. Yue B, Ye S, Liu F, et al. Bilateral lung transplantation for patients with destroyed lung and asymmetric chest deformity. Front Surg 2021;8:680207
13. Bello I, Sandiumenge A, Coll E, et al. Value of preoperative use of statins as a protective factor for severe graft dysfunction after lung transplantation: a multicenter propensity score analysis. Arch Bronconeumol (Engl Ed). 2021:S0300–2896(21)00137-X
14. Castleberry AW, Englum BR, Snyder LD, et al. The utility of preoperative six-minute-walk distance in lung transplantation. Am J Respir Crit Care Med 2015;192(7):843–852
15. Abu T, Levi A, Hasdai D, et al. Preoperative evaluation of pulmonary hypertension in lung transplant candidates: echocardiography versus right heart catheterization. BMC Cardiovasc Disord 2022;22(1):53
16. Weder MM, Aslam S, Ison MG. Lung Transplantation for COVID-19–related Lung Disease. Clinical Experience and Call for a Global Registry. Transplantation. 2023;107(1): 18–20

24

Perioperative Concerns for Lung Transplantation

Rashmi Singh, Poonam Malhotra Kapoor, Vishwas Malik, Neeti Makhija, and Sandeep Chauhan

Introduction

Lung transplantation constitutes definitive treatment option for patients suffering from end-stage lung disease. It is generally considered in patients who are having more than 50% risk of death from lung disease within 2 years but have high chances (>80%) of survival after 5 years of transplantation.[1] Currently, three most common indications of lung transplantation are idiopathic interstitial pneumonia, chronic obstructive pulmonary disease, and cystic fibrosis.

History

The very first attempt of lung transplantation in human was done by James Hardy in 1963. The patient survived lung transplantation, but he could not survive long and died after 18 days due to multiorgan failure.[2] Followed by him, multiple failed attempts of lung transplantation were done but none of them became clinically relevant. In 1983, Joseph Cooper reported the first successful series of lung transplant.[3] Presently, lung transplant has seen many changes in terms of technical aspects, immunosuppressive regimes, and understanding of lung physiology posttransplantation.

Donor Selection

A major setback in lung transplantation development is limited availability of donor lungs.

According to the definition of the Americian Society of Anesthesiologists (ASA) physical status, once the patient is declared brain dead, our aim is to maximize the preservation of organ function with hemodynamic goal which includes:

- Mean arterial pressure (MAP) >70 mmHg.
- Central venous pressure (CVP) up to 10 mmHg.
- Pulmonary capillary wedge pressure <12 mmHg.
- Lowest FiO_2 to maintain PaO_2 >100 mmHg and positive end-expiratory pressure (PEEP) <10.

Due to shortage of organ availability, donor criteria have been extended; however, strict ideal donor selection provides better graft survival.[4]

Ideal Donor Criteria

Ideal criteria for lung donors include the following:
- ABO compatibility.
- Age <55 years.
- No chest trauma, aspiration, or sepsis.
- Clear chest X-ray.
- Tabacco history of smoking less than 20 packs per year.
- No cardiothoracic surgery.
- Clear sputum.
- No purulent secretion.
- Size match.
- P/F ratio >400.

Extended Donor Criteria

Extended criteria for lung donors include the following:
- Age >55 years.
- Positive sputum.
- Localized chest trauma.
- Localized infiltrates on chest X-ray.
- Tobacco history >20 pack per year.
- History of asthma.
- Central nervous system (CNS) tumor.
- Intubation >48 hours.
- Size mismatch.
- P/F ratio <400.
- Donor characteristics with high risk include:
  - Female donor.
  - Male recipient.
  - Donor recipient weight ratio <0.7.
  - Donor recipient cytomegalovirus mismatch (donor positive/recipient negative).
- History of smoking/diabetes.

Selection and Preoperative Evaluation of Recipient

Ideal lung transplant recipient should be end-stage lung disease (NYHA class III and class IV), with a life expectancy of approximately 2 years, should not be having severe systemic disease, and should be psychologically stable with adequate social support.

Some of the contraindications for lung transplant include:

A. **Absolute contraindications**
- Malignancy within 2 years (preferably 5 y).
- Untreatable significant disease in another organ system.
- Uncorrected atherosclerotic disease.
- Acute medical instability: hepatic failure.
- Uncorrected bleeding disorder.
- *Mycobacterium tuberculosis* infection.
- Highly virulent or resistant microbial infection.
- Chest wall deformity.
- Obesity.
- Medical noncompliance.
- Psychiatric disease.
- Substance abuse.
- Absence of social support.

B. **Relative contraindications**
- Age >65 years with limited function reserve.
- Obesity.
- Malnutrition.

- Severe osteoporosis.
- Prior lung resection surgery.
- Mechanical ventilation or extracorporeal life support (ECLS)
- Highly resistant bacterial colonization.
- Hepatitis B and C.
- HIV infection.
- *Burkholderia* and *Mycobacterium abscessus* infection.

Disease-specific thresholds for referring and listing for patients have been provided by International Society for Heart and Lung Transplantation:[5]

A. Referral criteria
- NYHA class III or IV.
- Rapidly progressive disease.
- Optimized use of targeted pulmonary hypertension treatment.

B. Listing criteria
- NYHA functional class III or IV without improvement after 3 months of combination therapy with prostanoids.
- Cardiac index <2 L/min/m².
- Mean right atrial pressure >15 mmHg.

Patient selected for lung transplantation undergo extensive clinical, physical, laboratory, and psychological assessment. All patients undergo ventilation/perfusion scan to identify functional status of lung, computed tomography (CT) scan to look for anatomy of pulmonary artery and to rule out malignancy, and transthoracic echocardiogram (TTE) to know the status of cardiac function and to document any pulmonary artery hypertension. Patient >40 years and with pulmonary hypertension should undergo left heart catheterization to exclude intracardiac shunt. Considering the emergent nature of procedure these results should readily be available to anesthetists all the time. Based on these results high-risk patients should be identified and proper planning should be made accordingly.

High-risk recipients include:
- Extracorporeal membrane oxygenation (ECMO) before surgery.
- O₂ requirement >5 L/min.
- Retransplantation.
- Age >70 years.
- Renal, hepatic impairment, severe pulmonary hypertension.
- High or low body mass index (BMI).
- Chronic use of corticosteroids.

Surgical Procedure

Although single lung transplant can provide sufficient exercise tolerance,[6] some clinical condition mandates double lung transplant. Suppurative infectious disease of lung with risk of contamination of newly implanted lung requires double lung transplant.

Single Lung Transplant

Single lung transplantation is technically simple to perform. Based on results of ventilation/perfusion mismatch, least functional lung is transplanted via thoracotomy. Most frequent indication of single lung transplant is chronic obstructive pulmonary disease (COPD) and interstitial lung disease.

Double Lung Transplant

Earlier double lung transplants were done using an en bloc technique via median sternotomy. However, results were not satisfactory as there were high incidence of postoperative airway dehiscence. Also to facilitate pulmonary artery and venous anastomosis, cardiopulmonary bypass (CPB) and cardioplegic arrest were mandatory in every case. With the subsequent development of clamshell thoracosternotomy, many problems of en bloc technique have been addressed successfully.[7,8] Clamshell is essentially sequential single lung transplant only, in which transplantation of both the lungs is done in supine position. Here, native lung with worst function should be implanted first.

Sequence of Anastomosis

Bronchus being the most posterior structure is anastomosed first. Followed by bronchus, pulmonary artery (PA) is anastomosed which is followed by pulmonary vein–left atrium cuff anastomosis. However, different institutes may follow different sequence of anastomosis. After completion of all anastomosis, vascular clamps are removed and allograft is reperfused. Now, reperfusion should be done gradually over time as rapid reperfusion has been associated with reperfusion injury in some animal models.[9]

On-Pump versus Off-Pump Surgery

Lung transplantation even bilateral one can be performed without bypass.[10,11] However, patients with severe pulmonary hypertension or those already on ECMO requires on-pump surgery.

Indications for CPB during transplant are:
- Cardiac index <2 L/min/m².
- SvO₂ <60%.
- Mean arterial pressure <50–60 mmHg.
- SaO₂ <85–90%.
- pH <7.

Institution of CPB provides stable hemodynamics and clear surgical field. However there had been increased requirement of blood transfusion.[12] Also incidences of graft dysfunction is more in patients with CPB.[13] Patients with on-pump surgery requires longer duration of mechanical ventilation.[10]

Anesthetic Management

Anesthetic evaluation should include fasting status, exercise capacity, airway assessment, and any previous exposure to anesthetic. As patients are on long waiting list, investigations are usually old, and depending on the patient clinical status, some of the investigations can be repeated. The first dose of immunosuppressive agents is taken preoperatively. Sedatives as premedication should be used cautiously as they may exacerbate hypercarbia and hypoxia. On the contrary, preoperative anxiety and catecholamines release may worsen right ventricular (RV) function in patients with pulmonary hypertension.

Timing

Anesthesia induction should be timed accordingly to minimize graft ischemia time. Graft ischemia time is the time from the cross clamping the aorta in donor to reperfusion of allograft in recipient. Graft ischemia time >5.5 hour is associated with increased risk of graft dysfunction.[14]

All emergency drugs and defibrillator should be kept ready. Induction should be started in the presence of surgeon and perfusionist with availability of CPB. Along with routine monitors, invasive arterial line, central venous catheter, PA catheter, transesophageal probe, and bronchoscope should be kept available.

Goals of anesthetic induction are:
- Airway should be secured.
- All myocardial depressants drugs should be avoided.
- Induction should be slow and gradual.
- Considering full stomach, rapid sequence induction with cricoid pressure should be done.
- Lung hyperinflation should be avoided.
- Large increase in intrathoracic pressure from large tidal volume, high PEEP should be avoided.

Traditionally, drugs having minimal myocardial depressant effects should be used. Examples are etomidate and high-dose narcotics.

One-Lung Ventilation

In order to perform lung transplantation without CPB, one-lung ventilation is required. This can be achieved by insertion of double lumen tube (DLT) or use of bronchial blockers. Generally left-sided DLT is preferred over right DLT, as it is technically easy to insert. Once inserted, its position should be confirmed through fiberoptic bronchoscope. One must be thorough with the physiology of one-lung ventilation during lung transplant.

Principles of One-Lung Ventilation during Lung Transplant

- Tidal volume and respiratory rate:
  - Should be maintained in patients with normal or decreased lung compliance (primary pulmonary hypertension).
  - Should be decreased in patients with increased lung compliance (obstructive lung disease).
- Adequate oxygenation should be maintained by:
  - 100% inspired oxygen.
  - Applying continuous positive airway pressure (CPAP) (5–10 cm H_2O) to nonventilated lung.
  - Applying PEEP to ventilated lung.
  - Intermittent lung reinflation if necessary.
  - Surgical ligation of pulmonary artery of nonventilated lung.

Usually most of the patients tolerate one-lung ventilation and PA clamping except those with pulmonary hypertension. Patients with diminished RV function can undergo severe RV dysfunction and intraoperative RV dysfunction should be managed aggressively.

Management of intraoperative RV failure includes:
- Large increase in intrathoracic pressure (high PEEP, large tidal volume) should be avoided.
- Adequate preload should be maintained.
- RV coronary perfusion pressure should be maintained with adrenergic agonist.
- Pulmonary vasodilators can be considered, provided hemodynamics are maintained, for example, prostaglandins E1 (0.05–0.15 µg/kg/min) and inhaled nitric oxide (NO) (20–40 ppm).

In cases of doubtful RV function, a trial of PA clamping can be done for 5–10 min and RV function can be measured by serial TEE. In patients who do not tolerate PA clamping, CPB should be instituted immediately.

Once all anastomosis are complete, weaning from CPB is started. Lung protective ventilation strategy with tidal volume of 6 to 8 mL/kg, respiratory rate of 12 to 14, and PEEP of 5 is instituted. Lowest FiO_2 to maintain saturation above 90% should be used. Special consideration should be given to support RV function as this period is prone to undergo RV dysfunction. Ionodilators like milrinone and dobutamine may be considered during weaning from CPB. Serial TEE should be done for assessment of RV function, pulmonary artery, and pulmonary venous anastomosis.

TEE features of adequate anastomosis includes:
- PA diameter should be greater than 1 cm.
- Pulmonary vein diameter should be at least 0.5 cm with presence of flow as measured by color-flow Doppler.

- Pulse wave Doppler interrogation should yield flow rate less than 100 cm/s.

Once patient achieves satisfactory hemodynamics with TEE features suggestive of adequate anastomosis, cardiac bypass is turned off and heparin is reversed with protamine.

Management after Allograft Implantation

Bleeding: Heparin should be adequately reversed with protamine. Fresh frozen plasma (FFP), platelets should be transfused according to thromboelastography (TEG) parameters.

Desaturation: Lung protective ventilation should be instituted. Kinking or blockage of tracheal tube should be ruled out. A gentle suction may be done in case of increased secretion. Frank blood may suggest pulmonary edema may be due to graft dysfunction or pulmonary venous obstruction. If hypoxia persisted, institution of veno-venous (VV) ECMO should be considered.

Hemodynamic instability: Most common cause of perioperative hemodynamic instability is RV dysfunction. Other reason can be due to hypovolemia, arrhythmia, vasoplegia, or cardiac tamponade.

Postoperative Management

Goals of postoperative management include adequate ventilation of newly implanted lungs, early extubation, fluid restriction, routine immunosuppressive antibiotics, pain management, and thromboprophylaxis.

Typical combination of immunosuppressants used in these subsets are:

- Calcineurin inhibitors (tacrolimus or cyclosporin).
- Antiproliferative agents (azathioprine or mycophenolate).
- Corticosteroids.

Postoperative Complications

Primary Graft Dysfunction (PGD)

It affects almost 30% of patients and is commonly associated with pulmonary hypertension.[15] It can occur up to 3 days after allograft reperfusion and is characterized by impaired gas exchange in newly implanted lung.[16] Chest X-ray shows diffuse alveolar opacities in bilateral lung fields. Occurrence of PGD increases the chances of early and late mortality.[17]

Management of PGD is mainly supportive and includes lung protective ventilation, inhaled NO, and VV ECMO.

Acute Rejection

Rejection episodes are characterized by the presence of new infiltrates in chest X-ray along with poor gas exchange. Episodes of rejection may occur immediately after transplant to many days after that. Treatment includes large pulse of corticosteroids such as methylprednisolone or changing the immunosuppressive agents.

Bronchiolitis Obliterans

It is one of the most serious late complications of lung transplantation. Clinically patient presents with cough and progressive dyspnea with chest X-ray showing diffuse interstitial infiltrates. There occurs immune-mediated injury, which leads to small airway obstruction and fibrous scarring. A trail of augmentation of immunosuppressants may be tried but refractory cases require retransplantation as definitive option.

Other postoperative complications include RV failure, pneumothorax, pulmonary embolism, and acute kidney injury.

Conclusion

Patients undergoing lung transplant are generally old and have multiple comorbidities. Thorough knowledge of pulmonary physiology, one-lung ventilation, its successful implication, and TEE guidance for adequate anastomosis play a key role in the management of patients undergoing lung transplantation. These patients require a very meticulous postoperative care in terms of immune suppressants, antibiotics, mobilization, and early detection of transplant-related complications. Thus, balanced involvement of multidisciplinary team and its coordination can lead to successful outcome of patients following lung transplantation. Some respiratory multidrug-resistant (MDR) pathogen, especially Burkholderia Cepacia is a relative contraindication for lung transplant.[18,19] To date, cystic fibrosis patients infected with Burkholderia cepacia are regarded as high risk for post-transplantation mortality.[20] Considering that the proportion of patients requiring pre-transplantation intensive care unit (ICU) stay is increasing due to organ donor shortage and urgency-based organ allocation systems,[21] preoperative respiratory microbial colonization and resistant organisms are expected to become more common. However, it is unclear which pathogens or pattern of resistance impacts post-transplantation pneumonia (PTP). Perioperative colonization of recipients was a powerful predictive factor for PTP, which was associated with 1-year mortality in patients subjected to lung transplantation has recently been studied by T. Kim et al. on 76 lung transplant patients. They suggested that donor acceptance criteria may change to better address potential shortages in organ donation.[22]

References

1. Weill D, Benden C, Corris PA, et al. A consensus document for the selection of lung transplant candidates: 2014—an update from the Pulmonary Transplantation Council of the International Society for Heart and Lung Transplantation. J Heart Lung Transplant 2015;34(1):1–15

2. Hardy JD. The first lung transplant in man (1963) and the first heart transplant in man (1964). In: Transplantation proceedings 1999 Feb 1. Elsevier; (Vol. 31, No. 1–2, pp. 25–29)

3. Toronto Lung Transplant Group. Unilateral lung transplantation for pulmonary fibrosis. N Engl J Med 1986;314(18):1140–1145

4. Pierre AF, Sekine Y, Hutcheon MA, Waddell TK, Keshavjee SH. Marginal donor lungs: a reassessment. J Thorac Cardiovasc Surg 2002;123(3):421–427, discussion, 427–428

5. Lund LH, Edwards LB, Kucheryavaya AY, et al. The registry of the International Society for Heart and Lung Transplantation: thirty-second official adult heart transplantation report—2015; focus theme: early graft failure. J Heart Lung Transplant 2015;34(10):1244–1254

6. Low DE, Trulock EP, Kaiser LR, et al. Morbidity, mortality, and early results of single versus bilateral lung transplantation for emphysema. J Thorac Cardiovasc Surg 1992;103(6):1119–1126

7. Kaiser LR, Pasque MK, Trulock EP, Low DE, Dresler CM, Cooper JD. Bilateral sequential lung transplantation: the procedure of choice for double-lung replacement. Ann Thorac Surg 1991;52(3):438–445, discussion 445–446

8. Bisson A, Bonnette P. A new technique for double lung transplantation. "Bilateral single lung" transplantation. J Thorac Cardiovasc Surg 1992;103(1):40–46

9. Pierre AF, DeCampos KN, Liu M, et al. Rapid reperfusion causes stress failure in ischemic rat lungs. J Thorac Cardiovasc Surg 1998;116(6):932–942

10. Myles PS, Weeks AM, Buckland MR, Silvers A, Bujor M, Langley M. Anesthesia for bilateral sequential lung transplantation: experience of 64 cases. J Cardiothorac Vasc Anesth 1997;11(2):177–183

11. Triantafillou AN, Pasque MK, Huddleston CB, et al. Predictors, frequency, and indications for cardiopulmonary bypass during lung transplantation in adults. Ann Thorac Surg 1994;57(5):1248–1251

12. Quinlan JJ, Buffington, CW. Deliberate hypoventilation in a patient with air trapping during lung transplantation. Anesthesiology 1993;78(6):1177–1181

13. Aeba R, Griffith BP, Kormos RL, et al. Effect of cardiopulmonary bypass on early graft dysfunction in clinical lung transplantation. Ann Thorac Surg 1994;57(3):715–722

14. Thabut G, Mal H, Cerrina J, et al. Graft ischemic time and outcome of lung transplantation: a multicenter analysis. Am J Respir Crit Care Med 2005;171(7):786–791

15. Lee JC, Diamond JM, Christie JD. Critical care management of the lung transplant recipient. Curr Respir Care Rep 2012;1(3):168–176

16. Snell GI, Yusen RD, Weill D, et al. Report of the ISHLT Working Group on primary lung graft dysfunction, part I: definition and grading—a 2016 Consensus Group statement of the International Society for Heart and Lung Transplantation. J Heart Lung Transplant 2017;36(10):1097–1103

17. Christie JD, Sager JS, Kimmel SE, et al. Impact of primary graft failure on outcomes following lung transplantation. Chest 2005;127(1):161–165

18. Coiffard B, Prud'Homme E, Hraiech S, et al. Worldwide clinical practices in perioperative antibiotic therapy for lung transplantation. BMC Pulm Med 2020;20:109

19. Lund LH, Edwards LB, Dipchand AI, et al. The Registry of the International Society for Heart and Lung Transplantation: Thirty-third Adult Heart Transplantation Report-2016; Focus Theme: Primary Diagnostic Indications for Transplant. J Heart Lung Transplant 2016;35:1158–69

20. Murray S, Charbeneau J, Marshall BC, et al. Impact of burkholderia infection on lung transplantation in cystic fibrosis. Am J Respir Crit Care Med 2008;178:363–71

21. Kotloff RM, Thabut G. Lung transplantation. Am J Respir Crit Care Med 2011;184:159–71

22. Kim T, Yeo HJ, Jang JH, et al. Prognostic impact of preoperative respiratory colonization on early-onset pneumonia after lung transplantation. J Thorac Dis. 2022;14(6):1900–1908

25

Postoperative Considerations in Lung Transplant

Randeep Guleria, Vijay Hadda, Saurabh Mittal, Tejas Suri, Iti Shri, and Poonam Malhotra Kapoor

Introduction

Lung transplantation is an art that begins from patient selection to organ acceptance and prevention of allograft dysfunction. Approximately 4600[1] lung transplantation has been performed worldwide, with 339[2] in India itself till now. With the ushering in of innovative surgical techniques and immunosuppressive therapy, improved preservation of donor organs, optimized allocation, timely recognition of complications, and late recipient management, median survival time following a lung transplant has improved to 6.2 years[1] with enhanced quality of life. At 1 year of transplant, median survival was 8.0 years.[3]

Indications for lung transplantation can be broadly divided into obstructive, suppurative, vascular, and interstitial diseases.[4] Apart from the underlying proximate condition, age and associated comorbidities in the recipient, donor characteristics, and recipient–donor interaction have a profound bearing on perioperative outcome.

Postoperatively a myriad of complications ranging from mechanical problems to graft dysfunction and rejection may occur, knowledge of which is fundamental for proper diagnosis and management of the patient.

The postoperative problems can be categorized as per **Table 25.1**.[5-7]

A comprehensive and dedicated intensive care is critical to improving outcomes after lung transplant. Though evidence-based guidelines are still lacking, principal areas for postoperative management can be categorized into:

- Postoperative ventilation strategy.
- Postoperative fluid and hemodynamics management.
- Postoperative neurologic dysfunction management.

Table 25.1 Postoperative complications after lung transplant

Type	Postoperative complications
Graft related	• Primary graft dysfunction • Acute rejection • Donor-associated pneumonia
Respiratory	• Ventilator-associated pneumonia • Pulmonary embolism • Hemothorax • Lung torsion • Phrenic nerve injury • Native lung complications (viz., hyperinflation, infection, malignancy)
Mechanical	• Bronchial or pulmonary vein anastomotic complications (dehiscence) • Dislodgement or malpositioning of tubes and lines
Shock	• Distributive, cardiogenic, or obstructive
Cardiac	• Cardiogenic pulmonary edema • Right or left heart failure • Arrhythmias • Postoperative pericarditis

- Immunosuppressive and antibiotic therapy.
- Nutritional support.

Postoperative Ventilation Strategy

It is the cornerstone of intensive care unit (ICU) management in lung transplant patient for the ability to reduce not only ventilator-associated lung injury but also primary graft dysfunction (PGD). Large atelectasis may result from implantation of a large donor lung with contralateral edema in the central lung.

Recipient and Donor Size Mismatch

Size differences of 10 to 25% between a donor lung and a recipient lung are acceptable. Therefore, donor lung size within 10 to 25% of recipient size is considered to be acceptable for grafting.[4] As per the 2003 consensus of the International Heart and Lung Transplantation Association, the acceptable donor predicted total lung capacity (pTLC) is 75 to 125% of recipient pTLC for a bilateral lung transplantation.[8]

Since guidelines on optimal mechanical ventilation strategy in lung transplant are still lacking, principles of lung protective mechanical ventilation as in adult respiratory distress syndrome (ARDS) are applied here too:[7] tidal volume (TV) to 6 mL/kg of donor body weight, minimal inspired oxygen (FiO_2), titrating positive end-expiratory pressure (PEEP) according to FiO_2 (avoiding high levels to allow for bronchial healing), targeting a plateau pressure (PP) <30 cm H_2O, pH > 7.25, and oxygen saturation (SpO_2) > 90% so as to prevent oxidative stress and shear-stress injury.[7,9] If it was fibrotic disease or if an undersized graft, TVs of 4 to 6 mL/kg donor predicted body weight should be used to reduce the risk of overdistension, while in cases of obstructive disease, aim is to maximize the expiratory time.[4,10]

Following uncomplicated lung transplantation, postoperative elective ventilation is usually continued for 2 to 3 days after which the patient can undergo spontaneous breathing trial and extubation. The postextubation period can be covered with noninvasive ventilation or high-flow nasal cannula (HFNC) for a smooth transition to spontaneous breathing aided by chest physiotherapy, bronchoscopies and postural drainage, and early mobilization.[11-13] However, avoid the use of cough assist as to prevent injury to bronchial anastomosis. Donor lung size should ideally be within 10 to 15% of the size of the recipient lung.[4] As early as 2003, the national consensus of International Heart and Lung Transplantation, the acceptable donor pTLC should be 75 to 125% of the recipient.[8]

In cases of respiratory complications (e.g., PGD, infection, leaks, and rejection), increased duration of protective mechanical ventilation targeting even lower inspiratory PP (less than 25 cm H_2O), driving pressure less than 14 cm H_2O, and airway occlusion pressure of the first 100 ms less than 4 cm H_2O becomes more crucial.[14,15] Repeated bronchoscopies may be needed to rule out anastomotic complications.

Inhaled Pulmonary Vasodilators

Inhaled nitric oxide (iNO) in the range 10 to 40 ppm may attune inflammation and oxidative stress, coagulopathy, and hence mitigate effects of ischemia-reperfusion injury.[16,17]

Primary Graft Dysfunction (PGD)

It is acute lung injury with continuum of spectrum from moderate to severe. It is an early cause of longer postoperative ventilation, longer intensive care unit stay, and a greater predisposition to renal replacement therapy, reoperation, lung allograft dysfunction and mortality following lung transplant. The International Society for Heart and Lung Transplantation (ISHLT) 2005 (updated in 2016, **Table 25.2**) defined PGD as the PaO_2/FiO_2 (P/F) ratio and the presence of bilateral infiltrates on chest radiograph, at 100% FiO_2 and PEEP of 5 cm H_2O, at specific time points after reperfusion (i.e., within 6, 24, 48, and 72 hours).[18,19]

Diamond et al. demonstrated an incidence of 16.8% of grade III PGD in 1255 lung transplant recipients at 48 or 72 hours after reperfusion, contributing to a significant 90-day and 1-year mortality (18 and 23%, respectively).[20] Similarly Whitson et al reported a 17% incidence of 90-day mortality rate in grade III PGD within the first 48 hours following transplantation versus 9% without grade III PGD.[21] Not only the survival rate is decreased but there is a notable negative impact on quality of life due to poor functional status and an incremental risk of developing bronchiolitis obliterans syndrome (BOS), a major cause of dwindled long-term survival.[22]

Risk Factors for PGD[18]

Preoperative stage:
- Brain death compromising hemodynamic and hormonal status causes hypothermia and release of inflammatory mediators.
- Warm and cold ischemia impacts tissue oxygenation.
- Donor after circulatory death (DCD) versus donor after brain death (DBD): higher use of extracorporeal membrane oxygenation (ECMO) after DCD.

Intraoperative and postoperative stage:
- Donor's age: Extremes of age, with donor age between 55 and 64 not significantly associated with PGD, African American race, female gender, tobacco use/smoking/alcohol use, head trauma.
- Recipient risk factors: Obesity, COPD, pulmonary fibrosis, cystic fibrosis, sarcoidosis, idiopathic pulmonary arterial hypertension (every 10-mmHg elevation in mean pulmonary artery pressure [PAP] increases the risk of PGD by 30%).
- Excessive blood transfusion (>4 units).
- Fat embolism.
- Use of cardiopulmonary bypass (CPB).
- Reperfusion FiO_2 > 0.4 (increases risk by 6%).
- Prolonged mechanical ventilation.
- Aspiration, pneumonia.
- Higher levels of interleukin (IL)-8, macrophage colony stimulating factor, and growth-related oncogene-α.

Pathophysiologically, PGD is a consequence of ischemia-reperfusion injury (IRI) and subsequent release of inflammatory mediators.[18]

Treatment of PGD[7,18]

Since PGD resembles acute respiratory distress syndrome (ARDS), its treatment is an extrapolation from the same. Protracted protective mechanical ventilation strategy and sedation is continued in patients suspected to be at risk of PGD, along with rescue treatments such as prone positioning, iNO, and muscle relaxation. In very severe graft dysfunction and refractory hypoxemia, venovenous or venoarterial extracorporeal membrane oxygenation (ECMO) should be instituted within 24 hours of onset of severe PGD.

Normothermic ex vivo lung perfusion (EVLP) is an emerging technology that allows for delivery of potential therapeutic agents, as well as perfusing and ventilating ex vivo to maintain lung tissue viability.[18,23]

Prevention of PGD[18]

- Improving donor selection process and use of normothermic EVLP.
- Use of cytoprotective substances (e.g., prostaglandins, iNO, surfactant, adenosine).
- Inhibition of proinflammatory mediators (e.g., platelet-activating factor 1 inhibitor).

Table 25.2 ISHLT PGD definition and severity grading

PGD stage	P/F ratio (mmHg)	Chest radiography
0	>300	Normal
1	>300	Infiltrates consistent with noncardiogenic pulmonary edema
2	200–300	Infiltrates consistent with noncardiogenic pulmonary edema
3	<200	Infiltrates consistent with noncardiogenic pulmonary edema

Abbreviations: ISHLT, International Society for Heart and Lung Transplantation; PGD, primary graft dysfunction.

- Inhibition of polymorphonuclear leukocytes (PMNs) and derived factors (e.g., TNF-α, IL-1β, complement factors).

Postoperative Fluids and Hemodynamics Management

Of these, soluble complement receptor 1 inhibitor, plasminogen activating factor antagonist, and exogenous surfactant have demonstrated beneficial effects in improving oxygenation levels in PGD.

Decreased fluid and hemodynamics management: Lymphatic drainage disruption makes grafts sensitive to large volume fluid administration and vulnerable to injury and PGD.

A dedicated protocol for fluid management with the maintenance of specific hemodynamic targets (central venous pressure [CVP] $\leq$ 7 mmHg, mean arterial pressure [MAP] = 65–75 mmHg, and a cardiac index [CI] 2.2–2.5 L/min/m^2) with the end points of adequate tissue perfusion, viz., lactate, urine output, and mixed venous oxygen saturation (ScVO$_2$), is associated with better graft function.[7] A restrictive fluid strategy is not associated with increased use of vasopressors or any end-organ dysfunction.[7] Bedside ultrasound for determining volume status is challenging. Use of coagulation factors, antifibrinolytic agents, and point-of-care transfusion strategies may effectively reduce blood transfusion, an important factor implicated in severe PGD.[24]

Use of Swan-Ganz catheter or transpulmonary thermodilution or continuous left atrial pressure monitoring helps in meeting optimal fluid management targets.[4,25]

Pericarditis, supraventricular tachyarrhythmias (atrial fibrillation [AF] to the tune of 20–39%), and pulmonary edema may complicate postoperative course.

Treatment of AF involves correction of underlying cause like electrolyte abnormalities, fluid overload, pain. β-Blockers are first-line choices in hemodynamically stable patients and sotalol replaces amiodarone in view of inducing lung injury. Electrical cardioversion is reserved for unstable patients or those refractory to medical therapy. Anticoagulation is generally started if atrial fibrillation persists longer than 48 hours.[26]

Postoperative Management of Neurological Dysfunction: Prevention and Management of Neurologic Complications

Lung transplant recipients may encounter a myriad of postoperative neurological complications ranging from delirium (40%), stroke (4–10%), posterior reversible encephalopathy syndrome (PRES; 25%), immunosuppressive drug–induced encephalopathy, infections, seizures, phrenic and recurrent laryngeal nerve injury, and ICU acquired weakness.[7]

Risk factors are chronic hypoxia and hypercapnia, hypertension and diabetes, arrhythmias, use of CPB or ECMO, intraoperative hypotension, bleeding, and severe PGD.[27,28]

Early detection and prevention of delirium is mainstay of management and includes benzodiazepine-free sedation, adequate pain control by applying opioid-sparing techniques, early weaning and mobilization, maintaining nutrition, and preventing muscle weakness.

Posterior reversible encephalopathy syndrome, immunosuppressive drug–induced encephalopathy can be treated by substituting calcineurin inhibitors with basiliximab, and drug concentration monitoring.[29]

Phrenic nerve injury may occur due to stretching or direct surgical injury resulting in early extubation failure in absence of PGD or paradoxical breathing patterns. Phrenic nerve reconstruction and diaphragm pacing may be required.[30]

Hyperammonemic encephalopathy (1–4%) is a fatal complication. It is prudent to monitor plasma ammonia concentration, and if found higher than 100 µmol/l consider hemodialysis and antimicrobial therapy targeting urea plasma species.[31]

Immunosuppressive and Antibiotic Therapy

Immunosuppressive regimen may be a varying combination of induction therapy (basiliximab, antithymocyte globulin, and alemtuzumab being the most common) and triple-drug immunosuppression with a calcineurin inhibitor (cyclosporine A or tacrolimus), a cell-cycle inhibitor (azathioprine or mycophenolate mofetil/mycophenolic acid), and a corticosteroid.[7,32]

Pretransplant sensitization of the recipient to donor human leukocyte antigens (HLAs) increases mortality. Also risk of kidney injury due to calcineurin inhibitors should be duly addressed.

Reasons for rejection:

1. Hyperacute rejection results from preformed antibodies against the HLA of the donor.
2. Acute cellular rejection (ACR) is T-lymphocyte mediated. It is diagnosed by a combination of worsening of symptoms and lung function, imaging, antibodies, and tissue biopsy (perivascular and peribronchial lymphocytic infiltration). Mild rejection is usually treated with high-dose corticosteroids while more severe forms require immune-suppressing drugs (e.g., rabbit antithymocyte globulin [RATG] or alemtuzumab).[33]

In about one-third of transplant patients, antibody-mediated reaction (AMR) is directed against major histocompatibility complex antigens in the donor's lung occurring in second postoperative week to within first year of transplant. Repeated episodes may form a platform for chronic rejection or BOS. Treatment of AMR is challenging and includes intravenous immunoglobulin, plasmapheresis, or anti-CD20 monoclonal antibodies.[34]

The common risk factors include:
- Infections that involve the lung (e.g., cytomegalovirus [CMV], *Aspergillus, Pseudomonas* sp.).
- PGD.
- Irregular immunosuppressive medications.
- Gastroesophageal reflux disease (GERD).

Postoperative Infections

Since these patients are already immunocompromised and undergo immunosuppressive therapy, empiric and broad-spectrum antibiotics are mainstay of therapeutics, with prophylaxis continued for 2 to 7 days.

Pseudomonas aeruginosa followed by *Staphylococcus aureus* are the commonest causes of bacterial pneumonia, which in itself has an incidence reaching up to 44%. Duration of antibiotic therapy is at least for 10 to 14 days.[35]

Postoperative Risk of Pneumonia

Some factors enhancing the risk of pneumonia are:
1. Graft exposure to external environment.
2. Lack of nerve innervation impairs cough reflex and mucociliary clearance.
3. Paucity of adequate lymphatic drainage.
4. Risk of aspiration.
5. Anastomotic complications.

Opportunistic infections such as *Burkholderia cepacia* complex and *Mycobacterium abscessus*, CMV, or multidrug-resistant bacteria (e.g., *P. aeruginosa*) jeopardize long-term lung transplantation survival. In fact patients harboring *Burkholderia cenocepacia* are not considered fit to receive lung transplantation.

CMV infection is implicated in acute and chronic graft rejection, and exerts immunomodulatory effects as well, promoting other opportunistic infections.

Pneumocystis jirovecii is implicated as a common cause of severe pneumonia in lung transplantation recipients mandating prophylactic trimethoprim–sulfamethoxazole course.

Aspergillus followed by *Candida* species are often isolated as colonizing fungal species in the lung transplantation recipients' bronchoalveolar lavage while invasive fungal infections in lung transplantation have been associated with high morbidity and mortality. Although empirical antifungal coverage is widely practiced, ISHLT does not recommend the same.

Reported risk factors for invasive fungal infection include fungal colonization, idiopathic pulmonary fibrosis, geriatric age, obesity, airway ischemia, single-lung transplantation, and major construction projects around the hospital center.

Pneumonia and indwelling catheters are also major reason for blood stream infection that is associated with graft failure and survival.

Other infective complications are surgical wound infection, mediastinitis, empyema, and pericarditis that considerably cost the graft survival and impact overall mortality.

Unfortunately, no standard guideline or recommendation exist regarding the choice of perioperative antibiotic in lung transplantation, but regular prophylaxis is recommended (**Table 25.3**).[36]

Nutritional Support

Adequate nutrition is necessary to prevent infection, promote wound healing by supporting metabolic demands, and helps in mediating the immune response.[37]

The current literature lacks any specific guidelines on nutritional support to lung transplant recipients; nonetheless, the type of support is largely guided by the underlying

Table 25.3 Infectious organism and antibiotics

Infectious organism	Antibiotics recommended
Fungal infection	- Heterogenous practice - Duration of prophylaxis usually 6–12 mo - Systemic azole and inhaled liposomal amphotericin B
Tracheobronchial *Aspergillus* sp.	Voriconazole with nebulized amphotericin B
Mucormycosis	- IV liposomal amphotericin B followed by oral posaconazole - Surgical debridement
Pneumocystis sp.	- Lifelong prophylaxis with trimethoprim-sulfamethoxazole - Alternative is pentamidine
Cytomegalovirus	Ganciclovir IV followed by oral valganciclovir for 1–3 mo
Community-acquired respiratory viruses	Oseltamivir, Zanamivir
Clostridium difficile	Metronidazole along with vancomycin if complicated
Mycobacterium tuberculosis	Two-phase antibiotics
Nontubercular mycobacterium	Two-phase antibiotics

disease and occurrence of complications. As in other solid organ transplants, a daily caloric intake of 25 to 30 kcal/kg is recommended and resumption of early enteral feeding is the priority.[38]

According to most of the global literature, the use of pre-operative ECMO is also a challenge. In cases of cystic fibrosis, due to associated pancreatic insufficiency and malabsorption, elemental or semielemental feed formulations along with pancreatic enzymes are also enterally supplemented.

GERD commonly occurs in view of vagal nerve dysfunction, immunosuppressive therapy, and altered thoracic mechanics. Its management is critical for a propensity to chronic graft dysfunction, and involves head elevation at 30 degrees, proton pump inhibitors, and prokinetic agents.[39]

Vomiting, dyspepsia, and diarrhea may require laxatives or prokinetics while oropharyngeal dysphagia and reduced motility warrant early imaging with contrast and prompt surgical intercession. The most frequent causes of early post–lung transplantation abdominal surgery are bowel ischemia and bowel perforation.[40]

It is worth mentioning that early postoperative gastrointestinal (GI) complications are more frequent in β-1-antitrypsin–deficiency lung transplantation recipients, and hence polyethylene-glycol electrolyte solutions or N-acetylcysteine are enterally given in cystic fibrosis patients.

The 1-month mortality was higher in those lung transplant patients who were managed on intraoperative ECMO than those lung transplant patients on an off-CPB mode.

Other Complications

Postoperative hemorrhage: Its incidence has reduced with improved surgical techniques along with the use of ECMO for hemodynamic support.

Large airway complications such as bronchial stenosis may occur later on due to bronchial circulation interception and airway infection.

Vascular anastomotic complications: Both donor–recipient size mismatch, the twisting or thrombosis may compromise pulmonary artery and atrium anastomosis. These are dealt with either surgical revision or stenting or ballooning.

Rahulan et al., in a recent write-up on setting up a separate lung transplant ICU, in Bengaluru, Chennai, and Mumbai, retrospectively, in 132 lung transplant patients over 3 years, reported distal airway stenosis in 21.97%, bacteremia in 10.61%, and PGD grade 3 in 12.1% of the population. In India, gram-negative sepsis, the authors quoted was a major problem postoperatively, as was multi-drug resistant (MDR) pseudomonas and fungal airway infection, chiefly with *Aspergillus*. The authors have tried to overcome the same, by the postoperative use of antibiotics and antifungal agents.[42]

Role of Extracorporeal Membrane Oxygenation (ECMO) in Lung Transplant Patient

Perioperative use of ECMO has lessened the morbidity and mortality in lung transplant patients by providing cardiopulmonary support, and depending on the purpose, it could be venovenous (VV), venoarterial (VA), or venovenous-arterial (VVA).

ECMO currently has been employed in all the three phases of the lung transplant, viz., as a bridge to transplantation, intraoperatively to maintain hemodynamics that can be continued postoperatively, or for managing severe graft dysfunction, hyperacute rejection, or circulatory dysfunction.[4,7,10]

Postoperatively ECMO not only supports gas exchange and averts ventilator-associated lung injury, it also offloads right ventricle and provides hemodynamic support. It has been demonstrated, particularly in cases with pulmonary hypertension, that VA-ECMO by unloading and relaxing left ventricle helps reducing reperfusion injury.

However, the best strategy for ECMO remains controversial. VA-ECMO unloads both cardiopulmonary circulation and the left ventricular and, it is associated with more severe complications than VV ECMO in which the risk of perfusion injury is less affected. Weaning from VV-ECMO is contemplated once the patient's respiratory parameters improve and the patient tolerates protective ventilation. Similarly weaning from VA-ECMO is initiated once the patient has acceptable hemodynamics and perfusion at modest doses of inotropes. An acceptable 5-year survival rate has been reported after postoperative use of ECMO for PGD and the patients remained free of BOS at 3 years.[41]

Conclusion

The postoperative management of a lung transplant patient is complex and calls for an integrated and dedicated team approach. The outcome is highly dependent on interplay between various intricate perioperative complex processes. With the advancements in the technology, surgical processes, immunosuppressive drug therapy, and enhanced longevity, the desideratum is to standardize and continuously evolve lung transplantation techniques and guidelines so as to enhance the standard of care and recuperation of these patients. Recent studies in India have demonstrated that selected patients with end-stage lung disease who are in the early phase referred to an experienced transplant recipients centre.[42] Hundred percent survival has recently been reported in lung transplant patients who had COVID-19 infection as well[43–45] and than underwent a transplant.

Other potential complications in the postoperative period include atrial arrhythmias and neurologic complications such as stroke.[46] Atrial arrhythmias including atrial fibrillation, atrial tachycardia, and atrial flutter are common after lung transplantation. They occur in 19–46% of patients in the early postoperative period with a peak onset between 2 and 7 days after transplant. Risk factors for early postoperative atrial tachyarryhthmias include age, history of pre-transplant atrial tachyarrhythmia, male gender, hypertension, hyperlipidemia, coronary artery disease, left atrial enlargement, pulmonary fibrosis, and postoperative vasopressor use. The impact of pulmonary artery pressures and type of transplant (single versus double) remain controversial. Potential mechanisms of early postoperative atrial tachyarrhythmia include operative trauma with systemic inflammation and pericarditis, fluid shifts, electrolyte abnormalities, autonomic triggers, and hemodynamic changes.[47]

References

1. van der Mark SC, Hoek RAS, Hellemons ME. Developments in lung transplantation over the past decade. Eur Respir Rev 2020;29(157):190132

2. Sunder T. The evolution of lung transplantation in India and the current scenario. Indian J Thorac Cardiovasc Surg 2021;1–18

3. Yusen RD, Edwards LB, Dipchand AI, et al; International Society for Heart and Lung Transplantation. International Society for Heart and Lung Transplantation: The Registry of the International Society for Heart and Lung Transplantation: Thirty-third adult lung and heart-lung transplant report-2016; Focus theme: Primary diagnostic indications for transplant. J Heart Lung Transplant 2016;35(10):1170–1184

4. Nicoara A, Anderson-Dam J. Anesthesia for lung transplantation. Anesthesiol Clin 2017;35(3):473–489

5. Garrido G, Dhillon GS. Medical course and complications after lung transplantation. Psychosocial Care of End-Stage Organ Disease and Transplant Patients. 2018; 279–288

6. Soetanto V, Grewal US, Mehta AC, et al. Early postoperative complications in lung transplant recipients. Indian J Thorac Cardiovasc Surg 2021;1–11

7. Di Nardo M, Tikkanen J, Husain S, et al. Postoperative management of lung transplant recipients in the intensive care unit. Anesthesiology 2022;136(3):482–499

8. Orens JB, Boehler A, de Perrot M, et al; Pulmonary Council, International Society for Heart and Lung Transplantation. A review of lung transplant donor acceptability criteria. J Heart Lung Transplant 2003;22(11):1183–1200

9. Barnes L, Reed RM, Parekh KR, et al. Mechanical ventilation for the lung transplant recipient. Curr Pulmonol Rep 2015;4(2): 88–96

10. Kao CC, Parulekar AD. Postoperative management of lung transplant recipients. J Thorac Dis 2019;11(Suppl 14):S1782–S1788

11. Masclans JR, Zapatero A, Sacanell J. High flow therapy in post-lung transplant patients. Arch Bronconeumol 2017;53(4): 182–183

12. Wahidi MM, Ernst A. The role of bronchoscopy in the management of lung transplant recipients. Respir Care Clin N Am 2004;10(4):549–562

13. Downs AM. Physical therapy in lung transplantation. Phys Ther 1996;76(6):626–642

14. Bellani G, Grassi A, Sosio S, et al. Driving pressure is associated with outcome during assisted ventilation in acute respiratory distress syndrome. Anesthesiology 2019;131(3):594–604

15. Duncan SR, Kagawa FT, Kramer MR, Starnes VA, Theodore J. Effects of pulmonary restriction on hypercapnic responses of heart-lung transplant recipients. J Appl Physiol (1985) 1991;71(1):322–327

16. Khan TA, Schnickel G, Ross D, et al. A prospective, randomized, crossover pilot study of inhaled nitric oxide versus inhaled prostacyclin in heart transplant and lung transplant recipients. J Thorac Cardiovasc Surg 2009;138(6):1417–1424

17. Moreno I, Vicente R, Mir A, et al. Effects of inhaled nitric oxide on primary graft dysfunction in lung transplantation. Transplant Proc 2009;41(6):2210–2212

18. Morrison MI, Pither TL, Fisher AJ. Pathophysiology and classification of primary graft dysfunction after lung transplantation. J Thorac Dis 2017;9(10):4084–4097

19. Christie JD, Carby M, Bag R, Corris P, Hertz M, Weill D; ISHLT Working Group on Primary Lung Graft Dysfunction. Report of the ISHLT Working Group on Primary Lung Graft Dysfunction part II: definition. A consensus statement of the International Society for Heart and Lung Transplantation. J Heart Lung Transplant 2005;24(10):1454–1459

20. Diamond JM, Lee JC, Kawut SM, et al; Lung Transplant Outcomes Group. Clinical risk factors for primary graft dysfunction after lung transplantation. Am J Respir Crit Care Med 2013;187(5):527–534

21. Whitson BA, Nath DS, Johnson AC, et al. Risk factors for primary graft dysfunction after lung transplantation. J Thorac Cardiovasc Surg 2006;131(1):73–80

22. Daud SA, Yusen RD, Meyers BF, et al. Impact of immediate primary lung allograft dysfunction on bronchiolitis obliterans syndrome. Am J Respir Crit Care Med 2007;175(5):507–513

23. Cypel M, Yeung JC, Liu M, et al. Normothermic ex vivo lung perfusion in clinical lung transplantation. N Engl J Med 2011;364(15):1431–1440

24. Pena JJ, Bottiger BA, Miltiades AN. Perioperative management of bleeding and transfusion for lung transplantation. Semin Cardiothorac Vasc Anesth 2020;24(1):74–83

25. Mercier O, Lenavec J, Langer N. Left atrial pressure continuous monitoring improves early postoperative outcomes after double lung transplantation for pulmonary hypertension. J Heart Lung Transplant 2017;36(4):S407

26. Waldron NH, Klinger RY, Hartwig MG, Snyder LD, Daubert JP, Mathew JP. Adverse outcomes associated with postoperative atrial arrhythmias after lung transplantation: a meta-analysis and systematic review of the literature. Clin Transplant 2017;31(4):1–10

27. Mateen FJ, Dierkhising RA, Rabinstein AA, Van De Beek D, Wijdicks EFM. Neurological complications following adult lung transplantation. Am J Transplant 2010;10(4):908–914

28. Zivković SA, Jumaa M, Barisić N, McCurry K. Neurologic complications following lung transplantation. J Neurol Sci 2009;280(1-2):90–93

29. Chen S, Hu J, Xu L, Brandon D, Yu J, Zhang J. Posterior reversible encephalopathy syndrome after transplantation: a review. Mol Neurobiol 2016;53(10):6897–6909

30. LoMauro A, Righi I, Privitera E, et al. The impaired diaphragmatic function after bilateral lung transplantation: a multifactorial longitudinal study. J Heart Lung Transplant 2020;39(8): 795–804

31. Anwar S, Gupta D, Ashraf MA, et al. Symptomatic hyperammonemia after lung transplantation: lessons learnt. Hemodial Int 2014;18(1):185–191

32. Ailawadi G, Smith PW, Oka T, et al. Effects of induction immunosuppression regimen on acute rejection, bronchiolitis obliterans, and survival after lung transplantation. J Thorac Cardiovasc Surg 2008;135(3):594–602

33. Shyu S, Dew MA, Pilewski JM, et al. Five-year outcomes with alemtuzumab induction after lung transplantation. J Heart Lung Transplant 2011;30(7):743–754

34. Kulkarni HS, Bemiss BC, Hachem RR. Antibody-mediated rejection in lung transplantation. Curr Transplant Rep 2015; 2(4):316–323

35. Alsaeed M, Husain S. Infections in heart and lung transplant recipients. Crit Care Clin 2019;35(1):75–93

36. Nosotti M, Tarsia P, Morlacchi LC. Infections after lung transplantation. J Thorac Dis 2018;10(6):3849–3868

37. Hasse JM. Nutrition assessment and support of organ transplant recipients. JPEN J Parenter Enteral Nutr 2001;25(3):120–131

38. Jomphe V, Lands LC, Mailhot G. Nutritional requirements of lung transplant recipients: challenges and considerations. Nutrients 2018;10(6):E790

39. Castor JM, Wood RK, Muir AJ, Palmer SM, Shimpi RA. Gastroesophageal reflux and altered motility in lung transplant rejection. Neurogastroenterol Motil 2010;22(8):841–850

40. Miller CB, Malaisrie SC, Patel J, Garrity E, Vigneswaran WT, Gamelli RL. Intraabdominal complications after lung transplantation. J Am Coll Surg 2006;203(5):653–660

41. Vicente R, Moreno I, Soria A, Ramos F, Torregrosa S. Extracorporeal membrane oxygenation in lung transplantation. Med Intensiva 2013;37(2):110–115

42. Rahulan V, Shah U, Yadav P, et al. Challenges, experiences, and postoperative outcomes in setting up first successful lung transplant unit in India. Lung India 2021;38(3):216–222

43. Kurihara C, Manerikar A, Querrey M, et al. Clinical characteristics and outcomes of patients with COVID-19-associated acute respiratory distress syndrome who underwent lung transplant. JAMA 2022;327(7):652–661

44. Kotecha S, Ivulich S, Snell G. Review: immunosuppression for the lung transplant patient. J Thorac Dis 2021;13(11): 6628–6644

45. Tang C, Wang W, Xue Y, Yang J. Effect of MMF immunosuppression based on CNI reduction on CNI-related renal damage after lung transplantation. J Healthc Eng 2022;2022:8099684

46. Kao CC, Parulekar AD. Postoperative management of lung transplant recipients. J Thorac Dis. 2019;11(Suppl 14):S1782–S1788

47. Roukoz H, Benditt DG. Atrial arrhythmias after lung transplantation. Trends Cardiovasc Med 2018;28:53–61

26

Extracorporeal Membrane Oxygenation as a Bridge to Transplant

Poonam Malhotra Kapoor, Pranay Oza, Venkat Goyal, Mohit Prakash, Rajiv Gupta, and Ritu Airan

Heart Failure Management

Many cardiac diseases, coronary artery disease, and some viral cardiomyopathies over a period of time lead to heart failure (HF). More than 2 million Indians suffer from HF today. The first line of management includes lifestyle modification as well as medical therapy. The latter involves the usage of blocker drugs such as β-blockers, angiotensin-converting enzyme (ACE) inhibitors, angiotensin receptors, aldosterone antagonists, diuretics, digoxin, and many others. There is frequent addition to this list of drugs with more research and development (R&D). Salt and fluid restriction too plays a pivotal role. Patients with a wide Q wave, R wave, and S wave (QRS) complex in their electrocardiogram (ECG) and those having moderate-to-severe symptoms of HF need to have a cardiac resynchronization therapy (CRT), whereas patients with fatal arrhythmias need an implantable defibrillator inserted as a therapy. So, the use of advanced mechanical therapies is a necessity in HF patients.

Most Indians complaining of HF have either Class III or Class IV symptoms of dyspnea at rest. It may be for a short duration and may also be of a recent origin. Such scenarios in which HF patients require advanced mechanical support, the two definitive therapies, nearly 6,000 in number and still on the increase, are the use of ventricular-assist devices (VAD) and heart transplant, which have met with some success.

Extracorporeal Membrane Oxygenation

Extracorporeal membrane oxygenation (ECMO) is used in cardiac or pulmonary failure in moribund patients, wherein supraoptimal medical therapy does not work at all (**Figs. 26.1–26.3**). There are two types of ECMO, namely, venovenous (VV) and venoarterial (VA) ECMO. VV ECMO provides adequate oxygenation and carbon dioxide removal in isolated refractory respiratory failure while VA ECMO is used when support is required for cardiac and/or respiratory failure.[1,2] **Flowchart 26.1** will help the cardiologist in choosing the right kind of ECMO for their patients.

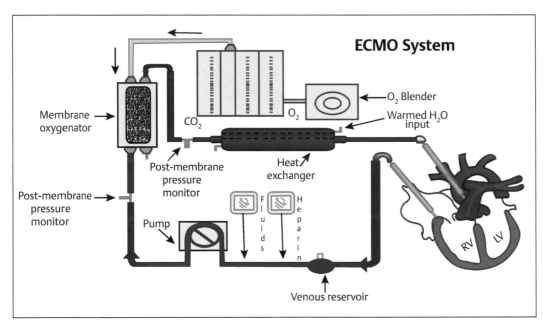

Fig. 26.1 Typical extracorporeal membrane oxygenation (ECMO) circuit.

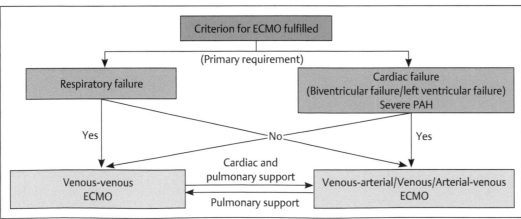

Flowchart 26.1 Choice of ECMO in different clinical scenarios. Abbreviations: ECMO, extracorporeal membrane oxygenation; PAH, pulmonary arterial hypertension.

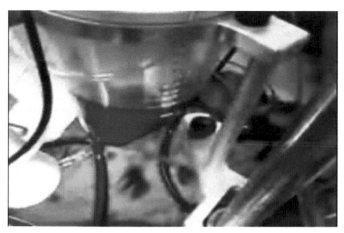

Fig. 26.2 The first venoarterial extracorporeal membrane oxygenation (VA ECMO) done at AIIMS, using a roller pump in a dextrotransposition of the great arteries (d-TGA) neonate.

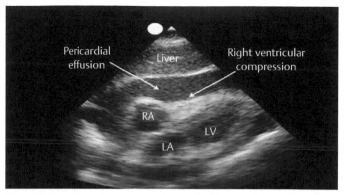

Fig. 26.3 Use of transesophageal echocardiography in an extracorporeal membrane oxygenation (ECMO) patients, aids in monitoring ECMO and bettering the results, when a significant MR comes up and there is stasis of blood in ascending aorta, when VA ECMO is 3–4 days ongoing 2022. Abbreviations: LA, left atrium; LV, left ventricle; RA, right atrium; VA ECMO, venoarterial extracorporeal membrane oxygenation.

AIIMS Experience on ECMO (2000–2022)

Till 2010, a total of 94 patients received ECMO support following cardiac surgery for repair of congenital heart disease (CHD) during the 10-year period (2000–2022) of study with survival to discharge of 61 patients (64.8%).[2] Patient's median age and weight were 53 days (range 29 d–4 y) and 3.41 kg (range 2.1–12.9 kg), respectively. Eighty-five children had an ascending aortic cannula and a single venous cannula in the right atrium in situ for cardiac surgery, which were connected to the ECMO circuit in the operating room. Nine patients required ECMO support in the postoperative period in the ICU, which was initiated by insertion of ascending aortic cannula and single venous right atrial cannula after removal of sternal sutures in the ICU. **Tables 26.1** to **26.3** show the result of patients on ECMO for different surgeries and their outcomes in term of mortality.[1]

Patient on VA ECMO with Severe Systolic and Diastolic MR ECMO Complications has Immense ECMO Complications

The complications may be a rupture or obstruction of any part of the ECMO circuit as shown in **Fig. 26.4**. The side effects of ECMO are seen to vary from bleeding to sepsis and thrombosis. **Fig. 26.5** shows a thrombus in the septum, following a myocardial infarction (MI), or there may be obstruction to flow in the superior vena cava (SVC) or inferior vena cava (IVC) as shown in **Fig. 26.6**.

At AIIMS, definitive surgical correction may be done in pediatric cardiac surgical patients of dextro-transposition of great arteries (DTGA), anomalous left coronary artery from the pulmonary artery (ALCAPA), etc., preemptively, using an ECMO circuit and coming off on an ECMO machine rather

Table 26.1 Outcome by diagnosis: AIIMS experience 2000–2022

Diagnosis	Survived n (%)	Died n (%)
TGAaq11 with IVS/TGA with VSD	51 (70.8)	21 (29.1)
VSD	3 (50)	3 (50)
TOF	3 (42.8)	4 (57.2)
ALCAPA	1 (25)	3 (75)
Truncus arteriosus	1 (50)	1 (50)
AVSD	2 (66.6)	1 (33.3)

Abbreviations: ALCAPA, anomalous left coronary artery from the pulmonary artery; AVSD, atrioventricular septal defect; VSD, ventricular septal defect; TGA, transposition of the great arteries; TOF, tetralogy of Fallot.

Table 26.2 AIIMS experience 2000–2022: using ECMO with high and low flows is compared

Patients receiving extracorporeal membrane oxygenation (ECMO) support (2011–2021)[3]		
	Flow given	No. of patients
Low-flow ECMO	50 mL/kg/min	60 patients
	100 mL/kg/min	40 patients
High-flow ECMO	150 mL/kg/min	70 patients
	200 mL/kg/min	30 patients

Note: Median age and weight of the patients were in the range of 29 days to 4 years and 3.5 kg (range of 2.1–12 kg) approximately. Low flow was given up to 100 mL/min, but in case of high flow, 150 mL/kg/min or more was given. This difference of 50 to 60 mL good outcome was in case of low-flow ECMO. The total number of patients receiving low-flow ECMO support was around 250 in AIIMS study with a 10-year period (2011–2021).[3]

Table 26.3 Adverse effects of LVAD

	CF LVAD (n = 133) [211 pt-years] Events/pt yr	CF LVAD (n = 59) [41 pt-years] Events/pt yr
Pump replacements	0.06	0.51
Stroke	0.13	0.22
• Ischemic	0.06	0.10
• Hemorrhagic	0.07	0.12
Device-related infection	0.48	0.90
Local non-device infection	0.76	1.33
Sepsis	0.39	1.11
Bleeding		
• Bleeding requiring PRBC	1.66	2.45
• Bleeding requiring surgery	0.24	0.29
Other neurological	0.17	0.29
Right heart failure		
• Extended inotropes	0.14	0.46
• RVAD	0.02	0.07
Cardiac arrhythmias	0.69	1.31
Respiratory failure	0.31	0.80
Renal failure	0.10	0.34
Hepatic dysfunction	0.01	0.00
Device thrombosis	0.02	0.00
Re-hospitalizations	2.64	4.25

Abbreviations: CF, continuous-flow; LVAD, left ventricular-assist device; PRBC, packed red blood cell; RVAD, right ventricular-assist device.

than the cardiopulmonary bypass (CPB) roller pump. This reduces complications and has advantages (**Box 26.1**).[4]

The use of integrated extracorporeal membrane oxygenator circuit benefits the patients well (**Box 26.2**).[4]

Whenever using ECMO as a bridge to transplant or a bridge to recovery or a bridge to VAD or a bridge to nowhere, it is important to remember that ECMO is a transient and not the definitive therapy—thus used as a bridge.

When weaning from ECMO, although no definitive weaning guidelines exist, we do the following, that is, we follow clinical judgment, hemodynamic parameters, and calculate the ECHO variables before weaning. It is important to monitor on ECMO (**Box 26.2**), and also follow closely the advantages of ECMO in the acute decompensated heart failure (ADHF) patient, in whom an intra-aortic balloon pump (IABP) may already be in place, and a portable ECMO may add benefit to act as bridge to VAD or recovery (**Box 26.3**).[5]

Box 26.1 Integrated ECMO circuit: Clinical uses and benefits—AIIMS experience

- Integrated ECMO circuitry was established along with CPB circuit and primed with blood
- Advantages of integrated circuit:
  ➤ No time is lost from decision to initiation of ECMO
  ➤ Early initiation may prevent end organ damage
  ➤ With a use of integrated ECMO, surgical asepsis is maintained
  ➤ The procedure is cost-effective
  ➤ Increasing survival in these critically ill patients

Abbreviations: CPB, cardiopulmonary bypass; ECMO, extracorporeal membrane oxygenation.

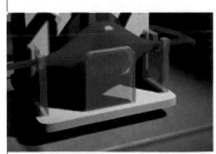
Circuit

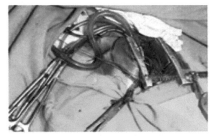
Cannulas

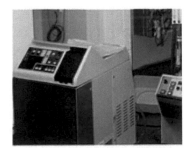
Bleeding

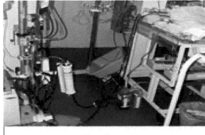
Bladder

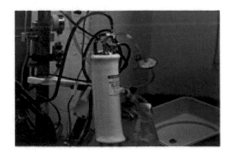
Oxygenator

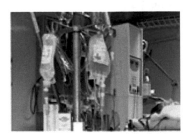
Heat exchanger

Fig. 26.4 Complications of extracorporeal membrane oxygenation (ECMO) may vary from bleeding to thrombosis and sepsis. It may result from rupture or dysfunction of any ECMO circuit component.

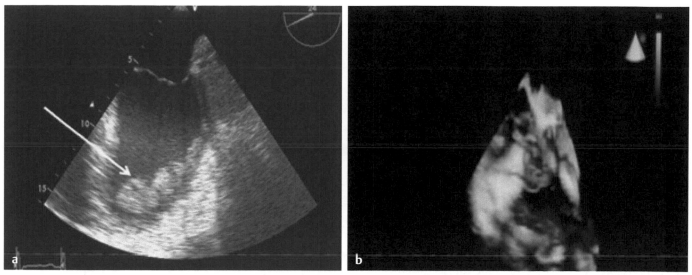

Fig. 26.5 Intraventricular thrombosis is a well-known complication of myocardial infraction. **(a)** Extracorporeal membrane oxygenation (ECMO) and left ventricle (LV) akinesis can increase this risk of thrombosis. **(b)** An embolus from right atrium (RA) to right ventricle (RV).

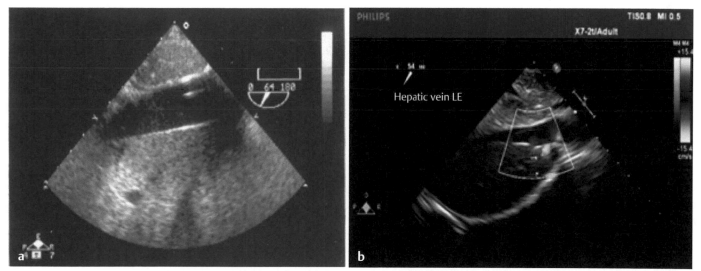

Fig. 26.6 Obstruction of the inferior vena cava (IVC) seen on a transesophageal echocardiography (TEE) in lower hepatic vein view.

Box 26.2 Objective parameters to target of cardiogenic shock on ECMO

- $ScVO_2 > 70\%$
- MAP > 60 mmHg (in case of full support with nonpulsatile flow)
- MAP > 70 mmHg (in case of partial support with pulsatile flow)
- Avoid full flow and give partial flow about 2/3 through ECMO
- Maintain oxygen saturation of 90% or PaO_2 of >50 mmHg (in young patient) and >60 (in elderly and with CAD or CVA)
- Maintain coronary saturation of >70%

Abbreviations: CAD, coronary artery disease; CVA, cardiovascular accident; ECMO, extracorporeal membrane oxygenation; MAP, mean arterial pressure; $ScVO_2$, central venous saturation.

Box 26.3 Advantages of ECMO in ADHF patients

- ECMO can be inserted at the bedside
- It is relatively cheap (as compared to the implantable LVAD)
- Gives the treating physicians some time to wait for recovery or a more stable condition
- Portable, can be inserted in Cath lab
- 17–21 Fr cannulas
- IABP to reduce afterload
- Centrifugal pump at 2–4 L/min
- Bridge to surgical VAD, transplant, or recovery

Abbreviations: ADHF, acute decompensated heart failure; ECMO, extracorporeal membrane oxygenation; IABP, intra-aortic balloon pump; LVAD, left ventricular assist device; VAD, ventricular assist device.

Future of ECMO

Applications for ECMO may expand in the future to include percutaneous temporary left ventricular assistance and low-flow ECMO for CO_2 removal (ECOOR). If new, miniature equipment of ECMO machinery, like oxygenators, pump, and surface coatings, are developed, there will be improvements in ECMO procedure, making it simpler and safer.

CARDIOHELP System

The modern CARDIOHELP machine is an upgraded form of an ECMO. It is lightweight and sleek for easy portability and can be easily used in changing scenarios in a hospital set-up. This new machine is most suitable in providing all of patients' needs for ECMO and in one single platform; it carries all range of ECMO features for cardiac insufficiency as well as respiratory distress.

In both VV and VA types of ECMO and also in percutaneous as well as centrally cannulated patients of ECMO, the CARDIOHELP works well to remove carbon dioxide efficiently and provide ideal "Protective Ventilation Protocols" (**Box 26.4**). Cost efficiency, improved mobility and portability, and improved clinical performance are the advantages of CARDIOHELP (**Fig. 26.7** and **Box 26.5**). The CARDIOHELP system delivers optimal care for the ECMO patients, with the improved features of protective ventilation and carbon dioxide removal.

Ventricular-Assist Devices

If ECMO is inserted then it must be remembered that it is a temporary device, the heart can be supported with a permanent therapy in the form of a VAD which is inserted surgically or percutaneously in the thoracic cavity or externally

by an expert cardiac surgeon. The indications for insertion of VAD are detailed in **Box 26.6**.

A VAD is a mechanical pump that is surgically attached to one of the heart's ventricles to augment or replace native ventricular function. It can be used for the left (LVAD), right (RVAD), or both ventricles (Bi-VAD). They are provided with external power sources that connect to the implanted pump

---

Box 26.4 Pump-assisted protection

- Possible fields of application: respiratory failure, such as ARDS, ALI, VILI
- Patient and user values: extracorporeal CO_2 removal enables protective ventilation
- Special feature: support of gas exchange for up to 30 d without exchanging components with focus on low flow and CO_2 removal instead of oxygenation
- Cannulation: percutaneous cannulation of either jugular, subclavian, or femoral vein

Abbreviations: ALI, acute lung injury; ARDS, acute respiratory distress syndrome; VILI, ventilator-induced lung injury.

Box 26.5 CARDIOHELP bedside adaption and transportation

- Different windows for optimized visualization enable the user to only see what he wants to see; separate lab value screen displaying hemoglobin, venous saturation, hematocrit, and temperature readings (venous and arterial)
- All alarms are indicated with colors and sound patterns, enabling the user to identify different alarm priorities
- The CARDIOHELP device alarm header will tell the user what the problem is, no hidden views, windows for fastest reaction time and maximum patient safety. The ward call allows alarms to be indicated even in remote locations
- Continuous storage of data in 3 s to 10 min steps
- Fast and simple start-up procedure with automated self-test and calibration
- User defined start-up configuration

Box 26.6 The need for a ventricular assist device (VAD) in heart disease patients

- Heart disease is the leading cause of death in the Western world:
  - ~5 million people in the US have congestive heart failure (CHF)
  - 250,000 are in the most advanced stage of CHF
  - ~500,000 new cases each year
  - ~50,000 deaths each year
  - Only effective treatment for end stage CHF is heart transplant

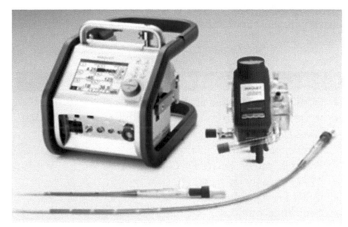

Fig. 26.7 The CARDIOHELP device.

via a percutaneous lead (driveline) that exits the body on the right abdomen. Pump output flow can be pulsatile or nonpulsatile (**Fig. 26.8**). The need for a VAD in heart disease patients is felt even more acutely today than ever before because the number of patients with heart disease is rising (**Boxes 26.6** and **26.7**).[5]

Left Ventricular-Assist Devices (LVAD)

LVADs are increasingly used as a bridge to transplantation. It remains unclear whether the use of pretransplant LVADs adversely affects short-term survival after cardiac transplantation (**Box 26.8** and **Table 26.3**).[6]

Components of an LVAD

The LVAD consists of a pump with controller, cannulas, and power source as explained in **Box 26.9**. Each component has its own sets on complications.

LVAD vs. Transplant

Malignancy is typically a contraindication for heart transplantation, but LVAD may be a consideration. No strict age limit for LVAD and no immunosuppressive therapy for LVAD are advised. If there are psychosocial factors that make the patient ineligible for transplant, it is unlikely that the patient will be an LVAD candidate.

Advances in VAD technology have made durable mechanical assist therapy available for select severely symptomatic HF patients. These pumps are surgically implanted at some tertiary care centers. To demonstrate mortality and QOL benefit, patients must undergo selection similar to heart transplant evaluation. Devices may become an important component in the management of acute HF. Although devices improve hemodynamic and metabolic parameters, there is currently no proven mortality benefit. These devices are not without complication; therefore, patient and device selection is key, requiring an integrated stepwise approach. ECMO in ADHF serves as a bridge to LVAD.[6]

Box 26.7   Indications for ventricular assist device

- Bridge to transplant (BTT):
  - ➤ Most common
  - ➤ Allow rehab from severe CHF while awaiting donor
- "Destination" therapy (DT):
  - ➤ Permanent device, instead of transplant
  - ➤ Currently only in transplant-ineligible patients
- Bridge to recovery (BTR):
  - ➤ Unload heart, allow "reverse remodeling"
  - ➤ Can be short or long term
- Bridge to candidacy (BTC)/Bridge to decision (BTD):
  - ➤ When eligibility unclear at implant
  - ➤ Not true "indication" but true for many patients

Box 26.8   Categorizing left ventricular assist device (LVAD) therapy by intent

- Bridge to transplant (BTT):
  - ➤ Intention is for patient to go to transplant
  - ➤ May prevent death on the wait list
- Destination therapy (DT):
  - ➤ Heart Mate XVE and Heart Mate II are the only LVADs approved for this purpose
  - ➤ Intention is for LVAD therapy to be indefinite
- Bridge to recovery:
  - ➤ Usually difficult to predict with certainty
- Bridge to decision

Box 26.9   Components of an LVAD

- Cannula
- Pump:
  - ➤ Internal
- Controller (computer)
- Power source:
  - ➤ Always external
  - ➤ Batteries
  - ➤ Wall unit

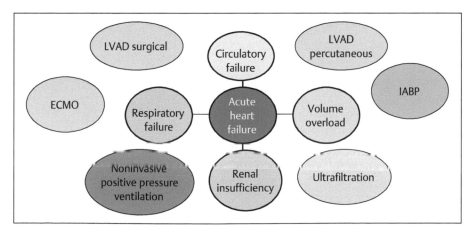

Fig. 26.8   The mechanical assist devices available for patients with heart failure. Abbreviations: ECMO, extracorporeal membrane oxygenation; IABP, intra-aortic balloon pump; LVAD, left ventricular assist device.

Conclusion

Presently, ECMO is viewed as an invasive procedure with significant risks, and should be used only after careful evaluation of risks/benefits and discussion with the family. However, it continues to represent an important support option in select critically ill infants and children. In the future, with increased experience, this procedure will become an even safer, more effective alternative to many less efficacious conventional therapies.

Awake ECMO is the new norm in bridge to lung transplant.[7] The benefits and favorable outcomes of awake ECMO for those awaiting organs for lung transplant is a new dimensions to healthcare. However, the use of ECMO as a bridge to lung/heart transplant is contraindicated when there is a neurological deficit, multidrug resistant infection and multiorgan failure.[8]

Keshavmurthy et al, have recently shown that ambulatory ECMO shows promise as a bridge to lung transplant. Ambulatory extracorporeal membrane oxygenation (ECMO) has shown promise as a bridge to lung transplantation. The primary goal of ambulatory ECMO is to provide enough gas exchange to allow patients to participate in preoperative physical therapy. Various strategies of ambulatory ECMO are utilized depending upon patients' need. A wide spectrum of ECMO configurations is available to tackle this situation Tachycardia is treated with B-blockade to decrease native cardiac output and thereby decrease shunting. VV ECMO with either two cannulae (IJ-Fem or Fem-Fem) dual-site access or dual-lumen and single cannula (IJ) single site access are the best options for acute respiratory failure. If no plans to initiate ECMO had been in place, emergent percutaneous cannulation at the bedside via the IJ and femoral vein or femoral-femoral veins may be required.[9]

References

1. Chauhan S, Subin S. Extracorporeal membrane oxygenation, an anesthesiologist's perspective: physiology and principles. Part 1. Ann Card Anaesth 2011;14(3):218–229
2. Chauhan S, Subin S. Extracorporeal membrane oxygenation—an anaesthesiologist's perspective—Part II: clinical and technical consideration. Ann Card Anaesth 2012;15(1):69–82
3. Airan R, Sharan S, Malhotra Kapoor P, Chowdhury U, Devagourou V, John A. Low flow venoarterial ECMO support management in postcardiac surgery patient. J Cardiac Crit Care 2021;5(2):103–107
4. Malhotra Kapoor P, Hasija S. Manual of extracorporeal membrane oxygenation (ECMO) in the ICU. 1st ed. Jaypee Publishers; 2014:243–248
5. Spielmann H, Seemann M, Friedrich N, et al. Self-management with the therapeutic regimen in patients with ventricular assist device (VAD) support: a scoping review. Heart Lung 2021;50(3):388–396
6. Ben Gal T, Ben Avraham B, Milicic D, et al. Guidance on the management of left ventricular assist device (LVAD) supported patients for the non-LVAD specialist healthcare provider: executive summary. Eur J Heart Fail 2021;23(10): 1597–1609
7. Lee SH. Awakening in extracorporeal membrane oxygenation as a bridge to lung transplantation. Acute Crit Care. 2022; 37(1):26–34
8. Vayvada M, Uygun Y, Cıtak S, Sarıbas E, Erkılıc A, Tasci E. Extracorporeal membrane oxygenation as a bridge to lung transplantation in a Turkish lung transplantation program: our initial experience. J Artif Organs. 2021;24(1):36–43
9. Keshavamurthy S, Bazan V, Tribble TA, et al. Ambulatory extracorporeal membrane oxygenation (ECMO) as a bridge to lung transplantation. Indian J Thorac Cardiovasc Surg. 2021;37(Suppl 3):366–379

27

Critical Care and Cardiac Services in the Current COVID Crisis (2020–2022)

Pradeep Narayan, Shashank Viswanathan, Russell D'Souza, and Muralidhar Kanchi

Introduction

With lifting of the lockdown and gradual resumption of prelockdown activities, a second, perhaps even bigger, wave of severe acute respiratory syndrome coronavirus 2 (SARS-CoV-2) or COVID-19-infected patients is expected. In the ensuing period it is extremely important for healthcare establishments to plan and prepare themselves from infrastructure and manpower perspectives. Development of evidence-based treatment protocols for COVID-19 patients as well as meeting the critical care needs of non-COVID patients and procedures was essential. It is therefore vital to develop local strategies and standard operating procedures (SOPs) to cater to the needs of the ongoing pandemic and at the same time prevent any collateral damage to patients suffering from other non-COVID ailments.

Challenges for the Critical Care Services Post Lockdown

The healthcare workers being the frontline defense in the pandemic were exposed to the detrimental hazards of infection. The World Health Organization (WHO) released guidelines highlighting the key duties of health workers.[1] SOPs had to be developed which clearly define entry criteria to the hospital in general and critical care unit in particular. Screening, triage, and limiting entry therefore had to start before entry to hospital premises. The only group of people who should be allowed to enter the hospital include infected patients, and those who definitely have not had the infection along with (attendants of patient and healthcare workers).

Clear-cut policies had to be formulated for movement and isolation of suspected COVID-19 patient. Structural changes had to be brought about in the critical care areas designated to cater to the COVID-19 patients. The institutions should aim for critical care isolation facilities to be equipped with negative air pressure with air change cycles >12/h and aerosol containment equipment. Besides, training of all healthcare professionals must be mandatory especially in donning and doffing of personal protection equipment (PPE). Use of PPE by all medical and paramedical personnels (**Fig. 27.1**) made tackling of COVID-19 easier in the second and third COVID waves.[2]

Current Critical Care Resources

There are 69,265 hospitals in India (43,487 in the private sector and 25,778 in the public) providing 94,961 critical care beds, majority of which are in the private hospitals estimated at 59,262 opposed to 35,699 in the public sector. The number of ventilators available is estimated at 47,481 (17,850 in the public sector and 29,631 in the private sector). The top three states with the highest number of critical care

resources in India were Uttar Pradesh (14.8%), Karnataka (13.8%), and Maharashtra (12.2%).[3] While shortages in PPE were reported in the early part of the pandemic, India is currently the second largest manufacturer of PPE and is not really a limiting factor in most healthcare facilities.

SARS-CoV-2 and the Critical Care Needs

Experience from other centers in the world suggests that almost 20% of infected patients may eventually require critical care.[4] Admission of infected patients to the intensive care units depends on a number of factors and includes the severity of illness as well as the critical care capacity of the facility.[5] The volume of people needing ICU care can be estimated by assessing the number of people getting infected as well as the number of patients requiring hospital admissions. The denominator had to be specified to make a valid comparison of admission rates. There is wide variation in the ICU admission rate with respect to both the measures. In Italy, ICU admissions represented 12% of the total positive

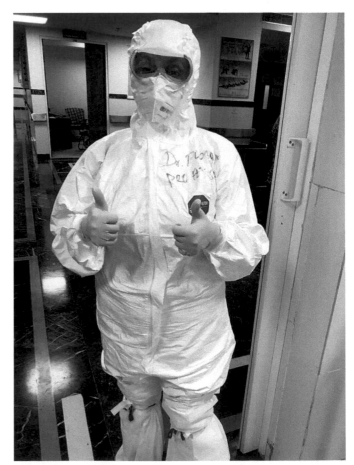

Fig. 27.1 Healthcare professionals with level 3 personal protection equipment (PPE) in the COVID-19 intensive care unit (ICU).

cases in the community which was significantly higher than that reported in China where only 5% of positive patients required ICU admission.[4]

Similar variations exist when the denominator is taken as patients admitted into the hospital who end up needing ICU beds. Among patients requiring hospitalization, admission rate was reported to be 16% of all hospitalized patients in Italy,[6] 25% in China,[7] and as high as 80% in the United States.[8] This wide variation is a result of regional factors, study sample size, as well as admission policies in different units. It is therefore extremely difficult to accurately predict the resource requirement in this pandemic. Every hospital depending on its catchment area and the population type (urban, rural, slum-dwellers) will have to work out its own expected requirements. In one of the largest studies on hospitalized patients in New York, it was seen that 14% needed ICU admission. The commonest reason for ICU admission in this and other studies is need for mechanical ventilation.[9] Apart from hypoxemic respiratory failure leading to intubation, inotropic support was another reason for admission. In patients needing mechanical ventilation, the mortality is in excess of 80%.[8]

Models of Provision of Critical Care at the Local/Regional Level

Segregation of COVID and non-COVID patients is perhaps the most important part of critical care management. This segregation of COVID and non-COVID patient care can occur at different levels depending on the existing facilities. At a regional level, entire hospitals ("hub-and-spoke" model) can be segregated into COVID and non-COVID hospitals. At a local level, hospitals must segregate different buildings or different floors or even different critical care units as COVID and non-COVID buildings, floors, or units.[2]

The hub-and-spoke model was adopted by some countries like Italy and the United Kingdom. In Lombardy, Italy, this model was successful in providing the increased demand for ICU beds for the COVID patients and at the same time managing non-COVID care.[6] This model was especially useful in providing cardiac surgical care during this pandemic. In Lombardy, 16 hospitals stopped cardiovascular surgical services (spokes) and 4 hospitals formed "the hub." In this hub-and-spoke system, all urgent and emergency cases were sent to these 4 units while the spokes continued to provide care to the COVID patients.[10] A similar model for redistribution of critical care beds and services in the context of cardiac surgery had been adopted in London and had been known as the Pan London Emergency Cardiac Surgery SOP (PLECS) COVID-19. However, even in these countries with a well-organized national health service, this had only been feasible on a regional basis.

In India with the absence of a nationalized robust healthcare system, a hub-and-spoke model was difficult to be adopted and hospitals had to develop policies and SOPs to provide ICU beds for the COVID as well as for the non-COVID patients. In hospitals equipped with more than one ICU unit, COVID and non-COVID units were clearly demarcated. In hospitals with a single ICU, a decision was taken to cater to either COVID or non-COVID patients but under no circumstances should they be mixed. This was done in all hospitals across the country.

Managing Volume in Critical Care with Respect to Cardiac Surgery

Critical care unit is the final common pathway for a large section of COVID and non-COVID medical and surgical emergencies as well as high-risk or complicated elective surgery. Unfortunately, it is extremely unlikely to see an increase in critical care beds in hospitals in the immediate future. Since a significant number of COVID patients require critical care beds and mechanical ventilation, this is bound to impact upon the requirement for critical care unit beds for non-COVID conditions. For specialties like cardiac surgery routine elective cases required critical care beds too; hence, this demand on critical care beds by the COVID pandemic was likely to affect the cardiac surgical workload in particular, which it did! Therefore, it is paramount that a clear balance is struck between the needs for caring for COVID patients and the needs for managing non-COVID patients.

While most hospitals hope to resume normal function in terms of case-mix return to the pre-COVID era, this is unlikely to happen anytime soon. A number of strategies for balancing these needs were proposed by different bodies. The operating capacity in cardiac surgery for instance is to be dictated by the COVID load of the hospital. For this purpose, the hospitals were classified into four tiers with a proposed reduction in operative capacity. Tier 1 hospitals with less than 30% infected patients would only require mild decrease in operating work; Tier 2 hospitals with more than 30% but less than 60% infected patients would require further decrease in operating work; Tier 3 hospitals with in between 60 and 80% infected patients would require significant decrease; and Tier 4 hospitals with above 80% infected patients should have negligible non-covid workload during this time of pandemic outbreak.[11]

Vulnerability of Critical Care Workers

This crisis led to health concerns as well as a psychosocial burden on the healthcare workers. Healthcare workers were found to be at high risk of acquiring nosocomial acquisition of infection. However, with increasing awareness and availability of PPE as well as implementation of policies and structural changes, the infection rate is now not dissimilar to the general population. Surprisingly, it was observed that healthcare workers working in lower risk areas experienced more infections. This could be secondary to lack of awareness, nonstringent protocols, and lesser utilization of PPE.[12,13] COVID-19 itself may cause a multitude of panic attacks, anxiousness, obsession, hysteria, depression, and other stress disorders. This infodemic was driven by various social media platforms. There is also detailed coverage of outbursts of sexism, bigotry, and xenophobia toward individual populations. However, forefront healthcare hands who were exposed more often were at greater risk of exposure to the virus and faced psychosomatic events which surfaced as burnout, anxiety, fear of transmission, depression, and substance abuse. The psychological health was the focus of another report from Singapore. The key finding was a significant incidence of depression, fatigue, anxiousness, and stress disorders in hospital workers.[14] Vicarious treatment of the healthcare workers had been reported and measures to prevent this had to be developed.[15]

Current Management Strategies and Future Perspectives of COVID-19

Management of COVID-19 is primarily supportive. Drugs such as remdesivir, lopinavir–ritonavir, corticosteroid, chloroquine, convalescence plasma, and Bacillus Calmette-Guérin vaccine (BCG) all had been part of critical care management with limited success. Vaccines breakthrough as preventive future strategy is also being researched upon. Respiratory support (continuous positive airway pressure [CPAP], intubation and mechanical ventilation, tracheostomy; **Figs. 27.2** and **27.3**), hemodynamic support using vasopressors, and renal support with renal replacement therapy may all be required depending on the clinical need (**Table 27.1**).

Drug Therapy

No antiviral drug is at present had an approval by the Food and Drug Administration (FDA) for COVID.[16]

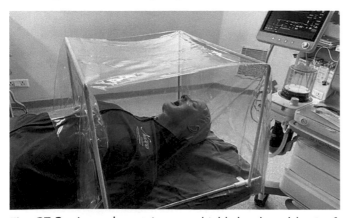

Fig. 27.2 Aerosol containment shield developed by Prof. Baljit Singh, Professor of Anesthesia, Shri Guru Gobind Singh Tricentenary University, Gurugram.

Remdesivir (GS-5734; Gilead Sciences, Inc.) is a nucleoside analogue that inhibits the virus in vitro. This property is to assess if remdesivir ameliorates the symptoms. Currently conflicting reports exist regarding benefit of remdesivir. A study involving 253 participants confirmed the benefit of remdesivir over placebo; however, there was no statistically significant clinical benefits.[17] The study was though underpowered. In contrast, another randomized trial published more or less at the same time with over thousand hospitalized infected patients reported faster recovery with remdesivir. Also, there was a much lower mortality rate at 14 days (7.1%) compared to 11.9% in patients on placebo.[18]

Another drug that had been tried to treat SARS-CoV-2 patients includes a **lopinavir and ritonavir** combination. Lopinavir is a human immunodeficiency virus (HIV) type 1 aspartate protease inhibitor which has in vitro inhibitory activity against SARS-CoV. Ritonavir inhibits cytochrome P-450 and is used along with lopinavir and the combination was assessed in the LOTUS China (Lopinavir Trial for Suppression of SARS-CoV-2 in China) study but was not found to be better than standard treatment.[19]

Another drug that has been discussed extensively is hydroxychloroquine prophylaxis. The rationale behind using chloroquine or the more potent hydroxychloroquine is its ability to affect glycosylation of the receptor and prevent the binding of the virus. Hydroxychloroquine was not found to be effective in preventing illness compatible with COVID-19 when initiated within 4 days after a high-risk or moderate-risk COVID-19 exposure.[20]

In critical care setting especially with regard to cardiac surgery the potential interaction between lopinavir/ritonavir and warfarin had to be borne in mind. This is especially important in patients with prosthetic valves who were on warfarin as there is a complex, multidrug interaction between warfarin and ritonavir leading to precipitous changes in international normalized ratio (INR) levels on initiation as well as discontinuation of ritonavir.[16]

Convalescent Plasma Therapy

Convalescent plasma therapy is another treatment modality that had seen a recent resurgence.[21] Use of convalescent plasma reduces both viral load and mortality. However, the benefit had only been reported in small case series.[22,23] Larger trials to decide on the dosage, the time points of administration and the clinical benefit were currently underway.

Role of BCG in Protection Against COVID-19

Countries that do not have policy of BCG vaccination for all such as Italy and the United States had higher mortality after infection. This supports the belief that BCG is protective in patients who were vaccinated, leading to a lower number of cases where BCG vaccination is given to all.[24]

This led to the inception of the BRACE trial (NCT04327206). In this trial BCG vaccination was used as an early intervention

Table 27.1 Management strategies of Covid-19

	Group 0	Group 1	Group 2	Group 3
Case definition	Mild disease/no testing for Covid	I. (a) Mild disease or where the report is not available II. (b) Mild disease/report positive	I. (a) Moderate disease/report awaited II. (b) Moderate disease/report negative III. Moderate disease/report positive	I. Severe disease/ report awaited II. Severe disease/report negative III. Severe disease/report positive
Investigations	No investigation to be done unless recommended by Covid physician	No investigation to be done unless recommended by Covid physician	CBC, CRP, renal and liver function, procalcitonin, blood culture, serum ferritin, ABG, chest X-ray, ECG, 2D echocardiography, urine, urine culture Optional: Creatine kinase, creatine kinase: MB, troponin-I, brain natriuretic peptide, D-dimer, IL-6	CBC, CRP, renal and liver function, procalcitonin, blood culture, serum ferritin, ABG, chest X-ray, ECG, 2D echocardiography, urine routine, urine culture Optional: Creatine kinase, creatine kinase: MB, troponin-I, brain natriuretic peptide, D-dimer, IL-6
Treatment	Desloratadine 5 mg or levocetrizine 5 mg OD paracetamol 650 mg (15 mg/kg) if febrile Salt water gargle 1-1-1-1 Report physician/pulmonologists consultation if worsening	Oseltamivir 75 mg bd × 5 d Azithromycin 500 mg OD × 3 d Desloratadine 5 mg / Levocetrizine 5 mg OD Paracetamol 650 mg (15 mg/kg) if febrile	(a) Supportive: O_2 via nasal prongs if $SpO_2 < 93\%$ IV antibiotics: Inj. ceftriaxone 1 g IV q 12h or Inj. amoxiclav 1.2 g IV q 8h Desloratadine 5 mg/Levocetrizine 5 mg OD MDI: ipratropium + levosalbutamol MDI Budesonide (200 µg) 2 puffs q12h via spacer (b) Specific oseltamivir 75 mg bd × 5 d Azithromycin 500 mg OD × 3 d HCQ 400 mg bd × 1 d; 200 mg bd × 5 d Covid specific: IV Remdesivir 200 mg on day 1 F/B 100 mg for 5 d IV Dexamethasone 6 mg once daily for 10 d -T. Hydroxychloroquine 400 mg 1-0-1 on first day and then 400 mg 1-0-0 for 4 d OR -T. Lopinavir + Ritonavir (200 mg + 50 mg) 2-0-2 for 10 d Note: HCQs/Lopinavir + Ritonavir may be withdrawn once the Covid test report is negative	(a) Supportive: O_2 via nasal prongs if $SpO_2 < 93\%$ and ventilator management as per ICU Team Oseltamivir 75 mg bd × 5 d -Prophylactic UFH or LMWH (Enoxaparin 0.5 mg/kg SC twice daily IV antibiotics Inj. Ceftriaxone 1 g IV q 12h, or Inj. Amoxiclav 1.2 g IV q 8h (may be modified based on culture reports after 48–72 h) Desloratadine 5 mg/Levocetrizine 5 mg OD MDI: ipratropium + levosalbutamol MDI Budesonide (200 µg) 2 puffs q 12h via spacer Covid specific: IV Remdesivir 200 mg on day 1 F/B 100 mg each day for 5 d: IV Dexamethasone 6 mg once daily for 10 d -T. Hydroxychloroquine 400 mg 1-0-1 on day 1, followed by 200 mg 1-0-1 for 5 d OR -T. Lopinavir+Ritonavir (200 mg + 50 mg) 2-0-2 for 10 d Special consideration Azithromycin 500 mg OD × 3 d HCQ 400 mg bd × 1 d; 200 mg bd × 5 d

Abbreviations: ABG, arterial blood gas; CBC, complete blood count; CRP, C-reactive protein; ECG, electrocardiogram; HCQ, hydroxychloroquine; ICU, intensive care unit; LMWH, low-molecular-weight heparin; MDI, metered-dose inhaler; UFH, unfractionated heparin.

to protect healthcare workers and other high-risk groups. It was a collaboration between Murdoch Children's Research Institute (MCRI), Melbourne University, and the Royal Children's Hospital. In this trial 10,078 healthcare workers received either BCG vaccine or placebo.[25]

Vaccines and the Future Perspective

Currently, a number of vaccines are in different phases of clinical evaluation. Vaccine development goes through a four-step stringent test before being approved by the regulatory bodies (**Flowchart 27.1**): (1) preclinical testing; (2) phase I for safety; (3) phase II trials to check the safety in a larger population; (4) phase III to test if the vaccine is effective. After the vaccine shows efficacy and little or almost no side effect, it is approved by the regulatory board for mass production and distribution to combat the disease. Ten vaccines are currently being clinically evaluated and another 123 are in preclinical stage.[26] Vaccine platforms were being utilized to expedite the search for a vaccine against the Sars-CoV-2. This includes nonreplicating viral vector, inactivated, RNA, and DNA vaccine platforms. The two important nonreplicating viral vector platforms include the AZD1222 (previously ChAdOx1) and the Adenovirus Type 5 vector platform (Ad5-nCoV). While the AZD1222 at the time of publication is in phase 2b/3, the Ad5-nCoV is in phase 2 (ChiCTR2000031781); AZD1222 is being carried out by the Jenner Institute at The University of Oxford and the vaccine in the rhesus macaques showed a "humoral and cellular immune response after a single dose."[27] The Ad5-nCoV vaccine trial is being carried out by China's CanSino Biologics. The findings of their phase 1 (ChiCTR2000030906; NCT04313127) clinical trial carried out in 108 participants between 18 and 60 years old who received low, medium, and high doses of Ad5-nCoV showed both T-cell responses and humoral responses.

Apart from these, a randomized trial is currently being carried out by researchers at Sinopharm and the Wuhan Institute of Virology.[28] Another randomized phase 2 trial among 600 healthy participants was fast-tracked by FDA on 12th May 2020. mRNA-1273 successfully produced neutralizing antibody titers similar to people who had recovered from the infection.[29]

Innovations in the Critical Care Area in the COVID Era

The requirement for isolation ward for COVID-19-infected and suspected patients emerged with an increasing demand for medical equipment such as indigenous ventilators and PPEs. To address this shortage, many scientists and engineers focused their work on developing various innovative designs for ventilators and diagnostics devices which will help in battling the pandemic. The Centre for Medical Innovation at the University of Utah, USA, developed droplet/aerosol containment tents, reusable face shields, powered air purifying respirator (PAPR), and 3D printed PARP adapters to help protect the hospital staffs.[30] Anesthesiologists and biomedical engineers at the Memorial Sloan Kettering Cancer Center, USA, modified the protective boxes used in intubation of infectious patients. The changes made in the box includes multiple access points that allow procedures such as intubation, bronchoscopy, and tracheostomy[31] (**Figs. 27.3 and 27.4** and **Flowchart 27.2**). The Indian scientists are developing a prototype for an electromechanical ventilator design made with components found in India and which complies with the guidelines of UK medicine and Healthcare Products Regulatory Agency. ICU protocols were introduced according to the structure and function of the coronavirus (**Fig. 27.5a**) and most such as membrane fusion of coronavirus (**Fig. 27.5b**) are still evolving.

Conclusion

The COVID-19 pandemic is here to stay like the influenza pandemic. It will be an endemic virus afflicting millions globally as we are seeing in mid 2022. As cardiac critical care intensivists new future directions in tackling this deadly endemic will help us overcome outcomes and limitations of this virus.

Implementation of scalable models for critical care delivery and cultivating education tools for team training and embracing newer technology like telemedicine with effective collaboration with social distancing at time of pandemic crisis are here to stay with us globally. Implement scalable models for critical care delivery, cultivate educational tools for team training, and embrace technologies (e.g., telemedicine) to enable effective collaboration despite social distancing imperatives.[32]

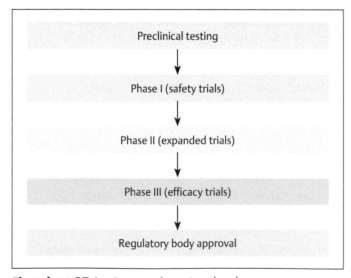

Flowchart 27.1 Stages of vaccine development.

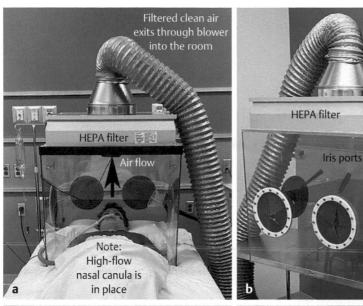

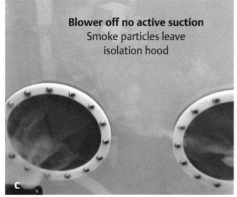

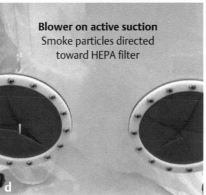

Filtered clean air exits through blower into the room

HEPA filter

Air flow

Note:
High-flow nasal canula is in place

a

HEPA filter

Iris ports

b

Blower off no active suction
Smoke particles leave isolation hood

c

Blower on active suction
Smoke particles directed toward HEPA filter

d

Fig. 27.3 Aerosol hood: **(a)** Rear view (caudal) images of the aerosol hood, showing all iris port and the high-efficiency particulate absorbing (HEPA) filter. **(b)** Images 30 to 40 seconds after igniting a smoke candle within the hood: left: no active suction. **(c)** Right: active suction at 10,000 L/min. **(d)** Active suction directs smoke particles toward the HEPA filter and releases clean air into the room.

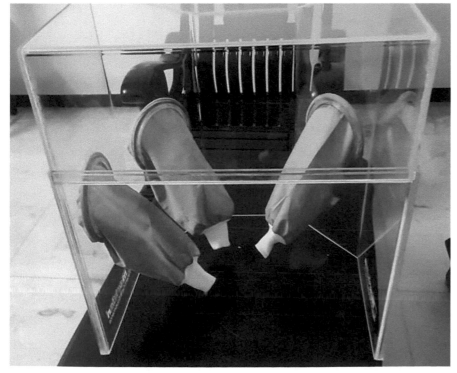

Fig. 27.4 "Negative pressure intubation bay" developed by Ganga Hospital, Coimbatore, was in much use during the three phases of COVID-19 in most major COVID centers in India for intubations of COVID cases.

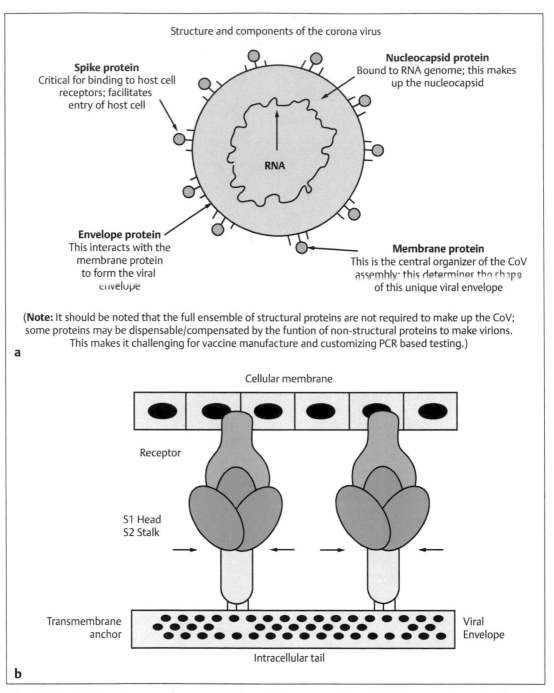

Fig. 27.5 (a) Structure and components of the coronavirus. **(b)** Structural mechanism for membrane fusion by coronavirus spikes.

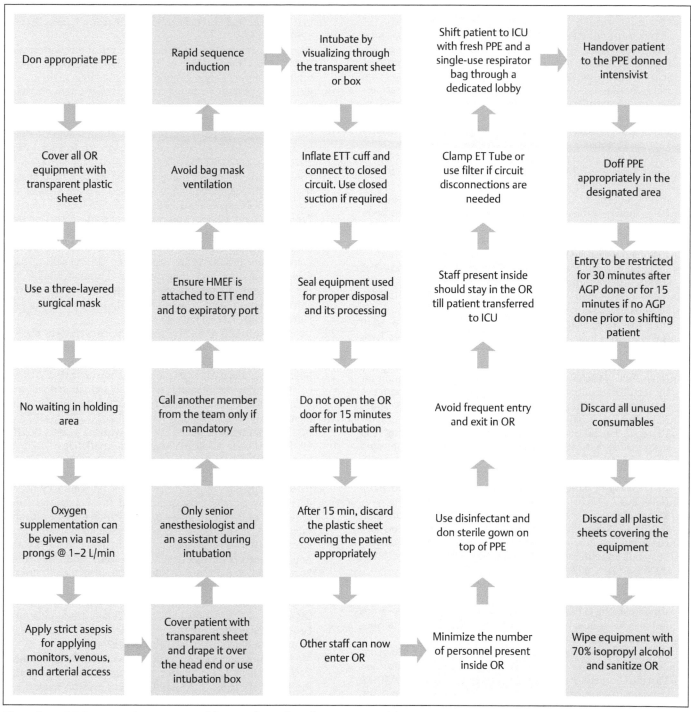

Flowchart 27.2 Anesthetic protocol for conduct of cardiac surgery. Abbreviations: AGP, aerosol generating procedures; ETT, endotracheal tube; HMEF, heat and moisture exchanger filters; ICU, intensive care unit; OR, operating room; PPE, personal protection equipment.

References

1. Coronavirus disease (COVID-19) outbreak: rights, roles and responsibilities of health workers, including key considerations for occupational safety and health [Internet]. [cited 2020 Jun 12]. https://www.who.int/publications/i/item/coronavirus-disease-(covid-19)-outbreak-rights-roles-and-responsibilities-of-health-workers-including-key-considerations-for-occupational-safety-and-health

2. Christopher DJ, Isaac BTJ, Rupali P, Thangakunam B. Health-care preparedness and health-care worker protection in Covid-19 pandemic [Internet]. Lung India: Official Organ of Indian Chest Society; 37:2020 [cited 2020 Jun 12]. https://.ncbi.nlm.nih.gov/32367846/

3. Kapoor G, Sriram A, Joshi J, Nandi A, Laxminarayan R. COVID-19 in India: state-wise estimates of current hospital beds, intensive care unit (ICU) beds and ventilators. https://cddep.org/publications/covid-19-in-india-state-wise-estimates-of-current-hospital-beds-icu-beds-and-ventilators/

4. Guan W, Ni Z, Hu Y, et al. Clinical characteristics of coronavirus disease 2019 in China. N Engl J Med [Internet]. 2020 Feb 28 [cited 2020 Jun 7]. https://www.nejm.org/doi/10.1056/NEJMoa2002032

5. Intensive care management of coronavirus disease 2019 (COVID-19): challenges and recommendations. Lancet Resp Med [Internet]. [cited 2020 Jun 7]. https://www.thelancet.com/journals/lanres/article/PIIS2213-2600(20)30161-2/fulltext

6. Grasselli G, Pesenti A, Cecconi M. Critical care utilization for the COVID-19 outbreak in Lombardy, Italy: early experience and forecast during an emergency response. JAMA 2020;323(16):1545–1546

7. Wang D, Hu B, Hu C, et al. Clinical characteristics of 138 hospitalized patients with 2019 novel coronavirus-infected pneumonia in Wuhan, China. JAMA 2020;323(11):1061–1069

8. Arentz M, Yim E, Klaff L, et al. Characteristics and outcomes of 21 critically ill patients with COVID-19 in Washington State. JAMA 2020;323(16):1612–1614

9. Richardson S, Hirsch JS, Narasimhan M, et al; the Northwell COVID-19 Research Consortium. Presenting characteristics, comorbidities, and outcomes among 5700 patients hospitalized with COVID-19 in the New York City Area. JAMA 2020;323(20):2052–2059

10. Bonalumi G, di Mauro M, Garatti A, Barili F, Gerosa G, Parolari A; Italian Society for Cardiac Surgery Task Force on COVID-19 Pandemic. The COVID-19 outbreak and its impact on hospitals in Italy: the model of cardiac surgery. Eur J Cardiothorac Surg 2020;57(6):1025–1028

11. Haft JW, Atluri P, Ailawadi G, et al; Society of Thoracic Surgeons COVID-19 Task Force and the Workforce for Adult Cardiac and Vascular Surgery. Adult cardiac surgery during the COVID-19 pandemic: a tiered patient triage guidance statement. Ann Thorac Surg 2020;110(2):697–700

12. Lai X, Wang M, Qin C, et al. Coronavirus Disease 2019 (COVID-2019) infection among health care workers and implications for prevention measures in a tertiary hospital in Wuhan, China. JAMA Netw Open 2020;3(5):e209666

13. Cheng VC-C, Wong S-C, Yuen K-Y. Estimating coronavirus disease 2019 infection risk in health care workers. JAMA Netw Open 2020;3(5):e209687

14. Tan BYQ, Chew NWS, Lee GKH, et al. Psychological impact of the COVID-19 pandemic on health care workers in Singapore. Ann Intern Med 2020;173(4):317–320

15. Li Z, Ge J, Yang M, et al. Vicarious traumatization in the general public, members, and non-members of medical teams aiding in COVID-19 control. Brain Behav Immun 2020;88:916–919

16. Knoell KR, Young TM, Cousins ES. Potential interaction involving warfarin and ritonavir. Ann Pharmacother 1998;32(12):1299–1302

17. Wang Y, Zhang D, Du G, et al. Remdesivir in adults with severe COVID-19: a randomised, double-blind, placebo-controlled, multicentre trial. Lancet 2020;395(10236):1569–1578

18. Jh B, Km T, Le D, et al. Remdesivir for the treatment of Covid-19: preliminary report [Internet]. New Engl J Med. 2020 [cited 2020 Jun 9]. https://.ncbi.nlm.nih.gov/32445440/

19. Cao B, Wang Y, Wen D, et al. A trial of Lopinavir-Ritonavir in adults hospitalized with severe Covid-19. N Engl J Med 2020;382(19):1787–1799

20. Boulware DR, Pullen MF, Bangdiwala AS, et al. A randomized trial of hydroxychloroquine as postexposure prophylaxis for Covid-19. N Engl J Med 2020;383(6):517–525

21. Tanne JH. Covid-19: FDA approves use of convalescent plasma to treat critically ill patients. BMJ 2020;368:m1256

22. Mair-Jenkins J, Saavedra-Campos M, Baillie JK, et al; Convalescent Plasma Study Group. The effectiveness of convalescent plasma and hyperimmune immunoglobulin for the treatment of severe acute respiratory infections of viral etiology: a systematic review and exploratory meta-analysis. J Infect Dis 2015;211(1):80–90

23. Duan K, Liu B, Li C, et al. Effectiveness of convalescent plasma therapy in severe COVID-19 patients. Proc Natl Acad Sci U S A 2020;117(17):9490–9496

24. Miller A, Reandelar MJ, Fasciglione K, Roumenova V, Li Y, Otazu GH. Correlation between universal BCG vaccination policy and reduced morbidity and mortality for COVID-19: an epidemiological study. medRxiv. 2020 Mar 28; 2020.03.24.20042937

25. BCG vaccination to protect healthcare workers against COVID-19: full text view. ClinicalTrials.gov [Internet]. [cited 2020 Jun 8]. https://clinicaltrials.gov/ct2/show/NCT04327206

26. Draft landscape of COVID-19 candidate vaccines [Internet]. [cited 2020 Jun 8]. https://www.who.int/who-documents-detail-redirect/draft-landscape-of-covid-19-candidate-vaccines

27. University of Oxford. A phase I/II study to determine efficacy, safety and immunogenicity of the candidate coronavirus disease (COVID-19) vaccine ChAdOx1 nCoV-19 in UK Healthy Adult Volunteers [Internet]. clinicaltrials.gov; 2020 May [cited 2020 Jun 4]. Report No.: NCT04324606. https://clinicaltrials.gov/ct2/show/NCT04324606

28. China Clinical Trial Registration Center-World Health Organization International Clinical Trial Registration Platform Level 1 Registration Authority [Internet]. [cited 2020 Jun 9]. http://www.chictr.org.cn/showproj.aspx?proj=53003

29. Moderna Announces Positive Interim Phade 1 Data for its mRNA Vaccine (mRNA-1273) Against Novel Coronavirus | Moderna, Inc. [Internet]. [cited 2020 Jun 9]. https://investors.modernatx.com/news-releases/news-release-details/moderna-announces-positive-interim-phade-1-data-its-mrna-vaccine/

30. Innovation in Response to COVID-19: innovation; Utah; Covid-19; University of Utah, School of Medicine [Internet]. [cited 2020 Jun 12]. https://uofuhealth.utah.edu/center-for-medical-innovation/blogs/2020/03/covid-update.php

31. COVID-19 Safety Innovations. Intubation-extubation boxes v3: thinking inside the box | Memorial Sloan Kettering Cancer Center [Internet]. [cited 2020 Jun 12]. https://www.mskcc.org/clinical-trials-updates/msk-covid-19-innovation-hub/covid-19-safety-innovations-intubation-extubation-boxes

32. Katz JN, Sinha SS, Alviar CL, et al. COVID-19 and Disruptive Modifications to Cardiac Critical Care Delivery: JACC Review Topic of the Week. J Am Coll Cardiol. 2020;76(1):72–84

28

Cardiac, Vascular, and Thrombotic Involvement in COVID-19 Infection

Rohan Kapur, Naveen Garg, K. K. Kapur, Pranav Kapoor, and Poonam Malhotra Kapoor

Introduction

The ongoing coronavirus 2019 pandemic (abbreviated as COVID-19), which originated in Wuhan, China toward the end of 2019, has strained the health care facilities in every corner of the world. This virus is spread by droplets. These droplets gain access into the mouth, eyes, and nose of the patient when an infected person coughs or sneezes. Angiotensin-converting enzyme (ACE-2) receptors mainly exist in the lungs and enable the entrance of this virus into the pneumocytes.[1]

Morphology

COVID-19 virus is an encapsulated RNA virus having only a single strand. It belongs to the beta-coronavirus subfamily of coronavirus. It has a positive sense, linear genome. It is a relatively large virus among the RNA viruses, with a size of about 60 to 140 nm. The structure of the virus is rather complex, consisting of nucleocapsid phosphoproteins, glycoproteins, and spike proteins, as shown in **Fig. 28.1**. Research has shown that it is the spike proteins which got mutated and led to the virus jumping from animals to humans.[2]

Pathogenesis

As shown in **Fig. 28.1**, the spike protein is sliced at S1/S2 region and later at S2′ site. The TMPRSS2 (transmembrane protease serine 2) enzyme facilitates this slicing, which then allows COVID-19 virus to attach to ACE-2 receptors in the respiratory tract columnar cells, type 2 pneumocytes, and cardiomyocytes. This binding is akin to a lock-and-key mechanism. On gaining entry into the cell via a process of endocytosis, the virus uncoats to release the RNA, and this RNA then replicates the RNA-dependent RNA polymerase which is present in the virus. This forms more copies of viral RNA, which are translated to viral proteins in the ribosome and are rearranged to form new copies of the virus

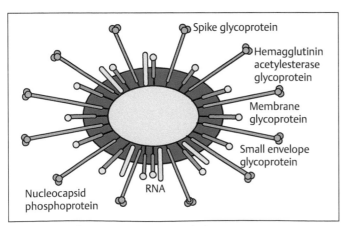

Fig. 28.1 The coronavirus morphology.

which then infect other cells as well as macrophages and T-lymphocytes. These macrophages and T-lymphocytes are primed. They release cytokines, such as interleukin-6 (IL-6) and tumor necrosis factor (TNF). Overproduction of these cytokines causes a "cytokine storm" which results in severe systemic inflammation and multiorgan failure.[3,4]

Cardiac Involvement

In young (<40 y) asymptomatic patients, cardiac involvement is quite rare. However, in high-risk patients (e.g., elderly, diabetic, and hypertensive patients) with pre-existing cardiac diseases, the heart gets increasingly involved. This involvement may require ICU facility including the use of noninvasive and invasive ventilation.[5-7] In such patients the cardiac involvement could be in the range of 50 to 60% and usually the mortality rate is quite high. This was elegantly demonstrated in a series of 150 patients with documented COVID-19 infection. Of the 68 nonsurvivors, cardiac involvement was observed in 13 patients, while in 82 survivors there was no cardiac involvement.[8]

Pathophysiology of Cardiac Involvement

- Patients having pre-existing comorbidities are likely to decompensate with the stress of COVID-19 infection. These include coronary artery disease, diabetes, hypertension, valvular heart disease, congenital heart disease, as well as chronic kidney disease and chronic liver dysfunction. Patients with end-stage cardiomyopathy requiring left ventricular-assist device (LVAD) and cardiac transplantation (issues of maintenance of immunosuppression and LVAD settings) can worsen their clinical status with COVID infection (**Fig. 28.2**).[6,7]
- Direct/Indirect involvement of myocardium (myocarditis):
  - On the other hand, myocardium is involved **indirectly** due to a severe inflammatory response resulting in release of proinflammatory markers, which include IL-1β, IL-6, C-reactive protein (CRP), ferritin, tumor necrosis factor (TNF), etc. These cytokines (or chemokines) are excessively produced and lead to "cytokine storm," which leads to multiorgan failure.
  - The presence of myocardial injury is an independent risk factor associated with increased mortality in COVID patients.[6,7]
- In a patient with pre-existing coronary artery diseases (critical/noncritical); the acute stress of COVID-19 infection could result in rupture of a vulnerable atherosclerotic plaque. This leads to ST-segment elevation myocardial infarction (STEMI).
  - The choice of treatment strategy in patients with STEMI is centered on either fibrinolytic therapy (if no contraindications) or an invasive

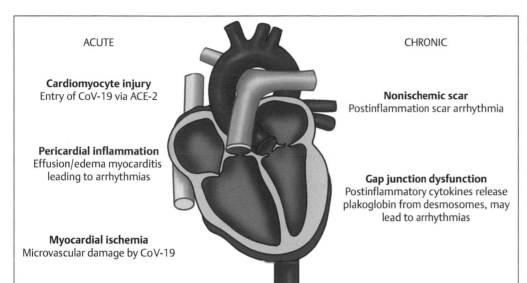

Fig. 28.2 Various acute and chronic cardiac manifestations and its sequels in COVID-19.

strategy (percutaneous coronary intervention [PCI]). However, the latter strategy entails referral of the patient to a PCI center.[8–11] The former strategy (fibrinolytic therapy) is cost effective, easily available, and transmission of COVID-19 infection to the interventional service providers is obviated. However, the invasive approach has the advantage of avoiding delays because of delayed ECG manifestation of STEMI.

➢ In a series of 18 patients with ST-segment elevation due to COVID-19 infection, 8 patients developed myocardial infarction while the remaining 10 patients had only myocardial injury (noncoronary). High mortality was observed in both these subsets. Nine out of 10 patients with noncoronary myocardial injury did not survive and only 4 out of 8 patients with MI survived.[12]

• A mismatch between myocardial blood supply and myocardial oxygen demand could result in significant **ischemia** to the myocardial cells. The causes of increased demand could be systemic inflammation, hypoxia, fast heart rate, and increased body temperature. This ischemia could result in severe LV dysfunction.[13,14]

• A wide spectrum of **cardiac arrhythmias** some of which could be just benign atrial or ventricular ectopics, while malignant arrhythmias such as Torsades de pointes could also result from myocardial inflammation. Furthermore, the commonly used anti-COVID-19 medications (chloroquine, hydroxychloroquine [HCQ], azithromycin, and antiviral drugs) could also precipitate life-threatening arrhythmias. Presence of congenital diseases of conduction system, such as long-QT syndrome and Brugada syndrome, predispose to the occurrence of malignant arrhythmias in COVID-19 patients. Similarly, dyselectrolytemia and

Table 28.1 Drug-related arrhythmias occurring in COVID-19

Arrhythmia in COVID-19	Precipitating drugs
Prolonged QT interval, short QT interval, ARVD, Brugada syndrome	Hydroxychloroquine Azithromycin Chloroquine Lopinavir/Ritonavir
Torsades de pointes related to catecholamines	Adrenaline, isoprenaline, dobutamine, and dopamine

Abbreviation: ARVD, arrhythmogenic right-ventricular cardiomyopathy.

arrhythmogenic right-ventricular (RV) cardiomyopathy (ARVD) could also facilitate the occurrence of such arrhythmias (**Table 28.1**).[15,16]

• Pericardial involvement, although uncommon, could manifest as significant (moderate to large) pericardial effusion; however, the occurrence of cardiac tamponade is rare.

• Different kinds of **stress cardiomyopathies** have been reported in COVID-19 patients. These include takotsubo cardiomyopathy, which is more common than the rather rare reverse takotsubo variant. Occasionally, a diffuse global involvement of myocardium could occur (nonischemic myopathy).[17,18]

• Vascular complications of COVID-19 include arterial thrombosis and venous thromboembolism including deep venous thrombosis (DVT).

➢ Acute vascular thrombosis including DVT is more likely to occur in patients with severe COVID infection.

➢ In a series of 184 COVID-19 patients with proven pneumonia admitted to ICU and given standard doses of thromboprophylaxis, the incidence of venous thromboembolism was 27% and arterial thrombosis was observed in 3.7%. Among the thrombotic complications, the most common was pulmonary embolism which was seen in 81% of patients with venous thromboembolism.

The presence of thrombotic complications was more likely if there was spontaneous elevation of prothrombin time (PT) by more than 3 seconds and partial thromboplastin time (PTT) by more than 5 seconds.[19]

- Cardiac involvement due to pulmonary embolism:
  - ➢ The prevalence of pulmonary embolism is much higher in patients with COVID-19 infections of the lungs as compared to non-COVID viral infections such as influenza.[20]
  - ➢ About 20 to 30% of patients with COVID-pneumonia are likely to develop pulmonary embolism.
  - ➢ The chances of developing venous thrombosis and pulmonary embolism are greatly increased if there is a significant elevation in D-dimer levels (2–3 times normal).[21]
  - ➢ Significant pulmonary artery hypertension leading to RV dysfunction could be either due to the development of pulmonary embolism or due to significant hypoxemia in a patient with COVID-pneumonia.
  - ➢ A timely diagnosis of pulmonary embolism allows appropriate management of critically ill patients, especially with the use of anticoagulation (either a low-molecular-weight heparin or unfractionated heparin).

Use of Cardiac Imaging in the Management of COVID Patients

Guidelines and Protocols

- Echocardiography is most cost-effective and reliable, noninvasive cardiac imaging modality. Most of the echocardiographic machines are capable of portable studies in critically ill patients. However, the performance of this procedure in COVID patients imposes a high risk of infection to the echocardiography service providers. Moreover, the equipment itself could be easily contaminated during its use on COVID patients[22] (**Box 28.1**).

- A judicious use of the echocardiographic procedure is advisable such that it is only utilized in case of incremental advantage, while managing COVID-19 patients with a probable cardiac involvement. Moreover, echocardiography should only be used if it is likely to lead to a significant change in the therapeutic management, for example, if this procedure could effect a change (in drug therapy or indicate a likelihood of interventional therapy or cardiac surgery). Therefore, this technique should be used only in the following situations:
  - ➢ Hemodynamically compromised patients.
  - ➢ Patients with overt congestive cardiac failure.
  - ➢ Patients with pre-existing congenital heart disease/valvular heart disease or known patients with ischemic heart disease.
  - ➢ Patients having a significant cardiac murmur.[22,23]

- Detailed appropriate precautionary measures should be instituted especially with regard to the protection of the echocardiography service providers, who should be given adequate personal protective equipment (PPE). Moreover, the echocardiography equipment itself should be protected from contamination using preventive measures as described below.

- Prior to the performance of echocardiography procedure:
  - ➢ There should be systematic and meticulous sanitization of the entire echocardiographic equipment. This should include cleaning of transducers, cables, monitors, knobs, etc., with sodium hypochlorite solution.
  - ➢ After cleaning and drying, the transducers, cables, and monitor should be completely covered with transparent polythene, as shown in **Fig. 28.3**.
  - ➢ The echocardiographic machine itself including the transducer-connecting cords as well as electrical wires are also covered in an outer polythene covering.

- While performing echocardiographic procedure, the covering over the main body of echomachine is removed but the transducer, monitor, and knobs remain covered with polythene.

- Postechocardiographic procedure: After the completion of echo examination the equipment is sent back to the heart station where all polythene coverings are

---

Box 28.1 Salient technical guidelines while performing echocardiography in COVID-19 patients

- Rapid echocardiography using POCUS or FOCUS views should be performed while assessing cardiac function in such patients
- Significant time efficiency can be achieved by performing offline measurements of cardiac chambers as well as evaluation of LV/RV functions
- As far as possible, TTE should be the imaging modality of choice and TEE should be avoided even in patients with suboptimal windows. Contrast-enhanced studies are recommended in such patients
- Use of CT or MRI may be preferred over TEE to confirm the diagnosis of LA-Appendage clot

Abbreviations: CT, computed tomography; FOCUS, focused cardiac ultrasound; LA-appendage, left atrial appendage; LV, left ventricle; MRI, magnetic resonance imaging; POCUS, point-of-care ultrasound; RV, right ventricle; TTE, transthoracic echocardiography; TEE, transesophageal echocardiography.

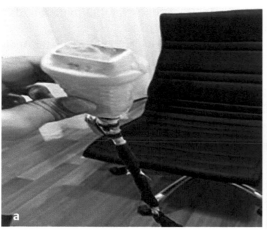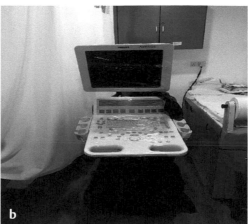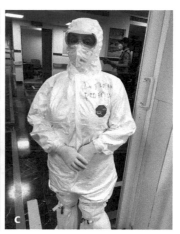

Fig. 28.3 (a, b) Transparent plastic coverings over transducer and machine. All wires are also wrapped over with plastic coverings after sanitization. **(c)** Use of personal protective equipment (PPE) by echocardiography providers and safety measures for echoequipment.

removed and machine is again meticulously sanitized and draped again for the examination of COVID or suspected COVID patients.

- Personal protective equipment (PPE)**:** The echocardiographic personnel should be provided with high-quality PPE which completely covers the face, especially eyes with suitable protective glasses and headgears (as shown in **Fig. 28.3**).
- ECG leads need not be attached to the echocardiographic equipment. The examination should consist of four or five basic views (parasternal LA/SA, apical 4C/2C, and subcostal or hypochondrial views). The basic aim of the imaging should be:
  - ➤ Determination of LV size and assessment of LV function.
  - ➤ Qualitative assessment of RV size and function.
  - ➤ Quick and accurate analysis of cardiac valves.
  - ➤ Detection and semiquantitative evaluation of pericardial/pleural effusion.
  - ➤ Quick evaluation of fluid status using the inferior vena cava (IVC) size to quantify the CVP (central venous pressure).
  - ➤ Hemodynamic evaluation of cardiac status using mitral inflow and LV outflow (**Box 28.2**).
- Echocardiography service providers are prone to acquiring infection while performing transesophageal echocardiogram (TEE) procedure on COVID-19 patients. The TEE procedure is therefore best avoided.
- Among the indications for a transesophageal study is to establish the presence of left atrial (LA) appendage clot in patients with atrial fibrillation (AF) or those who have had cardioembolic stroke. In this aspect, cardiac magnetic resonance imaging (MRI) or computed tomography (CT) scan could be utilized and the TEE obviated. The probability of transmitting COVID-19 infection to the MRI/CT personnel is extremely small

Box 28.2 Summary of the POCUS evaluation in critical care examination of COVID-19 patients

Echocardiographic examination using POCUS protocol:
- Left ventricle (LV) systolic dysfunction
- Right ventricle (RV) dysfunction
- Assessment of valvular stenosis/regurgitation
- Pulmonary embolism
- Pericardial effusion
- Vascular Doppler study to diagnose/exclude DVT
- IVC for fluid status
- Regional wall motion abnormality

Abbreviations: DVT, deep vein thrombosis; IVC, inferior vena cava; POCUS, point-of-care ultrasound.

owing to their distance from the patient. However, it is imperative that the MRI/CT equipment should be protected from contamination by meticulous sanitization.
- In continuation of the efforts to avoid infection to the echocardiographic personnel, following additional precautions should be observed:
  - ➤ The echocardiographic procedure could be avoided if troponin and N-terminal (NT)-prohormone B-type natriuretic peptide (NT-pro-BNP) levels are within the normal range.
  - ➤ If PCI procedure is contemplated, additional LV angiogram could be performed to assess regional and global LV systolic function.
  - ➤ Moreover, if a CT angiogram is planned to establish the diagnosis of pulmonary embolism, additional CT angiographic imaging of coronary arteries and cardiac chambers can be included in the CT angiostudy and thus the echocardiographic procedure could be avoided.

- If the CT angiographic procedure cannot be performed owing to the critical status of the patient then echocardiography procedure using the point-of-care ultrasound (POCUS) protocol should be performed to make a direct diagnosis of pulmonary embolism (presence of PA clot) or more commonly to provide an indirect diagnosis (large RV with low flow state in pulmonary arteries).

BP 90/60 mmHg, respiratory rate 32/min, and SPO_2 92% at room air (**Fig. 28.4a, b**).
- Case 2: COVID-19-positive elderly diabetic male with breathing difficulty admitted with hemodynamic instability. His HR is 140/min, BP 80/60 mmHg, SPO_2 85% at room air. Chest X-ray showed bilateral consolidation. Echocardiography was performed in emergency to rule out myocarditis (**Fig. 28.5**).

Authors' Experience with COVID-19 (Case Studies)

- Case 1: An elderly diabetic and hypertensive male; diagnosed as having COVID-19-pulmonary pneumonia; admitted in ICU. His heart rate (HR) is 120/min,

Cardiac Management

If cardiac complications are detected in a patient with COVID-19 infection, the management of such a patient requires a meticulous approach for the treatment of congestive cardiac failure, shock, hypotension; management of

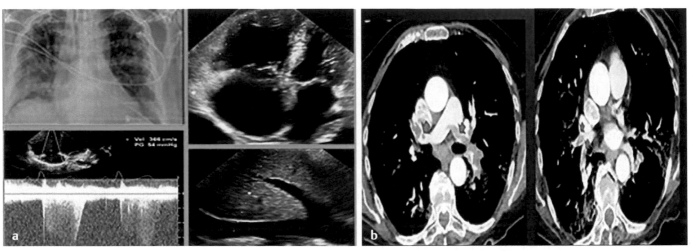

Fig. 28.4   (a, b) Chest X-ray depicts pulmonary pneumonia, and echocardiography revealed dilated right ventricular (RV), right artery (RA), and inferior vena cava (IVC) with pulmonary artery systolic pressure (PASP) >54 mmHg. This was consistent with pulmonary embolism which was confirmed in computed tomography (CT) scan (*blue arrows* point emboli in pulmonary segmental arteries).

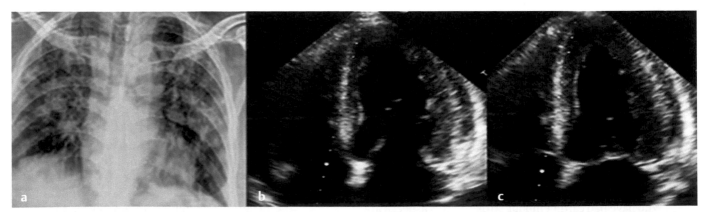

Fig. 28.5   (a–c) Chest X-ray depicts B/L consolidation and echocardiography showed normal functioning cardiac chambers with left ventricular ejection fraction (LVEF) 55% with no wall motion abnormality. Although blood reports showed leukocytosis and lymphopenia, emergency point-of-care ultrasound (POCUS) protocol ruled out any direct or indirect involvement of heart in this patient. Later, troponin and N-terminal (NT)-prohormone B-type natriuretic peptide (NT-proBNP) levels also came out to be normal.

malignant cardiac arrhythmia, as well as associated electrolyte imbalance. This could involve intensive monitoring in the ICU or using the telemetric approach for the detection and appropriate therapy of such dysrhythmias. In addition, the various cardiac diagnostic imaging may also be indicated such as echocardiography and cardiac CT/MRI. Besides the use of antiarrhythmic drugs, use, wherever appropriate, antiviral drugs, vasopressors, inotropes, diuretics, and treatment of associated dyselectrolytemia.

Specific Therapy for COVID-19

The specific therapy for COVID-19 include the following (**Table 28.2**):
- HCQ and azithromycin: In a small observational non-randomized study in France, use of HCQ and azithromycin has shown a significantly rapid clearance in nasal swab as compared to a control group of patients from a different hospital.[24] In vitro effect of HCQ has

Table 28.2 Various candidate drugs used in COVID-19

Drugs	Mechanism	Remarks
Chloroquine/Hydroxychloroquine	Blockade of viral entry by inhibiting glycosylation of host receptors; makes cell organelles alkaline and dysfunctional; acts as a zinc ionophore; anti-inflammatory action could help in cytokine storm	Used earlier in SARS/MERS. No authoritative RCT for COVID, only observational studies[24]
Azithromycin	Antibacterial with antiviral action; inhibits protein synthesis	No authoritative RCT; undergoing studies in combination with hydroxychloroquine[24]
Ritonavir/Lopinavir	Anti-HIV drugs: protease inhibitors	Works better in combination with ribavirin and interferon-β as a triple therapy vs. ritonavir/lopinavir combination alone[25]
Remdesivir	Nucleotide analog which inhibits viral RNA polymerase and viral replication	Highly promising drug with randomized study showing significant reduction in duration of active disease in severely ill patients[26,27]
Tocilizumab/Sirolumab	Monoclonal antibody to the IL-6 receptor	No RCT at present. Potential benefit in seriously ill COVID patients with cytokine storm. Often used with methylprednisolone
Ivermectin	Broad-spectrum antiprotozoal drug which reduces COVID-19 replication in vitro	In vivo effect not confirmed. Studies show in vitro effect[28]
Plasma therapy	Antibodies in plasma of recovered patients	Promising therapy undergoing trials. At present only anecdotal reports[29]
Favipiravir	Nucleotide analog which inhibits viral RNA polymerase and viral replication	Comparative randomized study with umifenovir showed earlier symptomatic improvement[30]
Umifenovir (Arbidol)	S protein/ACE 2 membrane fusion inhibitor	Comparative randomized study with favipiravir showed fairly good results[30]
Imatinib	Tyrosine kinase inhibitor; used in cancer therapy including leukemias	At present only speculative. Randomized trials are planned
Toll-like receptor 4 agonist	Immunomodulators which could boost innate as well as adaptive immunity	At present only speculative. No definite in vitro, in vivo studies in COVID patients
K11777, camostat, nafamostat	Cysteine protease (TMPRSS2) inhibitors which prevents the viral entry into the host cell	At present only speculative. No definite in vitro, in vivo studies
Cepharanthine, selamectin, mefloquine	Group of antimalarial drugs with potential for repurposing to fight COVID	Only in vitro studies, no in vivo studies[31]
BCG vaccination	Induces cell-mediated immunity against mycobacterium tuberculosis. Could potentially improve overall innate/adaptive immunity	At present, no conclusive evidence. Several trials are underway
Killed suspension of *Mycobacterium* W.	Safe, killed suspension of *Mycobacterium* W (Sepsivac). Being used as a repurposed immunomodulator	Potentially likely to be developed earlier as compared to regular vaccines for COVID CSIR trials are likely to get underway

Abbreviations: ACE, angiotensin-converting enzyme; CSIR, Council of Scientific and Industrial Research; RCT, randomized controlled trials.

also been shown in a study.[33] However, current evidence does not favor the use of HCQ.

- Triple therapy: lopinavir/ritonavir + ribavirin + interferon-β. A randomized study of 120 people done between February and March 2020; 86 to combination group and 41 to control group (who received lopinavir/ritonavir combination). Primary end point is the time required to provide a negative nasopharyngeal swab. Combination group had a significantly shorter median time to negative nasopharyngeal swab than the control group (7 vs. 12 d; $p = 0.001$).[25–27]
- Remdesivir: It is an antiviral drug which acts by inhibiting the action of RNA polymerase, thus preventing viral replication. Two important studies have been performed.
  - ➢ Between January and March, 61 patients received remdesivir. Thirty of these patients were on mechanical ventilation and 4 were on extracorporeal membrane oxygenation (ECMO). At the end of a median follow-up of 18 days, 36 patients out of 61 had an improvement of oxygen-support class, including 17 patients on ventilator (57%), who were extubated.[27]
  - ➢ In a study of 237 patients between February and March 2020, patients were randomized into a 2:1 ratio with 158 in remdesivir group and 79 in placebo group. Although it was not statistically significant, patients in remdesivir group showed numerical reduction in time to clinical improvement.[26] Remdesivir therefore appears to be a promising drug requiring larger randomized studies to confirm its efficacy in the treatment of COVID-19 patients.

Latest antiviral drugs used in COVID-19:

- Although remdesivir was the antiviral drug used maximally, for COVID-19, during the first and second wave, newer combinations have come up in 2022. These are briefly mentioned below:
  - ➢ Nirmatrelvir-ritonavir and molnupiravir should be considered for patients with symptoms of COVID-19 who test positive for SARS-CoV-2 and either are an older adult (aged 65 y or older) or are aged 12 y or older with an underlying condition that increases risk of severe outcomes of COVID-19 (such as cancer, heart disease, diabetes, and obesity). Nirmatrelvir-ritonavir and molnupiravir reduce the ability of SARS-CoV-2 to multiply and spread through the body. While these drugs may not shorten the duration of symptoms, they decrease the need for hospitalization and work best when taken early in the course of COVID-19. Molnupiravir should not be prescribed to patients who are pregnant or attempting to become

pregnant. Men who have sexual contact with individuals of childbearing age should use a reliable method of contraception consistently while taking molnupiravir and for 3 months afterward. Use of molnupiravir is not authorized for patients younger than 18 years due to potential effects on bone and cartilage. Details of antiviral drugs are discussed in another chapter of this book.[29]
  - ➢ Convalescent plasma therapy aims at using antibodies from blood of recovered COVID-19 patients and use these passive antibodies in infective patients with COVID-19 in advance stages of the disease. Such treatment has been used earlier to treat severe viral infections. This therapy can also be used to immunize those at high risk for contracting the virus, such as health workers, families of patients, and other high-risk contacts. A sufficient amount of antibody must be administered.[30,32]
  - ➢ Favipiravir is an antiviral drug and inhibitor of RNA polymerase. Preliminary results show a moderate antiviral effect on COVID-19. It was earlier used for influenza virus and its status is investigational for COVID-19.

An in vitro study demonstrated moderate antiviral effect on COVID-19 in China. In a recent randomized study comparing two antiviral drugs: favipiravir and umifenovir ("Arbidol"), the favipiravir group showed relatively early symptomatic recovery (pyrexia and cough), although the rate of recovery and need for noninvasive ventilation as well as auxiliary oxygen therapy was in the same range.[31]

- BCG: Owing to a general observation that patients in tuberculosis endemic areas who receive BCG vaccination have a lower prevalence of respiratory influenza virus infections, including COVID-19 and have a faster recovery, it was proposed that BCG vaccination induces a nonspecific improvement in the adaptive immunity. Based on this, clinical trials have been started on the use of BCG vaccination, including a large proposed trial to be conducted by ICMR.[34]

Vaccines against SARS-CoV-2

Genetic sequence of SARS-CoV-2 was unraveled in January 2020 and this triggered a global intense R&D activity to develop a vaccine against this disease. Vaccines against coronavirus are available for safe clinical use in 2022 globally. These vaccines could be:

- Complete live attenuated vaccines (e.g., COVAXIN—undergoing Phase III trial developed by Bharat Biotech in collaboration with ICMR).
- Vector viral vaccine: The genetic material of COVID-19 is inserted into attenuated adenovirus. For example, COVISHIELD, Oxford-Astra Zeneca. This marketed by

Serum Institute of India and approved for emergency use by DCGI. Sputnik-5 marketed by Dr. Reddy's Lab. It was manufactured by Gamaleya Research Institute-Moscow and is approved for distribution in Russia. ZydusCov-D, manufactured by Cadilla in Ahmedabad.

- mRNA Vaccine: These are based on a novel concept of using mRNA to stimulate the synthesis of spike proteins in the injected human subjects, which then induce the antibody response. Therefore, these vaccines cannot cause corona disease itself. The two vaccines in this group (Pfizer and Moderna) have completed Phase III trials and the Pfizer vaccine (Pfizer and Biotech) has been accorded accelerated approval in the United Kingdom and has just been granted approval by FDA. However, both these vaccines require extremely low temperature for distribution and storage (−70°C for the Pfizer vaccine and −20°C for Moderna vaccine). The third mRNA vaccine by Genova Biopharmaceuticals in Pune in collaboration with HDT-biotech Corporation Seattle, USA, is undergoing Phase II trials in India.
- Plasmid DNA vaccine (BIO-E vaccine): Developed by Bio-E (Hyderabad) in collaboration with Johnson & Johnson is based on transferring the genetic material to the plasmid bacterial DNA (*E. coli*).

The Moderna and Pfizer vaccines have a reported efficacy rate of 90 to 95% in Phase III trials while the COVISHIELD has reported efficacy of 70 to 80% and COVAXIN has efficacy rate of 60 to 65%.

Though now, in 2022 with nearly 95% vaccination done in india, with approach vaccines with made in India mark as well, still research is on market as more various come to the, there will be an effective vaccine available from several of the above companies. Moreover, these vaccines will definitely be very useful in case of re-emergence of COVID infection in subsequent months or years and could potentially stop its spread before it devastates the social fabric and causes economic havoc as seen in the present outbreak. The lessons learnt from generation of these vaccines may also aid in the development of future vaccines against known or mutated coronaviruses.[35]

Development of vaccines to induce protective antibodies against COVID-19 infection has taken place at a relatively rapid pace over the last 8 to 10 months. Several vaccines are undergoing Phase II/III trials and few of them have been given accelerated approval for use after successful completion of Phase III trials. Most of these vaccines are based on live attenuated coronaviruses or vector-associated adenoviruses. However, recently a path-breaking technology based on mRNA which stimulates production of spike proteins in the injected humans, appears to be very promising and exciting. It is quite possible that many of these vaccines would be available for immunization to millions of individuals all over the globe, over the next few years to come as was seen last 24 years.

COVID Vaccinations in the Last 2 Years

In all, vaccine development continued apace, and by February 2021 Kyriakidis et al[36] described 64 candidate vaccines, developed using different technologies (mRNA, replication-defective viral vector, virus-like particle, inactivated virus, and protein subunit), as they entered Phase III clinical trials. By May 2021, McDonald et al[37] were able to compile a systematic review and meta-analysis that compared reactogenicity, immunogenicity, and efficacy of 18 candidate vaccines based on studies in nonhuman primates and humans. Not surprisingly, the different vaccines varied in their abilities to induce antibodies (including neutralizing antibodies), T-cell responses, and their reactogenicity and efficacy.

Kreps et al[38] investigated attitudes of the general public toward COVID-19 vaccination and identified that the public were confused in their understanding of the differences between "Emergency Use Authorization" and conventional "licensure." The findings of studies such as this one have implications regarding public health strategies for implementation of many vaccines, not only COVID, to increase levels of vaccination in the general public. Another concern of the public is around the safety and efficacy of vaccines in special populations. For example, Low et al[39] undertook an important study that demonstrated codominant IgG and IgA expression with minimal vaccine mRNA in milk of lactating women who received the Pfizer-BioNTech BNT162b2 and no adverse events in infants who breastfed from these vaccinees. Finally, the COVID pandemic has identified the need for pandemic preparedness in the future for other pathogens, and Monrad et al[40] discuss the important issues of how we could finance such activities moving forward.

Does This World Still Need New COVID-19 Vaccines?

As in the efficacy trials of the vaccines already in use, estimates of omicron-specific vaccine efficacy are lacking, as well as data on durability of protection and safety in subpopulations such as older persons, pregnant women, and persons with immunosuppression. The first COVID-19 vaccines used during the pandemic may not be the best long-term solution. The next generation of COVID-19 vaccines will need to have broader epitope coverage to provide cross-immunity against SARS-CoV-2 variants, confer a longer duration of protection, and be easy to update in a timely manner for protection against any new variants. We may increasingly need to mix and match vaccines to leverage the benefits of each of these platforms. Finally, currently available vaccines have only modest effectiveness against mild infection and transmission, which is further reduced in the context of the newly emerging omicron subvariants (**Box 28.3**).[41]

Box 28.3 Important factors of COVID-19 vaccines

- Ease of schedules
- Vaccine effectiveness when used in routine programs
- Need and frequency of boosters
- Cost
- Considerations regarding cold-chain logistics
- Manufacturing scalability
- Acceptability by communities
- Scope for local or regional production

Conclusion and Summary

Cardiac complications in COVID-19 infections are relatively rare in young individuals with no associated pre-existing comorbidities. However, in the middle-aged/elderly patients with associated cardiac, pulmonary, renal, or hepatic disease, cardiovascular complications are not uncommon and their management could be quite challenging. In such patients, a cautious use of echocardiography using the POCUS protocol is advised. However, in patients with normal troponin and NT-proBNP levels, the use of this technique could be avoided. The echocardiographic procedure could also be obviated if the patients are undergoing CT evaluation for suspected pulmonary embolism and a cardiac CT could be included in the same sitting. Moreover, if coronary angiography or PCI is being contemplated, an additional LV angiogram could also avoid an echocardiographic procedure. However, in critically ill patients who cannot be transported for CT/angiography, bedside echocardiography could be critical for diagnosis and management of such patients. When such echocardiography studies are indicated, adequate draping of the echocardiography equipment is essential to avoid contamination. In addition, appropriate protection of echocardiographic personnel with high-quality PPE kits is extremely important. In hemodynamically unstable and decompensated patients, intensive monitoring in the ICU and an appropriate use of vasopressor, inotropes, diuretics, as well as antiarrhythmics are required. The use of antiviral drugs in patients with COVID-19 infections has been largely empirical with very few adequately controlled randomized studies being available. However, at present remdesivir is an extremely promising antiviral drug for COVID-19 infections and is in widespread use. The evidence for the use of other drugs (many of them being repurposed therapies) is quite scanty, and in some cases only in vitro studies have been performed. Although the use of convalescent plasma therapy is quite prevalent, the results are inconsistent. Considerable controversy exists on the use of immunomodulators (BCG Vaccination, mycobacterium W) to stimulate nonspecific immunity, and authoritative randomized studies are not available.

Targeting inflammation to prevent thrombosis leaves haemostasis mainly unaffected, circumventing the risk of bleeding associated with current approaches. Considering the growing number of anti-inflammatory therapies, it is crucial to appreciate their potential in covering therapeutic gaps in cardiovascular diseases.[42]

References

1. Guzik TJ, Mohiddin SA, Dimarco A, et al. COVID-19 and the cardiovascular system: implications for risk assessment, diagnosis, and treatment options. Cardiovasc Res 2020;116(10):1666–1687
2. Cascella M, Rajnik M, Cuomo A, et al. Features, evaluation and treatment coronavirus (COVID-19) [Updated 2020 Apr 6]. In: StatPearls [Internet]. Treasure Island, FL: StatPearls Publishing; 2020
3. Ye Q, Wang B, Mao J. The pathogenesis and treatment of the "Cytokine Storm" in COVID-19. J Infect 2020;80(6):607–613
4. Hoffmann M, Kleine-Weber H, Schroeder S, et al. SARS-CoV-2 cell entry depends on ACE2 and TMPRSS2 and is blocked by a clinically proven protease inhibitor. Cell 2020;181(2):271–280.e8
5. Kuster GM, Pfister O, Burkard T, et al. SARS-CoV2: should inhibitors of the renin–angiotensin system be withdrawn in patients with COVID-19? Eur Heart J 2020;41(19):1801–1803
6. Basu-Ray Indranill, Soos Michael P. Cardiac manifestations of coronavirus (COVID-19). NCBI Bookshelf. A Service of the National Library of Medicine, National Institutes of Health.
7. Zheng Y-Y, Ma Y-T, Zhang JY, Xie X. COVID-19 and the cardiovascular system. Nat Rev Cardiol 2020;17(5):259–260
8. Ruan Q, Yang K, Wang W, Jiang L, Song J. Clinical predictors of mortality due to COVID-19 based on an analysis of data of 150 patients from Wuhan, China. Intensive Care Med 2020;46(5):846–848
9. Liu Y, Yan LM, Wan L, et al. Viral dynamics in mild and severe cases of COVID-19. Lancet Infect Dis 2020;20(6):656–657
10. Kwong JC, Schwartz KL, Campitelli MA, et al. Acute myocardial infarction after laboratory-confirmed influenza infection. N Engl J Med 2018;378(4):345–353
11. Smeeth L, Thomas SL, Hall AJ, Hubbard R, Farrington P, Vallance P. Risk of myocardial infarction and stroke after acute infection or vaccination. N Engl J Med 2004;351(25):2611–2618
12. Bangalore S, Sharma A, Slotwiner A, et al. ST-segment elevation in patients with Covid-19: a Case Series. N Engl J Med 2020;382(25):2478–2480
13. Shi S, Qin M, Shen B, et al. Association of cardiac injury with mortality in hospitalized patients with COVID-19 in Wuhan, China. JAMA Cardiol 2020;5(7):802–810
14. Guo T, Fan Y, Chen M, et al. Cardiovascular implications of fatal outcomes of patients with coronavirus disease 2019 (COVID-19). JAMA Cardiol 2020;5(7):811–818
15. Prutkin JM, Knight BP, et al. Coronavirus disease 2019 (COVID-19): Arrhythmias and conduction system disease. https://www.uptodate.com/contents/coronavirus-disease-2019
16. Lakkireddy DR, Chung MK, Gopinathannair R, et al; Guidance for Cardiac Electrophysiology During the Coronavirus (COVID-19) Pandemic from the Heart Rhythm Society COVID-19 Task Force. Guidance for Cardiac Electrophysiology During the COVID-19 Pandemic from the Heart Rhythm Society COVID-19 Task Force; Electrophysiology Section of the American College of Cardiology; and the Electrocardiography and Arrhythmias

Committee of the Council on Clinical Cardiology, American Heart Association. Circulation 2020;141(21):e823–e831

17. Ezad S, McGee M, Boyle AJ. Takotsubo syndrome associated with ST elevation myocardial infarction. Case Rep Cardiol 2019;2019:1010243

18. Roca E, Lombardi C, et al. Takotsubo syndrome associated with COVID-19. https://www.ejcrim.com/index.php/EJCRIM/article/view/1665/2065

19. Klok FA, Kruip MJHA, van der Meer NJM, et al. Incidence of thrombotic complications in critically ill ICU patients with COVID-19. Thromb Res 2020;191:145–147

20. Danzi GB, Loffi M, Galeazzi G, Gherbesi E. Acute pulmonary embolism and COVID-19 pneumonia: a random association? Eur Heart J 2020;41(19):1858

21. Tang N, Li D, Wang X, Sun Z. Abnormal coagulation parameters are associated with poor prognosis in patients with novel coronavirus pneumonia. J Thromb Haemost 2020;18(4): 844–847

22. Kirkpatrick J, Mitchell C, Taub C, et al. ASE statement on protection of patients and echocardiography service providers during the 2019 novel coronavirus outbreak. https://www.asecho.org/wp-content/uploads/2020/03/COVIDStatementFINAL4-1-2020_v2_website.pdf. Acccessed April 13, 2020.

23. Peng Q-Y, Wang X-T, Zhang LN; Chinese Critical Care Ultrasound Study Group (CCUSG). Using echocardiography to guide the treatment of novel coronavirus pneumonia. Crit Care 2020;24(1):143

24. Gautret P, Lagier JC, Parola P, et al. Hydroxychloroquine and azithromycin as a treatment of COVID-19: results of an open-label non-randomized clinical trial. Int J Antimicrob Agents 2020;56(1):105949

25. Hung IF, Lung KC, Tso EY, et al. Triple combination of interferon beta-1b, lopinavir-ritonavir, and ribavirin in the treatment of patients admitted to hospital with COVID-19: an open-label, randomised, phase 2 trial. Lancet 2020;395(10238):1695–1704

26. Wang Y, Zhang D, Du G, et al. Remdesivir in adults with severe COVID-19: a randomised, double-blind, placebo-controlled, multicentre trial. Lancet 2020;395(10236):1569–1578

27. Grein J, Ohmagari N, Shin D, et al. Compassionate use of remdesivir for patients with severe Covid-19. N Engl J Med 2020;382(24):2327–2336

28. Leon C, Druce J, et al. The FDA-approved drug ivermectin inhibits the replication of SARS-CoV-2 in vitro. Antiviral Res 2020;178:104787

29. Gandhi RT, Malani PN, Del Rio C. COVID-19 therapeutics for nonhospitalized patients. JAMA 2022;327(7):617–618

30. Shen C, Wang Z, Zhao F, et al. Treatment of 5 critically ill patients with COVID-19 with convalescent plasma. JAMA 2020;323(16):1582–1589

31. Chen C, Huang J, Cheng Z, Wu J, Chen S, Zhang Y, Chen B, Lu M, LuoY, Zhang J, et al. Favipiravir versus Arbidol for COVID-19: a randomized clinical trial. medRxiv 2020. doi: https://doi.org/10.1101/2020.03.17.20037432

32. Fan H-H, Wang L-Q, Liu WL, et al. Repurposing of clinically approved drugs for treatment of coronavirus disease 2019 in a 2019-novel coronavirus-related coronavirus model. Chin Med J (Engl) 2020;133(9):1051–1056

33. Liu J, Cao R, Xu M, et al. Hydroxychloroquine, a less toxic derivative of chloroquine, is effective in inhibiting SARS-CoV-2 infection in vitro. Cell Discov 2020;6:16

34. Curtis N, Sparrow A, Ghebreyesus TA, Netea MG. Considering BCG vaccination to reduce the impact of COVID-19. Lancet 2020;395(10236):1545–1546

35. Le TT, Cramer JP, Chen R, Mayhew S. Evolution of the COVID-19 vaccine development landscape. Nat Rev Drug Discov 2020;19(10):667–668

36. Kyriakidis NC, López-Cortés A, González EV, Grimaldos AB, Prado EO. SARS-CoV-2 vaccines strategies: a comprehensive review of phase 3 candidates. NPJ Vaccines 2021;6(1):28

37. McDonald I, Murray SM, Reynolds CJ, Altmann DM, Boyton RJ. Comparative systematic review and meta-analysis of reactogenicity, immunogenicity and efficacy of vaccines against SARS-CoV-2. NPJ Vaccines 2021;6(1):74

38. Kreps S, Dasgupta N, Brownstein JS, Hswen Y, Kriner DL. Public attitudes toward COVID-19 vaccination: the role of vaccine attributes, incentives, and misinformation. NPJ Vaccines 2021;6(1):73

39. Low JM, Gu Y, Ng MSF, et al. Codominant IgG and IgA expression with minimal vaccine mRNA in milk of BNT162b2 vaccinees. NPJ Vaccines 2021;6(1):105

40. Monrad JT, Sandbrink JB, Cherian NG. Promoting versatile vaccine development for emerging pandemics. NPJ Vaccines 2021;6(1):26

41. World Health Organization. WHO SAGE Roadmap for prioritizing uses of COVID-19 vaccines. January 21, 2022. https:// www.who.int/publications/i/item/WHO-2019-nCoV-Vaccines-SAGE-Prioritization-2022.1

42. Stark K, Massberg S. Interplay Between Inflammation and Thrombosis in Cardiovascular Pathology. Nat Rev Cardiol. 2021 Sep;18(9):666–682

29

Hemostasis in COVID-19 Infection: Learnings So Far!

Ajay Gandhi, Klaus Gorlinger, and Poonam Malhotra Kapoor

Introduction

In the last 20 years, several viral epidemics, such as the severe acute respiratory syndrome coronavirus (SARS-CoV) in 2002, and H1N1 influenza in 2009, have been recorded. The Middle East respiratory syndrome coronavirus (MERS-CoV) was first identified in Saudi Arabia in 2012. Recently, an epidemic with unexplained low respiratory infections began in Wuhan, China, and the first case was reported on December 31, 2019. Published literature can trace the beginning of symptomatic individuals to the beginning of December 2019. This SARS-CoV-2 virus, which causes COVID-19, is very contagious and it quickly spread globally. On January 30, 2020, as per the International Health Regulations, the outbreak was declared by the WHO a Public Health Emergency of International Concern (PHEIC) as it had spread to 18 countries with four countries reporting human-to-human transmission.

Pathogenetic Mechanism of Action

The SARS-CoV-2 virus passes through the mucous membranes, especially nasal and laryngeal mucosa, and then enters the lungs through the respiratory tract. It enters the cells via the angiotensin-converting enzyme 2 (ACE2) receptors, which are most commonly found in the alveolar epithelial cells, followed by endothelial cells. Other organs having these receptors are the renal and the gastrointestinal tracts.

The pathogenic mechanism that produces pneumonia seems to be particularly complex. Among the known mechanisms, the viral infection is capable of triggering an excessive immune reaction in the host. In some cases, a reaction takes place which as a whole is labeled a "cytokine storm."[1,2] The effect is extensive tissue damage. The protagonist of this storm is interleukin 6 (IL-6). IL-6 is produced by activated leukocytes and acts on multiple cells and tissues. Physiologically, IL-6 increases during inflammatory diseases, infections, autoimmune disorders, cardiovascular diseases, and some types of cancer. It is also implicated into the pathogenesis of the cytokine release syndrome (CRS), which is an acute systemic inflammatory response syndrome (SIRS), characterized by fever and multiple organ dysfunction. Regarding the cardiovascular system, the virus can bind to the endothelial cells and may cause damage to the blood vessels, in particular to the microcirculation of the small blood vessels, which can lead to platelet activation and aggregation.

Hence, the human coronavirus HCoV-19 infection can cause acute respiratory distress syndrome (ARDS), hypercoagulability, hypertension, and extrapulmonary multiorgan dysfunction.

Clinical Course

The clinical phase is divided into three parts: the viremia phase, the acute phase (pneumonia phase), and the recovery phase. If the immune function of patients in the acute phase (pneumonia phase) is effective, and there are no more basic diseases, the virus can be effectively suppressed and then comes the recovery phase. If the patient is older, or in an immune-impaired state, combined with other basic diseases such as hypertension and diabetes, the immune system cannot effectively control the virus in the acute phase (pneumonia phase), then the patient will become severe or critical type.

COVID-19 and Changes in Hemostasis

The characteristic clinicopathologic manifestations in patients infected by SARS-CoV-2 virus are as follows:

1. Hypercoagulability: Although the incidence of thrombosis in patients with COVID-19 has not been statistically determined, about 50% of patients with COVID-19 are accompanied by elevated D-dimer levels during disease progression, and this proportion is as high as 100% in death cases. The level of D-dimer in severe patients is significantly higher than that in mild patients. Accordingly, elevated D-dimers (>1 mg/mL; 18.42; 95% confidence interval [CI], 2.64–128.55; p = 0.0033) have to be considered as a marker of poor outcome in patients with COVID-19 infection.[2-6] Hence admission to hospital should be considered in patients with raised D-dimer even in the absence of other severity symptoms since this clearly signifies *increased thrombin generation.*

COVID-19 pathological changes are mainly focused on the lungs; alveolar septal blood vessels are congested. Edema and clear thrombus formation in the blood vessels can be seen; therefore, this fibrin thrombus is different from white thrombus in the lungs of SARS patients.

Taking into account hemoconcentration, vascular endothelial injury, and hypercoagulable state of patients with COVID-19, in combination with bedridden, obesity, advanced age, and other risk factors, risk of thrombosis is increased in this patient population. Therefore, the risk of venous thromboembolism (VTE) cannot be ignored during the course and treatment of COVID-19.

2. Diffuse microvascular damage: Multiple organ failure caused by diffuse microvascular damage is an important cause of death in critically ill patients with COVID-19 and may be related to CRS caused by immune imbalance. In severe cases, the final result is either septic shock or ARDS. About 80% of patients meet the diagnostic criteria for disseminated intravascular coagulation (DIC), and most of them are in the DIC hypercoagulable stage, and some even have gangrene.

3. Bleeding risk: Interestingly, COVID-19 patients *may* also have an increased risk of bleeding due to *imbalances in platelet production and consumption*, and disorders of the coagulation system.[7] Coagulation dysfunction is found in almost all severe and critically ill patients. Consumption of platelets and coagulation factors may increase the risk of bleeding, which is not helpful to the control of primary disease and anticoagulation, intubation, and other treatments.

Laboratory Examination of Coagulopathy in Patients with COVID-19

- Elevated D-dimers can occur in 50% of patients with COVID-19, and fibrinogen degradation products (FDPs) and D-dimers are *significantly higher* in severe patients and nonsurvivors compared to mild patients and survivors.[2-6]
- As an acute response protein, fibrinogen may be *increased in the course of mild disease* and in the early stages of severe patients and can be *significantly reduced in the late stages* of severe patients. However, this increase is usually less pronounced in viral compared to bacterial sepsis.
- Prothrombin time (PT) and activated partial thromboplastin time (APTT) is *shortened* in a good number of cases, although *prolonged* results can also be seen in a proportion of the patients, particularly in the late stages and nonsurvivors.
- Most patients with COVID-19 have platelet count in the normal range, although the incidence of thrombocytopenia varies, the numbers falling with increasing severity.

Causes and Mechanisms of COVID-19 Coagulation Dysfunction

- **Viral infection:**
  - Both 2019-nCoV and SARS-CoV infect humans with angiotensin-converting enzyme 2 (ACE2), but the binding ability of former is 10 to 20 times that of latter.
  - After 2019-nCoV enters the body, it can be quickly recognized by the pathogen-associated molecular patterns (PAMPs) in the body, activating the innate immune system to clear the virus, but excessive activation can cause a cytokine storm, cause damage to the microvascular system, and inhibit anticoagulation system. DIC results in extensive microthrombosis in small vessels, leading to microcirculation disorders, which can cause severe multiple organ dysfunction syndrome (MODS).

- **Cytokine release syndrome:**
  - IL1β, IL6, IL12, IFNγ, IL-10, and monocyte chemokine 1 in patients with SARS are associated with pulmonary inflammation and severe lung injury.
  - IL-6 plays an important role in the network of inflammatory mediators. It can cause coagulation disorders through multiple pathways, such as stimulating the liver to synthesize more thrombopoietin, fibrinogen, etc., and destroying it by up-regulating the expression of vascular endothelial growth factor.

- **Immune-mediated damage to hematopoietic system:**
  - Coronavirus receptors include CD13, and human hematopoietic stem cells, megakaryocytes; platelets usually express high CD13. The virus can directly damage megakaryocytes and platelets by binding to CD13, invade hematopoietic stem cells, or infect bone marrow stromal cells and cause hematopoietic inhibition, resulting in reduced platelet production, or immune pathway activation of complement leading to increased platelet destruction.
  - The lung is one of the organs from which mature megakaryocytes release platelets. Lung damage reduces the division of megakaryocytes in the lungs, resulting in a decrease in platelet production. The inflammatory damage caused by this causes lung platelets to aggregate and cause thrombosis, leading to increased platelet depletion and destruction.

- **Ischemic hypoxia-reperfusion injury:**
  - Normal endothelial cells have anticoagulant properties. Hypoxia can reduce the anticoagulant properties of endothelial cells, increase permeability and leukocyte adhesion, and blood vessels are dominated by proinflammatory properties.
  - Endothelial cells express ACE2. Therefore, 2019-nCoV may aggravate endothelial cell damage, up-regulate tissue factor expression on the cell surface, and lose antithrombin, tissue factor pathway inhibitor (TFPI), and protein C, thereby damaging the overall endogenous anticoagulant system.

- **Drugs and operating factors:**
  - Certain antiviral drugs (α-interferon, ribavirin, abidol, oseltamivir, etc.), certain antibacterial drugs (moxifloxacin, etc.) can directly inhibit the hematopoietic system or induce liver injury, thereby reducing the synthesis of coagulation factors.

> During extracorporeal pulmonary oxygenation (ECMO) therapy, apart from additional release of inflammatory mediators such as IL-6, the artificial biological materials on the surface of extracorporeal circulation circuits can trigger activation of the coagulation system.[8–10]

- **Inappropriate use of blood products:**
  > As an immediate control measure to shock, a large amount of packed red blood cells may be transfused within a short time, which will dilute other blood components, may cause hypothermia, and may affect the coagulation system.
  > Platelets, plasma, and cryoprecipitate should ideally be administered according to relevant indicators such as clinically relevant bleeding and coagulation testing.

Treatment of Coagulopathy in COVID-19

1. Dynamic monitoring, early detection, and prevention of coagulopathy: COVID-19-induced coagulopathy is a dynamic process. Dynamic monitoring of hemostasis, rational use of viscoelastic testing (TEG, ROTEM) and other technologies, and the use of the Clinical Decision Support System (CDSS) for the detection of SIRS, sepsis, and septic shock, sepsis-induced coagulopathy (SIC), and the ISTH DIC score can be helpful in early detection, early diagnosis, and prevention of coagulopathy.[11–21]

2. Prevention and treatment of venous thrombosis: Most patients with COVID-19 have a hypercoagulable state. VTE risk assessment should be performed as soon as possible, and thromboembolic-related examinations should be performed, if necessary.

3. Stratified treatment of DIC: Early identification of DIC, classification or staging, and stratified treatment based on DIC clinical stage is recommended. It is not appropriate to simply supplement platelets and coagulation factors. Use of antifibrinolytic drugs in sepsis and DIC should be rationalized and considered cautiously.

4. Prevention of bleeding: Ideally, the first aim should be to treat the primary disease and to decrease the activation and consumption of platelets, coagulation inhibitors, and coagulation factors by the infection. Furthermore, risks and benefits of platelet transfusion have to be considered carefully, since it may trigger further inflammation and may increase mortality in nonbleeding patients.[22–25]

5. Supportive therapy and other treatments: Patients with severe pneumonia need oxygen, positive end expiratory pressure (PEEP)/respiratory therapy, and prone positioning.[10,26–31] Thromboprophylaxis, drugs to improve microcirculation, and vascular permeability should be considered.[32–38] Supplements, such as high-dose vitamin C, enhance immunity and may be beneficial.[39–41]

Some bullet points related to hemostasis in COVID-19
- Patients on chronic anticoagulant therapy are not considered "high risk" for COVID-19.[42]
- Fibrinogen, being an acute phase reactant, can rise with many infections due to different causes (bacterial more than viral sepsis). In case of COVID-19 patients, it rises in the early phase.
- D-dimer is a nonspecific marker of inflammation or infection and is a good predictor of poor outcome in patients with COVID-19 infections.
- Although elevated D-dimer levels have been interpreted as indicating thrombosis, they are elevated in many other disorders including infection. Therefore, an elevated D-dimer level in patients with COVID-19 infection *alone* does not provide evidence for thrombosis.
- The risk factors of older age, high sequential organ failure assessment (SOFA) score, and D-dimers higher than 1 mg/mL are most prominently associated with poor course and increased mortality.[3,43,44] D-dimer actually provides value in prognostication of outcome in hospitalized patients with or without sepsis and with or without COVID-19.

Conclusion

A relevant cause of hemostasis disorders is inflammation and cytokine storms, which cause, for example, endothelial dysfunction in blood vessels. In order to prevent and treat states of hypercoagulability and thrombosis, the administration of anticoagulants, e.g., heparin, is recommended.[45] Recently, there have been studies involving combination therapy with nafamostat and heparin. Nafamostat is a serine proteinase inhibitor used, among other factors, in treating disseminated intravascular coagulation (DIC). A study was conducted in a patient with COVID-19 pneumonia, hypoxemia and pulmonary embolism. The use of a combination of heparin and nafamostat resulted in significant improvements, which is promising for the effective treatment of severely ill COVID-19 patients. The advantage of nafamostat is that it does not cause bleeding as a side effect—unlike heparin, it also has antiviral effects and could be effective in treating DIC in patients with COVID-19.[46]

References

1. Ruan Q, Yang K, Wang W, et al. Clinical predictors of mortality due to COVID-19 based on an analysis of data of 150 patients from Wuhan, China. Intensive Care Med. 2020 Mar 3. doi:

10.1007/s00134 -020- 05991-x. [Epub ahead of print] https://link.springer.com/content/pdf/10.1007/s00134-020-05991-x.pdf

2. Gao Y, Li T, Han M, et al. Diagnostic utility of clinical laboratory data determinations for patients with the severe COVID-19. J Med Virol 2020;92(7):791–796

3. Zhou F, Yu T, Du R, et al. Clinical course and risk factors for mortality of adult inpatients with COVID-19 in Wuhan, China: a retrospective cohort study. Lancet 2020;395(10229):1054–1062

4. Wu C, Chen X, Cai Y, et al. Risk factors associated with acute respiratory distress syndrome and death in patients with coronavirus disease 2019 pneumonia in Wuhan, China. JAMA Intern Med 2020;180(7):934–943

5. Tang N, Li D, Wang X, Sun Z. Abnormal coagulation parameters are associated with poor prognosis in patients with novel coronavirus pneumonia. J Thromb Haemost 2020;18(4):844–847

6. Han H, Yang L, Liu R, et al. Prominent changes in blood coagulation of patients with SARS-CoV-2 infection. Clin Chem Lab Med 2020;58(7):1116–1120

7. Magdi M, Rahil A. Severe immune thrombocytopenia complicated by intracerebral haemorrhage associated with coronavirus infection: a case report and literature review. Eur J Case Rep Intern Med 2019;6(7):001155

8. MacLaren G, Fisher D, Brodie D. Preparing for the most critically ill patients with COVID-19: the potential role of extracorporeal membrane oxygenation. JAMA 2020;323(13):1245–1246

9. Henry BM. COVID-19, ECMO, and lymphopenia: a word of caution. Lancet Respir Med 2020;8(4):e24

10. Yang X, Yu Y, Xu J, et al. Clinical course and outcomes of critically ill patients with SARS-CoV-2 pneumonia in Wuhan, China: a single-centered, retrospective, observational study. Lancet Respir Med 2020;8(5):475–481

11. Boscolo A, Spiezia L, Campello E, et al. Whole-blood hypocoagulable profile correlates with a greater risk of death within 28 days in patients with severe sepsis. Korean J Anesthesiol 2020;73(3):224–231

12. Müller MCA, Meijers JC, van Meenen DM, Thachil J, Juffermans NP. Thromboelastometry in critically ill patients with disseminated intravascular coagulation. Blood Coagul Fibrinolysis 2019;30(5):181–187

13. Schmitt FCF, Manolov V, Morgenstern J, et al. Acute fibrinolysis shutdown occurs early in septic shock and is associated with increased morbidity and mortality: results of an observational pilot study. Ann Intensive Care 2019;9(1):19

14. Koami H, Sakamoto Y, Ohta M, et al. Can rotational thromboelastometry predict septic disseminated intravascular coagulation? Blood Coagul Fibrinolysis 2015;26(7):778–783

15. Andersen MG, Hvas CL, Tønnesen E, Hvas AM. Thromboelastometry as a supplementary tool for evaluation of hemostasis in severe sepsis and septic shock. Acta Anaesthesiol Scand 2014;58(5):525–533

16. Müller MC, Meijers JC, Vroom MB, Juffermans NP. Utility of thromboelastography and/or thromboelastometry in adults with sepsis: a systematic review. Crit Care 2014;18(1):R30

17 Adamzik M, Schafer S, Frey UH, et al. The NFKB1 promoter polymorphism (-94ins/delATTG) alters nuclear translocation of NF-κB1 in monocytes after lipopolysaccharide stimulation and is associated with increased mortality in sepsis. Anesthesiology 2013;118(1):123–133

18. Adamzik M, Görlinger K, Peters J, Hartmann M. Whole blood impedance aggregometry as a biomarker for the diagnosis and prognosis of severe sepsis. Crit Care 2012;16(5):R204

19. Brenner T, Schmidt K, Delang M, et al. Viscoelastic and aggregometric point-of-care testing in patients with septic shock - cross-links between inflammation and haemostasis. Acta Anaesthesiol Scand 2012;56(10):1277–1290

20. Adamzik M, Langemeier T, Frey UH, et al. Comparison of thrombelastometry with simplified acute physiology score II and sequential organ failure assessment scores for the prediction of 30-day survival: a cohort study. Shock 2011;35(4):339–342

21. Adamzik M, Eggmann M, Frey UH, et al. Comparison of thromboelastometry with procalcitonin, interleukin 6, and C-reactive protein as diagnostic tests for severe sepsis in critically ill adults. Crit Care 2010;14(5):R178

22. Warner MA, Chandran A, Frank RD, Kor DJ. Prophylactic platelet transfusions for critically ill patients with thrombocytopenia: a single-institution propensity-matched cohort study. Anesth Analg 2019;128(2):288–295

23. Schmidt AE, Henrichs KF, Kirkley SA, Refaai MA, Blumberg N. Prophylactic preprocedure platelet transfusion is associated with increased risk of thrombosis and mortality. Am J Clin Pathol 2017;149(1):87–94

24. Zakko L, Rustagi T, Douglas M, Laine L. No benefit from platelet transfusion for gastrointestinal bleeding in patients taking antiplatelet agents. Clin Gastroenterol Hepatol 2017;15(1):46–52

25. Baharoglu MI, Cordonnier C, Al-Shahi Salman R, et al; PATCH Investigators. Platelet transfusion versus standard care after acute stroke due to spontaneous cerebral haemorrhage associated with antiplatelet therapy (PATCH): a randomised, open-label, phase 3 trial. Lancet 2016;387(10038):2605–2613

26. Kluge S, Janssens U, Welte T, et al. Recommendations for critically ill patients with COVID-19. Med Klin Intensivmed Notfmed. 2020 Mar 12. Doi: 10.1007/s00063-020-00674-3. [Epub ahead of print] https://link.springer.com/article/10.1007/s00063-020-00674-3

27. Li T. Diagnosis and clinical management of severe acute respiratory syndrome Coronavirus 2 (SARS-CoV-2) infection: an operational recommendation of Peking Union Medical College Hospital (V2.0). Emerg Microbes Infect 2020;9(1):582–585

28. He F, Deng Y, Li W. Coronavirus disease 2019: What we know? J Med Virol 2020;92(7):719–725

29. Wang D, Hu B, Hu C, et al. Clinical characteristics of 138 hospitalized patients with 2019 novel coronavirus-infected pneumonia in Wuhan, China. JAMA 2020;323(11):1061–1069

30. Huang C, Wang Y, Li X, et al. Clinical features of patients infected with 2019 novel coronavirus in Wuhan, China. Lancet 2020;395(10223):497–506

31. Clerkin KJ, Fried JA, Raikhelkar J, et al. Coronavirus disease 2019 (COVID-19) and cardiovascular disease. Circulation. 2020 Mar 21. doi: 10.1161/CIRCULATIONAHA.120.046941. [Epub ahead of print] https://www.ahajournals.org/doi/pdf/10.1161/CIRCULATIONAHA.120.046941

32. Lin L, Lu L, Cao W, Li T. Hypothesis for potential pathogenesis of SARS-CoV-2 infection-a review of immune changes in patients with viral pneumonia. Emerg Microbes Infect 2020;9(1):727–732

33. Tang N, Bai H, Chen X, et al. Anticoagulant treatment is associated with decreased mortality in severe coronavirus

disease 2019 patients with coagulopathy. J Thromb Haemost. 2020 Mar 27. doi: 10.1111/jth.14817. [Epub ahead of print] https://onlinelibrary.wiley.com/doi/epdf/10.1111/jth.14817

34. Murao S, Yamakawa K. A systematic summary of systematic reviews on anticoagulant therapy in sepsis. J Clin Med 2019;8(11):E1869

35. Boddi M, Peris A. Deep vein thrombosis in intensive care. Adv Exp Med Biol 2017;906:167–181

36. Hanify JM, Dupree LH, Johnson DW, Ferreira JA. Failure of chemical thromboprophylaxis in critically ill medical and surgical patients with sepsis. J Crit Care 2017;37:206–210

37. Branchford BR, Carpenter SL. The role of inflammation in venous thromboembolism. Front Pediatr 2018;6:142

38. Iba T, Gando S, Thachil J. Anticoagulant therapy for sepsis-associated disseminated intravascular coagulation: the view from Japan. J Thromb Haemost 2014;12(7):1010–1019

39. Iglesias J, Vassallo AV, Patel VV, Sullivan JB, Cavanaugh J, Elbaga Y. Outcomes of metabolic resuscitation using ascorbic acid, thiamine, and glucocorticoids in the early treatment of sepsis: the ORANGES trial. Chest 2020;158(1):164–173

40. Marik PE. Vitamin C: an essential "stress hormone" during sepsis. J Thorac Dis 2020;12(Suppl 1):S84–S88

41. Belsky JB, Wira CR, Jacob V, Sather JE, Lee PJ. A review of micronutrients in sepsis: the role of thiamine, l-carnitine, vitamin C, selenium and vitamin D. Nutr Res Rev 2018; 31(2):281–290

42. https://www.worldthrombosisday.org/news/post/anticoagulation-forum-managing-anticoagulation-during-covid-19-pandemic-frequently-asked-questions/

43. Ferreira FL, Bota DP, Bross A, Mélot C, Vincent JL. Serial evaluation of the SOFA score to predict outcome in critically ill patients. JAMA 2001;286(14):1754–1758

44. Vincent JL, de Mendonça A, Cantraine F, et al. Use of the SOFA score to assess the incidence of organ dysfunction/failure in intensive care units: results of a multicenter, prospective study. Working group on "sepsis-related problems" of the European Society of Intensive Care Medicine. Crit Care Med 1998;26(11):1793–1800

45. Ulanowska M, Olas B. Modulation of Hemostasis in COVID-19; Blood Platelets May Be Important Pieces in the COVID-19 Puzzle. Pathogens. 2021;10(3):370

46. Asakura H., Ogawa H. Potential of heparin and nafamostat combination therapy for COVID-19. J. Thromb. Haemost. 2020;18:1521–1522

30

Antiviral Drugs

Poonam Malhotra Kapoor, Mohit Prakash, Pranav Kapoor, and Omer Mohammed Mujahid

Introduction

Viruses versus Microbes: Are They Alike?

Viruses are different from microbes. The many differences seen are briefly discussed in this chapter.

First, viruses do not self-multiply, which is unlike microbes. It has to attach to and enter a host cell to synthesize proteins like DNA and RNA. Thus, it replicates only with the help of a host cell. Second, viruses are difficult to kill as they live within a host cell. An antiviral drug that kills the virus will also kill the host cells. Some viruses that are prevalent in the environment are easily controlled by available antiviral therapy. These are listed in **Box 30.1**.

The action of antiviral drugs is transient. As soon as these drugs are stopped, the viral growth surfaces again. The viruses need to be phosphorylated by enzymes in order to remain active. Acyclovir, which is a prototype of antiviral drugs, and other antiviral drugs inhibit active multiplication within the host cells; thus the antiviral effect is nullified on the removal of these drugs.

Antiviral Drugs in the ICU

Post-COVID in 2020–21, the role of antiviral drugs has come to the forefront. A large number of viruses (**Box 30.1**) can be controlled by antiviral drugs, with excellent outcomes. Antiviral drugs such as remdesivir, hydroquinone, lopinavir, and interferon were removed from the list of essential anti-COVID drugs by the WHO in 2020–21 as these drugs had less effect on the hospital/ICU length of stay in a sick COVID-19 patient during the pandemic.[1,2]

Pathophysiology of Antiviral Drugs

It is important to know that viruses have no cell wall and no metabolic machinery of their own; they use host enzymes to multiply either in the cytoplasm or nucleus of the host cells. Thus, most viruses are made up of nucleic acid components (DNA/RNA) and all viruses are obligate parasites.

The chemical structure of antiviral drugs is either purine or pyrimidine in nature. As shown in **Figs. 30.1** and **30.2**,

viruses differ from bacteria and infect all parts of the human body.

Viruses attack each and every organ system of the human body, as shown in **Fig. 30.3**. Polio, influenza, herpes, cytomegalovirus (CMV), hepatitis, varicella, etc., are all virus-borne diseases, afflicting different organ systems.

Important things to note here are that:

Current antiviral agents do not eliminate nonreplicating or latent virus. Effective host immune response is essential for recovery from viral infection. Clinical efficacy depends on achieving inhibitory concentration at the site of infection within the infected cells. The antiviral drugs block or inhibit the virus within the cells by transcript or genome translation and also by early and late protein synthesis.[3,4]

Antiherpes Viral Agents

Antiherpes viral agents are a major group of antiviral drugs, which are in use since long. They are enlisted in **Box 30.2** with their prototypes and their pharmacology.

Acyclovir Antiviral Activities

The action of acyclovir is highly selective. It activates only those cells that are infected by herpes virus. Uninfected cells do not phosphorylate, with a half-life of 4 to 5 hours and about 80% renal exception. Acyclovir can be given orally, intravenously, or topically (**Tables 30.1** and **30.2**; **Box 30.3**).

Acyclovir and Its Congeners Against Herpes

Valacyclovir is a prodrug of acyclovir with better bioavailability. Famciclovir is hydrolyzed to penciclovir and has greatest bioavailability. Penciclovir is used only topically whereas famciclovir can be administered orally. Acyclovir, valacyclovir, ganciclovir, famciclovir, penciclovir all are guanine nucleoside analogs.

Box 30.1 Antivirals available for many viral infections
Viruses controlled by current antiviral therapy are: • Cytomegalovirus (CMV) • Hepatitis viruses • Herpes viruses • Human immunodeficiency virus (HIV) • Influenza viruses (the "flu" viruses) • Respiratory syncytial virus (RSV)

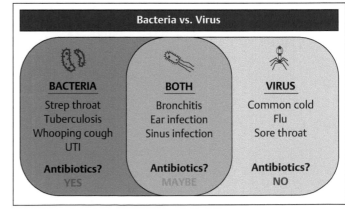

Fig. 30.1 Use of antibiotics in bacterial versus viral infections.

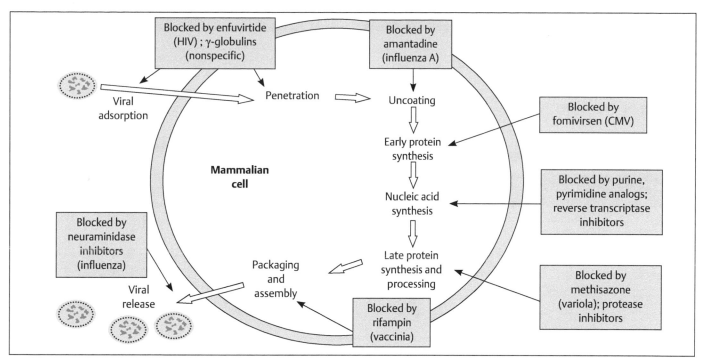

Fig. 30.2 Stages of viral replication in a mammalian cell. Abbreviations: CMV, cytomegalovirus; HIV, human immunodeficiency virus.

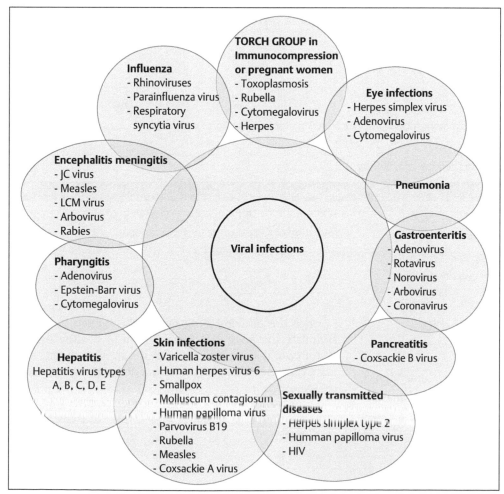

Fig. 30.3 Overview of viral infections. Abbreviations: HIV, human immunodeficiency virus; JC virus, John Cunningham virus; LCM, lymphocytic choriomeningitis virus.

Box 30.2 Antiherpes virus agents

- Acyclovir/Valacyclovir
- Famciclovir/Penciclovir
- Ganciclovir/Cidofovir
- Foscarnet
- Trifluridine/Idoxuridine/Vidarabine

Box 30.3 Pharmacokinetics of acyclovir

- Oral bioavailability ~20–30%
- Distribution: in all body tissues including CNS
- Renal excretion is more than 80%
- Half-life of 2–5 h
- Administration: topical, oral, IV

Table 30.1 Antiherpes antiviral drugs

Name of drugs	Bioavailability	Prodrugs	Guanine analogs	Oral bioavailability	Topical administration	Adverse events
Acyclovir	Nucleotide analog		+	20–30% +	Oral, ½ and topical	Renal excretion
Valacyclovir	Nucleotide analog	+ of Acyclovir	+	++	−	80% N, V, D
Ganciclovir	Nucleotide analog		+	+++	−	Neutropenia thrombocytopenia
Famciclovir	Hydrolyzed to penciclovir		+	++++	−	
Penciclovir	Hydrolyzed to penciclovir		+	++	Topical only ++	
Foscarnet	Hydrolyzed to penciclovir	Alternative drug for HSV infected			10 ± 20%	Hypomagnesemia, nephrotoxicity, neurotoxicity
Trifluridine/ Idoxuridine	Pyrimidine nucleoside DNA synthesis				Topical only	
Vidarabine	Nucleoside analog					Ophthalmic ointment, anemia, SIADH

Abbreviations: HSV, herpes simplex virus; SIADH, syndrome of inappropriate secretion of antidiuretic hormone.

Table 30.2 Different viscoelastic tests and their interpretations

Acyclovir	Ganciclovir
HSV genital infections	CMV retinitis in immunocompromised patient
HSV infections in immunocompromised patient	Prevention of CMV disease in transplant patients
Side effects: Nausea, vomiting, diarrhea, nephrotoxicity, myelosuppression, and neutropenia	

Abbreviations: CMV, cytomegalovirus; HSV, herpes simplex virus.

Action Mechanism of Acyclovir and Its Congeners

All drugs are phosphorylated by a viral thymidine-kinase, then metabolized by host cell kinases to nucleotide analogs. The analog inhibits viral DNA-polymerase. Only actively replicating viruses are inhibited.

Once the antiviral drug enters the human body, they stimulate the body's immune system. A healthy immune system works synergistically with the antiviral drug to eliminate the virus (**Box 30.4**). Antiviral drugs are classified into two categories:

- Retroviral antiviral drugs: used to treat HIV infections.
- Nonretroviral antiviral drugs: used to treat non-HIV infections.

Antiretroviral Drugs

Highly active antiretroviral therapy (HAART) includes at least three medications. These medications work in different ways to reduce the viral load.

Neuraminidase Inhibitors: Influenza Antiviral Drugs

Oseltamivir/Zanamivir: Influenza contains an enzyme neuraminidase which is essential for the replication of the virus. Oseltamivir and zanamivir are effective against both influenza A and B. These drugs do not interfere with the immune response to influenza A vaccine and can be used for both prophylaxis and acute treatment. Oseltamivir is administered orally and zanamivir intranasally. The risk of bronchospasm exists with zanamivir. It prevents the release of new virions and their spread from cell to cell (**Box 30.5**).

The nonretroviral drugs inhibit viral replication. They are generally used to treat non-HIV viral infections. A brief summary is provided in **Box 30.6**.

Cidofovir Antiviral Drugs: Against CMV Antiviral Actions

Cidofovir is used for the treatment of CMV retinitis in immunocompromised patients. It is a nucleotide analog of cytosine—no phosphorylation is required and it inhibits viral DNA synthesis. It is available for intravenous (IV), intravitreal injection, and also topical usage. However, nephrotoxicity is a major disadvantage.

Vidarabine Antiviral Drugs

This drug is converted to its triphosphate analog which inhibits viral DNA-polymerase. Oral bioavailability is ~2% administration: ophthalmic ointment. It is used for the treatment of herpes simplex virus (HSV) keratoconjunctivitis in immunocompromised patients. Anemia and SIADH (syndrome of inappropriate secretion of antidiuretic hormone) are its adverse effects (**Table 30.3**).

Foscarnet Antiviral Drugs

Therapeutic uses of foscarnet antiviral drugs are seen in:
- HSV infections
- CMV retinitis.

Adverse effects of foscarnet antiviral drugs include hypocalcemia, hypomagnesemia, neurotoxicity, nephrotoxicity, and interstitial nephritis.

Anti-influenza Antiviral Drugs

Two groups of RNA-containing viruses, influenza A and influenza B, are etiologic causes of influenza. When the RNA is released into the cell, it gets replicated and makes protein that forms new viral particles as well (**Box 30.7**).

Box 30.4 How do the antiviral drugs act?

Key characteristics of antiviral drugs are:
- Virus infects the cell and replicates there
- Interfere with the nucleic acid synthesis of the virus
- Binds to the cell
- Work synergistically with a healthy immune system to eliminate the virus

---

Box 30.5 Protease inhibitors (PIs) antiretroviral drugs

- Inhibit the protease retroviral enzyme, preventing viral replication. A few examples are:
  - Amprenavir (Agenerase)
  - Indinavir (Crixivan)
  - Nelfinavir (Viracept)
  - Ritonavir (Norvir)
  - Saquinavir (Inverse)

Box 30.6 Antiviral drugs: Nonretroviral group

Mechanism of action:
- Inhibit viral replication

Used to treat non-HIV viral infections:
- Influenza viruses
- Herpes simplex virus (HSV), varicella zoster virus (VZV)
- Cytomegalovirus (CMV)
- Hepatitis A, B, C (HAV, HBV, NCV)

Adverse effects:
- Vary with each drug on an individual basis
- Healthy cells also are often killed, resulting in serious toxicities

---

Box 30.7 Antiviral drugs for respiratory viral infections

- Amantadine/Rimantadine
- Oseltamivir/Zanamivir (Neuraminidase inhibitors)
- RSV bronchiolitis
- Ribavirin

Table 30.3 Difference between trifluridine and vidarabine antiviral drugs

Pharmacology of trifluridine	Pharmacology of vidarabine
• Trifluridine is a pyrimidine nucleoside analog • Inhibits viral DNA synthesis	• Vidarabine is a nucleoside analog • Inhibits stress-induced cardiomyopathy

Pharmacokinetics of Amantadine Antiviral Drugs

Amantadine with oral bioavailability ~50 to 90% extensively crosses the blood–brain barrier but rimantadine does not cross extensively.

Interferon Antiviral Drugs

Interferons (IFNs) are natural proteins produced by the cells of the immune systems in response to challenges by foreign agents such as viruses, bacteria, parasites, and tumor cells. It has antiviral, immune-modulating, and antiproliferative actions.

There are three classes of interferons: α, β, and γ. α- and β-interferons are produced by all the cells in response to viral infections. γ-interferons are produced only by T-lymphocyte and NK-cells in response to cytokines—immune-regulating effects. γ-Interferon has less antiviral activity compared to α- and β-interferon.[6-9] The action of these enzymes leads to an inhibition of translation (**Table 30.1**).

Adverse Effects of Interferon Antiviral Drugs

Some side-effects of interferons are acute flu-like syndrome, bone marrow suppression, neurotoxicity, and cardiotoxicity.

The antiviral drugs inhibit viral fusion, preventing viral replication. Enfuvirtide (Fuzeon) is one of the newest class of antiretroviral drugs. Combinations of multiple antiretroviral medications are common. Adverse effects vary with each drug and may be severe; hence, it is important to monitor for dose in order to limit toxicities. It is important to monitor for signs of opportunistic diseases when on antiviral drugs (**Table 30.4**).

Oseltamivir

This newer anti-influenza virus drug is a sialic acid analog with broad spectrum activity covering influenza A (amantadine sensitive as well as resistant), H5N1 (bird flu), nH1N1 (swine flu) strains and influenza B. It is an ester prodrug that is rapidly and nearly completely hydrolyzed during absorption in intestine and by liver to the active form oseltamivir carboxylate with an oral bioavailability of ~80%. The active metabolite is not further metabolized and is excreted by the kidney with a t½ of 6–10 hours. It acts by inhibiting influenza virus neuraminidase enzyme which is needed for release of progeny virions from the infected cell. Spread of the virus in the body is thus checked. Resistance can develop by mutation of the viral neuraminidase enzyme. In many areas, oseltamivir-resistant H1N1 (seasonal influenza) and H5N1 have been encountered, though swine flu (nH1N1) is still mostly sensitive. Some oseltamivir-resistant strains remain susceptible to zanamivir and vice versa.

Oseltamivir is indicated both for prophylaxis as well as treatment of influenza A, swine flu, bird flu and influenza B. Started at the onset of symptoms, it is the most effective drug; reduces the severity, duration, and complications of the illness. Prophylactic use for 5–10 days prevents illness in contacts of influenza patients.

Side effects are nausea and abdominal pain due to gastric irritation (reduced by taking the drug with food), headache, weakness, sadness, diarrhea, cough, and insomnia. Skin reactions have been reported.

Zanamivir

Another influenza A (including amantadine-resistant, nH1N1, H5N1 strains) and influenza B virus neuraminidase

Table 30.4 Summary of antiviral drugs

FDA approval status	Drug name	Mode of action	Anti-infective mechanism	Target disease
Approved	Lopinavir/Ritonavir	Protease inhibitors	Inhibit HIV-1 protease for protein cleavage	HIV/AIDS, SAR, MERS
Approved	Remdesivir (GS-5734)	Nucleotide analog prodrugs	Interfere with virus post entry	Ebola, SARS, MERS
Approved, investigational	Chloroquine	9-amonoquinoline neuraminidase inhibitor	Increasing endosomal pH, immunomodulating, autophagy inhibitors	Malaria, autoimmune disease
Approved	Oseltamivir		Inhibiting the activity of the viral neuraminidase enzyme preventing budding from the host cell, viral replication, and infectivity	Influenza virus A
Approved, investigational	Ganciclovir	Nucleoside analog	Potent inhibitor of the herpes virus family	AIDS associated cytomegalovirus infections

Abbreviations: AIDS, acquired immunodeficiency syndrome; HIV, human immunodeficiency virus; MERS, Middle East respiratory syndrome; SARS, severe acute respiratory syndrome.

inhibitor that is administered by inhalation as a powder due to very low oral bioavailability.

The inhaled powder can induce bronchospasm in some individuals. This may be severe in asthmatics; contraindicated in them. Headache, dizziness, nausea, and rashes are mild and infrequent side effects.

After i.m./s.c. injection, interferon is distributed to tissues. It is degraded mainly in liver and kidney and remains detectable in plasma for 24 hours. However, cellular effects are longer lasting because the interferon induced proteins persist, so that IFN is generally administered thrice weekly. Complexed with polyethylene glycol (peginterferon), it is absorbed more slowly—exerts more sustained effects, permitting weekly administration and improving clinical efficacy.

Anti-COVID Antiviral Drugs

Mortality in case of interferon use remains unaffected with simultaneous glucocorticoid use.[10]

Remdesivir is the only FDA-approved drug for COVID-19 pandemic. It causes a shortening of recovery time, by around 5 days, so it has a modest antiviral effect. Molnupiravir is a nucleoside analog, mimicking RNA action. It duplicates its RNA genome and forms new virus, upon a COVID-19 infection. Molnupiravir works inside the cell whereas remdesivir is a chain terminator. Molnupiravir with a 5-day duration course has to be used cautiously in pregnancy.

Paxlovid inhibits the enzyme needed to process viral proteins to its ultimate form. The drug is a combination of an antiviral, dubbed PF-07321332, and another drug called ritonavir, which helps to prevent the breakdown of the antiviral by the liver enzymes before it has a chance to disable the coronavirus.

Could the Coronavirus Become Resistant to Antivirals?

Drug resistance is a familiar problem and is the reason that some viral infections, such as HIV and hepatitis C, are treated using combinations of antivirals. So far, molnupiravir and Paxlovid have been tested only as single therapies. It will be important to look at people who don't respond to molnupiravir or Paxlovid to find out whether viral resistance is a factor. **Box 30.8** lists the effective management strategies for COVID-19.

Conclusion

Most studies have shown that some new antiviral drugs like molnupiravir, fluvoxamine, and Paxlovid are effective in reducing the mortality and hospitalization rates in COVID-19 patients.[11] They cause less side effects are thus safe with

Box 30.8   Management strategies for COVID-19
• Remdesivir is promising
• Lopinavir has lower efficacy
• Oseltamivir has shown no clear benefit
• Favipiravir: useful in mild-to-moderate cases
• Molnupiravir could be the definitive treatment for all COVID-19 variants, in a 5-day treatment regimen

a breakthrough potential against viruses like COVID-19,[12,13] despite the global, inequality for access to these drugs. Innovation and trends in the development and approval of antiviral medicines continue.[14] Using host cells targeting or oral antiviral drugs to prevent pandemics, is feasible and hence imperative for promoting public health, which would bring about transformational changes[15] as shown by the Solidarity Trial of WHO[16] and is using emerging antiviral strategies and drug delivering systems like RIBOTAC and PROTAC for future drug discovery.[17]

The present's antiviral drugs still do not prepare us for the next pandemic. There needs to be continued surveillance and modeling to support the prediction of which deadly virus will be the next to emerge into the human population. Of critical importance is directing research effort and investment into the development of broadly acting antivirals that can be mobilized as the first line of defense upon emergence of new viral pathogens.[18]

References

1. World Health Organization. A coordinated global research roadmap: 2019 novel coronavirus. March 2020. https://www.who.int/publications/m/item/a-coordinated-global-research-roadmap

2. Axfors C, Schmitt AM, Janiaud P, et al. Mortality outcomes with hydroxychloroquine and chloroquine in COVID-19: an international collaborative meta-analysis of randomized trials. October 22, 2020. https://www.medrxiv.org/content/10.1101/2020.09.16.20194571v2. preprint

3. Venisse N, Peytavin G, Bouchet S, et al; ANRS-AC43 Clinical Pharmacology Committee, SFPT Therapeutic Drug Monitoring and Treatment Personalization group. Concerns about pharmacokinetic (PK) and pharmacokinetic-pharmacodynamic (PK-PD) studies in the new therapeutic area of COVID-19 infection. Antiviral Res 2020;181:104866

4. Buchwalder PA, Buclin T, Trinchard I, Munafo A, Biollaz J. Pharmacokinetics and pharmacodynamics of IFN-beta 1a in healthy volunteers. J Interferon Cytokine Res 2000;20(10):857–866

5. Beigel JH, Tomashek KM, Dodd LE, et al; ACTT-1 Study Group Members. Remdesivir for the treatment of Covid-19: final report. N Engl J Med 2020;383(19):1813–1826

6. Flammer JR, Dobrovolna J, Kennedy MA, et al. The type I interferon signaling pathway is a target for glucocorticoid inhibition. Mol Cell Biol 2010;30(19):4564–4574

7. Jalkanen J, Hollmén M, Jalkanen S. Interferon beta-1a for COVID-19: critical importance of the administration route. Crit Care 2020;24(1):335

8. Jalkanen J, Pettilä V, Huttunen T, Hollmén M, Jalkanen S. Glucocorticoids inhibit type I IFN beta signaling and the upregulation of CD73 in human lung. Intensive Care Med 2020;46(10):1937–1940

9. World Health Organization. Corticosteroids for COVID-19: living guidance. November 28, 2021. https://apps.who.int/iris/handle/10665/334125

10. FDA Center for Drug Evaluation and Research. FDA's approval of Veklury (remdesivir) for the treatment of Covid-19: summary review. https://www.accessdata.fda.gov/drugsatfda_docs/nda/2020/214787Orig1s000Sumr.pdf

11. Wen W, Chen C, Tang J, et al. Efficacy and safety of three new oral antiviral treatment (molnupiravir, fluvoxamine and Paxlovid) for COVID-19: a meta-analysis. Ann Med 2022;54(1):516–523

12. Takashita E, Yamayoshi S, Simon V, et al. Efficacy of antibodies and antiviral drugs against Omicron BA.2.12.1, BA.4, and BA.5 subvariants. N Engl J Med 2022;387(5):468–470

13. Plata GG. The black market for covid-19 antiviral drugs. BMJ 2022;377:o1282

14. Chaudhuri S, Symons JA, Deval J. Innovation and trends in the development and approval of antiviral medicines: 1987–2017 and beyond. Antiviral Res 2018;155:76–88

15. Dwek RA, Bell JI, Feldmann M, Zitzmann N. Host-targeting oral antiviral drugs to prevent pandemics. 2022;399(10333):1381–1382

16. WHO Solidarity Trial Consortium. Repurposed antiviral drugs for Covid-19—interim WHO solidarity trial results. N Engl J Med 2021;384(6):497–511

17. Xu S, Ding D, Zhang X, et al. Newly emerging strategies in antiviral drug discovery: dedicated to Prof. Dr. Erik De Clercq on occasion of his 80th anniversary. Molecules 2022;27(3):850

18. Adamson CS, Chibale K, Goss RJM, Jaspars M, Newman DJ. Dorrington RA. Antiviral drug discovery: preparing for the next pandemic. Chem Soc Rev. 2021;50(6):3647–3655

31

ECMO in COVID-19

Poonam Malhotra Kapoor, Yatin Mehta, and Pranav Kapoor

Introduction

Extracorporeal membrane oxygenation (ECMO) as a rescue therapy to treat refractory acute respiratory distress syndromes (ARDS) has been in use during the last two decades.[1-4] In the COVID-19 pandemic too ECMO was tried in the COVID-affected patients. In both first and second COVID waves, mortality on ECMO was experienced, with more cases in the second wave. Rescue utilization and local networking is essential for optimizing ECMO in COVID-19. Most centers did not use ECMO in the first wave, due to lack of awareness, fear of complications, lack of availability of both equipment and expertise, or no availability of bed or machine. During the COVID-19 pandemic, in India, we faced a shortage of equipment, ICU beds, and expert ICU personnel, which prevented ECMO use in many cases. Thus, at the end of the second wave of COVID-19 meticulous and careful planning was recommended.[5]

During the COVID-19 pandemic, utilization of ECMO was less due to shortage of ECMO machine. Scarcity was also seen in the knowledge of handling ECMO in COVID-19 patients specifically the pathophysiological consideration of ECMO coagulation and inflammation and their interactions with each other. Kowalewski et al have discussed strategies of ECMO use in COVID-19, of when to insert ECMO, who to treat on ECMO and availability of cost effective strategies (**Box 31.1** and **Fig. 31.1**).[6]

Early VV ECMO in COVID-19

The use of venovenous (VV) ECMO early in COVID-19 ARDS refractory to all other treatment gives good outcomes in following aspects:

- Minimizes respiratory driver pressure.
- Reduces both pulmonary and systemic inflammation.
- Timely ECMO overcomes multipulmonary and cardiac support organ dysfunction as well.
- It is certain now, after phase second and third of COVID-19 pandemic, that VV ECMO is a suitable option in COVID-19 patients. ECMO helps in carbon dioxide removal as well.

Mechanical ventilation strategies should have VV ECMO inserted as soon as possible. ECMO is useful, in cardiac patients as well, in whom a venoarterial (VA) ECMO may be preferred to VV ECMO as shown in **Box 31.2** and **Fig. 31.2**.

Since this requires expertise, timeliness, and appropriate protocols, which were most often missed in COVID-19, the results were not so satisfactory at first.

Monitoring Lymphocyte Count Was a Disruptor in the Treatment of COVID-19 with ECMO

There are many advantages of monitoring lymphocytes in ECMO-administered COVID-19 patients, as shown by Putowski et al.[7] These authors observed a drop in the lymphocyte count while monitoring six COVID-19 patients who were on ECMO. They observed a similarity between the lymphocyte count and disease severity of the new COVID-19 virus. Interleukin 6 levels were different, between survivors and nonsurvivors of COVID-19.[7]

It is important to keep in mind that for ECMO to act as a bridge to lung transplant, right selection and timely ECMO insertion is most essential. Thus, ARDS patients mandating the need for lung transplant are exceedingly sick and need immense support with or without ECMO. It is thus imperative to choose the right patient and correct time of starting

---

Box 31.1	Indications for ECMO in COVID-19

- Severe pneumonia in COVID-19 patient with ARDS, not responding to all conventional treatments such as prone positioning, lung protective ventilation (LPV), neuromuscular blockade, and adequate hydration
- $PaO_2/FiO_2 < 100$ mmHg
- Arterial pH < 7.2
- $PaCO_2 > 60$ mmHg

Abbreviations: ARDS, acute respiratory distress syndrome; ECMO, extracorporeal membrane oxygenation; FiO_2, fraction of inspired oxygen; PaO_2, partial pressure of oxygen; $PaCO_2$, partial pressure of carbon dioxide.

Box 31.2	Conditions mandating a venoarterial ECMO

- Pneumonia associated with right heart failure or congestive heart failure
- Fulminant myocarditis
- Myocardial infarction
- Sepsis-related cardiomyopathy

Abbreviation: ECMO, extracorporeal membrane oxygenation.

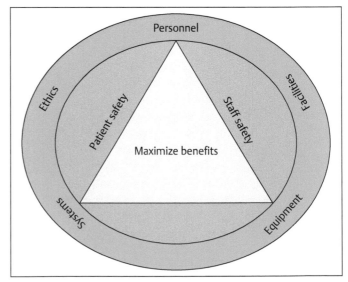

Fig. 31.1 Safety of the use of extracorporeal membrane oxygenation (ECMO) in COVID-19 patients requires the right equipment, personnel, and teamwork.

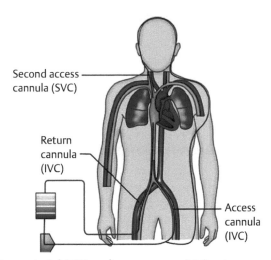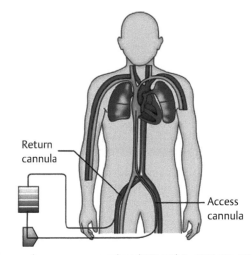

Second access cannula (SVC)

Return cannula (IVC)

Access cannula (IVC)

Return cannula

Access cannula

Fig. 31.2   Venoarterial (VA) and venovenous (VV) extracorporeal membrane oxygenation (ECMO) in COVID-19 patients.

Box 31.3   Indications of ECMO in lung transplant

- Pulmonary consolidation, secondary to severe COVID-19 infection, exhaustion of all conservation treatment options
- No recovery of the COVID-19 damaged lungs despite at least 4 weeks of ventilation/ECMO
- Evidence of advanced and irreversible lung damage in several consecutive CT scans
- Age less than 65 years and no relevant comorbidities; patient should be in good physical condition and have a good chance of complete physical rehabilitation following the transplant
- Pulmonary fibrosis with secondary bacterial pneumonia responding to conventional treatment of SARS COVID-19
- Lung tissue bronchoscopic sampling biopsy depicting irreversible damage to the lungs
- Due to SARS COVID-19 where there is loss in normal alveolar architecture, extensive cysts lined with squamous cuboidal epithelium and hemosiderin deposits need an ECMO
- Lung transplant should only be considered when sufficient time has elapsed to exclude possible recovery
- Two negative PCR test of bronchoalveolar fluid or nasopharyngeal swabs in all intubated patients is a must to ensure viral clearance before lung transplant

Abbreviations: ECMO, extracorporeal membrane oxygenation; PCR, polymerase chain reaction; SARS, severe acute respiratory syndrome.

Box 31.4   Contraindications for lung transplant

Presence of one of the following precluded the insertion of lung transplant:
- Multiorgan failure
- Mental assessment not feasible in unresponsive or not awake patient, no clear consciousness level seen in patients
- Stroke
- Sepsis and bacteremia
- Severe fragility (relative contraindications)
- Consent not given
- Contraindications to systemic anticoagulation
- Uncontrolled metastatic disease or a terminate illness
- Inability for transplant according to standard criteria

Box 31.5   Important precautions during ECMO as a bridge to transplant

- Imperative to remember that the waitlist is influenced by the blood group and type, body size, and antibodies of the patients
- This phase is crucial as exacerbations may be observed.
- These patients would require some form of ventilation in case the patients worsen while awaiting a donor, then we may use ECMO as a bridge to transplant or decision-making
- ECMO for either should not be delayed, and it should be expedited using a multidisciplinary team approach

---

Box 31.6   ICU conditions for ECMO during COVID-19

- Pre-ECMO apply best conventional intensive care before inserting an ECMO
- Use artificial intelligence for patient selection
- Reorganize ICU staffing
- Be a part of the solution by contributing to research

Abbreviations: ECMO, extracorporeal membrane oxygenation; ICU, intensive care unit.

ECMO. There is no recovery of COVID-19-damaged lungs for at least 4 weeks. So ECMO and ventilation can be continued for the same period. Lung transplant should be considered only when sufficient time has elapsed post-COVID-19 (**Boxes 31.3–31.5**).

Two negative polymerase chain reaction (PCR) tests of bronchial fluid or nasopharyngeal swabs in all nonintubated patients is a must, to ensure that the virus has completely cleared before the lung transplant is done. In a pandemic, it is best to create conditions for ECMO preparation before its use in the ICU. Everything begins as listed in **Box 31.6**, by providing the best conventional intensive care measures before an ECMO pump is inserted. Artificial intelligence aids in careful faltering/selection of patients. For optimal ECMO outcomes, resource utilization and expertise in ECMO insertion, maintenance, and weaning are as important as research and evidence-based medicine practice.[7]

Management of ECMO in COVID-19

The management of ECMO procedures during COVID-19, whether VV or VA ECMO, entails (**Box 31.7**) maintaining pulmonary, hemodynamic, hematological, as well as general measures to ensure adequate ventilation. ECMO mandates provisioning blood transfusions, using coagulopathy strategies, timing tracheostomy, and maintaining goal-directed hemodynamic monitoring. According to Abrams et al, ECMO utilization during COVID-19 pandemic is a burden-based approach. Due to a high number of cases in a pandemic there will be decreased ECMO utilization as resources will be inadequate to provide optimal ECMO care. Bigniew et al in 2020 gave an extended view that systems should be optimized for ECMO initiation and maintenance when considering ECMO in COVID-19 patients (**Box 31.8**).[8]

Supady et al in January did retrospective analysis on 133 COVID-19 patients on VV ECMO for predicting their outcome measures.[9] They concluded that 30-day survival, in COVID-19 patients, treated with VV ECMO is around 54 percent, encouraging more research. The use of scores such as state of the art analysis (SOTA), acute physiology and chronic health evaluation (APACHE), respiratory ECMO survival prediction (RESP), and predicting death for severe ARDS on VV ECMO (PRESERVE), developed long ago, cannot be recommended for treatment decisions in severe COVID-19 ARDS. Also VV ECMO should be considered, if deemed beneficial, as long as resources are available. A score above or below a cut-off value is an additional advantage for evaluation of prognostic value, but cannot be used for triaging these patients.

Transporting Patients on ECMO in COVID-19

Recently, Javidfar et al conducted a retrospective trial of 113 patients with diagnosis of COVID-19 on VV ECMO[10] and another study in Qatar on 113 mobile patients. COVID-19 patients on invasive mechanical ventilation can be successfully transported on ECMO, which can be ground and air. This group did not report any adverse events, including pump failures, cannulation complications, and decannulation or dislodgement outside the hospital or in transit. No instances were found of transport team members also contracting COVID-19 after contacting COVID patients during transportation care. Airborne contact precautions with eyewear was adhered to by all ECMO team personnel, with weaning of the

---

Box 31.7 Optimization strategy in ECMO for COVID-19

- Neuromuscular blockade, high PEEP strategy, inhaled pulmonary vasodilators, recruitment maneuvers, and high-frequency oscillatory ventilation
- Recommend early ECMO as per EOLIA trial criteria; salvage ECMO, which involves deferral of ECMO imitation until further decompensation (as in the crossovers to ECMO in the EOLIA control group), is not supported by the evidence but might be preferable to not initiating ECMO at all in such patients
- Neuromuscular blockers
- High PEEP strategy
- Inhaled pulmonary vasodilators
- Recruitment measures
- High-frequency oscillatory ventilation

Abbreviations: ECMO, extracorporeal membrane oxygenation; PEEP, positive end-expiratory pressure.

Box 31.8 Optimization of ECMO in COVID-19

- Neuromuscular blockers
- High PEEP strategy
- Inhaled pulmonary vasodilators
- Recruitment measures
- High-frequency oscillatory ventilation

Abbreviations: ECMO, extracorporeal membrane oxygenation; PEEP, positive end-expiratory pressure.

---

standard. Personal protective equipment was used as well. Following airborne, contact, and eye (ACE) protection precautions, these authors could safely transport a COVID-19 patient on ECMO to a specialized ECMO center in their country. ECMO is not a therapy to be rushed to the frontline, when all resources are stretched in a pandemic. In 2020, the role of ECMO in COVID-19 was unclear. The Extracorporeal Life Support Organization (ELSO) registry has been at the frontline in providing new information about COVID-19 during the last 2 years, and many prospective, observational studies are under way under its leadership. Roberto Lorusso, during EuroELSO conference in 2021, called for close cooperation and further research on VV ECMO for COVID-19 patients.[13]

ECMO in Children with COVID-19

Conventional selection criteria for COVID-19–related ECMO should be used; however, when resources become more constrained during a pandemic, more stringent contraindications should be implemented. Rarely, children may require ECMO support for COVID-19–related ARDS, myocarditis, or multisystem inflammatory syndrome in children (MIS-C); conventional selection criteria and management practices should be the standard. Authors strongly encourage participation in data submission to investigate the optimal use of ECMO for COVID-19.

Duration on ECMO (>90% VV) for COVID-19 from three large observational studies was median 13.9 days (interquartile range [IQR], 7.8–23.3 d),[11] median 20 days (IQR, 10–40 d),[12] and mean 18 days.[13] It is important to note that successful native lung recovery has been reported after prolonged (>28 d) VV ECMO support.[14] The role of chest imaging in determining futility while on VV ECMO is unknown. Patients with COVID-19 initially exhibited similar mortality when supported with VV ECMO as compared to historical data in patients with other causes of acute severe respiratory failure.

Barbaro and colleagues show that, later in the pandemic, patients more often had noninvasive ventilation before ECMO and were given steroids or other specific COVID-19 therapies. The latter is probably reflected in the increased burden of coinfections reported in the post-May 1 cohorts.[15] Clinicians rely on experience that they do not yet have to allocate patients to ECMO and therefore might miss important characteristics. It is not surprising that outcomes are changing as the pandemic is progressing. In the report by Barbaro and colleagues, no one knows if some patients survived despite ECMO they did not need, or if some died just because of ECMO, or what happened to those who were denied ECMO—this is still the conundrum to clarify before we decide if ECMO is worth using. ECMO cannot be blamed for the increased mortality; it is merely a tool and clinicians still need to understand when to use it for the greatest benefit. Barbaro and colleagues should be commended for scratching the surface and reporting honestly and openly. To date, thousands of patients with COVID-19 have been ventilated in intensive care and a proportion had access to ECMO. Collating and analyzing their clinical journeys might help to clarify if ECMO is a tool to keep.

The inflexion point at which one is better than the other is unknown, even if criteria are well defined and regularly reviewed.[16] Clinicians sometimes select patients who have so much lung damage by the time ECMO is started that there is no possible recovery.

Extracorporeal Life Support

The largest ELSO data from 213 centers and 36 countries, of nearly 1035 ECMO, showed an overall mortality of nearly 37% (95% CI 34-40) from all centers.[1] **Box 31.9** shows increased incidence of newer changes in COVID-19 mortality, which is seen in all COVID-19 patients on ECMO with all indications, and not just ARDS.[17,18]

Optimization of ECMO in COVID-19 requires a thorough pre-ECMO, during ECMO run, and post-ECMO open strategy (**Box 31.10** and **Table 31.1**) to improve the ECMO outcomes.

Conclusion

It is important to look for long-term outcomes with COVID-19 patients on ECMO. Routine or systematic use of screening

---

Box 31.9 Newer changes reported in ECMO for COVID-19

- Increased incidence of thrombotic complication
- Increased bleeding incidence (42%) of total patients
- Increased incidence of mortality
- Increased incidence of nosocomial infections
- Like the EOLIA trial nearly 94% of patients were put in the prone position for management
- Increased use of novel therapies like bundled treatment, seen trailed more specifically in COVID-19, undergoing ECMO
- Use of prone positioning in ECMO for COVID-19 showed lesser mortality
- Use of the Protek-duo tandem heart cannula (cardiac assist increased, Pittsburgh, PA) which uses a right heart support and returns oxygenated blood, via the dual lumen cannula directly into the pulmonary artery, under echocardiography guidance
- Early weaning using this cannula, with the mechanical-assist device in situ the right heart, within 13 days was reported with a discharge to survival of 73%

Abbreviation: ECMO, extracorporeal membrane oxygenation.

Box 31.10 Future factors to optimize ECMO in COVID-19 to improve the outcomes

- Prone positioning
- Optimal anticoagulation
- Early extubation
- Use of mechanical right ventricular support

Abbreviation: ECMO, extracorporeal membrane oxygenation.

Table 31.1 Preoperative vs. perioperative strategies to improve ECMO outcomes

Preoperative	Perioperative
- Use of immune modulators (steroids ± antiviral drugs) - Timing of ECMO imitation. Same as EULIA trial? - ECPR: does it have a role here?	- Longer ECMO runs means more morbidity - Increase in bleeding/thrombin ECMOs - Screening for DVT: is it a must? - Full-dose anticoagulation, prone-positioning awake ECMO, or use of mechanical right heart-assist device: are these interventions essential? - If tracheostomy is needed in these patients, then what is its optimal timing?

Abbreviations: DVT, deep vein thrombosis; ECMO, extracorporeal membrane oxygenation; ECPR, extracorporeal cardiopulmonary resuscitation.

for deep vein thrombosis/pulmonary embolism (DVT/PE) post-ECMO insertion in COVID-19 patients with maximum ECMO duration, when recovery of patients is still possible should be discussed and implemented by the ECMO team.

To conclude that early cannulation (≤4 days) of younger patients (≤55 years) may improve overall survival and that a history of IHD might indicate a reduced prognosis.[19]

References

1. Brodie D, Slutsky AS, Combes A. Extracorporeal life support for adults with respiratory failure and related indications: a review. JAMA 2019;322(6):557–568

2. Abrams D, Ferguson ND, Brochard L, et al. ECMO for ARDS: from salvage to standard of care? Lancet Respir Med 2019;7(2): 108–110

3. Fan E, Brodie D, Slutsky AS. Acute respiratory distress syndrome: advances in diagnosis and treatment. JAMA 2018;319(7): 698–710

4. Combes A, Hajage D, Capellier G, et al; EOLIA Trial Group, REVA, and ECMONet. Extracorporeal membrane oxygenation for severe acute respiratory distress syndrome. N Engl J Med 2018; 378(21):1965–1975

5. Li Bassi G, Suen J, Barnett AG, et al; COVID-19 Critical Care Consortium Investigators. Design and rationale of the COVID-19 Critical Care Consortium international, multicentre, observational study. BMJ Open 2020;10(12):e041417

6. Kowalewski M, Fina D, Słomka A, et al. COVID-19 and ECMO: the interplay between coagulation and inflammation-a narrative review. Crit Care 2020;24(1):205

7. Henry BM. COVID-19, ECMO, and lymphopenia: a word of caution. Lancet Respir Med 2020;8(4):e24. Published Online March 13, https://doi.org/10.1016/ S2213–2600(20)30119–3

8. Putowski Z, Szczepańska A, Czok M, Krzych ŁJ. Veno-Venous Extracorporeal Membrane Oxygenation in COVID-19-Where Are We Now? Int J Environ Res Public Health 2021;18(3):1173

9. Supady A, DellaVolpe J, Taccone FS, et al. Outcome Prediction in Patients with Severe COVID-19 Requiring Extracorporeal Membrane Oxygenation-A Retrospective International Multicenter Study. Membranes (Basel) 2021;11(3):170

10. Javidfar J, Labib A, Ragazzo G, et al. Covid-19 Critical Care Consortium. Mobile Extracorporeal Membrane Oxygenation for Covid-19 Does Not Pose Extra Risk to Transport Team. ASAIO J 2022;68(2):163–167

11. Barbaro RP, MacLaren G, Boonstra PS, et al; Extracorporeal Life Support Organization. Extracorporeal membrane oxygenation support in COVID-19: An international cohort study of the Extracorporeal Life Support Organization registry. Lancet 2020;396(10257):1071-1078

12. Schmidt M, Hajage D, Lebreton G, et al; Groupe de Recherche Clinique en Ren animation et Soins intensifs du Patient en Insuffisance Respiratoire aiguE (GRC-RESPIRE) Sorbonne Université; Paris-Sorbonne ECMO-COVID investigators. Extracorporeal membrane oxygenation for severe acute respiratory distress syndrome associated with COVID-19: A retrospective cohort study. Lancet Respir Med 2020;8(11):1121-1131

13. Lorusso R, Combes A, Lo Coco V, De Piero ME, Belohlavek J; EuroECMO COVID-19 Working Group; Euro-ELSO Steering Committee. ECMO for COVID-19 patients in Europe and Israel. [published online ahead of print January 9, 2021]

14. Dreier E, Malfertheiner MV, Dienemann T, et al. ECMO in COVID-19—prolonged therapy needed? A retrospective analysis of outcome and prognostic factors. Perfusion 2021;36(6):582-591

15. Camporota L, Meadows C, Ledot S, et al. Consensus on the referral and admission of patients with severe respiratory failure to the NHS ECMO service. Lancet Respir Med 2021;9(2):e16-e17

16. Vuylsteke A. Ecmo in covid-19: do not blame the tool. Lancet 2021;398(10307):1197–1199

17. Friedrichson B, Kloka JA, Neef V, et al. Extracorporeal membrane oxygenation in coronavirus disease 2019: A nationwide cohort analysis of 4279 runs from Germany. Eur J Anaesthesiol 2022; 39(5):445–451

18. Assouline B, Assouline-Reinmann M, Giraud R, et al. Management of high-risk pulmonary embolism: what is the place of extracorporeal membrane oxygenation? J Clin Med 2022;11(16):4734

19. Makhoul M, Keizman E, Carmi U, et al. Outcomes of Extracorporeal Membrane Oxygenation (ECMO) for COVID-19 Patients: A Multi-Institutional Analysis. Vaccines. Vaccines 2023; 11(1): 108

32

Extracorporeal Membrane Oxygenation in Cardiac ICU

Poonam Malhotra Kapoor, Manoj Sahu, and Sarvesh Pal Singh

Background

Extracorporeal membrane oxygenation (ECMO) is an extracorporeal technology where an artificial surface maintains physiological gas exchange of the patient oxygenator incorporated in the ECMO circuit, oxygenates the blood, removes carbon dioxide, and returns to the patient.

Despite best mechanical ventilation, hypoxemic patients in cardiogenic shock or lung failure are generally candidates for ECMO support. ECMO in respiratory failure helps reduce mechanical ventilator support, thus allowing time for lung recovery (**Fig. 32.1**).

Types of ECMO

The decision to use ECMO is confirmed on the basis of the factors listed in **Box 32.1**. Depending upon the draining and returning vessels, ECMO is chiefly divided into two main categories: venoarterial (VA) ECMO and venovenous (VV)

Box 32.1 Factors to be considered before deploying ECMO
• Is the organ likely to recover: Reversible disease with treatment, using ECMO only as rest, is an important consideration before initiating ECMO
• Consider options for cardiac recovery: To use ECMO as a bridge to further cardiac recovery or a bridge to VAD or bridge to transplant
• Metastatic malignancy: It is an absolute contraindication
• Advanced age
• Consider graft reactions and rejections
• Cerebral injury to be ruled out
• Rule out history of a cardiac arrest witnessed or unwitnessed
• Rule out aortic dissection and aortic regurgitation

Abbreviations: ECMO, extracorporeal membrane oxygenation; VAD, ventricular assist device.

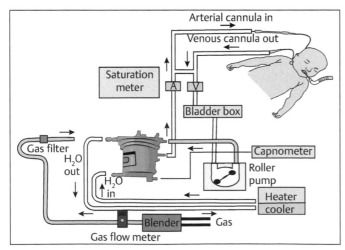

Fig. 32.1 A diagram of extracorporeal membrane oxygenation (ECMO) machine.

ECMO. Sometimes, we need additional cannula either at arterial side or at venous end for adequate support. Depending upon the additional cannula required for drainage or returning purpose, both VA and VV ECMO are subclassified into their variants as described below.

ECMO can be broadly categorized into two types:
- *Venovenous ECMO (VV ECMO):* It is appropriate only for respiratory failure.
- *Venoarterial ECMO (VA ECMO):* It is used for cardiogenic shock and is currently the fastest growing indication for ECMO worldwide.

Extracorporeal Membrane Oxygenation Machine

The machine components include:
- TUBINGS which act as pathway to take blood from the patient to the machine and back to the patient.
- PUMP to take and give blood to the patient.
- MEMBRANE to which the pump pushes blood for removing carbon dioxide and adding oxygen.
- HEMOTHERM to warm the blood to maintain body temperature.

Patients who are hypoxemic despite maximal conventional ventilatory support, who have significant ventilator-induced lung injury, or who are in reversible cardiogenic shock may be considered for ECMO support. For respiratory failure, the basic premise is that ECMO will allow the level of ventilatory support to be reduced, which may allow time for recovery from the underlying pathology and recovery from ventilator-induced lung injury to occur.

The type of ECMO performed will depend on the patient's underlying cardiac function. Venovenous (VV) ECMO is usually performed for isolated respiratory failure, whereas venoarterial (VA) ECMO (full cardiopulmonary bypass [CPB]) is performed for combined cardiac and respiratory failure.

The term "extracorporeal membrane oxygenation (ECMO)" was initially used to describe a long-term extracorporeal support that focused on the function of oxygenation. Subsequently, in some patients, the emphasis shifted to carbon dioxide removal. In recent times, keeping the variations of ECMO circuitry (**Fig. 32.2**) use in different clinical scenarios (e.g., bridge to multiple organ support: brain, lungs, heart, and kidney), the term ECMO has been replaced with extracorporeal life support (ECLS) to describe the ECMO technology. The two terms are synonymous; ECLS can be used for mechanical assistance during cardiac or pulmonary failure occurring in neonates, children, or older adults.

ECMO versus CPB

ECMO is different from CPB. To quote Dr. Robert Bartlett on what ECLS is:[1] "ECLS is a cousin, but not a twin to operating room cardiopulmonary bypasses." It is a teamwork. The differences between ECLS/ECMO and CPB are well laid out in **Table 32.1**, but it is important to remember that extensive training is required to perform both ECLS and CPB. A diagram of ECMO is shown in **Fig. 32.3**.

Is Extracorporeal Membrane Oxygenation (ECMO) Safe?

Changes in the ECMO circuitry materials, with the addition of biocompatible and heparin-bonded circuits, have made ECMO a safe option today. These materials are longer lasting, preventing frequent ECMO changes. The latter also decreases the complications of bleeding and need for unnecessary

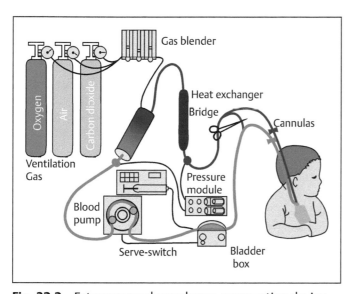

Fig. 32.2 Extracorporeal membrane oxygenation device.

blood and blood components transfusion. ECMO training from centers of excellence recognized by ELSO like RVCC or TSS (AIIMS Delhi) also helps minimize ECMO components in the last decade.

History of Extracorporeal Membrane Oxygenation (ECMO)

In May 1953, Gibbon used artificial oxygenation and perfusion support for the first successful open heart operation.[3] In 1954, Lillehei developed the cross-circulation technique by using slightly anesthetized adult volunteers as live CPB apparatuses during the repair of certain congenital cardiac disorders.[4] In 1955, at the Mayo clinic, Kirklin et al improved on Gibbon's device and successfully repaired an atrial septal defect[5] in a baby, who was suffering from meconium aspiration.

In 1965, Rashkind and coworkers were the first to use a bubble oxygenator as support in a neonate dying of respiratory failure.[6] In 1969, Dorson and colleagues reported the use of a membrane oxygenator for CPB in infants.[7]

It was in 1970, when Baffes et al reported the successful use of ECMO as support in infants with congenital heart defects, who were undergoing cardiac surgery.[8] In 1975 Bartlett et al were the first to successfully use ECMO in neonates with severe respiratory distress.[9]

Clear survival benefits published in many clinical trials showed enhanced survival infants with acute respiratory distress syndrome (ARDS) doing well on ECMO, but in the late 1960s this was not true for ARDS in adults, in whom ECMO was deployed. A survival of less than 50% had emerged in the above patients around that time.[10] The bedside use of ECMO as an extension of prolonged cardiopulmonary support was established in 1971.

Table 32.1 ECMO versus standard CPB

ECMO	Standard CPB
• Frequently used only using neck vessels in the cervical region	Uses transthoracic cannulation under the effect of general anesthesia
• ECMO bypass the lungs and heart, giving them "Rest," in critical care conditions when mortality is high • It is a partial CPB form	A route standard bypass, also provides rest to major organs, but for elective or emergency cardiac surgery; chances of surgical survival remains high
• Awake ECMO is a normal thing today	Awake CPB requires regional anesthesia; in most cases, CPB is done under general anesthesia only
• ECMO machine is a most advanced ventilator known	CPB alone is not a ventilator
• ECMO generally used after a CPB in lower states • ECMO can be used for prolonged duration from 1 day to over 107 days[2]	CPB is of a shorter duration (3–13 h) even though the flows are nonpulsatile in both ECMO and CPB
• ECMO tubes and circuitry can be placed in peripheral limbs as well in an emergency	CPB always requires a central RA and aortic cannulation for cardiac surgery

Abbreviations: CPB, cardiopulmonary bypass; ECMO, extracorporeal membrane oxygenation; RA, right artery.

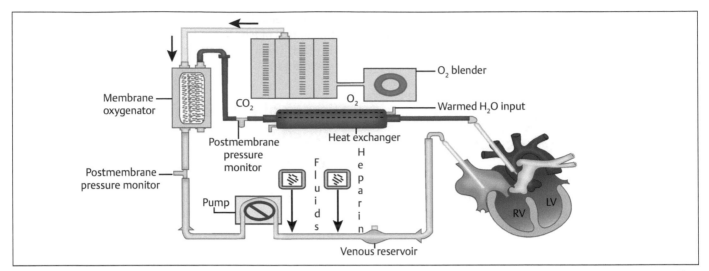

Fig. 32.3 Extracorporeal membrane oxygenation system Adapted with permission from Kapoor PM, Sethi BS. Introduction to Extracorporeal Membrane Oxygenation. In: Kapoor PM, ed. Manual Of Extracorporeal Membrane Oxygenation (ECMO) In The ICU, 1 ed. India: Jaypee Publication; 2014.

Before 1970, gas exchange in long-term cardiopulmonary support was with the use of oxygenators, which had blood-gas separation interface, leading to increased incidence of hemolysis, thrombocytopenia, and coagulopathy as shown by Kolobow et al when unanesthestized lambs were put on partial CPB, using the spiral membrane oxygenator.[11] In the ECMO one could either use a centrifugal or roller pump or it could be a pumpless ECMO, which utilizes the patient's own arteriovenous pressure gradient by using the patient's arteriovenous pressure gradient (pumpless).

Extracorporeal Membrane Oxygenation in India

In India, there are more than 105 centers, and more than 600 cases are managed every year on ECMO at AIIMS.[12] In the last 5 years Ridhi Vinayak Hospital, Mumbai dealt 200 cases with 45% mortality (70% respiratory, 20 pediatric. I neonatal PPIIN). AIIMS, New Delhi dealt 300 in cases eight past year, 290 cardiac, 10 respiratory. The BL Kapoor Hospital did 5 pediatrics in past year, 1 cardiac (survival), 4 respiratory (3 survived). KIMS Hyderabad, DMC Hospital, Ludhiana, MAX Super Specialty Hospital, New Delhi Apollo, MGM Chennai and many more hospitals handled ECMO cases deftly in the last 10 years and the number of ECMO centres doing successful ECMO, is on the rise.[13]

Venovenous Extracorporeal Membrane Oxygenation

In failing lungs, when there is no concomitant cardiac failure one can have access to a VV ECMO. In latter, i.e., venovenous ECMO, a drainage or access cannula from the large central veins of the patients (internal jugular vein [IJV], superior vena cava [SVC], or inferior vena cava [IVC]) drains patients' blood into the ECMO circuit, and the oxygenated blood is returned to the right atrium (via the return cannula). Whenever, ECMO flow is high, demand a second access cannula. In patients with severe respiratory failure, it is advisable to deploy a second access/drainage cannula for better ECMO flow. VV ECMO improves the patient's oxygenation by reducing the amount of blood that passes through the lung without being oxygenated and in addition removes CO_2 from the patient's blood. This allows the level of ventilatory support to be with high ECMO flow rate as is required in severe respiratory failure, this is when a second venous access cannula may be required making it a VVV ECMO.[14,15]

Relative to the patient's own native cardiac output and to the pump flow rate are the two determinants of the efficiency of the level of oxygenation achieved by the ECMO flow rates and the patients if by the latter two oxygenation are not adequate, then there is definitely recirculation of blood, between the inflow and the outflow cannulas.

VV ECMO is more efficient at removing CO_2 from the blood than delivering oxygen. The amount of CO_2 removal depends on the ECMO flow rate relative to the patient's cardiac output and also depends on the oxygen flow rate to the oxygenator. Increasing oxygen flow rate decreases the CO_2 in the blood leaving the oxygenator (analogous to the effect that increasing minute ventilation has on arterial pCO_2). The oxygen flow rate to the oxygenator should be roughly twice the ECMO flow rate. With an ECMO rate of approximately two-third the patient's cardiac output, and an oxygen flow rate of twice the pump flow, nearly all of the patient's CO_2 production can be removed by the oxygenator. The North-South syndrome or the Harlequin syndrome is a complication which can be easily overcome.

Venoarterial Extracorporeal Membrane Oxygenation

When the patient's venous blood is accessed from the large central veins and from ECMO circuit, oxygenated blood is returned to the major artery, then a VA ECMO is instituted. This form of ECMO provides support to a failing heart generally due to low cardiac output in a failing heart.

Low-Flow Venoarterial Extracorporeal Membrane Oxygenation

When smaller ECMO cannulas are inserted percutaneously, in an emergency situation, as in an ECMO cardiopulmonary resuscitation (ECPR), then ECMO is generally initiated and maintained on low flows. It is an emergency resuscitative intervention or ECMO CPR, with greater benefits than a high-flow ECMO.[14]

Venovenous or Venoarterial Extracorporeal Membrane Oxygenation

As shown in **Figs. 32.4** and **32.5** VV ECMO has many advantages over VA ECMO.[13] VV ECMO avoids risk of potential injury to the arterial vessels, avoids risk of air embolism from the circuit, and avoids stress as it has a low-pressure gradient circuit; thus, in doing this, VV ECMO promotes longer shelf-life of the ECMO oxygenator. The hemodynamic disturbances produced by the VV ECMO are also less (**Table 32.2**). VV ECMO in comparison to VA ECMO also preserves the pulmonary blood flow as seen in many animal studies.

Table 32.2   Cannulation options

Peripheral or central VA or VV ECMO	
Venous cannula locations	• RIJ RA, femoral vein • Pulmonary artery
Arterial cannula locations	• Carotid, aorta • Femoral artery, axillary, subclavian
Drainage line	• Left atrium, left ventricle
VA ECMO	• Femoral vein to femoral artery (peripheral) • Open chest—RA to aorta or LV (central)
VV ECMO	• Femoral vein to right IJ (peripheral) • Direct chest—RA to PA (central) • Avalon dual lumen—right IJ

Abbreviations: ECMO, extracorporeal membrane oxygenation; IJ, internal jugular; LV, left ventricle; PA, pulmonary artery; RA, right artery; RIJ, right internal jugular; VA, venoarterial; VV, venovenous.

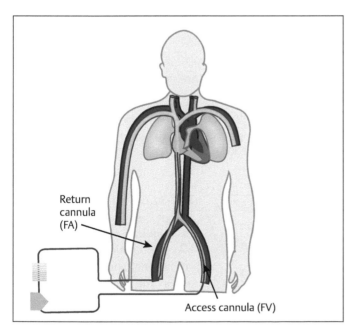

Fig. 32.4 Venovenous extracorporeal membrane. Abbreviations: FA, femoral artery; FV, femoral vein. Adapted with permission from Kapoor PM, Sethi BS. Introduction to Extracorporeal Membrane Oxygenation. In: Kapoor PM, ed. Manual Of Extracorporeal Membrane Oxygenation (ECMO) In The ICU, 1 ed. India: Jaypee Publication; 2014.

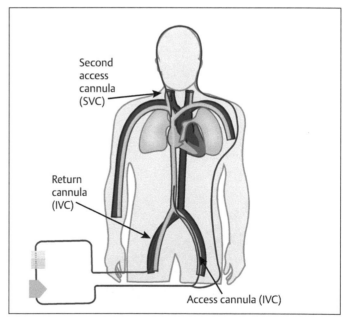

Fig. 32.5 Venoarterial extracorporeal oxygenation circuit membrane oxygenation circuit. Abbreviations: IVC, inferior vena cava; SVC, superior vena cava. Adapted with permission from Kapoor PM, Sethi BS. Introduction to Extracorporeal Membrane Oxygenation. In: Kapoor PM, ed. Manual Of Extracorporeal Membrane Oxygenation (ECMO) In The ICU, 1 ed. India: Jaypee Publication; 2014.

Is VA ECMO Without Any Advantage Over VV ECMO?

VA ECMO provides complete hemodynamics, cardiac output, and oxygenation support, when as a bridge to recovery or destination therapy. In poisoning, cardiogenic shock, myocarditis, and hypothermia, VA ECMO scores over VV ECMO (**Table 32.3**).

Traditionally, two sets of cannulas have been used for the drainage (typically 23–27 Fr) which is inserted in the IVC via the femoral vein (FV) and the returning cannula into one of the IJV, FV, or subclavian veins. This may cause recirculation especially when ECMO flows are high and also limits patient's mobility.

Bicaval dual lumen cannula with simultaneous drainage and reinfusion of the blood via the right IJV (**Figs. 32.6** and **32.7**).

As shown in **Fig. 32.8**, this peripheral VA ECMO may give rise to distal limb ischemia and need to insert a 9-Fr or 12-Fr drainage cannula at the same site to prevent hemolysis in the clot (**Fig. 32.9**).

Risk of Hemolysis during ECMO

- **Minimize**
  - ➤ Larger cannula size.
  - ➤ Lower flow.
  - ➤ Lowest possible to maintain adequate oxygenation.
  - ➤ Still >1.5 L/min to prevent circuit thrombosis.
- May need to insert one access cannula; high-flow ECMO.
- Change oxygenator if lots of clots exist in the oxygenator.
- Monitor[10] at least twice a day.
  - ➤ Dec. Hb.
  - ➤ Inc. plasma-free Hb.
  - ➤ Inc. bilirubin.
  - ➤ Urine color.
  - ➤ Renal function.

This is best done by the bedside nurse perfusionist both visually and with the help of a torch, with very vigilant monitoring on the development of clots, ischemia of distal limbs,

Table 32.3 Difference between VA ECMO and VV ECMO

Property	VA ECMO	VV ECMO
Cannulation site	IJV/FV and RCC/Ax/FA/Ao	IJV alone/IJV-FV/FV-FV/Saph-saph/RA
PaO$_2$	60–150 mmHg	45–80 mmHg
Indicator of O$_2$ sufficiency	Mixed venous saturation or PaO$_2$	Combination of SaO$_2$, PaO$_2$, cerebral venous saturation and premembrane saturation trend
Cardiac effect	↓ preload; ↑ afterload; pulse pr ↓; coronary oxygen by LV blood; Cardiac stun-like picture is seen	Negligible effects; may improve coronary oxygenation; may reduce RV afterload
O$_2$ delivery capacity	High	Moderate. ↑ cephalad drain
Circulatory support	Partial to complete	Indirect: ↑ delivery of O$_2$ to coronary and pulmonary circulation

Abbreviations: Ao, ascending aorta; ECMO, extracorporeal membrane oxygenation; FA, femoral artery; FV, femoral vein; IJV, internal jugular vein; LV, left ventricle; PaO$_2$, partial pressure of oxygen; RA, right atrium; RCC, right common carotid; RV, right ventricle; SaO$_2$, oxygen saturation; VA, venoarterial; VV, venovenous.

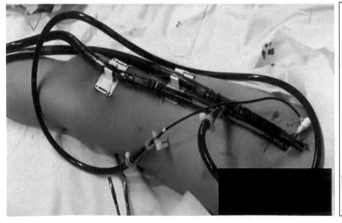

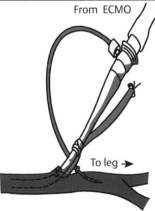

Fig. 32.6 Extracorporeal membrane oxygenation (ECMO) cannulation. This is peripheral VA cannulation wherein both the arterial and venous cannulas are in the same groin. Adapted with permission from Kapoor PM, Goyal V, Oza P, Hasija S. Complications of Extracorporeal Membrane Oxygenation. In: Kapoor PM, ed. Manual of ECMO in ICU, 1 ed. India: Jaypee Publication; 2014.

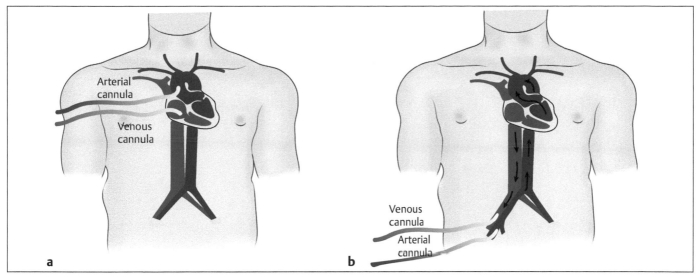

Fig. 32.7 **(a)** Central extracorporeal membrane oxygenation (ECMO) cannulation and **(b)** peripheral ECMO cannulation. Adapted with permission from Chopra HK, Kapoor PM. Role of Extracorporeal Membrane Oxygenation for Acute Decompensated Heart Failure: Kapoor PM, ed. Manual Of Extracorporeal Membrane Oxygenation (ECMO) In The ICU, 1 ed. India: Jaypee Publication; 2014.

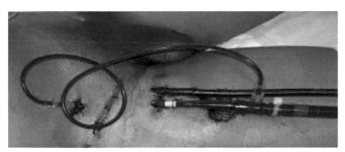

Fig. 32.8 Extracorporeal membrane oxygenation (ECMO) cannulation in the groin.

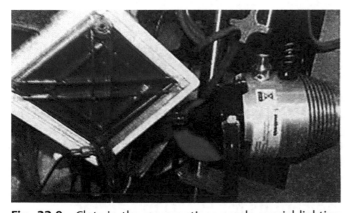

Fig. 32.9 Clots in the oxygenation; needs special lighting and continuous vigilance. Use of a torch to observe small clots is recommended. Adapted with permission from Kapoor PM, Airan R, Mandal B. Extracorporeal Membrane Oxygenation Circuit and Hardware. In: Kapoor PM, ed. Manual Of Extracorporeal Membrane Oxygenation (ECMO) In The ICU, 1 ed. India: Jaypee Publication; 2014.

thrombosis, DVT, etc., and a drop in PaO_2 and patient's saturation. The patient on VV and VA ECMO is most vulnerable to sudden arrest due to thrombosis, as seen during COVID-19 pandemic in recent times (**Fig. 32.10**).

It is now well established that VV ECMO has a major role to play in the treatment of ARDS.[16]

Thus, when one is on the threshold of initiating ECMO, it is imperative that one keeps not only the patients' indications, contraindications, and complications in mind, but must look at the entire aspect of it all together, in a patient population, which is at the threshold of a resource-limited pandemic.[17] So benefit to one patient of ECMO implementation must keep in mind the broader impact of ECMO use on other patients as two individuals would have separate indications for the same ECMO type inserted.

Coordinated Approaches by Healthcare Networks

Need of the hour is the use of coordinated approach to adhere to established ECMO practice, in order to optimize the provision of ECMO in a crisis/outbreak. The diffidence and inhibition of providing an essential life-saving tool like ECMO has to be overcome by the healthcare authorities and intensivists alike.[18]

ECMO Use in a Pandemic

It is essential to judiciously utilize resources by developing regional, national, and international networks, which serve

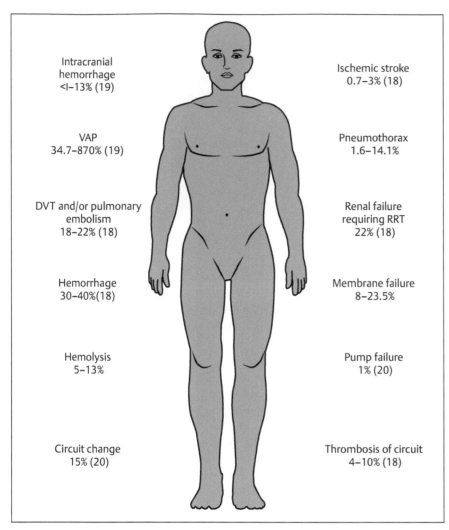

Intracranial
hemorrhage
<I–13% (19)

VAP
34.7–870% (19)

DVT and/or pulmonary
embolism
18–22% (18)

Hemorrhage
30–40%(18)

Hemolysis
5–13%

Circuit change
15% (20)

Ischemic stroke
0.7–3% (18)

Pneumothorax
1.6–14.1%

Renal failure
requiring RRT
22% (18)

Membrane failure
8–23.5%

Pump failure
1% (20)

Thrombosis of circuit
4–10% (18)

Fig. 32.10 Selected extracorporeal membrane oxygenation (ECMO)-related complications for patients with severe COVID-19-related acute respiratory distress syndrome (ARDS). Abbreviations: DVT, deep vein thrombosis; RRT, renal replacement therapy; VAP, ventilator-associated pneumonia.

to provide ECMO in a pandemic ECMO life support with ECMO. Increased mortality trends in COVID-19 patients, in many global ECMO centers in all three waves of COVID-19 pandemic, warrants judicious use of ECMO, universally.

Careful Patient's Selection is a Must Before Deploying ECMO

Patient's selection[19,20] as shown in most recent publications reveals that mortality was higher in COVID-19 than in HINI influenza-hit ARDS patients, who were treated with ECMO. Fanelli et al did a retrospective cohort study of these two diseases in patients from seven Italian centers. They concluded the differences between these two diseases. However, no significant after adjustments were made to advanced age and longer length of ICU stay in the two groups. Thus, COVID-19 patients who were older and had a longer length of stay in the ICU for ECMO-treated ARDS pneumonia were at greater risk of dying than the HINI influenza pneumonia patients on ECMO.[21] This mandates a careful evaluation and judicious selection of patients for ECMO insertion for higher benefits of this therapy.

COVID-19 witnessed the recruitment of new ECMO centers in the three waves of the pandemic globally, but particularly in the Middle East and India.

Rabie et al did a multicenter, retrospective analysis of patients from 19 ECMO centers in five countries in the Middle East and India. They concluded that during a pandemic use of ECMO shows favorable outcomes in highly selected patients as resources allow as resources were made available. The vast multitude of ECMO centers in COVID-19 globally (around 50 in India itself), with good expertise and expert supervision of ECMO, may provide immense positive ECMO outcomes in a ARDS pandemic.[22]

Indications for ECMO in Cardiac Surgery Patients

As outlined in **Box 32.2**, in cardiac patients with circulatory failure (e.g., advanced heart failure, myocarditis, and cardiogenic shock), and in patients with postcardiotomy low cardiac output when there is failure to wean from bypass, a VA ECMO is indicated.

Box 32.2   Indications for VA ECMO in cardiac surgical patients

- Patients of cardiogenic shock unresponsive to maximum inotropes and medical treatment
- Patients having failure to wean from cardiopulmonary bypass
- Advanced heart failure
- Patients unresponsive to intra-aortic balloon pump (IABP)
- VA ECMO as a temporary bridge to rest and recovery to the heart

Abbreviations: VA ECMO, venoarterial extracorporeal membrane oxygenation.

Box 32.3   Indications for ECMO in adults

- Presence of cardiorespiratory failure with an impending mortality of more than 90%. These may include patients with one or more of the following:
  - Unresponsive to conventional treatment
  - A transpulmonary shunt more than 30% at an FiO_2 of 0.6
  - Patients with static compliance of less than 0.5 mL/cm H_2O/kg
  - Abnormal chest X-ray in all four quadrants
  - Advanced heart failure
  - Cardiac arrest
  - Increase $PaCO_2$ with pulmonary hypertension <7.0

Abbreviations: ECMO, extracorporeal membrane oxygenation.; $FiO2$ fraction of inspired oxygen; $PaCO_2$, partial pressure of carbon dioxide.

Box 32.4   Contraindications of ECMO in adults

- Advanced age, more than 65 y
- Prolonged ventilation of more than 7 d, prior to ECMO insertion
- Irreversible pathology
- Presence of intracranial hemorrhage or even a closed space hemorrhage

Abbreviation: ECMO, extracorporeal membrane oxygenation.

ECMO indications are separate in adults and children, as outlined in **Box 32.3**.

There are contraindications to ECMO in adults as well, as outlined in **Box 32.4**.

All through the past four decades, ECMO has been shown to be more successful in children than adults. Broad indications and contraindications to ECLS in children are summarized in **Table 32.4**.

Contraindications to ECMO

- **Only absolute:**
  - Do not resuscitate.
- **"Relative" contraindications:**
  - Past contraindications.
  - Neurological compromise.
  - "Recent" surgery/trauma.
  - "Recent" neurosurgical procedures.
  - Acute multiorgan failure.
  - Chronic organ insufficiency.
  - Chronic respiratory insufficiency.
  - Immunosuppression.

ECMO as a Bridge

Today ECMO is used more as a "Bridge" that is a temporary life support till a definitive destination therapy is available. So, ECMO is sought to:

- Recovery.
- Ventricular-assist device.
- Cardiac or lung transplant.

Ethical Aspects of ECMO

Recent advances in ECMO technology allow for prolonged support with decreased complications. The development of mobile ECMO teams, the rapidity of initiation, and the

Table 32.4   Indications and contraindications to ECLS in children

Indications	Contraindications
- Unable to wean off CPB	- Low birth weight (<500 g)
- Presence of PAH with CHF	- Premature with gestational age less than 34 wk
- Malignant arrhythmias	- Irreversible pathology in a child
- Respiratory failure	- Intracranial hemorrhage
- Cardiogenic shock, not amenable to medical therapy	- Mechanical ventilation greater than 10 d
- Intracardiac shunting cyanosis	- Grade I IVH
- ECLS needed for support in Cath lab procedures as well	- Coagulation problems
- ECLS for bridge to recovery or cardiac lung transplant	

Abbreviations: CHF, cardiac heart failure; CPB, cardiopulmonary bypass; ECLS, extracorporeal life support; IVH, intraventricular hemorrhage; PAH, pulmonary arterial hypertension.

growing body of evidence, much of which remains controversial, have led to a significant increase in the use of ECMO worldwide. This increase in use of a technology that is not a destination device in itself introduces many ethical dilemmas specific to this technology.

ECMO and COVID-19

So ethically, commercial use of ECMO insertion for enhanced support should not be allowed early.[23,24] For commercial ECMO use, Maclaren et al reiterated that ECMO is not a therapy to be rushed to the frontline when all resources are stretched in a pandemic.[25]

As per Abrams et al in recent times, early extubation comes from the use of VV ECMO in COVID-19 patients. Most experts have observed that with the use of single access, dual-staged VV ECMO, in COVID-19 patients,[26,27] there were promising outcomes when early extubation was performed in these COVID-19 patients with respiratory failure on ECMO. Complications of ischemic strokes, thrombosis, and inotropic requirements were also minimal. In a recent, retrospective clinical trial conducted on 101 critically ill patients from Austria, Hermann et al also reiterated that prolonged invasive ventilation, prior to ECMO insertion in COVID-19, should be considered a contraindication for ECMO in patients with COVID-19-related ARDS.[28] Scrutinizing should be done on factors for ECMO, and it should be done on an individual patient's basis. In a pooled met analysis of pediatric cancer patients on ECMO, it was observed that the commonest indication for ECMO was respiratory failure, and pooled mortality in these cancer-ridden pediatric ECMO patients was around 55%.[29,30]

Some studies have shown that with an oxygenation index greater than 40, the mortality in pediatric ARDS patients on ECMO is very high. Thus, indications and contraindications before deploying an ECMO are essential, and these criteria should be meticulously met by all intensivists.[31,32]

Hemolysis and ECMO Pumps in the 21st Century

As experience grew during the first three decades of prolonged ECLS, hemolysis (PfHb > 15 mg/dL) was a rare complication. In most cases, elevated free hemoglobin resolved over time and, when it occurred, it was related to immediate postcraniotomy patients or circuit attachments like continuous renal replacement therapy (CRRT) or clotting in the circuit. Most centers used servoregulated roller pumps, and the centers that used conventional centrifugal pumps were careful to avoid high pump speeds.[33]

ECMO and Drainage Sufficiency

Drainage insufficiency occurring soon after ECMO initiation may be due to vasodilation, for instance, as occasionally seen with exposure of the blood to the ECMO circuit, or to cannulation issues, such as undersized or malpositioned cannulas or vascular injury.[34]

Later in the ECMO course, drainage insufficiency may be seen with agitation, as sedation is lightened, or with volume removal.

Conclusion

As concluded by Tongyoo, et al in 2022, in hospital mortality in RCMO supported patients in high around 69% with higher mortality when ECMO continuous beyond 2 hours. (35) In-hospital mortality among ECMO-supported patients was high at 69%. SOFA score >14, hospitalized >72 hours, PaO_2/FiO_2 ratio <60, and pH <7.2 were found to be independent predictors of in-hospital mortality.[35]

Summary

The management of advanced heart failure is a dynamic process that requires frequent re-evaluation timing of ECMO placement. ECMO for bridge to transplant and destination therapy (DT) has been shown to improve mortality rates and quality of life. There are short-term ECMO (ECPR) options available for emergent situations. A one size fits all model for initialing ECMO in a critical care patient, does not hold true today. Despite the increase in mortality over time, ECMO still serves an important role as supportive therapy for select patients. Physicians should carefully weigh the potential benefits and harms of ECMO for each patient in the context of resource availability, the individual's disease course, and local experience and mortality rates in order to decide on ECMO candidacy.

References

1. Zwischenberger JB, Bartlett RH. What is ECLS? An introduction to extracorporeal life support. https://www.med.umich.edu/ecmo/about/what.html. Accessed on March 11, 2022
2. Iacono A, Groves S, Garcia J, Griffith B. Lung transplantation following 107 days of extracorporeal membrane oxygenation. Eur J Cardiothorac Surg 2010;37(4):969–971
3. Gibbon JH Jr. Application of a mechanical heart and lung apparatus to cardiac surgery. Minn Med 1954;37(3):171–185
4. Lillehei CW. A personalized history of extracorporeal circulation. Trans Am Soc Artif Intern Organs 1982;28:5–16

5. Kirklin JW, Donald DE, Harshbarger HG, et al. Studies in extracorporeal circulation. I. Applicability of Gibbon-type pump-oxygenator to human intracardiac surgery: 40 cases. Ann Surg 1956;144(1):2–8

6. Rashkind WJ, Freeman A, Klein D, Toft RW. Evaluation of a disposable plastic, low volume, pumpless oxygenator as a lung substitute. J Pediatr 1965;66:94–102

7. Dorson W Jr, Baker E, Cohen ML, et al. A perfusion system for infants. Trans Am Soc Artif Intern Organs 1969;15:155–160

8. Baffes TG, Fridman JL, Bicoff JP, Whitehill JL. Extracorporeal circulation for support of palliative cardiac surgery in infants. Ann Thorac Surg 1970;10(4):354–363

9. Bartlett RH, Gazzaniga AB, Jefferies MR, Huxtable RF, Haiduc NJ, Fong SW. Extracorporeal membrane oxygenation (ECMO) cardiopulmonary support in infancy. Trans Am Soc Artif Intern Organs 1976;22:80–93

10. Hill JD, O'Brien TG, Murray JJ, et al. Prolonged extracorporeal oxygenation for acute post-traumatic respiratory failure (shock-lung syndrome). Use of the Bramson membrane lung. N Engl J Med 1972;286(12):629–634

11. Kolobow T, Spragg RG, Pierce JE, Zapol WM. Extended term (to 16 days) partial extracorporeal blood gas exchange with the spiral membrane lung in unanesthetized lambs. Trans Am Soc Artif Intern Organs 1971;17:350–354

12. Chauhan S, Subin S. Extracorporeal membrane oxygenation, an anesthesiologist's perspective: physiology and principles. Part 1. Ann Card Anaesth 2011;14(3):218–229

13. Kapoor P. Platform for students, clinicians and the common people. J Card Crit Care TSS 2018;2:1–2

14. Airan R, Sharan S, Malhotra Kapoor P, Chowdhury U, Velayoudam D, John A. Low flow venoarterial ECMO support management in post cardiac surgery patient. J Card Crit Care 2021;5:103–107

15. Keebler ME, Haddad EV, Choi CW, et al. Venoarterial extracorporeal membrane oxygenation in cardiogenic shock. JACC Heart Fail 2018;6(6):503–516

16. Short B, Abrams D, Brodie D. Extracorporeal membrane oxygenation for coronavirus disease 2019-related acute respiratory distress syndrome. Curr Opin Crit Care 2022;28(1): 90–97

17. Brodie D, Slutsky AS, Combes A. Extracorporeal life support for adults with respiratory failure and related indications: a review. JAMA 2019;322(6):557–568

18. Malhotra Kapoor P. ECMO in COVID-19—The diffidence has to be overcome by the intensivists and administrators in 2021. J Card Crit Care TSS 2021;5(2):79–81

19. Karagiannidis C, Slutsky AS, Bein T, Windisch W, Weber-Carstens S, Brodie D. Complete countrywide mortality in COVID patients receiving ECMO in Germany throughout the first three waves of the pandemic. Crit Care 2021;25(1):413

20. Supady A, Biever PM, Staudacher DL, Wengenmayer T. Choosing the right reference cohort for assessing outcome of venovenous ECMO. Crit Care 2022;26(1):17

21. Fanelli V, Giani M, Grasselli G, et al. Extracorporeal membrane oxygenation for COVID-19 and influenza H1N1 associated acute respiratory distress syndrome: a multicenter retrospective cohort study. Crit Care 2022;26(1):34

22. Rabie AA, Azzam MH, Al-Fares AA, et al. Implementation of new ECMO centers during the COVID-19 pandemic: experience and results from the Middle East and India. Intensive Care Med 2021;47(8):887–895

23. Abrams D, Lorusso R, Vincent J-L, Brodie D. ECMO during the COVID-19 pandemic: when is it unjustified? Crit Care 2020; 24(1):507

24. Heinsar S, Peek GJ, Fraser JF. ECMO during the COVID-19 pandemic: when is it justified? Crit Care 2020;24(1):650

25. MacLaren G, Fisher D, Brodie D. Preparing for the most critically ill patients with COVID-19: the potential role of extracorporeal membrane oxygenation. JAMA 2020;323(13):1245–1246

26. Mustafa AK, Alexander PJ, Joshi DJ, et al. Extracorporeal membrane oxygenation for patients with COVID-19 in severe respiratory failure. JAMA Surg 2020;155(10):990–992

27. Combes A, Hajage D, Capellier G, et al; EOLIA Trial Group, REVA, and ECMONet. Extracorporeal membrane oxygenation for severe acute respiratory distress syndrome. N Engl J Med 2018;378(21):1965–1975

28. Hermann M, Laxar D, Krall C, et al. Duration of invasive mechanical ventilation prior to extracorporeal membrane oxygenation is not associated with survival in acute respiratory distress syndrome caused by coronavirus disease 2019. Ann Intensive Care 2022;12(1):6

29. Slooff V, Hoogendoorn R, Nielsen JSA, et al; POKER (PICU Oncology Kids in Europe Research group) research consortium of ESPNIC (European Society of Paediatric Neonatal Intensive Care). Role of extracorporeal membrane oxygenation in pediatric cancer patients: a systematic review and meta-analysis of observational studies. Ann Intensive Care 2022; 12(1):8

30. Bayrakci B, Josephson C, Fackler J. Oxygenation index for extracorporeal membrane oxygenation: is there predictive significance? J Artif Organs 2007;10(1):6–9

31. Badulak J, Antonini MV, Stead CM, et al; ELSO COVID-19 Working Group Members. Extracorporeal membrane oxygenation for COVID-19: updated 2021 guidelines from the Extracorporeal Life Support Organization. ASAIO J 2021;67(5):485–495

32. Lebreton G, Schmidt M, Ponnaiah M, et al; Paris ECMO-COVID-19 investigators. Extracorporeal membrane oxygenation network organisation and clinical outcomes during the COVID-19 pandemic in Greater Paris, France: a multicentre cohort study. Lancet Respir Med 2021;9(8):851–862

33. Toomasian JM, Bartlett RH. Hemolysis and ECMO pumps in the 21st century. Perfusion 2011;26(1):5–6

34. Shaefi S, Brenner SK, Gupta S, et al; STOP-COVID Investigators. Extracorporeal membrane oxygenation in patients with severe respiratory failure from COVID-19. Intensive Care Med 2021; 47(2):208–221

35. Tongyoo S, Chanthawatthanarak S, Permpikul C, et al. Extracorporeal membrane oxygenation (ECMO) support for acute hypoxemic respiratory failure patients: outcomes and predictive factors. J Thorac Dis. 2022;14(2):371–380

33

Patient Blood Management in ECMO Cardiac Critical Care

Poonam Malhotra Kapoor, Vandana Bhardwaj, Ameya Karanjkar,
Sandeep Sharan, Mohit Prakash, and Omer Mohammed Mujahid

Introduction

The hematology laboratory–derived activated partial thromboplastin time (APTT) along with activated clotting time (ACT) is a major guide to heparin therapy in an extracorporeal membrane oxygenation (ECMO) patient. The normal range for APTT in ECMO patients is 45 to 55 seconds, with a platelet count, greater than 80,000/µL of blood. In India most ECMO centers perform both ACT and APTT on a daily basis as described in **Box 33.1**.

Plasma-free hemoglobin is checked, when we suspect hemolysis. Its normal range is less than 0.1 g/L. If the plasma-free hemoglobin is more than its normal range then a thorough re-evaluation should be done by the ECMO team. All parameters that are checked daily should be kept as near normal as possible.

The updated 2021 clinical (Society of Cardiovascular Anesthesiologists/Society of Thoracic Surgeons [SCA/STS]) practice guidelines on patient blood management (PBM) in cardiac surgery for anesthesiologists reiterated the importance of the use of an evidence-based, multimodal, and multidisciplinary approach, with top priority particularly to conserve the patient's blood and save resources, so as to have the best optimal results, within the available resources. This is a daunting task as the clinical practice in blood management is more toward liberal transfusion in the past few years.[1]

Risk Factors for Abnormal Bleeding on ECMO

Bleeding in patients on venoarterial (VA) ECMO is more than that in patients on venovenous (VV) ECMO because of an inherent or an iatrogenic cause. Some of the risk factors for increased bleeding in patients on VA ECMO are enlisted in **Box 33.2**.

There are many methods to overcome abnormal bleeding, which includes performing such procedures as much off-pump as possible, timely preoperative correction of the anemia, stopping antiplatelet drugs 3 to 5 days before surgery, keeping the comorbidities within control, and performing most therapeutic cardiac procedures as minimally invasive or noninvasive as feasible.

While working on 6,075 patients, authors gave enough evidence that a pragmatic, preoperative approach to treating anemia and iron deficiency with folic acid, vitamin B12, and oral/intravenous iron therapy can substantially decrease the intraoperative use of blood and blood products, and thus increase the postoperative hematocrit. Such approaches should be encouraged, especially in a developing country like ours.[2]

Do the International Patient Blood Management Guidelines Apply to the Indian Scenario?

A multidiversity expert group has enumerated the diverse healthcare facilities prevalent in different two- or three-tier urban cities as well as rural India. The expert panel finalized an urgent need for a holistic and multidisciplinary approach to management of abnormal bleeding. The Indian PBM management in ECMO patients emphasizes the following three factors: (1) Detailed clinical history, which is a more important guide than a preoperative bleeding time (BT) value. Changes in platelet functions should be picked up precariously. (2) The coagulation laboratory with the timely use of point-of-care viscoelastic (VET) tests is an important contributor to providing the right blood components. (3) Availability of resources for providing the equipment, reagents and blood products, and/or concentrates for the abnormal preoperative bleeding is equally important. These constitute a three-pillar approach to managing abnormal bleeding. In all cases of abnormal perioperative bleeding, a uniform validated protocol should be carried out in a timely manner to increase the patient safety at all costs.[2]

Box 33.1 Investigations for ECMO on a daily basis

- D-Dimer
- Blood culture twice a week
- ACT—twice a day or as indicated
- Chest X-ray
- Echocardiography (transthoracic echocardiograms [TTE] or transesophageal echocardiograms [TEE]) for monitoring biventricular position of ECMO cannulas
- Blood urea
- Coronary artery bypass grafting (CABG) for serum electrolytes like sodium, potassium, calcium, magnesium, chloride, and base excess
- Serum fibrinogen
- Plasma-free hemoglobin
- Liver function tests
- International normalized ratio (INR)
- Platelet count

Box 33.2 Risks factors for increased bleeding on VA ECMO

- Advanced age
- Anemia
- Thrombocytopenia
- Complex redo cardiac surgeries
- Redo valves/thoracic/aortic procedures
- Comorbidities

Problems with Blood Transfusion

Blood transfusion entails problems of finance, demand versus supply, and hazards of blood transfusion like anaphylaxis and massive transfusion giving rise to lung injury (TRALI) or hypocalcemia.[3] Today, most ECMO centers have moved toward a restricted blood transfusion therapy, moving away from undertaking liberal transfusion due to disadvantages of latter as mentioned above.

Stopping Antiplatelet Agents before Surgery

Following the European Association of Cardiovascular Thoracic Anesthesia (EACTA) guidelines, the expert panel has finalized that preoperatively (3–7 d) the antiplatelet drugs should be stopped (**Table 33.1**).[1]

Blood Storage at Appropriate Temperature

The blood should be stored at the right temperature, and all blood components like cryoprecipitate,[5] platelet, and fibrinogen concentrates should be stored in freezers in the blood bank and thawed before use. Pharmacological agents such as antifibrinolytics, tranexamic acid, factor VIIa, and epsilon aminocaproic acid also need proper room temperature for storage.

Ideal VET tests in cardiac surgical patients and ECMO patients are listed in **Table 33.2**.

Blood Products Available in Indian Blood Banks

Box 33.3 enumerates the common blood products available in most Indian blood banks for a daily basis management of postoperative bleeding and/or ECMO following cardiac surgery.

Coagulopathy Worsens the ECMO Run

It is important to rule out that the patient is not coagulopathic at all times, when on ECMO. This is particularly true in a pregnant cardiac patient put on ECMO or undergoing

Table 33.1 Appropriate timing for stopping antiplatelet agents before surgery

Antiplatelet drug	Days before stopping for surgery
Aspirin	Continue till day of surgery; to be stopped only if high risk of bleeding or patient refuses blood transfusion
P2Y12 receptor antagonists: • Ticagrelor • Clopidogrel • Prasugrel	Postpone surgery: • 3 d • 5 d • 7 d

Table 33.2 Different viscoelastic tests and their interpretation

Name of cardiac surgery	Best test/lab or VET to be done	Most appropriate POC/VET
Aortic dissection CABG ECMO Abnormal bleeding postoperative	Sonoclot: • PF • TEG • Verify now • ROTEM platelet count • Fibrinogen levels • PT • APTT	Sonoclot: • PF • EXTEM, INTEM, and FIBTEM • ACT • MCF • X angle • LY30
Residual effect	Anti-XA ACT	• ROTEM: INTEM and HEPTEM • TEG: Kaolin TEG • TEG: Heparinase teg • Sonoclot: CRT
Protamine overdose	Fibrinogen levels: • PT • APTT	ROTEM: INTEM, HEPTEM, CT ratio
DIC	Fibrinogen platelet count D-Dimer	• EXTEM, FIBTEM • Rapid TEG, TEG FF

Abbreviations: ACT, activated clotting time; APTT, activated partial thromboplastin time; CABG, coronary artery bypass graft; CRT, cardiac resynchronization therapy; DIC, disseminated intravascular coagulation; ECMO, extracorporeal membrane oxygenation; FF, functional fibrinogen; MCF, maximum clot firmness; ROTEM, rotational thromboelastometry; TEG, thromboelastography.

- Packed red blood cells (RBC)
- Fresh frozen plasma
- Platelet concentrates: Both random donor platelet and single donor platelet
- Cryoprecipitate
- Fibrinogen concentrates
- Prothrombin complex concentrates (PCC)
- Tranexamic acid
- Epsilon aminocaproic acid
- Recombinant factor VIIa prothrombin complex concentrate (PCC)
- Antidotes
- Desmopressin

Box 33.4 Is the patient coagulopathic?

- Normal intrauterine pregnancy: Hypercoagulable physiologically
- Fibrinogen in third trimester: 350–600 mg%
- All patients who are bleeding need not be coagulopathy
- Dilution coagulopathy: Later stage of resuscitation
- Consumption coagulopathy: Early in APH, AFE, AFLP, severe PIH, IUD
- Hypothermia, acidosis worsen coagulopathy

Abbreviations: APH, antepartum hemorrhage; AFE, amniotic fluid embolism; AFLP, fatty liver of pregnancy; IUD, intrauterine device; PIH, pregnancy-induced hypertension.

cardiac surgery in first, second, or third trimester of pregnancy (**Box 33.4**).

Is the Patient Hypovolemic?

It is also important to rule out that the cardiac patient is not volume depleted or hypovolemic. Visual appearance can lead to misjudgment, so checking parameters of Echo or right atrial (RA) pressures is essential, as is ruling out tachycardia, checking the presence of comorbidities, and preventing excessive increase in blood volume (**Fig. 33.1**). The preoperative, intraoperative, and postoperative checklist of the patient ensuring availability of blood and its products all are the necessary laboratory parameters, which should be crosschecked, by at least two OT personnel. This prevents complications later on and progression to disseminated intravascular coagulation (DIC) is prevented too.

The Backbone of PBM in ECMO in India are the Viscoelastic Tests—ROTEM, TEG, and Sonoclot for Faster Turn Around Tune Before Correct Transfer

Anticoagulation monitoring in India is on a tight rope. Use of rotational thromboelastometry (ROTEM) or a thromboelastography-based point-of-care testing done on the patient in a timely manner prevents excessive postoperative bleeding.[6] The point-of-care tests should be implemented at the ground level (in the OT and ICU), with patient notes on the machine as a sticker for all to observe and enacting communication at shift change is most important (**Fig. 33.2a–d**).[6,7]

All OT and ICU personnel should be well versed with the interpretation of different point-of-care test results. Point-of-care tests such as ROTEM, thromboelastography (TEG), and Sonoclot systems give reliable information on the development of hypofibrinogenemia or hyperfibrinolysis in an ECMO patient. The "MCF" (maximum clot firmness) on

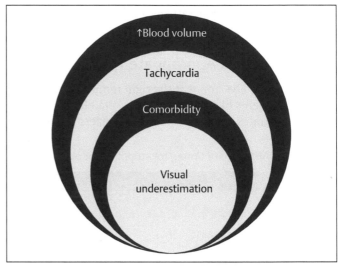

Fig. 33.1 Hypovolemia on extracorporeal membrane oxygenation (ECMO) brings about tachycardia and altered hemodynamics.

ROTEM with the "FIBTEM" is the most reliable marker for hyperfibrinogenemia, respectively. The turnaround time for test result is only 15 minutes, which is a signature graph that shows the result of anticoagulant used, as against the conventional APTT and fibrinogen which take hours in a laboratory (**Fig. 33.3**). The preemptive tests to thus control bleeding are also much faster. Qualitative and quantitative platelet dysfunction on cardiopulmonary bypass (CPB) and ECMO[8] is well seen on the ROTEM or multiple or Sonoclot PF results. Any one monitor can give accurate results of platelet function. ROTEM with its ADPTEM, ARATEM, and TRAPTEM platelet aggregometry parameters could be the answer for rapid prediction of coagulopathy or hyperfibrinolysis on ECMO. Following an algorithm in the OT/ICU in a bleeding patient gives best results. The All India Institute of Medical Sciences (AIIMS) algorithm used in cyanotic cardiac surgery and in coronary artery bypass graft (CABG) surgery has helped authors manage bleeding better in ECMO patients and in the OT/ICU (**Flowchart 33.1**).

So, best practice is to follow an algorithm as the authors have done in AIIMS Cardiac Centre since 2016.

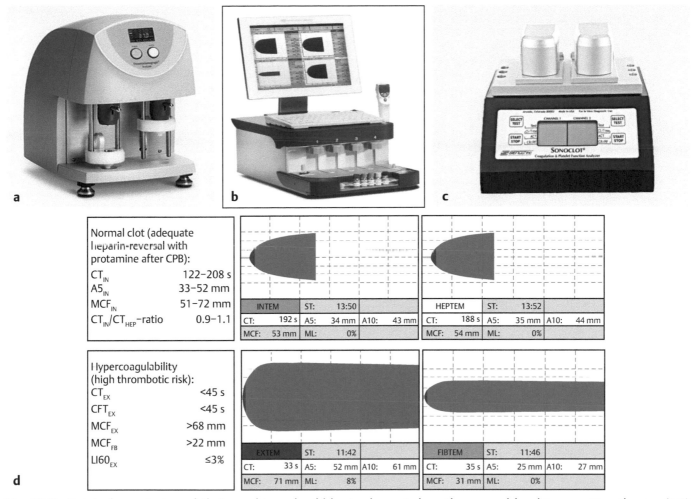

Normal clot (adequate heparin-reversal with protamine after CPB):		
CT_{IN}	122–208 s	
$A5_{IN}$	33–52 mm	
MCF_{IN}	51–72 mm	
CT_{IN}/CT_{HEP}–ratio	0.9–1.1	

INTEM	ST:	13:50
CT: 192 s	A5: 34 mm	A10: 43 mm
MCF: 53 mm	ML: 0%	

HEPTEM	ST:	13:52
CT: 188 s	A5: 35 mm	A10: 44 mm
MCF: 54 mm	ML: 0%	

Hypercoagulability (high thrombotic risk):	
CT_{EX}	<45 s
CFT_{EX}	<45 s
MCF_{EX}	>68 mm
MCF_{FB}	>22 mm
$LI60_{EX}$	≤3%

EXTEM	ST:	11:42
CT: 33 s	A5: 52 mm	A10: 61 mm
MCF: 71 mm	ML: 8%	

FIBTEM	ST:	11:46
CT: 35 s	A5: 25 mm	A10: 27 mm
MCF: 31 mm	ML: 0%	

Fig. 33.2 Point-of-care tests and their machines should be implemented on the ground level in operation theater (OT) and intensive care unit (ICU). **(a)** Thromboelastography machine. **(b)** Rotational thromboelastometry (ROTEM) machine. **(c)** Sonoclot (activated clotting time machine). **(d)** Hypercoagulability and normal clot.

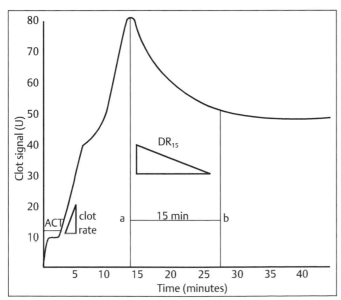

Fig. 33.3 Normal Sonoclot curve result after an anticoagulant is used.

Correlation between Rotational Thromboelastometry (ROTEM) and Bleeding on VA ECMO

TEG and standard tests are used for evaluating platelet dysfunction and hypofibrinogenemia in patients on VA-ECMO. Managing bleeding using AIIMS algorithm in cyanotic patients and performing ROTEM platelet function tests in CABG patients helped authors as intensivists at AIIMS to use the right blood component product in most patients and correct the bleeding (**Flowchart 33.1**).

Flowchart 33.2 depicts whether platelet aggregometry in on-pump CABG is a game changer to improve outcomes.[11]

ECMO Centers in India

In December 2021 India had 110 dedicated ECMO centers. These centers are actively involved in ECMO work in the

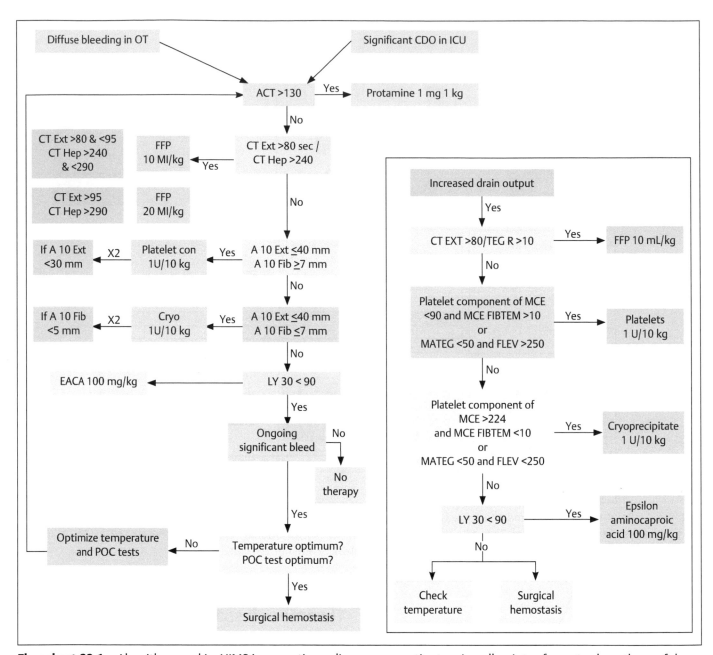

Flowchart 33.1 Algorithm used in AIIMS in cyanotic cardiac surgery patients using all points of care to show the usefulness of giving blood component therapy first, instead of fresh whole blood as a part of restricted blood transfusion while on extracorporeal membrane oxygenation (ECMO).[9,10] Abbreviations: EACA, epsilon aminocaproic acid; FFP, fresh frozen plasma; FLEV, functional fibrinogen; ICU, intensive care unit; MCE, maximum clot elasticity; OT, operation theater; POC, point-of-care testing; TEG, thromboelastography.

cardiac, pediatric trauma, obstetric, and pulmonary areas, and in poisoned patients in the ICU. Out of these 110 centers 25 are registered to ELSO, the global registry of ECMO centers, situated in the United States (**Table 33.3**).

Steps to be taken to prevent patient bleeding and its management on ECMO and cardiac surgery are enumerated as 21 points in **Box 33.5**.

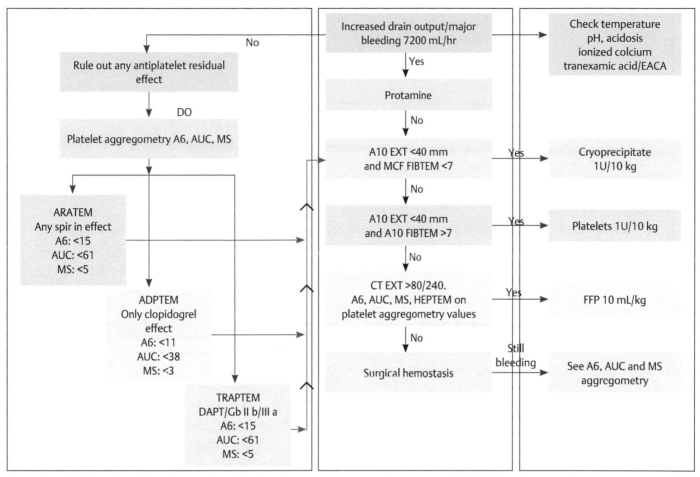

Flowchart 33.2 Algorithm for testing platelets in coronary artery bypass graft (CABG) patients going on extracorporeal membrane oxygenation (ECMO). Abbreviations: ADPTEM, adenosine disphosphate thromboelastometry; AUC, area under the curve; FFP, fresh frozen plasma; MCF, maximum clot firmness; MS, maximum slope of the aggregation curve; TRAPTEM, thrombin activating peptide thromboelastometry.

Box 33.5 Steps to be taken to prevent patient bleeding and its management on ECMO and cardiac surgery

- Correction of anemia and diagnosis of its etiology
- Minimizing phlebotomy and volume and frequency of blood samples taken on the ECMO patient
- Preoperative correction of anemia and thrombocytopenia in the cardiac surgical/ECMO patient
- Withdrawing antiplatelet drugs as follows before elective surgery:
  - Aspirin: To continue till day of surgery
  - Clopidogrel: 3 days before surgery
  - Ticagrelor: 5 days before surgery
  - Prasugrel: 7 days before surgery
- Utilization of laboratory and point-of-care tests judiciously and optimally with all expertise and cost-effectiveness
- Restarting antiplatelet and oral anticoagulants until all bleeding has finished
- Prothrombin concentrate is recommended if the antidote for a specific non-vitamin-K oral anticoagulant (NOAC) is not available
- Use of synthetic antifibrinolytic agents like EACA, tranexamic acid to be used as first choice, after surgery in case of excessive oozing, to reduce blood loss and also blood transfusion
- Tranexamic acid and normothermia prevent excessive bleeding in off-pump procedures
- Topical application of antifibrinolytic agents and surface sealants like fibrin glue, gel foams, thrombin, etc., to be used
- Alternate excessive bleeding with the use of desmopressin, von Wille brand and factor 13 concentrates especially in ECMO patients

(Continued)

Box 33.5 (*Continued*)

- In HIT patients, antithrombin III concentrates are encouraged
- Fresh frozen plasma transfusion is feasible in patients with single or multiple factor deficiencies
- Cell salvage and autologous predonation may be practiced in Jehovah Witness, along with extracorporeal circulation and plasmapheresis
- Prevent and treat hypothermia and acidosis at all times, while on ECMO[11,12]
- Restrictive blood transfusion in 2022[11,12]
- There is a role of factor concentrates in patient blood management while on ECMO
- Factor concentrate acts faster than individual blood component therapy
- ROTEM platelet function–based testing, which is algorithm based and is done in a goal-directed transfusion strategy model, gives the best guidance to the correct blood product usage of excessive red blood and yellow blood products
- The three pillars of PBM, involving a multimodal, multidisciplinary approach with the aim to resuscitate early, needs preoperative implementation
- Implementing guidelines on the ground in the operating room and intensive care units are to be enacted fast with discipline and teamwork[11,12]

Abbreviations: EACA, epsilon aminocaproic acid; ECMO, extracorporeal membrane oxygenation.

Table 33.3 Extracorporeal membrane oxygenation (ECMO) centers of India.[12]

No.	Hospital/Institute Name	City	No.	Hospital/Institute Name	City
North Zone			13	SDM College Of Medical Sciences and Hospital	Dharward
1	AIIMS	New Delhi	14	Kovai Medical Centre and Hospital	Coimbatore
2	Sir Ganga Ram Hospital	New Delhi	15	Manipal Hospital, Hal	Bangalore
3	Medanta—The Medicity	Gurgaon	16	Manipal Hospital Whitefield	Bangalore
4	Max Hospital	Saket, New Delhi	17	Narayan Hrudayalay/Narayana Institute of Cardiac Sciences	Bangalore
5	Fortis Hospital	Gurgaon	**West Zone**		
6	Fortis Hospital	Mohali	1	Fortis Hospital	Mumbai
7	Dayanand Medical College And Hospital Unit Hero—DMC Heart Institute	Ludhiana	2	Kokilaben Dhirubhai Ambani Hospital	Mumbai
South Zone			3	Riddhivinayak Critical Care & Cardiac Centre	Mumbai
1	KIMS Hospital	Hyderabad	4	Sir H N Reliance Foundation Hospital and Research Centre	Mumbai
2	Virinchi Hospital	Hyderabad	5	Sunshine Global Hospital	Surat
3	Apollo Health City Jubilee Hills	Hyderabad	6	CIMS Hospital	Ahmedabad
4	Star Hospital	Hyderabad	**East Zone**		
5	Yashoda Hospital	Hyderabad	1	Rabindranath Tagore International Institute of Cardiac Sciences	Kolkata
6	Fortis Malar Hospital	Chennai			
7	Apollo Hospital	Chennai	2	Medica Superspecialty Hospital	Kolkata
8	Fortis Hospital	Chennai	3	Nh Narayana Superspeciality Hospital	Howrah
9	Kauvery Hospital	Chennai			
10	MGM Healthcare Private Limited	Chennai			
11	Global Hospital	Chennai			
12	Velammal Hospital	Madurai			

Conclusion

The three pillars of PBM, involving a multimodal, multidisciplinary approach with the aim to resuscitate early, needs preoperative implementation with the correct defect shown early. Implementing guidelines on the ground in the operating room and intensive care units are to be enacted fast with discipline and teamwork. tests are available, which confuse the intensivists, so their detailed knowledge and correct information is important at early stage, for a successful patient blood management strategy on ECMO.

Many barriers, such as dogmatic ideas, logistics and lack of support from the medical and administrative departments need to be overcome and each center must find solutions to their specific problems. In this paper we present a narrative overview of the challenges and updated recommendations for the implementation of a PBM program in cardiac surgery.[13,14]

References

1. Tibi P, McClure RS, Huang J, et al. STS/SCA/AmSECT/SABM update to the clinical practice guidelines on patient blood management. Ann Thorac Surg 2021;112(3):981–1004
2. Gandhi A, Görlinger K, Nair SC, et al. Patient blood management in India: review of current practices and feasibility of applying appropriate standard of care guidelines. A position paper by an interdisciplinary expert group. J Anaesthesiol Clin Pharmacol 2021;37(1):3–13
3. Huang J, Firestone S, Moffatt-Bruce S, Tibi P, Shore-Lesserson L. 2021 clinical practice guidelines for anesthesiologists on patient blood management in cardiac surgery. J Cardiothorac Vasc Anesth 2021;35(12):3493–3495
4. Pagano D, Milojevic M, Meesters MI, et al. 2017 EACTS/EACTA guidelines on patient blood management for adult cardiac surgery. Eur J Cardiothorac Surg 2018;53(1):79–111
5. García-Roa M, Del Carmen Vicente-Ayuso M, Bobes AM, et al. Red blood cell storage time and transfusion: current practice, concerns and future perspectives. Blood Transfus 2017;15(3):222–231
6. Shaydakov ME, Sigmon DF, Blebea J. Thromboelastography. [Updated 2021 Apr 20]. In: StatPearls [Internet]. Treasure Island, FL: StatPearls Publishing; 2021 Jan. https://www.ncbi.nlm.nih.gov/books/NBK537061/. Accessed on 15 December 2021.
7. Kapoor PM. Patient blood management in cardiac surgery and ECMO: the Indian scenario in 2021. J Card Crit Care 2021;5:181–183
8. Balle CM, Jeppesen AN, Christensen S, Hvas A-M. Platelet function during extracorporeal membrane oxygenation in adult patients. Front Cardiovasc Med 2019;6:114
9. Bhardwaj V, Kapoor PM, Karanjkar AA, et al. Congenital cyanotic cardiac surgery in children: is algorithm-based point-of-care testing essential to prevent bleeding? J Card Crit Care TSS 2018;2:84–90
10. Karanjkar A, Malhotra Kapoor P, Sharan S, et al. A prospective randomized clinical trial of efficacy of algorithm-based point of care guided hemostatic therapy in cyanotic congenital heart disease surgical patient. J Cardiac Crit Care TSS 2019;3(1):8–16
11. Sharan S, Kapoor PM, Choudhury M, Devagourou V, Kumar Choudhury U, Ravi V. Role of platelet function test in predicting postoperative bleeding risk after coronary artery bypass grafting: a prospective observational study. J Card Crit Care 2021;5:88–96
12. Kapoor PM, Ed. Evoluation of extracorporeal membrane oxygenation. In: Textbook of extracorporeal membrane oxygenation. 2nd ed. Chapter 4. Jaypee Publishers; 2018:13-18
13. Rancati V, Scala E, Ltaief Z, et al. Challenges in Patient Blood Management for Cardiac Surgery: A Narrative Review. J Clin Med. 2021;10(11):2454
14. Bolliger D, Lancé MD. Factor Concentrate-Based Approaches to Blood Conservation in Cardiac Surgery: European Perspectives in 2020. Curr. Anesthesiol. Rep. 2020;10:137–146

34

Simulation on Extracorporeal Membrane Oxygenation

Poonam Malhotra Kapoor, Sindhuja Ramarathinam, Nisha Shetty, Komal Purabiya, and Prajakta Davne

Introduction

Franklin said, "Tell me and I forget, show me and I remember, involve me and I learn".

The extracorporeal membrane oxygenation (ECMO) circuit simulator system is based on interconnected modules serving different functions required for simulation of ECMO emergencies. It includes simplified three-dimensional (3D) printed replicas of otherwise expensive consumable parts, such as the oxygenation membrane and the actual ECMO machine to enable the circulation of a thermochromic fluid simulating the patient blood. The simulation society has collaborated with the Indian Institute of Science (IIS) Bangalore ECMO simulation solutions to address the challenges of ECMO simulation. The team is developing a relatively low-cost yet high-fidelity or high-technology modular ECMO simulator. The work has been partially supported by some research grants.[1-5]

ECMO simulation training can be done through Water Drills, Wet labs, and online programs, but a continuous trend with hands-on experience of the clinical scenario is what makes simulation training complete and exhilarating. Until recent past the simulation training programs in the country were done through software-based systems along with low-fidelity mannequins. However currently we have a simulation system which is indigenously developed by IIS Bangalore for dedicated use in ECMO simulation. The mannequin is specially designed for ECMO cannulation as a task trainer and can also be used for clinical patient management with high-fidelity simulation pertaining to ECMO. All India Institute of Medical Sciences (AIIMS) has conducted many such workshops on this simulator training (**Fig. 34.1**).

The entire data in the simulator monitor is got together and then projected on to the big screen, such that many more students may visualize the same (**Fig. 34.2**). An imitating ICU setup should be available with simulation props to give it a proper simulation lab look.

Considering the multimodality approach and the complexities involved, it is necessary to have a fully trained ECMO team in a hospital, including surgeons, doctors, perfusionist, and nurses. Multidepartment coordination is a prerequisite as intensive care, cardiac surgery, blood banks, nephrology, and pathology units are all involved in this procedure. ECMO training and simulation programs for hospitals help in addressing these challenges. It fills the gap in communication and coordination within a team when members of the team start working in fully controlled simulation environment. In addition, it overcomes the challenges in complication handling.

ECMO in the ICU saves lives, in case of both cardiac and pulmonary failure. Simulation-based ECMO training makes practice on ECMO technology and its complexities look simpler. Repetitive practice on the ECMO simulator confers precision and dexterity to the intensivist ECMO cannulation and perfusion technology skills, as mistakes made while practicing are not on the patient. Thus many complications while on ECMO are avoided. Post-COVID era, ECMO knowledge and use have increased significantly. A detailed knowledge of the ECMO components and hardware, and its assembly and complications, is provided during the simulation-based training by the educators, in a stepwise manner, thus allaying mistakes which could have fatal outcomes. Since 2021, in the post-COVID era, in every ICU, intensive simulation-based ECMO training is mandatory. Simulation-based ECMO training should generally show a continuous trend of the patient's clinical condition.

Generally simulation workshops involves series of lectures and water drills for cannulation techniques, but what is essentially needed is real-time problem-based clinical teaching of the ECMO technique, as it changes from time to time. There is also an urgent need to have hands-on experience on the ECMO machine and for cannula insertion and their maintenance and monitoring as well.

ECMO training usually consists of didactic lectures and water drill of ECMO circuit. However, the learners cannot experience the change in the clinical condition of the patient. Simulation-based learning provides participants an interactive, team-based training without risk to the real patients. Simulation-based ECMO programs aim to provide structural and standardized training opportunity for clinical staff member to gain hands-on experience in ECMO circuit management and troubleshooting technique.

Advantages of Simulation Programs

In the last 10 years and especially post-COVID, there is a voluminous increase in the number of ECMO centers in India and worldwide. ECMO procedure is complex and involves complications if done by a novice. Each ECMO team member requires a detailed knowledge of ECMO physiology, cannulations, and ECMO hardware and components involved. Skills for rapid response to ECMO failure, cardiac arrest, and pulmonary hemorrhage must be expedited with expertise. ECMO maintenance and weaning is a skillful art requiring intensive training. From cannulation to management of ongoing care of ECMO to successful weaning of ECMO support, each of these stages should be understood by the

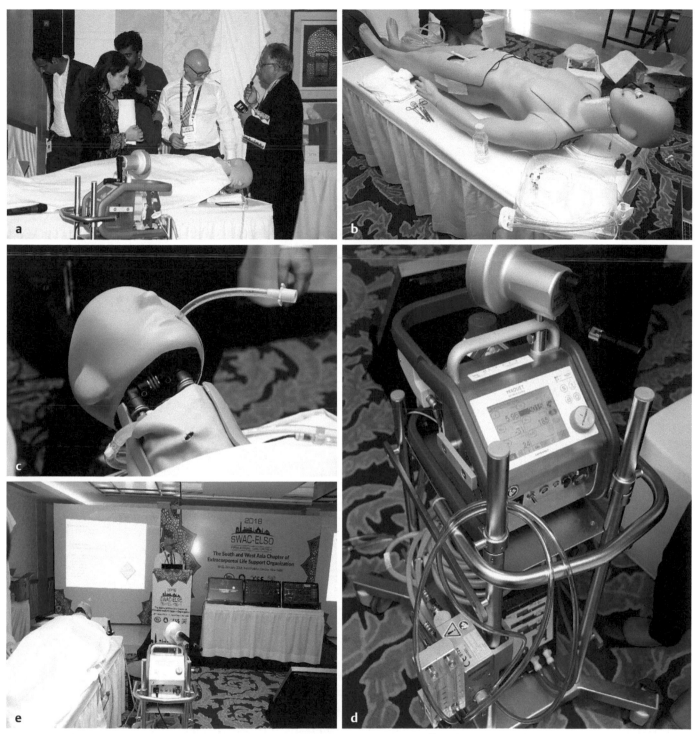

Fig. 34.1 **(a)** Extracorporeal membrane oxygenation (ECMO) mannequin. **(b)** Close-up of the mannequin. **(c)** A close-up of the mannequin's electrical connections. **(d)** The Cardiohelp ECMO machine which is portable. **(e)** All attachments to the mannequin (serves as the patient) and the monitoring screens assembled together.

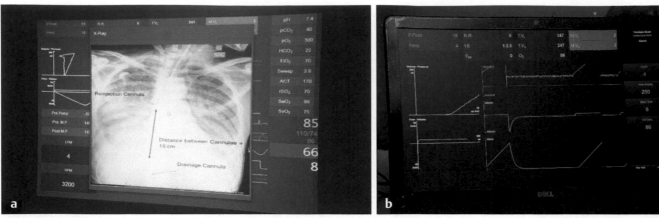

Fig. 34.2 **(a)** Data of the patient projected onto the big screen for bigger audience viewing. **(b)** Data on the computer monitor.

ECMO team members involved in the management of these patients.

Different ECMO centers have different case mix of indications due to various reasons including geography and specialization. Therefore some ECMO centers have more of venovenous (VV) ECMO cases while other centers have more of venoarterial (VA) ECMO cases.

Simulation-based training represents a valuable tool in intense education, to understand the objective and also measurable and clinically relevant long-term outcomes. It offers the opportunity to practice the technical skills repeatedly and to become proficient in high-risk low-frequency events while avoiding harm to the patients where errors may have direct consequences on mortality and morbidity. In addition to improving technical skills, simulation-based training has also been shown to provide essential cognitive and behavioral skills when compared to theoretical teaching, and most importantly, it enables the team to work toward quality and safety.

In general, simulators come with many advantages albeit with some limitations as well (**Box 34.1**). Providing sound, practical feedback helps in better designing of the simulator. A higher fidelity simulator provides more information and greater diversity of clinical scenarios[1] than low or medium fidelity simulators.[1] Use of animation and computer graphics on a big screen is an excellent tool for the students, to learn the complex nuances of ECMO—both venovenous and venoarterial.

ECMO Simulator Setup

The setup includes screen, simulation room, and simulation props. For bigger viewership, the entire data can be incorporated together and put up for viewing on to a bigger screen. While setting up an ECMO simulation scenario, it is essential to use simulation props and modules and recreate a

Box 34.1 Utility of ECMO simulators

Advantages

- Provide users with practical hands-on experience and feedback on real-time clinical scenarios
- Since there is feedback, the correctness and efficiency of a particular design can be refurbished
- High-fidelity ECMO simulators are more useful than the low-fidelity ones
- Simulator allows rapid prototyping in which the primary systems are designed in such a way that high-level training can be provided, with the designs being high end from the beginning so that they remain feasible and practical
- Simulators are good tools for teaching and demonstrating ECMO concepts to students from beginning to end
- Allows flexibility of slow and stable repetitive learning, avoiding complications
- Fast learning for the student

Limitations

- It is not real clinical setup but only a learning tool; it gives an idea but not accuracy

Abbreviation: ECMO, extracorporeal membrane oxygenation.

simulation room, like an ICU room to give a real live picture. Simulation props are essential while setting up simulation for ECMO (**Fig. 34.3** and **Box 34.2**).

Mannequin Design

The ECMO mannequin is designed to teach the details of both types of ECMO: venovenous and venoarterial. The distal limb ischemia perfusion cannulation can also be demonstrated. **Box 34.2** provides the list of ECMO kits with details of ECMO circuit, cannulas, and the ECMO reservoir, all of which are essential to set up any type of ECMO.

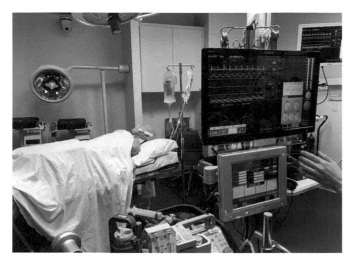

Fig. 34.3 The extracorporeal membrane oxygenation (ECMO) simulator setup.

Box 34.3   The cannulation task trainer is aimed at making the students understand the practical requirements (cannulation tray, cannula types) and developing confidence of students on

- Vessel identification
- Sizing
- Seldinger technique
- Positioning
- De-airing

ECMO Cannulation Task Trainer

The ECMO mannequin is designed for an adult ECMO. The percutaneous cannulation technique for both femoral and jugular route is nicely taught on this mannequin. All ultrasound-guided cannulations are feasible, and all central and peripheral pulses can be palpated with variable simulated intensity (**Box 34.3**, **Figs. 34.4** and **34.5**).

ECMO Circuit and ECMO Cannulas

The ECMO circuit is connected to the inserted ECMO cannulas (**Fig. 34.6a–d**) such that we have the drainage or access cannula from the patient to the ECMO machine, and the return cannula oxygenated blood from the ECMO machines back to the patient.

The Use of ECMO Simulator

The ECMO mannequin simulation circuit and external reservoir are designed to mimic an ECMO patient. The simulation circuit flow can be controlled from the trainer tabs through wireless protocol. Also the LED lights fixed onto the tubing help in simulating blood color change.

Box 34.2   ECMO kit for teaching simulation on ECMO

- Cardiohelp full system
- HLS kit
- Air and oxygen source
- Ventilator
- ICU environment props
- Vitals virtual monitor
- ECMO virtual monitor
- SimCast (for projection)
- Trainer iPad
- Trainee iPad

Abbreviations: ECMO, extracorporeal membrane oxygenation; HLS, heart lung support; ICU, intensive care unit.

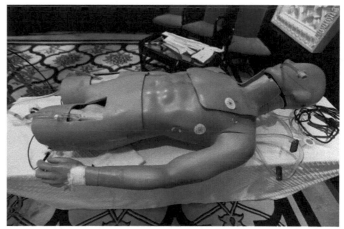

Fig. 34.4 The Indian Institute of Science Bangalore Simulator—marketed by Maquet—used for teaching simulation all over different extracorporeal membrane oxygenation (ECMO) centers in India.

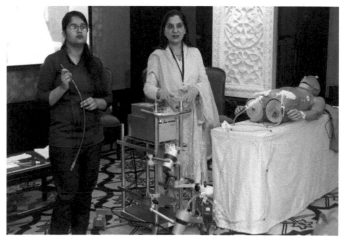

Fig. 34.5 The Maquet Rotaflow connected to the extracorporeal membrane oxygenation (ECMO) simulator in real time. ECMO scenarios like ECMO cannulation, priming, ventilation, and hemodynamics can all be done on this simulator. Teamwork in ECMO simulation is essential.

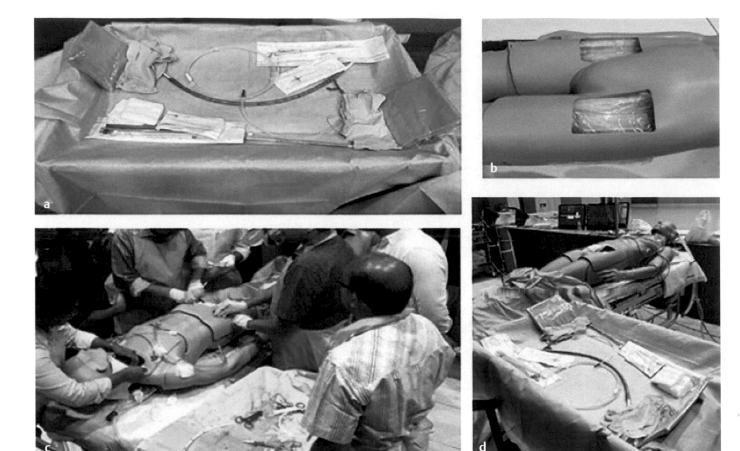

Fig. 34.6 **(a)** The cannulas used in extracorporeal membrane oxygenation (ECMO) tray; **(b)** access cannulas and their sites on the mannequin; **(c)** the process of ECMO cannulation; **(d)** the complete ECMO setup.

The virtual monitor presents all the clinical parameters. The ECMO monitor is fed with values replicating the Cardiohelp/Rotaflow parameters including ECMO flows, rotation per minute (RPM), three pressures P1, P2 and P3 before and after the oxygenator and mixed venous oximetry (SvO_2) and blender parameters. Both these monitors aid in creating the clinical picture of the patient pertaining to the scenario.

The trainer iPad controls the complete interface, and with a wireless system, it interacts with each device. This design allows preset scenarios as well as new flow change based on the participants' reaction to the scenario. The trainee iPads and the Sim cast are used to project patient investigations (X-ray, ultrasonography [USG], computed tomography [CT], Arterial Blood Gas [ABG], lab values) as per the request and scenario.

The clinical picture from the monitors, the investigations from the iPad, the ECMO parameters, and flow changes from the mannequin help in creating high-fidelity simulation (**Fig. 34.7**). This provides scope for creating various scenarios right from basic hypovolemia to advanced ECMO transport situations. This innovative indigenous system has vast scope to expand indications and application on need basis.

Debriefing and Briefing the Simulation Scenarios to the Students

The ECMO simulators are provided with animation and computer graphics such that dynamic flow exists between the different simulator components, such that the learner understands the current and the flows. Example of an ECMO circuit as simulator is a prototype. The student understands all about the ECMO circuit by understanding the difference between the input signal and its path and the output fan-out; thus, whatever is happening between the two points is understood by the learner as dynamics of the ECMO circuit. Thus ECMO circuit learning hastens or slows down according to the students' learning capability. Feedback loops are most important for better understanding.[6–8] The simulation rooms look like an ICU environment as the mannequin is intubated and then ventilated with IV access and all anesthesia drugs.

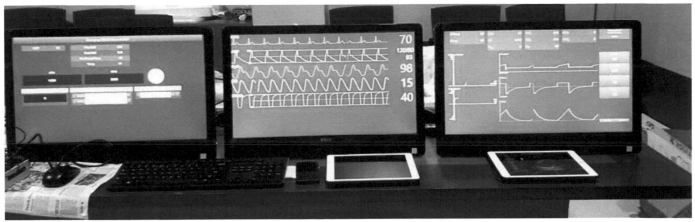

Fig. 34.7 The virtual monitors for extracorporeal membrane oxygenation (ECMO) hemodynamic measurements used as screening monitors.

Training Scenario in ECMO Simulation

A balloon is connected to the mannequin's trachea to simulate the lung functions and compliance and an infusion pump is attached to deliver intravenous fluids. Thus, patient's physiological parameters are displayed on a remote-controlled panel wherein pulse oximetry and bedside monitoring are observed on the screen. Fluid can be withdrawn to simulate hypovolemia and this hypotension and decrease in right atrial pressures is also displayed on the screen. Similarly, we can simulate air embolism by injecting air from a syringe into the ECMO circuit. At the headend of the patient, the main monitor displays essential parameters like mean arterial pressure, heart rate, electrocardiogram (ECG), and oxygen saturation of the patient. These are controlled remotely by a technician, who at the instruction of the main simulator tutor can change the parameters, according to the clinical scenario. The laboratory reading of the patient can be retrieved on request **(Box 34.4)**.

Participants are welcomed and registered before the starting of the training. They are introduced to one another and briefed about the simulation environment. They are informed that the training is only for learning purpose and is not used for assessment or punitive purposes.

When the scenario starts, the instructor introduces the patient's case history, present clinical status and issues, IV access, medications, and laboratory results (e.g., arterial blood gas, plasma-free hemoglobin level, and postoxygenator pO_2 level). On request, results of relevant imaging studies are provided (e.g., X-ray, CT scan, and ECG). In each scenario, participants in the group have to appoint one leader to lead the team. After the scenario training is complete, participants move to a separate cubicle for debriefing. Instructors have to debrief according to the manual with preset teaching objectives and debriefing notes. All learners are expected to actively participate in the discussion, and

> **Box 34.4** Components of the modular ECMO simulator to treat a VT/VF cardiac arrest on an ECMO patient
>
> - Real-life scenario is replicated
> - The tubing is pinched
> - Accidental recirculation is created
> - Pulmonary hypertension is transferred to the CT room
> - Differential hypoxia is detected upon transfer from another hospital
> - Hypovolemia is now detected due to a broken pigtail catheter
> - Hypothermia too is detected as the perfusionist saying "forgot to switch the heater on"
> - Oxygen tubing gets disconnected
> - Leading to limb ischemia
> - Air bubbles detected on access cannula ECMO site
> - Console also fails due to circuit problem
> - Accidental decannulation

Abbreviations: CT, computed tomography; ECMO, extracorporeal membrane oxygenation; VF, ventricular fibrillation; VT, ventricular tachycardia.

the facilitator serves as a guide for the discussion rather than a "lecturer." If the participants want to practice any technical issues again, then instructors will arrange the practice at the end of the debriefing session.

Debriefing

Participants in one room listen to the leader about ECMO scenarios as enumerated in **Table 34.1** and then move to another room for debriefing. The leader is a facilitator who explains the clinical scenarios during an ECMO run. This training and debriefing can be very often practiced again and again.

Table 34.1   Common ECMO clinical scenarios and simulation interventions on ECMO simulator

Clinical scenarios	Problem	Interventions
Low peripheral oxygen saturation	• Circuit flow is inadequate • Lung function worsens (VV) • Upper body desaturation (VA) • Increase oxygen requirements	• Increase ECMO flows • Look into the pathology • Cool the patient • Sedate the patient • Change to VA
High drainage limb oxygen saturation	• Recirculation (VV ECMO)	• Change cannula type • Adjust pump flows • Give IV fluids • Change to VA ECMO • Do an echocardiography: TTE or TEE
Loss of ECMO flows	• Pump failure • Circuit airlock • Circuit blood thrombosis • Obstruction in the circuit	• Replace the circuit • De-air the circuit • Check cannula and tube migration and kinks • Use manual hand crane • Do CPR
Low circuit flows, high negative drainage limb pressure	• Drainage cannula insufficiency	• Address cannula issues • Check blood volume/administer fluids

Abbreviations: CPR, cardiopulmonary resuscitation; ECMO, extracorporeal membrane oxygenation; IV, intravenous; TEE, transesophageal echocardiogram; TTE, transthoracic echocardiogram; VA, venoarterial; VV, venovenous.

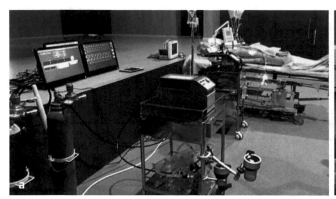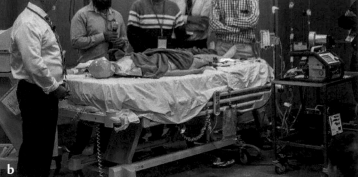

Fig. 34.8   **(a)** The simulation setup in a SIMLAB. **(b)** Simulation scenario being enacted on the fully computerized mannequin.

Tables 34.2 and **34.3** tell us about common complications of ECMO such as oxygenator failure, pump failure, clots in the oxygenator, and hypovolemia. The simulated scenarios enacted on the mannequin also tell the mode of treatment.

Box 34.5 provides us a detailed insight into the components of the ECMO simulator machine setup in the ICU and rechecks needed when ECMO flow drops and drainage insufficiency ensues. **Fig. 34.8** shows a SIMLAB with the entire ECMO setup.

Nontechnical Aspect

Appropriate team behaviors and clear communication are of utmost importance in caring for ECMO patients. Therefore, staff members that take care of ECMO patient should possess

Box 34.5   Simulated ECMO clinical scenarios and cross clamp in the ICU

Check the following:
• ECMO circuit
• ECMO console
• Oxygen source
• Patient clinical condition

Know the following terms:
• P Ventilation
• P Delta
• P Art
• P int

Know the chief cause of flow drop and the pressure alarms

Abbreviations: ECMO, extracorporeal membrane oxygenation; ICU, intensive care unit.

Table 34.2 Simulated ECMO scenarios, methods of simulation, induced cues, and gaps and drawbacks of ECMO simulation

Scenarios	Methods	Cues	Gaps and drawbacks
Pump or power failure	Confederate nurse turns off the pump	Loss in circuit flow and pump's rotation per minute	Checking the status of the pump is a part of troubleshooting pump failure Participants have to pretend the pump is not turned off
	Confederate nurse turns off the power	• Battery alarm triggers if the battery was drained beforehand • If the battery is completely drained, the pump and console will turn off	Similar to the above, participants have to pretend the power is not disconnected/turned off; furthermore, console battery must be drained before simulation and the scenario must begin shortly after to prevent it from charging back up
Oxygenator failure or membrane clots	Adding fluid into the circuit or partially clamp the arterial line. Injection of animal liver puree into the venous line of the circuit	Rise in pre- and postmembrane pressure and fall in circuit flow rate. Rise in trans-membrane pressure (rise in premembrane and fall in postmembrane pressure), fall in circuit flow rate, and the appearance of dark spots on the membrane	• Incorrect cues: the emergency is characterized by the rise of transmembrane pressure • Missing cues: visible clots on the membrane, no blood color change representing hypoxemia, unrealistic blood parameters (blood gases, hematocrit, hemoglobin, and activated clotting time) on modern ECMO consoles (e.g., Cardiohelp) or inline monitors
			• Contextual authenticity: rapid oxygenator failure is extremely rare. Clots typically build up, and hence, a more realistic scenario would start with indicators of oxygenator failure such as low oxygenation efficiency and high transmembrane pressure that are not sufficient to trigger alarms but still indicate potential failure • In addition, it is difficult to discretely clamp the circuit lines. Address the incorrect pressure cues and missing visible clots in the method above. However, it can be performed only once per oxygenator as the liver cannot be removed afterward. It is inconvenient and expensive to replicate

Abbreviation: ECMO, extracorporeal membrane oxygenation.

Table 34.3 Simulated ECMO scenario, methods of simulation, and probable diagnosis

Scenarios	Simulation methods	Probable diagnosis and limitations
Hypovolemia, on pressure monitor	• Simulated by the scrub nurse shaking the venous line[7–10] • Can also demonstrate visible bleeding by using a red-colored link in the chest drain	• Seen chattering of the venous line by the learner • Bleeding seen in chest drain is a cue to access cannula or drainage cannula insufficiency or hypotension

Abbreviation: ECMO, extracorporeal membrane oxygenation.

both technical (medical knowledge and technical skills) and nontechnical skills. Nontechnical skills include situation awareness, communication, teamwork, leadership, and decision-making. The importance of nontechnical skills is to increase the work safety and ensure effective working environment, with a minimum of technical errors (**Fig. 34.9**).

A Modern ECMO Simulation Setup

The ECMO troubleshooting remains as the nidus of each ECMO simulation scenario. Teamwork is followed as basic discipline with a leader chosen from the team. Data is obtained from the environment and each team member enacts it out (**Fig. 34.10**).

Besides discussing technical skills knowledge, instructors would also encourage group discussion on their nontechnical

skill performance.[10,11] They would be encouraged to express their views on issues such as any performance gaps, the reasons behind such gaps, what could have improved, and the relevance to their real-life experience. During the process, the instructors, apart from encouraging the participants to speak out, have to assist the participants to clarify issues, correct misunderstanding, and reinforce certain predefined teaching objectives.[12-16]

Conclusion

Developing a stand-alone ECMO simulator, which is cost-effective and delivers high-fidelity clinical case scenarios, with less limitations, is the need of the hour. A functioning ECMO machine and alternatives in the circuit, done manually to show circuit design and also showcase the complications,

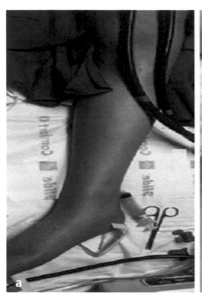
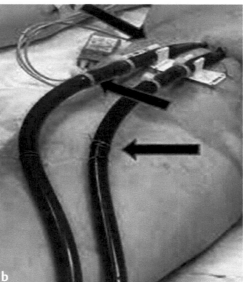
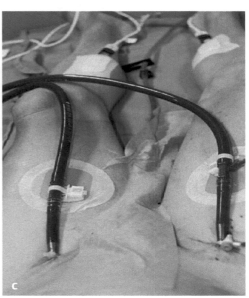

Normal circuit operation · Hypoxia · Recirculation

Fig. 34.9 **(a–c)** Components of the modular extracorporeal membrane oxygenation (ECMO) simulator.

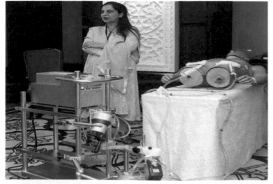
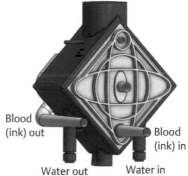
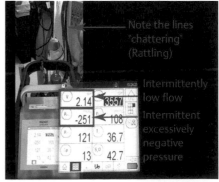

Fig. 34.10 A modern extracorporeal membrane oxygenation (ECMO) simulation setup. It is currently used with modern centrifugal pump-based ECMO circuits, such as the Maquet Rotaflow pump, the Maquet Cardiohelp system, Thoratec's CentriMag in addition to a plethora of basic to advanced mannequins, such as the Laerdal's Resuci Junior, SimMan, SimBaby and Nursing Kelly, CAE's PediaSim, and Gaumard's Hal.

is need of the hour. The IIS Bangalore ECMO simulator is one such ECMO simulator, with the software updated regularly to enhance the diverse ECMO complications for all of us to learn.

ECMO education and simulation delivered online is feasible, welcomed and supportive of a change in ECMO training course format. As we incorporate more innovative digital technologies, tele-simulation may further enhance the quality of future ECMO training.[16]

References

1. Kapoor PM. Simulation on extracorporeal membrane oxygenation. J Card Crit Care 2020;3:55–58
2. Brum R, Rajani R, Gelandt E, et al. Simulation training for extracorporeal membrane oxygenation. Ann Card Anaesth 2015;18(2):185–190
3. Alinier G, Hassan IF, Alsalemi A, et al. Addressing the challenges of ECMO simulation. Perfusion 2018;33(7):568–576
4. Al Disi M, Alsalemi A, Alhomsi Y, Bensaali F, Amira A, Alinier G. Extracorporeal membrane oxygenation simulation-based training: methods, drawbacks and a novel solution. Perfusion 2019;34(3):183–194
5. Alinier G. Cost-effective extracorporeal membrane oxygenation simulation. J Card Crit Care TSS 2018;2:5–9
6. Ng GWY, So EHK, Ho LY. Simulation training on extracorporeal membrane oxygenation. In: Firstenberg MS, ed. Extracorporeal Membrane Oxygenation—Advances in Therapy [Internet]. London: IntechOpen; 2016. Accessed March 22, 2022 at: https://www.intechopen.com/chapters/50706
7. Mendonca M. Simulation for ECLS. The Egyptian Journal of Critical Care Medicine 2016;4:17–23
8. Anderson JM, Boyle KB, Murphy AA, Yaeger KA, LeFlore J, Halamek LP. Simulating extracorporeal membrane oxygenation emergencies to improve human performance. Part I: methodologic and technologic innovations. Simul Healthc 2006;1(4):220–227
9. Nimmo GR, Wylie G, Scarth J, et al. Critical events simulation for neonatal and paediatric ECMO. Simulation 2008;4(5)
10. Burkhart HM, Riley JB, Lynch JJ, et al. Simulation-based postcardiotomy extracorporeal membrane oxygenation crisis training for thoracic surgery residents. Ann Thorac Surg 2013;95(3):901–906 © 2013 by The Society of Thoracic Surgeons
11. Anderson JM, Boyle KB, Murphy AA, Yaeger KA, LeFlore J, Halamek LP. Simulating extracorporeal membrane oxygenation emergencies to improve human performance. Part I: methodologic and technologic innovations. Simul Healthc 2006;1(4):220–227
12. Banfi C, Bendjelid K, Giraud R. High-fidelity simulation for extracorporeal membrane oxygenation training, utile or futile? J Thorac Dis 2017;9(11):4283–4285
13. Brum R, Rajani R, Gelandt E, et al. Simulation training for extracorporeal membrane oxygenation. Ann Card Anaesth 2015;18(2):185–190
14. Sin SWC, Ng PY, Ngai WCW, Lai PCK, Mok AYT, Chan RWK. Simulation training for crises during venoarterial extracorporeal membrane oxygenation. J Thorac Dis 2019;11(5):2144–2152
15. Puslecki M, Ligowski M, Kiel M, et al. Prototype of extracorporeal membrane oxygenation (ECMO) therapy simulator used in regional ECMO program. J Thorac Dis 2018;10(8):5073–5079
16. Wong AS, Marwali EM, Maclaren G, et al. ECMO simulation training during a worldwide pandemic: The role of ECMO telesimulation. Perfusion. 2022; 2676591221093868

35

ECMO and Sepsis

Yatin Mehta, Gaurav Kochhar, Ajmer Singh, Pravin Saxena, and Poonam Malhotra Kapoor

Sepsis and Septic Shock

Sepsis is defined as life-threatening organ dysfunction due to dysregulated host response to infection, and organ dysfunction is defined as an acute change in total Sequential Organ Failure Assessment (SOFA) score greater than 2 points secondary to the infection cause.[1] Septic shock occurring in patients with sepsis comprises of an underlying cellular/metabolic and circulatory abnormality that is associated with increased mortality. Septic shock is defined by persisting hypotension requiring vasopressors to maintain a mean arterial pressure of 65 mm Hg or higher, and a serum lactate level greater than 2 mmol/L (18 mg/dL) despite adequate volume resuscitation.[1] The new definition, also called sepsis 3, does away with the concept of systemic inflammatory response syndrome. The previous severe sepsis is now the new definition of sepsis. The 2018 update on surviving sepsis emphasizes the need of urgent/prompt treatment following detection of hypotension as "Hour 1 bundle" by starting immediate therapy with the right fluids, vasopressors, and appropriate antibiotics, in all cases of life-threatening hypotension instead of waiting or extending resuscitation measures over a larger time (**Flowchart 35.1**).[2]

A large number of factors too contribute to septic shock (**Box 35.1**).

Emerging Role of ECMO in Sepsis

Most critically ill patients are ailed by sepsis and septic shock.[6] As time goes on there is a compromise in organ perfusion and multiple organ failure sets in.[7,8] Extracorporeal membrane oxygenation (ECMO) has been suggested as a therapeutic therapy for neonates and pediatric patient, when all other therapies fail. Previously sepsis was once

considered as a contraindication for ECMO because microorganisms could easily inhabitate the artificial circuits and cause severe uncontrolled infection. Main concerns were cannula might perpetuate bacteremia, foreign membranes might aggravate inflammatory response, and preexisting coagulopathy might increase bleeding complications[6] and enhance mortality (**Box 35.1**). However, advances in ECMO management and circuit technology have made the indications for ECMO in sepsis possible and potentially a viable option. Septic patients are no longer excluded as candidates for ECMO. This was corroborated by the study findings showing a survival rate of up to 15% in some patients, especially in those adults who were 60 years and above, of which nearly 38% succumbed on ECMO. The outcomes of ECMO in adults with refractory shock remained dismissal, but pediatrics ECMO sepsis showed favorable results.[9–11] According to Ling et al,[12] venoarterial (VA) ECMO may be a suitable alternative to venovenous (VV) ECMO in septic shock. Majority of septic shock patients with sepsis induced myocardial damage were observed in those adults, receiving ECMO as circulatory support for refractory septic shock.[13]

Why is the Sepsis so Dreadful in ECMO?

There are two forms of septic shock which lead to mortality. These are either distributive shock, with low systemic vascular resistance (**Boxes 35.2** and **35.3**), or refractory

---

Box 35.1 Factors contributing to sepsis in adults due to prolonged extracorporeal membrane oxygenation (ECMO)

- High severity of underlying illness
- Disease-induced compromised immune system
- Advanced age
- Indwelling medical cannulas and devices[3,4]
- Presence of comorbidities[5]
- In adults, more than children, the femoral route of ECMO cannulation more than the IJV route or the double lumen cannula use increases the chances for ECMO

Box 35.2 Disease status and type of ECMO

- VV ECMO is used in case of:
  - ARDS
  - Hypoxemia
  - Respiratory failure
- VA ECMO is used in case of:
  - Hypoxemia RV dysfunction
  - Cardiomyopathy vasoplegia
  - RV and LV failure

Abbreviations: ARDS, acute respiratory distress syndrome; ECMO, extracorporeal membrane oxygenation; LV, left ventricle; RV, right ventricle, VA, venoarterial; VV, venovenous.

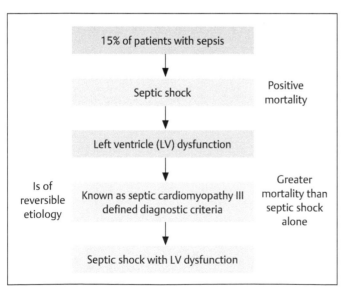

Flowchart 35.1 Consequences of extracorporeal membrane oxygenation (ECMO) sepsis.

hypotension but with preserved cardiac index.[14] Cardiac failure in sepsis is an inadequacy of cardiac output and oxygen delivery due to cardiac dysfunction. Cardiac dysfunction can be right ventricle (RV) or left ventricle (LV) or combined failure (**Box 35.4**). RV dysfunction can cause decreased venous return; LV diastolic dysfunction may cause impairment of LV preload. LV systolic dysfunction, also usually called "septic cardiomyopathy," is often present with LV diastolic dysfunction.

Prolonged ECMO Increases Sepsis in Adults

Patients on prolonged ECMO use do not have good outcomes as other complications invariably set in leading to increased mortality, ventilation-associated pneumonia, and blood stream infections. The latter constitutes major form of sepsis in adult patients.[14] Nearly 4 to 45% of patients on

---

Box 35.3 Presentation of sepsis in different age groups

- Newborn neonates: pulmonary arterial hypertension (PAH) and rectourethral fistula (RUF)
- Young children: left heart failure (LHF)
- Adults: distributive shock

Box 35.4 Depressed intrinsic myocardial performance (100%) on ECMO leads to both diastolic and systolic dysfunction

- LV diastolic dysfunction (50%)
  - ➤ Slight LV dilation LV compliance is impaired
  - ➤ LV Relaxation impairment
  - ➤ Tolerance to fluids may be modified
- BV Systolic dysfunction (30–50%)
  - ➤ Can be isolated or associated with acute lung injury (ALI)/acute respiratory distress syndrome (ARDS)
  - ➤ Is dependent on respiratory setting
  - ➤ Decrease venous return
- LV Systolic dysfunction (up to 60% at day 3)
  - ➤ Is afterload sensitive
  - ➤ Does not increase LV filling pressure
  - ➤ Is usually corrected by small dose of dobutamine

Abbreviations: BV, biventricular; ECMO, extracorporeal membrane oxygenation; LV, left ventricle.

ECMO do develop sepsis due to reasons listed in **Box 35.4**.[10] For patients in distributive shock, who present with lower normal or supranormal cardiac function, ECMO has less prognostic value (**Table 35.1**). ECMO has less prolonged value in patients with distributive shock, who remain with lower normal or supernormal cardiac function as listed in **Table 35.1**.

Phase B in ECMO of Septic Shock

ECMO provides time for recovery of the failing heart as it continues to provide perfusion to the other vital organs until voluntary and unsolicited cardiac recovery occurs; sepsis in this period can be prevented by using judicious antibiotics and preventing drainage insufficiency during ECMO.[9,10] In the second and third phase, ECMO may not show favorable results[10] (**Box 35.5**).

Respiratory Infections also Lead to Sepsis

Lung is the most common infection site affected in sepsis. Respiratory failure is an independent risk factor for hospital mortality, constituting about 40%. Hence, the treatment of severe respiratory failure constitutes a significant portion of the sepsis treatment regimen.

Apart from septic shock, acute respiratory distress syndrome (ARDS) may also warrant the use of ECMO. Acute lung injury and ARDS are very common manifestations of sepsis in critically ill patients. If conventional techniques, the use of inhaled nitric oxide, high-frequency oscillation, and prone positioning becomes inadequate to provide adequate ventilation then ECMO may have a role in maintaining arterial oxygenation and carbon dioxide clearance. ECMO specially the VV type is a rescue therapy for the failing lungs and ARDS. Many clinical trials such as the ECMO and EOLIA trials

---

Box 35.5 ECMO in sepsis: why use it at all?

- Temporary cardiovascular ECMO provides support
- Temporary lung support
- Temporary renal support
- Dilution of cytokines

Abbreviation: ECMO, extracorporeal membrane oxygenation.

Table 35.1 Phases in extracorporeal membrane oxygenation (ECMO) with septic shock

Early phase	Second phase	Third phase
• Low-flow state related to hypovolemia	• Hyperdynamic state	• Decreased cardiac output
• Volume expansion increases	• High cardiac output	• Increased systemic vascular resistance
• Cardiac output and improves patient's perfusion, when ECMO is begun	• Low systemic vascular resistance	• Progressive metabolic acidosis

have proved the sufficiency of VV ECMO for ARDS over the conventional ventilation mode.[11] Many studies have shown the effectiveness of ECMO for influenza A (H1N1)–related severe acute respiratory failure in 2009 to 2010.

Septic shock can have diverse manifestations hemodynamically, ranging from single or biventricular failure to vasodilation and impaired oxygen utilization. In the newborn, persistent pulmonary hypertension and RV failure are predominant. In infants and younger children, LV impairment and low cardiac output are common. In older children and adults, the pattern is usually that of vasoplegic or distributive shock or ventricular dysfunction. Fundamentally, if tissue oxygen delivery cannot be maintained despite aggressive medical management like optimal ventilation, inotropes, and intravenous fluids, then ECMO should be considered.

Left ventricular ejection fraction (LVEF) >35% or <20% shows a lack of longitudinal echocardiography data to find whether cardiac function is improving or worsening.

Which Modality in Sepsis—VV or VA ECMO?

VA ECMO in sepsis provides cardiac and respiratory support, decreases RV preload, has no risk of recirculation, and provides better oxygen delivery. However, VA ECMO can cause increased LV afterload, lowers pulse pressure, causes "Cardiac Stun," and decreases cerebral autoregulation.

VV ECMO avoids major arterial cannulation, provides direct pulmonary oxygenation, improves coronary oxygenation, limits neurological complications, and maintains patient pulsatility and cardiac output, but VV ECMO does not provide direct cardiac support and increased incidence of recirculation (**Box 35.6**).

VV Better in Low Output States

VV avoids arterial cannulation, utilizes patient plasticity, and is preferred in high output shock. VA may be better in low output shock as it provides better cardiac output, pulmonary oxygenation, and coronary oxygenation.

Box 35.6 Outcomes of septic patients with VA ECMO

- Preserved LVEF: worst outcomes
- Hyperdynamic LV function: worst outcomes
- Low LVEF first 4 days of VA ECMO: better outcomes

Abbreviations: LV, left ventricle; LVEF, left ventricular ejection fraction; VA ECMO, venoarterial extracorporeal membrane oxygenation.

What Is the Evidence which Depicts Pediatric and Adults in Sepsis Are Undergoing ECMO?

Pediatric Data for ECMO Sepsis

Recommendation for ECMO by Guidelines for the Management of Pediatric Severe Sepsis and Septic Shock: If the supraoptimal medical therapy and optimal ventilation, inotropes, vasodilators and intravenous fluids, tissue oxygenation is not maintained only then, ECMO is considered. The pattern of shock differs with age. In pediatric patients, there is a common feature of LV dysfunction and low cardiac output, whereas in young and old adults the shock features presented more as vasoplegia, distributive shock, or severe LV dysfunction. So we use ECMO in sepsis, as ECMO provides a source of bridge to recovery and dilution of cytokine.

ECMO has been suggested in refractory septic shock or with respiration-associated failure with sepsis (Grade 2C). Extracorporeal Life Support Organization Registry has shown survival rates of 73% for neonates and 39% for children after the use of ECMO for the treatment of sepsis. The survival rate was higher for those undergoing VV ECMO. A separate review of the database reported a 41% survival rate to discharge for those children undergoing ECMO for sepsis. A retrospective study, looking at the use of VA ECMO in refractory septic shock reported a 74% (17 patients) survival rate to discharge.[12] Because many centers are currently not capable of performing ECMO on children, it is important to remember that early transfer to an appropriate institution may be necessary for the survival of these patients.[4,12,15]

Central ECMO seems to be associated with better survival than conventional ECMO and should be considered by clinicians as a viable strategy in children with refractory septic shock.[5] In refractory septic shock in children, 47% of total patients supported on ECMO survived to hospital discharge.[16]

In a large, multicenter, pediatric sepsis pediatric intensive care unit (PICU) cohort study, it was found that ECMO use in pediatric sepsis has exceptionally increased since 2009. It is important to note that similarly significant increase in ECMO utilization after 2009 in patients with multiple organ dysfunction syndrome (MODS) was also seen. This may have been due to increasing support in the literature on successful use of ECMO in patients with comorbidities. The recommendations in the American Critical Care Medicine (ACCM) sepsis guidelines also support ECMO consideration. Mortality rates in pediatric sepsis patients receiving ECMO reduced over time and are comparable to the latest nationally published pediatric sepsis outcome data.[17]

Adult Data for ECMO Sepsis

Historically, ECMO has been notorious for high mortality and morbidity. However in the current era, survival after ECMO has improved to ~90% in neonates[18,19] and 75% in children.[5,16] Therefore, ECMO is a valuable therapeutic option for refractory septic shock in neonates and children. However, experience using ECMO is limited in adults with refractory septic shock. Two case series of adult patients who received ECMO for refractory septic shock showed conflicting results. The survival to hospital discharge was 71% (10/14) in Bréchot et al,[16] but only 15% (8/52) in Huang et al.[17] However, Huang et al specifically mentioned some important points: patient age of 60 years or older might be a contraindication and these patients might require central ECMO rather than peripheral VA ECMO. A recent study provided additional information regarding the efficacy and safety of ECMO in adult patients with refractory septic shock. Survival to hospital discharge was 22% (7/32) and remained low despite ECMO support.[18]

ECMO might be considered as a potentially valuable therapeutic option for patients with refractory cardiovascular dysfunction in the context of septic shock, although more data and larger patient cohorts are needed to confirm the findings presented herein as shown by Combes et al.[19] Delay in timely ECMO insertion often leads to adverse outcomes.

Conclusion

A high index of suspicion should be kept in mind regarding the prevalence of sepsis in ECMO, especially when (i) duration of ECMO is more than 12 days,[20] (ii) a high SOFA score before cannulation is present and there is dyselectrolytemia, like hyponatremia with seizures, etc., (iii) mechanical malfunction of the ECMO circuit, etc. Coagulase-negative staphylococcus-induced blood stream infection and in India prevalence of negative bacteria in the blood stream cause higher incidence in ICU too.[20] A procalcitonin (PCT) out of 1.83 ng/mL with clinical correlation.

ECMO is a valuable treatment for failing hearts and lungs, and patients in septic shock too benefit from ECMO. It is wise to conclude that in varied population of both distributive septic shock and septic shock with cytotoxic cardiac failure with high risk for mortality, a peripheral cannulation ECMO support may be beneficial for both hospital and long-term survival. More information is needed from septic shock patients before a consensus can be formed that ECMO should be definitely continued in experienced hands/at a high-volume center when sepsis occurs in both VA and VV ECMO. It cannot be emphasized enough that experience from septic shock patients is fundamental and that ECMO should be initiated by and/or at least continued at a high-volume

ECMO center with experience in both VV and VA ECMO for a dynamic approach to patient's need.[19]

Deviation from certain thresholds may justify escalating therapy, including invasive ECMO therapy even before intubation, and even before the Berlin definition informs us that PaO_2/FiO_2 is below 100. In this context, 'bridging-ECMO' allows time for the host to eliminate the pathogen and control the inflammatory response under the best protective ventilatory conditions.[20]

References

1. Singer M, Deutschman CS, Seymour CW, et al. The third International consensus definitions for sepsis and septic shock (Sepsis-3). JAMA 2016;315(8):801–810
2. Levy MM, Evan LE, Rhodes A. Surviving sepsis update campaign bundle: 2018 update. Crit Care Med June 2018;46(6):997–1000
3. Brierley J, Carcillo JA, Choong K, et al. Clinical practice parameters for hemodynamic support of pediatric and neonatal septic shock: 2007 update from the American College of Critical Care Medicine. Crit Care Med 2009;37(2):666–688
4. Ruth A, McCracken CE, Fortenberry JD, Hebbar KB. Extracorporeal therapies in pediatric severe sepsis: findings from the pediatric health-care information system. Crit Care 2015;19:397
5. Hocker JR, Simpson PM, Rabalais GP, Stewart DL, Cook LN. Extracorporeal membrane oxygenation and early-onset group B streptococcal sepsis. Pediatrics 1992;89(1):1–4
6. Ruokonen E, Takala J, Kari A, Alhava E. Septic shock and multiple organ failure. Crit Care Med 1991;19(9):1146–1151
7. Friedman G, Silva E, Vincent JL. Has the mortality of septic shock changed with time. Crit Care Med 1998;26(12): 2078–2086
8. Russell JA, Singer J, Bernard GR, et al. Changing pattern of organ dysfunction in early human sepsis is related to mortality. Crit Care Med 2000;28(10):3405–3411
9. Vieillard-Baron A, Cecconi M. Understanding cardiac failure in sepsis. Intensive Care Med 2014;40(10):1560–1563
10. Maclaren G, Butt W, Best D, Donath S, Taylor A. Extracorporeal membrane oxygenation for refractory septic shock in children: one institution's experience. Pediatr Crit Care Med 2007;8(5):447–451
11. Peek GJ, Clemens F, Elbourne D, et al. CESAR: conventional ventilatory support vs extracorporeal membrane oxygenation for severe adult respiratory failure. BMC Health Serv Res 2006;6:163
12. Ling RR, Ramanathan K, Poon WH, et al. Venoarterial extracorporeal membrane oxygenation as mechanical circulatory support in adult septic shock: a systematic review and meta-analysis with individual participant data meta-regression analysis. Crit Care 2021;25(1):246
13. Huang C-T, Tsai YJ, Tsai PR, Ko WJ. Extracorporeal membrane oxygenation resuscitation in adult patients with refractory septic shock. J Thorac Cardiovasc Surg 2013;146(5):1041–1046
14. Gopalakrishnan R, Vashisht R. Sepsis and ECMO. [published online ahead of print, 2020 May 14] Indian J Thorac Cardiovasc Surg 2021;37(Suppl 2):267–274

15. Domico MB, Ridout DA, Bronicki R, et al. The impact of mechanical ventilation time before initiation of extracorporeal life support on survival in pediatric respiratory failure: a review of the Extracorporeal Life Support Registry. Pediatr Crit Care Med 2012;13(1):16–21. (Registry review; 1325 subjects)

16. Bréchot N, Luyt CE, Schmidt M, et al. Venoarterial extracorporeal membrane oxygenation support for refractory cardiovascular dysfunction during severe bacterial septic shock. Crit Care Med 2013;41(7):1616–1626

17. Huang CT, Tsai YJ, Tsai PR, Ko WJ. Extracorporeal membrane oxygenation resuscitation in adult patients with refractory septic shock. J Thorac Cardiovasc Surg 2013;146(5): 1041–1046

18. Takauji S, Hayakawa M, Ono K, Makise H. Respiratory extracorporeal membrane oxygenation for severe sepsis and septic shock in adults: a propensity score analysis in a multicenter retrospective observational study. Acute Med Surg 2017;4(4):408–417

19. Combes A. Role of VA ECMO in septic shock: Does it work? Qatar Medical Journal, 4th Annual ELSO-SWAC Conference Proceedings 2017:24

20. Rau A, Moerer O, Winkler MS. Indications for extracorporeal membrane oxygenation in coronavirus disease 2019: is the Berlin definition still adequate to adjust therapeutic interventions? A case report. European Journal of Anaesthesiology and Intensive Care 2(1):p e0012, 2023

36

Indications and Contraindications of Extracorporeal Membrane Oxygenation

Poonam Malhotra Kapoor, Sandeep Chauhan, Neeti Makhija, Minati Choudhury, Sambhunath Das, Vishwas Malik, and Parag Ghardhe

Introduction

With the rise in extracorporeal membrane oxygenation (ECMO) globally, among diverse cohorts, the indications and contraindications for the ECMO has also undergone many changes. There is now an indication for ECMO use, particularly after the COVID-19 pandemic,[1] in each ICU. The temporary support of ECMO is used for oxygenation, carbon-dioxide removal, as well as for providing hemodynamic support.[2] Elective venoarterial (VA) ECMO is used today in the catheterization laboratory for high-risk patients undergoing ventricular tachycardia (VT) ablation, and in unanticipated intraoperative cardiac arrest, without preexisting organ failure.[3–5] Venovenous (VV) ECMO is used for respiratory support, for example, in COVID-19 adults and in acute respiratory distress syndrome (ARDS) patients with complex tracheobronchial and lung surgery and cases of refractory hypoxia, who are unresponsive to conventional treatment. **Box 36.1** shows previous indications of VA ECMO, while **Box 36.2** shows the newer indications of VA ECMO as it stands in 2022.[8–14]

VA ECMO can be used for diverse cardiac conditions as shown in **Flowchart 36.1** and **Boxes 36.1** and **36.2**.

VV ECMO for respiratory failure is used more in intensive care units (ICUs) for conditions indicated in **Boxes 36.3** and **36.4**, generally those wherein there are failing lungs.

A large number of publications and research have added newer indications of venovenous extracorporeal life support (VV ECLS) as summarized in **Box 36.4**.

Common Indications of Venovenous ECMO

Common indications for which VV ECMO was used previously are well laid out in **Box 36.3**. However today in 2022, the extent of VV ECMO use has extended particularly for lung

Box 36.1   Indications for VA ECMO
• Most importantly in cardiac or circulatory failure with patient in cardiogenic shock
• Peripartum cardiomyopathy
• Ventilator support as a bridge to transplant
• Massive pulmonary embolism
• Cardiac arrest
• Failure to wean from CPB after cardiac surgery
• Acute myocarditis
• Refractory ventricular arrhythmias
• Overdose of cardio toxic dose
• RV failure during LVAD support
• Trauma to great vessels: aorta and pulmonary artery
• Massive pulmonary bleeding
• Trauma to pulmonary trunk
• As integrated ECMO in pediatric cardiac surgery

Abbreviations: CPB, cardiopulmonary bypass; ECMO, extracorporeal membrane oxygenation; LVAD, left ventricular assist device; VA, venoarterial.

Box 36.2   Newer indications of VA ECMO
• Catheterization laboratory ventricular tachycardia (VT) ablation
• Unanticipated intraoperative cardiac arrest
• Complications of myocarditis and cardiogenic shock
• Sepsis-associated cardiomyopathy
• RV support during LVAD implantation
• Bridge to VAD or heart or lung transplant
• Pulmonary hypertension with RV failure
• Posttransplant graft failure
• Massive pulmonary embolism
• eCPR
• Refractory ventricular arrhythmias
• Postcardiotomy cardiomyopathy
• Fulminant myocarditis
• Catecholamine-induced cardiomyopathy
• Minimally invasive coronary cardiac surgery (MICCS)

Abbreviations: eCPR, extracorporeal cardiopulmonary resuscitation; LVAD, left ventricular-assist device; RV, right ventricle; VA ECMO, venoarterial extracorporeal membrane oxygenation.

Box 36.3   Common indications for VV ECMO
• Difficult airway
• Severe ARDS pneumonia
• Graft rejection following lung transplant
• Alveolar proteinosis
• Smoke inhalation
• Status asthmaticus
• Aspiration pneumonia
• Pulmonary trauma

Abbreviations: ARDS, acute respiratory distress syndrome; ECMO, extracorporeal membrane oxygenation; VV, venovenous.

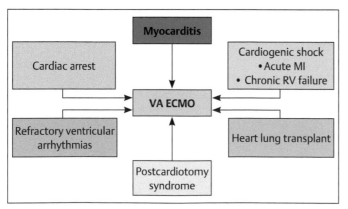

Flowchart 36.1 Uses of VA ECMO. Abbreviations: MI, myocardial ischemia; RV, right ventricle; VA ECMO, venoarterial extracorporeal membrane oxygenation.

- COVID-19 ARDS
- Complex tracheabronchial and lung surgery
- Refractory cases of hypoxemia, nonresponsive to conventional treatment
- Prolonged mechanical ventilation (less than a week), severe air leak syndrome
- Mortality risk is greater than 50%
- Early use of VV ECMO after respiratory failure sets in (within 1–2 d), benefits COVID-19 patients more
- Surgery for congenital airway abnormality
- Difficulty in the patient's airway ventilation
- Facilitate "AWAKE INDUCTION" in patients with severely compromised airway anatomy in adults
- Flexible bronchoscopy for placement removal of end bronchial stents
- Refractory bronchospasm
- Status asthmatics
- Rigid bronchoscopy for resection of tracheal tumor
- Surgery for tracheomalacia
- Management of patients with underlying lung pathology
- Large bronchopleural fistula
- Very low BMI
- Kyphosis
- Complex lung resections
- Intraoperative and postoperative lung transplantation
- Compression of mediastinal vessels
- Surgery for refractory bronchospasm
- Carinal resection with left pneumonectomy

Abbreviations: ARDS, acute respiratory distress syndrome; BMI, body mass index; ECMO, extracorporeal membrane oxygenation; VV, venovenous.

Box 36.5 2021 STS/SCA/AmSECT/SABM guidelines for perfusion interventions

- Retrograde autologous priming of the CPB circuit
- Reduced priming volume in the CPB circuit
- Reduces hemodilution
- Blood conservation (class I Level of Evidence B)
- Minimally invasive extracorporeal circulation
- Restrictive transfusion strategy as part of combined blood conservation approach (class IIA Level of Evidence B)

Abbreviations: AmSECT, American Society of ExtraCorporeal Technology; CPB, cardiopulmonary bypass; SABM, Society for the Advancement of Blood Management; SCA, Society of Cardiovascular Anesthesiologists; STS; Society for Thoracic Surgeons.

transplant thoracic and difficult airway surgery. VV ECMO is particularly useful in ARDS, when the PaO_2/FIO_2 ratio is less than 150 mmHg. According to the ELSO (Extracorporeal Life Support Organization) guidelines, ECMO should not be implanted in severe acute or multiple organ failure patients without any chance to recovery.[15] A strong recommendation

for ECMO is presence of ARDS with PaO_2/FIO_2 of less than 150 mmHg.[16] In pediatric patients, recommendations include inability to wean from cardiopulmonary bypass (CPB), cardiogenic shock both in and outside the hospital, and cardiac arrest. VA ECMO when used early and timely in children definitely improves outcomes.

As given by the Society for Thoracic Surgeons (STS), the guidelines to perfusion perspectives in ECMO show immense benefits of ECLS modality as outlined in **Box 36.5**.

Comparison of VV ECMO and VA ECMO

VA ECMO can provide support for both cardiac and pulmonary failures but VV ECMO cannot. The latter is used only for isolated oxygenation ventilation support, whereas VA ECMO provides both cardiac and respiratory support. Echocardiography is must in VA ECMO as it aids in quick decision-making. **Table 36.1** enumerates the differences between VA ECMO and VV ECMO, which seems to be important in the post-COVID era as the distinction between VA ECMO and VV ECMO is shrinking.

ECMO Circuit and Implantation Techniques in Pediatric Patients versus Adult

Are they different? Yes, ECMO circuits are different in adults and kids.

Pediatric patients may weigh from 4 to 50 kg, and thus the ECMO circuits, cannulas, and cannulation sites will differ. ECMO flows are dependent on weight (**Table 36.2**).[4] Also, the ECMO sites differ in the two populations (**Table 36.3**).

VA ECMO in the Setting of Cardiac Arrest

ECMO is a high-risk therapy that should be performed only in experienced centers having an expert, multidiscipline, well-equipped team for tackling ECMO patients. When cardiac arrest in a child or adult is refractory to support optimal treatment then an ECMO-based cardiopulmonary resuscitation (CPR), also known as eCPR, can be performed. The latter provides excellent cerebral perfusion. The incidence of cardiac arrest may be as low as 0.7 to 8%[7] but eCPR is a part of every congenital cardiac surgery protocol as well. Postcardiotomy cardiac arrest entails a resternotomy within 5 minutes of the arrest, according to the guidelines. It is imperative in all scenarios to have an expedited ECMO implantation done. In a cardiac arrest with no reversible cause, such as pericardial tamponade, ECMO should be quickly inserted, without any delay. Doubts exist at some ECMO points about the ECMO duration, the lowest pH to be

Table 36.1 Difference between VA ECMO and VV ECMO

Property	VA ECMO	VV ECMO
Cannulation site	IJV/FV and RCC/Ax/FA/Ao	IJV alone/IJV-FV/FV-FV/Saphsaph/RA
PaO$_2$	60–150 mmHg	45–80 mmHg
Indicator of O$_2$ sufficiency	Mixed venous saturation or PaO$_2$	Combination of SaO$_2$, PaO$_2$, cerebral venous saturation and premembrane saturation trend
Cardiac effect	↓ preload; ↑ afterload; pulse pr ↓; coronary oxygen by LV blood; cardiac stun	Negligible effects; may improve coronary oxygenation; may reduce RV afterload
O$_2$ delivery capacity	High	Moderate: ↑ cephalad drain
Circulatory support	Partial to complete	Indirect: ↑ delivery of O$_2$ to coronary and pulmonary circulation

Abbreviations: Ao, ascending aorta; ECMO, extracorporeal membrane oxygenation; FA, femoral artery; FV, femoral vein; IJV, internal jugular vein; LV, left ventricle; PaO$_2$, partial pressure of oxygen; RA, right atrium; RCC, right common carotid; RV, right ventricle, VA, venoarterial; VV, venovenous.

Table 36.2 Pediatric patients versus adult

Neonates and pediatric patients	Priming volume of ECMO circuit	ECMO flows
Up to 15 kg	250 mL	1.7 L/min
15 kg	750 mL	7.0 L/min

Abbreviation: ECMO, extracorporeal membrane oxygenation.

Table 36.3 Implantation sites: neck versus the femoral vessels

Patient group	Implantation sites
• Adult and emergency	• Femoral vessels
• Children before walking age	• Neck vessels
	• Flow limitation
	• Good in emergency
	• Easy to approach
	• Good even in CPR

Abbreviation: CPR, cardiopulmonary resuscitation.

Box 36.6 Summary of ELSO registry in 2020 on pediatric ECMO for cardiac arrest

- ECMO for cardiac arrest is on the rise (11%)
- Good teamwork, training on simulators with checklists facilitates interventions
- Pediatric eCPR in neonates (36%) and pediatric as (13%) population is on the rise
- Femoral vessels used for eCPR in adults, but not in children and neonates
- Neck cannulation in pediatric patients allow unhampered chest compressions during ECMO implantation in pediatric patients[10]
- Neck cannulation to prevent thromboembolism mandates presence of an intact circle of Willis or a ligation of the distal internal carotid artery for protection against thromboembolism and subsequent cerebral infarction

Abbreviations: ECMO, extracorporeal membrane oxygenation; eCPR, extracorporeal cardiopulmonary resuscitation; ELSO, Extracorporeal Life Support Organization.

achieved, the highest lactate on ECMO as these hypoperfusive states lead to neurological sequalae to develop till the pH normalizes. If all above doubts are cleared then ECMO for cardiac arrest is a wonderful tool for patient's outcomes. Algorithms for eCPR use are institutional dependent.

The ELSO Registry report in 2020 reiterated that in most pediatric patients, the use of eCPR is on the rise as shown in **Box 36.6**. When done with good teamwork, its results too are excellent.

Indications for ECMO in Sepsis

Septic shock is an indicator for ECMO in some patients, as listed in **Table 36.4**.

Box 36.7 shows the indications where different mechanical devices can be used judiciously.

Table 36.4 Proposed indications for ECMO in ARDS patients

Indications	Possible exclusion criteria
• Potentially reversible severe respiratory failure	• Age >70 y
• PaO$_2$/FiO$_2$ < 100 ratio, with a FiO$_2$ at 1.00	• Advanced lung disease
• Alveolar-arterial gradient (A-a DO$_2$) >600 mmHg	• Contraindication for anticoagulation
• Shunt fraction >30%	• Prolonged mechanical ventilation

Abbreviations: ARDS, adult respiratory distress syndrome; ECMO, extracorporeal membrane oxygenation; FiO$_2$ fraction of inspired oxygen; PaO$_2$, partial pressure of oxygen.

Box 36.7 Typical causes for use of mechanical devices

- Acute myocardial infarction
- Myocarditis
- Peripartum cardiomyopathy
- Decompensated chronic heart failure
- Postcardiotomy shock

Box 36.8 ECMO advantages over other mechanical support devices

ECMO provides the following over the mechanical support devices:

- Oxygenation and biventricular support
- Good recovery in an acute MI after revascularization
- ECMO used as a bridge to transplant in unrevascurizable acute MI
- ECMO as bridge to ventricular-assist device (VAD)

Abbreviations: ECMO, extracorporeal membrane oxygenation; MI, myocardial infarction.

Box 36.9 Indications of ECMO in neonates and pediatric patients

Cardiac indications
- Hypoplastic left heart syndrome
- Left ventricular outflow obstruction
- Right ventricular obstruction
- Septal defects
- Cardiomyopathy
- Myocarditis

Respiratory indications
- Meconium aspiration syndrome
- Persistent pulmonary hypertension of newborn/persistent fetal circulation
- Congenital diaphragmatic hernia
- Pneumonia

Cardiac and lung transplant-related indications
- Pretransplantation as bridge to transplant
- Primary graft dysfunction after a lung transplant
- Elective intraoperative
- Bridge to decision
- Air leak syndrome
- Failure to wean from CPB

Abbreviations: CPB, cardiopulmonary bypass; ECMO, extracorporeal membrane oxygenation.

Selecting the type of ECMO (i.e., VA or VV ECMO) is essential.

VA ECMO: It is used in cases of cardiorespiratory failure, and it is either central or peripheral.

Central VA ECMO: It is mainly given in patients undergoing cardiac surgery and also in cardiac failure patients. It is the most suited form of ECMO in pediatric patients with cardiac failure/arrest and in patients with poor lung function

(large shunt). Hypoxia from pulmonary veins to the brain is thus overcome.

Peripheral VA ECMO: This mode is excellent for those not requiring cardiac surgery and where lung function is good.

Box 36.8 lists how ECMO is more advantageous than the other mechanical intra-aortic balloon pump (IABP) or tandem heart.

VV ECMO: It is used in cases of respiratory failure but with good cardiac function.

Hi-flow VV ECMO is resorted to when the size of the access cannula is small (25 Fr PC cannulas). So, when greater oxygenation is required for a single access cannula, a second access cannula may be inserted via, for example, the internal jugular vein.

Guidelines on Relative Survival without Extracorporeal Membrane Oxygenation with Other Mechanical-Assist Devices

Use of an IABP or ventricular-assist device (VAD), on a temporary basis, can be considered as follows:[32]
- IABP postcardiotomy.
- Postcardiotomy using a Samuel score for a temporary circulatory support.
- Surgical temporary VAD: Abiomed, levitronix.
- Percutaneous VAD: Tandem heart, Impella.

Indications for Pediatric and Adult ECMO in Noncardiac Surgery

ECMO is primarily used in noncardiac surgery for respiratory failure (**Box 36.9**). *ARDS-Influenza H1N1 virus associated* with a respiratory indication for ECMO was only subcategorized recently. As mentioned, ECMO presents two modalities: VA ECMO and VV ECMO, which can be used separately or simultaneously (combined ECMO).[14]

Inclusion Criteria for Starting ECMO

Presence of any two of the following criteria observed over a period of 4 to 6 hours after maximum medical resuscitation:
- PaO_2/FiO_2 ratio of <75%.
- Oxygen index of >40%.
- Murray's score of >3.0.
- Alveolar-arterial (aA) gradient >600.
- Hypercapnia with pH of <7.2 observed over more than 3 hours.
- Lung compliance <0.5 mL/cm H_2O/kg.

Exclusion Criteria for ECMO

- Irreversible disease—like malignancy.
- Age >75 years.

- Patient on ventilator for >15 days.
- Intracranial bleeding.
- Active bleeding from no compressive site.
- Irreversible or indeterminate neurological status.
- Unwitnessed arrest or arrest lasting more than 30 minutes.
- Patient's gross multiorgan failure.

In the CAESAR trial at Glenfield, UK, patients with severe respiratory failure are shown by:[16]
- The mean pre-ECMO Murray Lung Injury Score of 3.4 (SD 0.5).
- PaO$_2$/FiO$_2$ ratio of 65 mmHg (SD 36.9) was included for ECMO.

Contraindications to ECMO

Contraindications to ECMO are listed in **Box 36.10**.
The three absolute contraindications are described in **Table 36.5**.
Absolute contraindications to all forms of ECMO are:
- Age > 65 years.
- Nonrecoverable cardiac disease.
- Nonrecoverable respiratory disease.

Box 36.10 ECMO contraindications
Relative contraindications
• Bleeding from many sites due to trauma
• Patient in multiple organ failure
Absolute contraindications
These can be further subdivided into:
• General absolute contraindications
• Absolute contraindications to VA ECMO
• Absolute contraindications to VV ECMO

Abbreviations: ECMO, extracorporeal membrane oxygenation; VA, venoarterial; VV, venovenous.

- Nonrecoverable central nervous system (CNS) disease.
- Chronic severe pulmonary hypertension.
- Active malignancy, graft versus host disease or significant immunosuppression:
  - Post bone marrow, renal, liver transplant or heart/lung transplant beyond 30 days.
- Weight > 140 kg.
- Advanced liver disease.
- AIDS as defined by:
  - Secondary malignancy, prior hepatic or renal (cardiac resynchronization therapy [CRT] >250 μmol/L) impairment or need for salvage antiretroviral therapy.
- Neurological impairment.
- End stage, inoperable, irreversible disease.
- Uncontrolled.
- During CPR no blood vessels are seen.
- Associated lesions not seen.
- If CPR goes beyond 60 min.
- If cardiac arrest is not witnessed by ECMO intensivist.

Relative contraindications to all forms of ECMO are:
- Trauma with multiple bleeding sites.
- Multiple organ failure.

Absolute contraindications to VV ECMO for respiratory failure are:
- Severe pulmonary hypertension (mean pulmonary arterial pressure [mPAP] > 50 mmHg).
- Severe right or left heart failure (EF < 25%).
- Cardiac arrest.

Absolute contraindications to VA ECMO are:
- Aortic dissection.
- Severe aortic valve regurgitation.
- High-pressure ventilation (peak inspiratory pressure >30 cm H$_2$O) for >7 days.
- High FiO$_2$ requirements (>0.8) for >7 days.
- Limited vascular access.

Table 36.5 Absolute contraindications to ECMO

General absolute contraindications	Absolute contraindications to VA ECMO	Absolute contraindications to VV ECMO

• Irreversible organ damage
• Multiple organ failure
• If heart/lung transplant is not to be considered, then starting an ECMO may not be beneficial
	• Aortic dissection
	• Severe AR
	• Prolonged pressure controlled ventilation
	• High FiO$_2$
	• Vascular access not available
	• Jehovah's witnesses refusing blood transfusion
	• If overall patient condition is such that there will not be any benefit from inserting a VA ECMO, e.g.,
	  ▷ Metastatic cancer
	  ▷ Cerebral injury not amenable to treatment
		• Severe PAH (mPAP more than 50 mmHg)
		• Severely low ejection fraction due to RV or LV failure
		• Cardiac arrest

Abbreviations: AR, aortic regurgitation; ECMO, extracorporeal mechanical ventilation; FiO$_2$, fraction of inspired oxygen; LV, left ventricle; mPAP, mean pulmonary arterial pressure; PAH, pulmonary hypertension; RV, right ventricle; VA, venoarterial; VV, venovenous.

- Refusal to accept blood products.
- Any condition or organ dysfunction that would limit the likelihood of overall benefit from ECMO such as severe, irreversible brain injury or untreatable metastatic cancer.[17–21]

Absolute Contraindications Include Contraindication to Anticoagulation

When considering ECMO as a bridge to lung transplant and if lung transplantation is not to be considered or the patient is in multiorgan failure or has irreversible organ damage, then in such patients who are not candidates for transplant ECMO support is of no benefit. ECMO is not generally recommended in patients who cannot be anticoagulated, but this is not an absolute contraindication.[22–23]

Severe aortic regurgitation or aortic dissections are contraindications for VA ECMO. ECMO therapy is continuously evolving and it is preferable to involve an ECMO specialist in discussing indications and contraindications in each instance.[26,27]

Indications for Venovenous Extracorporeal Life Support

When a lung failure patient on prolonged lung protective, mechanical ventilation (low VT; limited Pplat) continues to have worsened hemodynamics, then VV ECMO is indicated in patients with a potentially reversible lung pathology, like ARDS. Despite other associated therapies such as prone positioning, inhaled pulmonary vasodilator high-frequency oscillatory ventilation, and ECMO carbon dioxide removal, if patient continues to further deteriorate, then before further organ failure happens, it is wise to start VV ECLS, with the criteria laid down in **Box 36.11**.

A large number of pathological conditions, as listed in **Box 36.12**, may also require a VV ECLS.

Berlin Definition of ARDS and Ancillary Variables for ECMO[28]

The "Berlin definition of ARDS" paper describes severe ARDS as:

- Respiratory failure in patients within 1 week of a known clinical insult or new or worsening respiratory symptoms.
- Bilateral opacities on chest imaging, not fully explained by effusions, lobar/lung collapse, or nodules.
- Respiratory failure not fully explained by cardiac failure or fluid overload.
- Degree of hypoxemia (P/F < 13.5 [100 mmHg] with positive end-expiratory pressure [PEEP] > 5 cm H_2O).

Box 36.11   Criteria for initiating VV ECLS

- Murray score of 3 or 4
- P/F ratio less than 10, on an FiO_2 of 90% or more
- Hypercapnia in a patient with a $PaCO_2$ more than 11 or a pH less than 7.20
- If the corrected minute ventilation is more than 10 L/min, due to increased dead space
- Pplat is greater than 30 cm H_2O
- Static compliance of respiratory system is less than 20 mL/cm H_2O
- If patient is on mechanical ventilation of less than 7 days of duration

Abbreviations: ECLS, extracorporeal life support; FiO_2, fraction of inspired oxygen; $PaCO_2$, partial pressure of carbon dioxide; VV, venovenous.

Box 36.12   Pathological conditions requiring ECLS

- ARDS
- Air leak syndrome
- Pulmonary hemorrhage
- Injuries due to inhalation
- Status asthmaticus
- Alveolar proteinosis
- Acute graft failure after a lung transplant

Abbreviations: ARDS, acute respiratory distress syndrome; ECLS, extracorporeal life support.

Ancillary variables such as those given below are essential to note for ECMO:

- Radiographic severity: Opacities in 3 or 4 quadrants of the chest radiograph.
- PEEP > 10 cm H_2O.
- Static compliance of respiratory system <40 cm H_2O.

Minute ventilation standardized at $PaCO_2$ of 5.4 kPa: >10 L/min (Min ventilation × $PaCO_2$/5.4, surrogate marker for increased dead space) were not found to change the mortality prediction compared to using severe hypoxemia (P/F < 13.5) alone.

Contraindications for Extracorporeal Life Support in an Emergency Setting

Exclusion criteria for ECLS are given below. In an emergency setting, it may not be possible to identify all the conditions that would normally exclude patients from ECLS.[17] At the discretion of the consultant intensivist or cardiothoracic surgeon, ECLS may be commenced emergently and if contraindications become obvious at a later time, ECLS should be withdrawn.

Absolute contraindications for VV ECLS:

- Progressive nonrecoverable lung disease, not amenable to transplantation.

- Chronic severe pulmonary hypertension with right ventricular failure.
- Advanced malignancy.
- Chronic organ dysfunction.
- Lung failure associated with bone marrow transplantation.
- Contraindication to anticoagulation therapy.
- Recent spinal cord or central nervous system trauma or hemorrhage.

Relative contraindications for VV ECLS:
- Mechanical ventilation with FiO_2 > 0.9 and Pplat > 30 cm H_2O for >7 days.
- Age > 70 years.
- Body weight: >140 kg.
- Trauma with multiple bleeding sites.
- Significant immunosuppression.
- Recent diagnosis of hematological malignancy.

ICU Indications for Venoarterial Extracorporeal Life Support

ECMO is used only when short-term support is required in case of a failing heart or lung failure, when all else has failed (supraoptimal volume therapy, maximal inotropic support, and prolonged lung ventilator therapy along with an IABP or a CPR are inadequate to revive a patient). A review by an ECMO team of a cardiologist, an ECMO intensivist, and/or a cardiothoracic surgeon is mandatory, before a VA ECMO is initiated.

It is recommended to observe indices of tissue hypoperfusion, chiefly systemic hypotension, mental status changes, oliguria, skin mottling changes, alterations in temperature gradients, myocardial ischemia, and an increase in lactate clearance.[29] In patients with a good hematocrit (more than 35%) and adequate oxygenation, tissue hypoperfusion is seen with a mixed or central venous oxygenation of less than 70%.[30]

Peripheral VA ECLS
This can be inserted in:
- Rapidly, in an emergency.
- Femoral artery and femoral vein cannulation.
- Is good when native, lung function is appropriate.

Box 36.13 Central VA ECLS

Most often employed in patients with:
- Failure to wean off CPB during cardiac surgery
- Heart failure
- Poor native lung function
- Prefer central VA ECLS to peripheral ECLS when due to dysfunctional native lungs, deoxygenated blood from these lungs is pumped into the proximal aorta

Abbreviations: CPB, cardiopulmonary bypass; VA ECLS, venoarterial extracorporeal life support.

- To be used when a patient does not require sternotomy or cardiac surgery.
- In this form, deoxygenated blood is drained from the inferior or superior vena cava and oxygenated blood drains into the femoral artery (FA) or ascending aorta (central VA ECMO) (**Box 36.13** and **Flowchart 36.2**).

Pathologic conditions that may require VA ECLS:
- Postcardiotomy cardiogenic shock.
- Ischemic cardiogenic shock.
- Bridge to decision regarding suitability for therapy (e.g., revascularization) or for longer term support (e.g., VAD, transplantation).
- Acute decompensation of dilated cardiomyopathy.
- Peripartum cardiomyopathy.

Indications for Conversion from VA to VV ECMO

In a patient cannulated for VA ECMO, initially due to inadequate cardiac output, who subsequently regains cardiac function but cannot be decannulated due to continued pulmonary disease, the cannulation can be modified to facilitate continuation of extracorporeal support in VV ECMO.[18,19]

Ventilatory Support in VA ECMO

Aim is to achieve "rest settings" on VA ECMO. Inotropes should be weaned off to minimum or no inotropic support, preferably early as soon as ECMO is initiated. A partial CPB-like state so as to unload the heart pump is the basic premise in a VA ECMO patient. This ventricular unloading helps in remodeling and providing rest to the ventricle, not the empty heart.

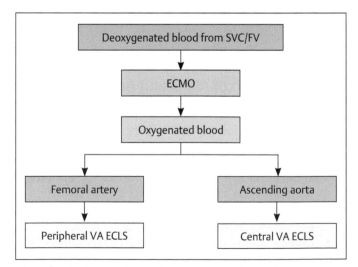

Flowchart 36.2 Central versus peripheral VA ECLS. Abbreviations: ECMO, extracorporeal mechanical ventilation; FV, femoral vein; SVC, superior vena cava; VA ECLS, venoarterial extracorporeal life support.

Box 36.14 Ideal extracorporeal flow
Ideal ECMO flow includes: • Adults: 3 L/min is good • 60–80% of resting predicted cardiac output • Important to insert a distal perfusion cannula distal to the ECMO flow with a minimal flow of 150 mL/min diverted to the distal limb, to prevent distal limb ischemia • Prevent cardiac stunning as much as possible by maintaining adequate coronary and central perfusion. This, if not done, gives rise to hypoxic perfusion, then it may require an additional cannula either in the IJV (V-AV ECMO) or rarely, in the axilla (V-AA ECMO). The latter is rarely reported

Abbreviations: ECMO, extracorporeal membrane oxygenation; V-AV, venoarterialvenous; V-AA, veno-arterio-arterial.

It is also important to use as much of pulsatile flow as possible, keep the inotropic score to less than 20, with pulsatile flow rather than no inotropes with nonpulsatile flow, always maintaining hemodynamics as given in **Box 36.14**.

Second, we should try to maintain pulsatile flow. Mild to moderate inotropic support is preferred (inotropic score <20) if required, with pulsatile flow rather than no inotropes with nonpulsatile flow. However, one should maintain the optimum vitals (ScvO$_2$ of >70% and mean arterial pressure [MAP] of 70 in adult) with the flow required (pulsatile or nonpulsatile). Ideally, extracorporeal flow is managed between 60 and 80% of predicted resting cardiac output (for adult, blood flow of ~3 L/min should be good enough). The other important factor one should keep in mind when returning cannula in femoral artery is to put distal perfusion cannula so as to prevent leg ischemia. Distal perfusion cannula is inserted distal to ECMO flow and approximately a minimal flow of 150 mL/min is diverted in that limb.

The cardiac stunning should be prevented and treated as discussed earlier and coronary perfusion should be maintained. If there is inadequate coronary and cerebral perfusion or if it is hypoxic perfusion then an additional return cannula should be inserted in internal jugular vein (V-AV ECMO) or rarely in axillary artery (V-AA ECMO).

Contraindications to lung transplantation are listed in **Box 36.15**.

Conclusion

The risk of death significantly increased when ECMO therapy became indicated after more than 3 days of invasive MV. The delay between intubation and ECMO cannulation, as a survival factor, presents a strong argument for early cannulation to allow protective ventilatory strategies to maintain high compliance by reducing the mechanical power.[31]

Box 36.15 Contraindications to lung transplantation[33]
Absolute contraindications • History of malignancy • Significant dysfunction of another major organ system (hear, liver, kidney, brain) • Severe thorax deformity • BMI > 35 kg/m^2 • Nonadherence to medical therapy (recent and history) • Active tuberculosis • History of illicit substance abuse • Inability to participate in rehabilitation • Poorly controlled infection/resistant microbes • Uncorrectable bleeding • Unstable medical condition • Uncorrected coronary artery disease **Relative contraindications** • Mechanical ventilation/extracorporeal life support • Controlled coronary artery disease • Significant osteoporosis • Colonization with resistant microbes • Infection liver cirrhosis • HIV infection (unless treated adequately) • Poorly controlled diabetes, hypertension, epilepsy, peptic ulcer disease, gastroesophageal reflux, central venous obstruction

Abbreviations: BMI, body mass index; HIV, human immunodeficiency virus.

Summary

Only potentially reversible, pathology which is life-threatening lung or cardiac failure patients, who are not improving with conventional management, need a VV or VA ECMO. Indications and contraindications for initiating the right ECMO is most essential.[32-34] All this is at the discretion of the ECMO intensivist with a coordinated teamwork from all in the ECMO team. Taking care of ECMO complications is as important as implanting an ECMO.

References

1. Hemmila MR, Rowe SA, Boules TN, et al. Extracorporeal life support for severe acute respiratory distress syndrome in adults. Ann Surg 2004;240(4):595–605, discussion 605–607
2. Thiagarajan RR, Barbaro RP, Rycus PT, et al; ELSO member centers. Extracorporeal Life Support Organization Registry International Report 2016. ASAIO J 2017;63(1):60–67
3. Wang CH, Chen YS, Ma MH. Extracorporeal life support. Curr Opin Crit Care 2013;19(3):202–207
4. Schmiady M, Döll C, Cavigelli-Brunner A, et al. Extracorporeal membrane oxygenation in neonates and children. Cardiovasc Med 2017;20:57–61
5. Kurkluoglu M, Hynes CF, Alfares FA, et al. Choice of peripheral venoarterial extra-corporeal membrane oxygenation cannu-

lation site in patients above 15 kilograms. J Card Surg 2015; 30(5):461–465

6. Martin GB, Rivers EP, Paradis NA, Goetting MG, Morris DC, Nowak RM. Emergency department cardiopulmonary bypass in the treatment of human cardiac arrest. Chest 1998;113(3): 743–751

7. Nagao K, Hayashi N, Kanmatsuse K, et al. Cardiopulmonary cerebral resuscitation using emergency cardiopulmonary bypass, coronary reperfusion therapy and mild hypothermia in patients with cardiac arrest outside the hospital. J Am Coll Cardiol 2000;36(3):776–783

8. Society of Thoracic Surgeons Task Force on Resuscitation After Cardiac Surgery. The Society of Thoracic Surgeons Expert Consensus for the resuscitation of patients who arrest after cardiac surgery. Ann Thorac Surg 2017;103(3):1005–1020

9. Truhlář A, Deakin CD, Soar J, et al; Cardiac Arrest in Special Circumstances Section Collaborators. European Resuscitation Council Guidelines for Resuscitation 2015: Section 4. Cardiac arrest in special circumstances. Resuscitation 2015;95:148–201

10. Erek E, Aydın S, Suzan D, et al. Extracorporeal cardiopulmonary resuscitation for refractory cardiac arrest in children after cardiac surgery. Anatol J Cardiol 2017;17(4):328–333

11. Tajik M, Cardarelli MG. Extracorporeal membrane oxygenation after cardiac arrest in children: what do we know? Eur J Cardiothorac Surg 2008;33(3):409–417

12. Barbaro RP, Paden ML, Guner YS, et al; ELSO Member Centers. Pediatric Extracorporeal Life Support Organization Registry International Report 2016. ASAIO J 2017;63(4):456–463

13. Hausmann H, Potapov EV, Koster A, et al. Prognosis after the implantation of an intra-aortic balloon pump in cardiac surgery calculated with a new score. Circulation 2002;106(12, Suppl 1):I203–I206

14. Samuels LE, Kaufman MS, Thomas MP, Holmes EC, Brockman SK, Wechsler AS. Pharmacological criteria for ventricular assist device insertion following postcardiotomy shock: experience with the Abiomed BVS system. J Card Surg 1999;14(4):288–293

15. Peek GJ, Moore HM, Moore N, Sosnowski AW, Firmin RK. Extracorporeal membrane oxygenation for adult respiratory failure. Chest 1997;112(3):759–764

16. Lewandowski K, Rossaint R, Pappert D, et al. High survival rate in 122 ARDS patients managed according to a clinical algorithm including extracorporeal membrane oxygenation. Intensive Care Med 1997;23(8):819–835

17. Peek GJ, Clemens F, Elbourne D, et al. CESAR: conventional ventilatory support vs extracorporeal membrane oxygenation for severe adult respiratory failure. BMC Health Serv Res 2006;6:163

18. Bacchetta M, Javidfar J, Sonett J, Kim H, Zwischenberger J, Wang D. Ease of conversion from venovenous extracorporeal membrane oxygenation to cardiopulmonary bypass and venoarterial extracorporeal membrane oxygenation with a bicaval dual lumen catheter. ASAIO J 2011;57(4):283–285

19. Kugelman A, Gangitano E, Pincros J, Tantivit P, Taschuk R, Durand M. Venovenous versus venoarterial extracorporeal membrane oxygenation in congenital diaphragmatic hernia. J Pediatr Surg 2003;38(8):1131–1136

20. Umei N, Ichiba S, Ujike Y, Tsukahara K. Successful application of venoarterial-venous extracorporeal membrane oxygenation in the reversal of severe cardiorespiratory failure. BMJ Case Rep 2015;2015:2015

21. Zangrillo A, Landoni G, Biondi-Zoccai G, et al. A meta-analysis of complications and mortality of extracorporeal membrane oxygenation. Crit Care Resusc 2013;15(3):172–178

22. Tsai HC, Chang CH, Tsai FC, et al. Acute respiratory distress syndrome with and without extracorporeal membrane oxygenation: a score matched study. Ann Thorac Surg 2015; 100(2):458–464

23. Ferguson ND, Fan E, Camporota L, et al. The Berlin definition of ARDS: an expanded rationale, justification, and supplementary material. Intensive Care Med 2012;38(10):1573–1582

24. Braune S, Sieweke A, Brettner F, et al. The feasibility and safety of extracorporeal carbon dioxide removal to avoid intubation in patients with COPD unresponsive to noninvasive ventilation for acute hypercapnic respiratory failure (ECLAIR study): multicentre case-control study. Intensive Care Med 2016;42(9): 1437–1444

25. Ouweneel DM, Schotborgh JV, Limpens J, et al. Extracorporeal life support during cardiac arrest and cardiogenic shock: a systematic review and meta-analysis. Intensive Care Med 2016;42(12):1922–1934

26. Grant C Jr, Richards JB, Frakes M, Cohen J, Wilcox SR. ECMO and right ventricular failure: review of the literature. J Intensive Care Med 2021;36(3):352–360

27. Debaty G, Babaz V, Durand M, et al. Prognostic factors for extracorporeal cardiopulmonary resuscitation recipients following out-of-hospital refractory cardiac arrest. A systematic review and meta-analysis. Resuscitation 2017;112:1–10

28. Matthay MA, Thompson BT, Ware LB. The Berlin definition of acute respiratory distress syndrome: should patients receiving high-flow nasal oxygen be included? Lancet Respir Med 2021;9(8):933–936

29. Ladha S, Kapoor PM, Singh SP, Kiran U, Chowdhury UK. The role of blood lactate clearance as a predictor of mortality in children undergoing surgery for tetralogy of Fallot. Ann Card Anaesth 2016;19(2):217–224

30. Agarwal Kumar N, Subramanian A. Central venous oxygenation for mixed venous oxygen saturation. J Card Crit Care TSS 2018;2:57–60

31. Lebreton G, Schmidt M, Ponnaiah M, et al. Extracorporeal membrane oxygenation network organisation and clinical outcomes during the COVID-19 pandemic in Greater Paris, France: a multicentre cohort study. Lancet Respir Med 2021; 9:851–862

32. Ohira S, Malekan R, Goldberg JB, Lansman SL, Spielvogel D, Kai M; Collaborators. Axillary artery cannulation for veno-arterial extracorporeal membrane oxygenation support in cardiogenic shock. JTCVS Tech 2020;5:62–71

33. Gajkowski EF, Herrera G, Hatton L, Velia Antonini M, Vercaemst L, Cooley E. ELSO guidelines for adult and pediatric extracorporeal membrane oxygenation circuits. ASAIO J 2022;68(2):133–152

34. Harnisch LO, Moerer O. Contraindications to the initiation of veno-venous ECMO for severe acute respiratory failure in adults: a systematic review and practical approach based on the current literature. Membranes (Basel) 2021;11(8):584

37

Monitoring of Extracorporeal Membrane Oxygenation

Poonam Malhotra Kapoor, Mohit Prakash, Devishree Das, Minati Choudhury, and Sarvesh Pal Singh

Introduction

In the past, the extracorporeal membrane oxygenation (ECMO) definition was used, according to some nomenclature, for venovenous (VV) ECMO and the term "extracorporeal life support" (ECLS) was used for the venoarterial (VA) form of ECMO. The term ECLS can be used for any type today, be it mechanical-assist device for circulatory or pulmonary failure occurring in neonates, infants, children, and adults. The above two words are acronyms for the use of cardiopulmonary bypass using portable mechanical devices.[1]

Adding oxygen and removing carbon dioxide is basis for VV ECMO, as well, but it is done for respiratory failure. As ECMO is generally performed in a portable machine, keep in mind that with a VV ECMO, complete cardiac support is not feasible. For an increase in cardiac output, a VA ECMO configuration is adopted, at the bedside in an ICU.[3,4]

The new term "mobile ECMO" is emerging. This type of ECMO encompasses placing ECMO on a patient while on road, such that no time is lost. As ECMO can easily be placed in expert hands even outside the hospital, treatment for a cardiac arrest patient begins early, thus improving outcomes in hemodynamic and neurological status and also mortality.

Application of ECLS Systems

The decision to start ECMO should be made only after all indications and contraindications have been discussed within the team. An expert team, skilled in ECMO, is required for individual ECMO decisions (**Box 37.1**).

Box 37.1 Indications and contraindications for use of ECLS[1,2]
Indications
• Resistant to treatment of ventricular arrhythmias
• ECPR
• Treatment resistant cardiogenic shock:
➢ MI
➢ Myocarditis not amenable to treatment
• Weaning from CPB not feasible
• Acute decompensated heart failure
• Acute decompensated valve not responding to dysfunction with CPR
Contraindications
• Intracranial hemorrhage or bleeding
• Advanced age or frailty
• Restricted access due to peripheral vascular disease
• Contraindications to any form of anticoagulation
• Severe neurological disorder
• Multiorgan failure

Abbreviations: CPB, cardiopulmonary bypass; ECPR, extracorporeal cardiopulmonary resuscitation; MI, myocardial ischemia.

Implantation and Components of ECLS Systems

A femorofemoral cannulation wherein peripheral inguinal vessels are used is preferred in an acutely sick patient, who is being taken up for ECMO (**Table 37.1** and **Fig. 37.1**). In this case the femoral vein is cannulated with a 19- to 23-Fr draining cannula via the femoral artery. With this cannulation technique, a right ventricular (RV) unloading is achieved. The amount of ECMO blood flow (EBF) is determined by the size of the cannula. This route is preferred in emergency ECMO (**Fig. 37.2** and **Table 37.2**).

Successful implantation of ECMO cannulas, should be cross checked using echocardiography (ECG) or radioscopy such as an X-ray or computed tomography (CT) scan. The ECLS device connects the femorofemoral vessels using cannulas connected to the ECMO machine and ECMO blood flow thus retrograde with both femoral cannulation.

Monitoring of Patient's Parameters

Monitoring of patient's parameters is vital (**Boxes 37.2–37.4** and **Table 37.3**). It helps in assessing the patient's progress and spotting signs of complications. Clinically, the efficacy of

Table 37.1 Acute case for ECMO femoral-VA

Type	Cases
A	• Prefer femorofemoral cannulation • RV unloading with femoral cannulation • Drainage cannula: 19–23 Fr in FV→ RA • Return cannula: 15–19 Fr in FA → iliac artery
B	• Central cannulation is surgical • Drainage cannula is in the RA
C	• Femorosubclavian: return cannula is in the ascending aorta • Femorosubclavian technique is also used. Both central and subclavian routes are not preferred in an acute emergency ECMO insertion scenario

Abbreviations: ECMO, extracorporeal membrane oxygenation; FV, femoral vein; FA, femoral artery; RA, right atrium; VA, venoarterial.

Table 37.2 Types of ECMO

Cannulation	Bad lung Good heart	Good lung Bad heart	Bad lung Bad heart
V-V	✓	X	X
V-A peripheral	X	✓	✓
V-A Central	✓ (not required)	✓	✓

Abbreviations: V-A, venoarterial; V-V, venovenous.

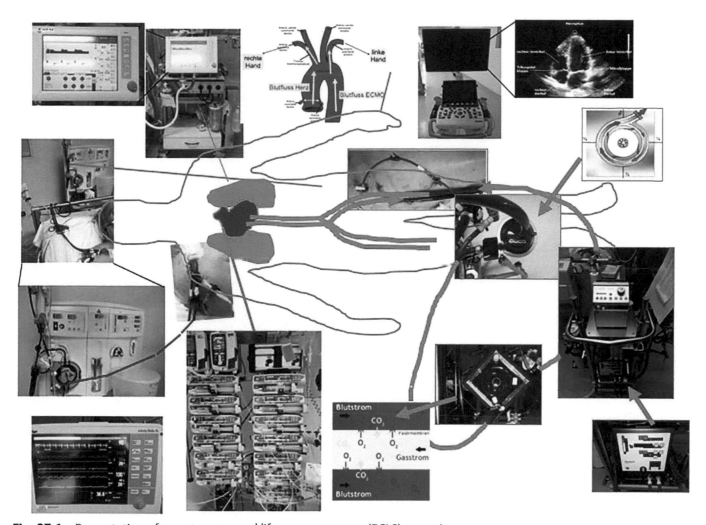

Fig. 37.1 Presentation of an extracorporeal life support system (ECLS) scenario.

Table 37.3 Integrative model for clinical monitoring

Physical examination is a must for hypoperfused state		What can we use?
Cool extremities	**Labs**	• Look at all the variables
Low urine output	• Increasing BUN/CR ratio	• SvO$_2$, urine output, acidosis (lactate)
Increasing CR	• LEFT	• CO/CI, filling pressures (PAD, CVP), SVR/SVRI
Confusion	• Coagulation abnormalities	• PA pressures, oxygenation
Nausea/Vomiting	• BNP	• Echocardiography
Peripheral edema	• Hyponatremia	
Ascites	• Acidosis	
SOB		

Abbreviations: BNP, B-type natriuretic peptide; CO, cardiac output; CI, cardiac index; CVP, central venous pressure; CR, creatinine; LFT, liver function test; PAD, pain, agitation, and delirium; PAP, pulmonary artery pressures; SOB; shortness of breath; SVR, systemic vascular resistance; SvO$_2$, central venous oximetry; SVRI, systemic vascular resistance index.

the system can be monitored by noting the vital parameters, oxygenation of the blood and tissue, urine, and monitoring laboratory parameters.[3]

It is essential to monitor vital parameters (i.e., ECG rhythm, pulse rate, invasive blood pressure, temperature, and respiratory rate), ECMO parameters (i.e., RPM, blood flow rate, gas flow rate, circuit pressure), and oxygenation status at arterial and venous end (i.e., SpO$_2$, SvO$_2$), and if possible cerebral oxygenation (rSO2 or BtO2).[5] Along with the regular monitoring of urine output and urine color

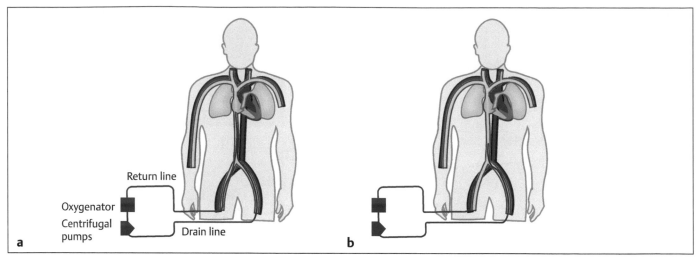

Fig. 37.2 Types of extracorporeal membrane oxygenation (ECMO), **(a)** Venovenous ECMO **(b)** Venoarterial ECMO.

Box 37.2 Components of an ECMO machine

- Membrane oxygenator
- Centrifugal pump
- Tubings and connectors
- Temperature device

Abbreviation: ECMO, extracorporeal membrane oxygenation.

Box 37.3 Importance of monitoring on ECMO ECLS

- Assess the accuracy of the system
- Monitor patient's progress
- Monitor efficacy of the system to maintain the safety of the system
- To rule out complications
- Monitoring of patient's parameters helps us in assessing the patient's progress

Abbreviations: ECLS, extracorporeal life support system, ECMO, extracorporeal membrane oxygenation.

Box 37.4 Success lies with vigilant monitoring

- Clinical parameters of patients
- Monitoring of accuracy of system and circuit
- Biochemical and laboratory parameters
- Radiologic monitoring
- Circuit monitoring
- Hemodynamic monitoring
- End-tidal carbon dioxide ($ETCO_2$) removal
- Anticoagulation monitoring

(1 hourly), vascular and neurological status (4 hourly) is equally important.

Various devices are available to monitor pressure, flow, and temperature of the ECMO blood and gas circuits, as well as physiological variables in the patient. However, there are currently limitations in measuring blood gases, which are required frequently in order to effectively monitor the

Box 37.5 Which patients need monitoring of gas exchanges[7]

Current guidelines suggest selective use in the following:
- Cardiogenic shock
- Acute on chronic heart failure
- Transplant/VAD patients
- Escalating inotropic supports
- Postprocedure/MI with heart failure
- At risk for RV/LV failure

Abbreviations: LV, left ventricle; MI, myocardial ischemia; RV, right ventricle; VAD, ventricular assist device.

adequacy of gas exchange support. In-line analyzers enable rapid and immediate assessment of blood gas results directly at the point of care. This aids in early decision-making and ensures closer control of therapy, besides conserving blood and minimizing any chance of infection from repetitive sampling.[6]

Monitoring of Gas Exchanges

In a critical care unit, it is essential to monitor the gas exchange. Methods of monitoring gas exchanges online include arterial saturation, mixed or central venous oxygenation, end tidal volume carbon dioxide ($ETCO_2$), and even blood gases such as pO_2, pCO_2, and pH (**Box 37.5**).

SpO_2

It measures the arterial saturation at the periphery with the help of pulse oximeter. It gives an idea about the peripheral perfusion. Saturation cannot be monitored in case of severe hypotension, vasoconstriction (due to high vasopressor shock state). It should be maintained above 90% and during VV ECMO even the saturation of 80 to 85% is acceptable. It is very important to monitor in VV ECMO but during VA ECMO mixed venous oxygen saturation is more important. During VA ECMO it is essential to intermittently monitor right-hand saturation, as it will tell you about the right brachiocephalic artery and indirectly coronary circulation (native circulation) in case of VA ECMO.

ScvO$_2$ or SvO$_2$

It is the most important indicator for managing critically ill patients. It represents the balance of systemic oxygen delivery and consumption. It is the current clinical standard for determination of oxygen adequacy on VA ECMO. It is also the current target for therapeutic interventions. However, it is unclear how well SvO$_2$ correlates with cerebral oxygenation.

It represents the adequacy of tissue perfusion and oxygen extraction. Usually ratio of O$_2$ consumption to O$_2$ delivery depends on oxygen extraction. Usually oxygen delivery is five times that of tissue oxygen extraction.

In case of a fully saturated, arterial blood, it is the proportion of oxygenation extracted from the arterial blood, which determines the decrease in venous saturation. The venous saturation will be seen as 80% if the oxygen extraction ratio is 20%. This follows the principles of normal human physiology.

True end-organ perfusion is measured with a "mixed venous" specimen taken from the pulmonary artery. Normal pulmonary artery saturation is 65 to 75%. Factors affecting the mixed venous saturation are cellular or metabolic demands, availability of oxygen, and ability of hemoglobin to unload oxygen and deliver oxygen to tissues. Premembrane saturations of the ECMO circuit do not represent true mixed venous saturations. It is the closest and most consistent indicator of oxygen delivery in VA ECMO. In VA ECMO, it is important to monitor premembrane saturations, and not patient arterial saturation or PaO2s, to evaluate adequate oxygen delivery, while during VV ECMO, premembrane saturation is not reliable due to recirculation factor.

The causes for decreased mixed venous saturation are decreased oxygen delivery or increased extraction. Decreased delivery is secondary to severe hypoxia, a low output state such as cardiogenic shock. Increased extraction can be due to increased metabolic activity such as sepsis. A transient or persistent increase in metabolic rate (e.g., fever, shivering, or seizures) will cause a major drop in venous saturation, with other parameters remaining unchanged. Low levels reflect inadequate perfusion. The basic principle of treatment is to increase supply to the tissue or decrease extraction or metabolic activity. The supply can be increased by maintaining adequate blood pressure, oxygenation, cardiac output, and hematocrit. Improved peripheral perfusion by using peripheral vasodilators like dobutamine, nitroglycerin or arginine vasodilator and increases cardiac output. If the patient is on ECMO then increase ECMO flow rate. Other alternative is to decrease the metabolic activity with sedation and hypothermia (**Fig. 37.3**).

Elevated levels represent diminished extraction by the tissue representing usually the dead tissue (e.g., severe central nervous system [CNS] injury, SvO$_2$ is high). Other reason for high venous saturation during VV ECMO is more recirculation (if premembrane venous saturation is used).

Cerebral Saturation

It is another most important parameter that needs to be monitored especially in patients with head injury or patients on VA and VV ECMO. Neurological outcome and complications are the major concern in ECMO. In severely critical patients even when on high ECMO support, sometimes the borderline hemodynamics and oxygenation parameters are accepted. Moreover, VA ECMO provides retrograde flow, and therefore with compromised hemodynamics whether the cerebral circulation is adequate or not always remains a question to ponder on. The usual trend is to monitor clinically by thorough neurological examination and sedation break period. Many of the times these parameters are not accurate so it is essential to monitor cerebral saturation. It provides clue about adequate cerebral perfusion.

Cerebral saturation can be monitored by brain tissue partial oxygen pressure (BtO2) or by regional oxygen saturation (rSO2) index.

BtO2 is used in adult traumatic brain injury (TBI) management. It is measured by Licox brain tissue oxygen monitoring system which can detect early changes in cerebral oxygenation, perfusion, and temperature. Low values have been shown to correlate with worse neurologic outcome.

rSO2 is measured by Somanetics INVOS cerebral oximeter and near-infrared spectroscopy (NIRS).[8] Factors affecting regional cerebral saturation are arterial pressure, carbon dioxide concentration, pump blood flow, arterial oxygen saturation (FiO$_2$), hematocrit, levels of anesthesia,

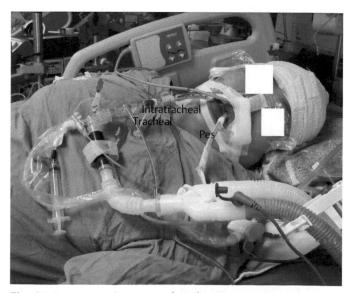

Fig. 37.3 Figure shows a sedated patient in the ICU.

and temperature. Low NIRS index has been associated with cerebral dysfunction in cardiac patients. Index <50 or index >20% decrease from baseline are significant values.[9,10] NIRS does not rely on pulse pressure. It can read at extremely low values and does not cut-out at value <35%. It is more accurate for targeting of cerebral perfusion.

Circuit Monitoring

This includes the following (**Fig. 37.4**):
- Circuit blood flow.
- Circuit gas flow.
- Circuit pressure.
- Circuit integrity.

End-Tidal Carbon Dioxide (ETCO$_2$)

The airway inlet measurement of the net tidal carbon dioxide levels is a good monitoring parameter of the native lung function. In the initial ECMO setting the ETCO$_2$ may be as low as 5 mmHg. As more functioning alveoli get recruited with ventilation or as there is an increase in the pulmonary blood flow levels (**Box 37.6**), the ETCO$_2$ gets increased. When ETCO$_2$ touches a level of 35 mmHg and remains there, along with other parameters, a weaning off ECMO may begin.

Vital Parameters

Routine monitoring of vital parameters such as blood pressure, heart rate, temperature, and respiratory rate reveals the patient's progress. During VA ECMO the target should be the mean arterial pressure and pulse pressure. Mean arterial pressure will indicate the adequacy of the perfusion pressure while pulse pressure reflects the native cardiac contribution. Decreased pulse pressure suggests less contribution from the heart and more contribution from the ECMO. Pulse pressure less than 10 signifies myocardial stunning.

Patient on ECMO has tachycardia but it usually settles once the hypoxia and perfusion improves. Persistent tachycardia can suggest inadequate flow or oxygenation. Sudden tachycardia during ECMO run can be due to arrhythmias due to electrolyte imbalance or occult bleeding.

Hourly urine output is another crucial factor that needs to be monitored in critical care. During ECMO run even the urine color is equally important as it suggests the beginning

Box 37.6 ETCO$_2$ levels as ECMO progresses
• ECMO beginning ETCO$_2$ < 5 mmHg
• ECMO ensues 210–215 mmHg
• ETCO$_2$, 35 mmHg insider weaning ECMO peak

Abbreviations: ECMO, extracorporeal membrane oxygenation; ETCO$_2$, end-tidal carbon dioxide.

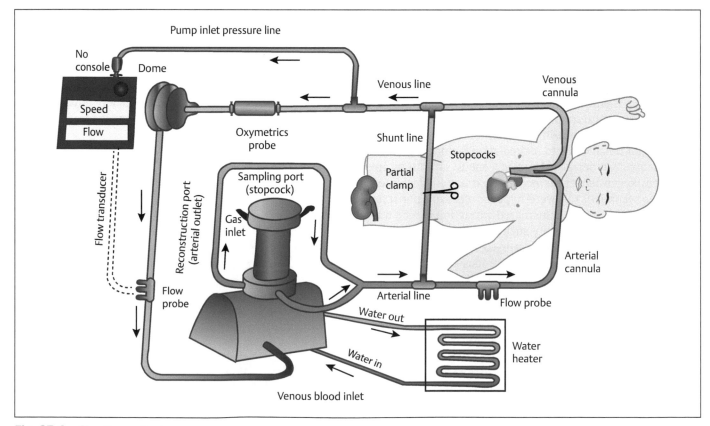

Fig. 37.4 Circuit monitoring.

of hemolysis. Usually during ECMO runs urine output is preferably maintained at more than 2 mL/kg/min.

Monitoring is required to assess the accuracy of the system, efficacy of the system, and also to watch for the safety of the system. Whenever the patient is on artificial life support, it is mandatory to know and establish the accuracy of the system per se. Secondly, it is essential to know whether the system is working efficiently to the desired level, and lastly we need to know whether it is working within the safe margin.

So, we divide the ECMO system monitoring into three categories, namely, monitoring the accuracy of the system, monitoring the efficacy of the system, and monitoring the safety of the system.

Gas Flow Rate

It is the amount of sweep gas passing through the membrane. It should be set in relation with blood flow and usually the ratio of gas flow:blood flow should be 0.5:1 and can go up to 1.5:1. Sweep gas helps in carbon dioxide removal, and it has to be adjusted as per carbon dioxide level.

A flow meter and blender are used to regulate gas flow to the membrane. In case if carbon dioxide level remains low even with minimal sweep gas then either a carbogen mixture or pure CO_2 can be added to sweep gas. With the addition of CO_2 continuous monitoring of postoxygenator blood gases is recommended to ensure that the pH and pCO_2 are in the target range.[12,13]

ECMO FiO_2 is usually adjusted to 100% to start with and then gradually weaned. Many of the centers always keep ECMO FiO_2 100% and they only wean sweep gas flow rate (**Box 37.7**).

Monitoring the Accuracy of System

This includes the monitoring of the ECMO machine and different components of the ECMO circuit. This is to ensure the proper functioning of the machine and the circuit components. The circuit check is done to look for any clot, air, leakage, etc., hourly. Pump is checked regularly to ascertain its proper functioning. One should know all the specifications of the components used (e.g., maximum blood flow rate of the tubing), and that oxygenator can be assessed by monitoring the delta pressure and postoxygenator blood gas. The accuracy of the machine can be monitored by checking the different parameters and revolution per minute (RPM; indirectly checks the blood flow rate), gas flow rate, and FiO_2 (**Box 37.8**).[4]

Blood Flow Rate

Blood flow rate cannot be adjusted directly but it is set by adjusting RPM. Usually blood flow rate can be adjusted between 60 and 150 mL/kg/min or 2.4 L/min/m². It should be adjusted depending upon pO_2 (in VV ECMO) and mean arterial pressure and mixed venous saturation (in VA ECMO).

The flow should be started at the rate of 20 mL/kg/min and then gradually increased by 10 mL/kg/min every 5 to 10 minutes till we get the desired result.[12,13]

Flow should not be increased suddenly except in case of extracorporeal cardiopulmonary resuscitation (ECPR). If there is rapid increase in flow then it can give rise to cardiac stunning. Blood flow rate should be kept at least acceptable so that it provides sufficient oxygen delivery to the tissue. High flow leads to increased resistance and suction effect which causes hemolysis. Blood flow rate depends on the RPM, preload to the circuit, and afterload to the circuit. It is directly proportional to RPM and preload of the circuit while inversely proportional to afterload (**Box 37.9** and **Table 37.4**).

Revolution per Minute (RPM)

What we can set is the RPM; the flow will depend on the preload and afterload condition of the circuit. Usually with the patient in stable condition a constant RPM will result in a constant blood flow. Under no circumstances should the RPM be set at 0 RPM, as the centrifugal pump is a nonocclusive device. Running at a too low RPM may result in backflow within the system from the arterial system into the venous system. If the flow needs to be stopped urgently, clamp the outflow line first before stopping the RPM (**Fig. 37.5**).

Box 37.7 Monitoring of gas exchanges

Gas exchanges can be monitored online by the following:
- Arterial saturation
- Mixed or central venous oxygenation
- End-tidal volume carbon dioxide ($ETCO_2$)
- Blood gases like pO_2, pCO_2, and pH

Box 37.8 Monitoring of accuracy of system during ECMO

- Circuit check
- Revolution per minute
- Blood flow rates
- ECMO FiO_2
- Delta pressure
- Postoxygenator blood gas
- Gas flow rates

Abbreviations: ECMO, extracorporeal membrane oxygenation; FiO_2, fraction of inspired oxygen.

Box 37.9 Precautions to be taken with ECMO flows

- Avoid sudden increases in ECMO flows, except in case of ECPR
- Rapid increase in ECMO flows gives rise to cardiac stunning
- ECMO blood flow rate should be kept at a minimum
- High ECMO flows cause suction effect or hemolysis

Abbreviations: ECMO, extracorporeal membrane oxygenation; ECPR, extracorporeal cardiopulmonary resuscitation.

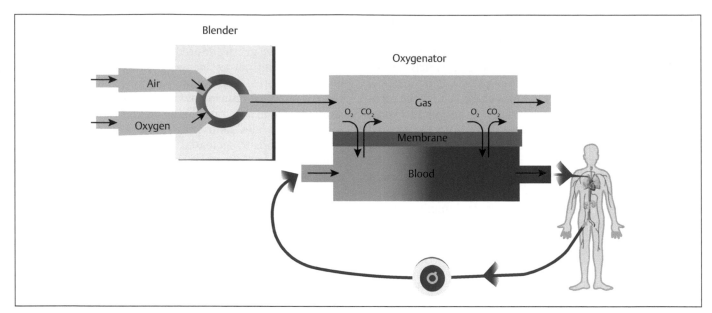

Fig. 37.5 Blender, pump, and oxygenator in the extracorporeal membrane oxygenation (ECMO) circuit for revolutions per minute.

Table 37.4 Factors affecting blood flow during ECMO

Increase flow on ECMO	Decrease flow on ECMO

• Increased RPM
• Decreased resistance (afterload):
  ➢ Vasodilation of the patient
  ➢ Improved arterial cannula positioning
• Increased preload:
  ➢ Increased patient filling
  ➢ Improved venous cannula position
	• Decreased RPM
	• Increased resistance (afterload):
	  ➢ Vasoconstriction
	  ➢ Kinking of tubing
	  ➢ Bad cannula position
	  ➢ Hypertension
	• Decreased preload:
	  ➢ Hypovolemic of the patient
	  ➢ Bad cannula positioning
	  ➢ Kinking of the tubing

Abbreviations: ECMO, extracorporeal membrane oxygenation; RPM, revolutions per minute.

Box 37.10 Delta pressure and drainage

• Impaired ECMO drainage is seen in hypovolemia and with low circuit flow, but high pump speed
• A normal pressure in the drainage cannula is between 50 and 80 mmHg
• A value less than 100 mmHg suggests impaired venous drainage
• Pressure drop difference if high between pressure at the inlet or outlet of the membrane lung suggests resistance inside the membrane oxygenator and causes obstruction to ECMO flows

Abbreviation: ECMO, extracorporeal membrane oxygenation.

Assessing Membrane Function

Membrane functions can be assessed by delta pressure and postmembrane blood gas. Membrane is much more efficient at exchanging CO_2 than O_2. The Delta pressure is defined as the difference between the pre- and postoxygenator pressure. It increases when the resistance in the oxygenator increases. It suggests clogging of the oxygenator. It is the earliest sign of membrane failure. It depends on the type of oxygenator; hollow fiber oxygenator has least delta pressure while silicon oxygenator has maximum delta pressure. It should be monitored continuously (**Box 37.10**).[14,15] Postoxygenator blood gas reflects the efficacy of the oxygenator. Ideally, it should be checked once daily and as and when required. Postoxygenator pO_2 should be at least more than 150 and CO_2 should be less than 40. Postoxygenator blood gas depends on the blood flow rate. If the blood flow rate is more than the capacity of the oxygenator then it will lead to hemolysis and postmembrane blood gas will show hypoxia. In this situation, one more oxygenator is added parallel to the previous one.

Monitoring of Efficacy

Once we know the accuracy of the machine function, its efficacy can be judged by the clinical and laboratory parameters. This will tell us about the adequacy of our support. Is our support adequate? Or, do we need to do something more? The ultimate goal of the ECMO is to maintain adequate tissue perfusion and minimize complications. The efficacy of VV ECMO is determined by the pO_2 and pCO_2 levels while the efficacy of VA ECMO is determined by mean arterial pressure, mixed venous saturations, and lactate levels. Mean arterial pressure and mixed venous saturation have already been discussed earlier.

Lactate levels suggest the tissue perfusion like mixed venous oxygen saturation. The normal range is 4.5 to 20 mg/dL or 0.5 to 2.2 mmol/L. Lactate levels go high whenever there is tissue hypoxia. Other causes of elevated lactates are acute or chronic renal failure, hepatic failure, and pseudo high levels can be secondary to adrenaline infusion. It should be monitored twice a day or frequently if not stable. The sample must be processed in 15 to 20 minutes of collection and should be sent on ice bag to retard glycolysis.

pO_2 and pCO_2 Measurement Are a Must

Blood gas needs to be monitored for the efficacy of the system. pO_2 and pCO_2 reflect the efficacy of VV ECMO. pO_2 should be more than 50 (for VV) and more than 60 (for VA) while pCO_2 should be less than 40. It should be monitored twice or thrice in a day. Again for VA ECMO mixed venous saturation is more important than arterial blood gas. Blood pH should also be monitored and tried to maintain in normal range.

Respiratory acidosis and hypercapnia can be corrected by increasing sweep gas flow and by decreasing restlessness and agitation. Metabolic acidosis usually reflects tissue hypoxia and can be corrected by increasing EBF and ECMO FiO2 (**Box 37.11**).

Monitoring of the Safety

Lastly, after the efficiency of our support is ensured, we need to know whether whatever we are doing is in the safe range and will have no or less adverse effects. The safety can be monitored by checking the ECMO parameters, hematological parameter, coagulative status, routine biochemical and radiological parameters, and last but not least clinical parameters. A high index of suspicion with imaging to rule out either thrombosis or should be rested with imaging view on ECHO or flouroscopy bleeding (**Box 37.12**).

Extracorporeal Membrane Oxygenation Parameters

ECMO parameters such as prepump pressure and pre- and postoxygenator pressure need to be monitored to prevent excessive hemolysis. Prepump pressure reflects the venous drainage pressure.

Acceptable limit is up to −20 mmHg. More negative pressure causes hemolysis and if pressure falls below −200 then it can lead to cavitation. It can also cause endothelial damage to right atrium or vena cava due to suction effect. The usual causes are low volume, poor catheter placement or inadequate cannula size pre- and postoxygenator pressures reflect the pressure on the arterial limb of the circuit. These pressures depend on the resistance of the circuit, RPM, systemic pressure, and systemic vascular resistance. Circuit factors include the size of cannula, size of tubing, and the type of oxygenator. Hollow fiber oxygenator has low pre- and postoxygenator pressures around 100 while silicon oxygenator has very high pressures around 300 mmHg. High pre- and postoxygenator pressures can damage the membrane fibers and cause hemolysis.

Coagulative Status

One of the major complications encountered during ECMO run is either thrombosis or bleeding. Hence, a strict control on anticoagulation is essential.[16]

Hematological Parameters

Hematological parameters monitored for safety purpose are hemoglobin level, plasma-free hemoglobin, and white blood cell counts.

Hemoglobin can decrease due to bleeding or hemolysis. It is essential to maintain hematocrit around 35 to 40% (for VA) and >40 (for VV) for effective ECMO run. It should be monitored twice daily. Plasma-free hemoglobin suggests the severity of hemolysis. The acceptable range when patient is on ECMO is less than 50 mg/dL. High bilirubin or lipemic plasma may cause falsely elevated values. It should be monitored on alternate days. White blood cell count needs to be monitored for the possibility of infection. ECMO patients are critically ill and have high chances of infections due to multiple lines.

Biochemical Parameters

Routine biochemical profile, such as electrolyte, calcium, creatinine, etc., needs to be monitored at least once or twice a day. Renal involvement during ECMO is common and, hence, creatinine and other renal function tests need to be closely monitored. Electrolyte imbalance can occur due to dilutional effect.[17] Serum calcium level can decrease due to the multiple citrated blood transfusions. All this can lead to cardiac stunning and cardiac arrhythmia.

Box 37.11 Respiratory acidosis

- Increase the sweep gas flow
- Decrease patient's restlessness and anxiety
- Increasing ECMO blood flow
- Increasing ECMO FiO_2

Abbreviations: ECMO, extracorporeal membrane oxygenator; FiO_2, fraction of inspired oxygen.

Box 37.12 Monitoring of safety on ECMO

- ECMO parameters
- Biochemical parameters
- Clinical parameters
- Radiological parameters

Abbreviation: ECMO, extracorporeal membrane oxygenation.

Hemolytic profile, such as bilirubin, lactate dehydrogenase (LDH), and urine for hemoglobinuria, needs monitoring and appropriate treatment to prevent renal failure and disseminated intravascular coagulation (DIC). Procalcitonin (PCT) and C-reactive protein (CRP) levels should also be monitored regularly as it can be the only sign of infection. Patient on ECMO may not have fever due to temperature regulation by heater unit. White blood cell count may not be reliable completely. PCT level more than 10 suggests the possibility of sepsis and may demand change of antibiotics. Ideally, serial monitoring of PCT and CRP is required to assess the antibiotic response.

Clinical Parameters

Clinical parameters pertaining to safety of ECMO are urine color and peripheral vascular status. Monitoring urine color is important as it could be the earliest signs to indicate hemolysis and hematuria. It is very important to assess peripheral circulation especially in cases of VA ECMO with groin cannulation. The leg should be checked every hour to verify sufficient perfusion and drainage. Look for peripheral pulsation, color of the limb, capillary refill, and edema. Both the limbs should be monitored for ischemic signs (due to thromboembolic phenomena).

Box 37.13 Radiological parameters defining the safety of ECMO

- Echocardiography opening of aortic valve LVOT VTI <10 cm$_2$ EF >40%
- CT of the head for any cerebral infarcts/hemorrhage
- CT angiogram for pulmonary embolism

Abbreviations: CT, computed tomography; ECMO, extracorporeal membrane oxygenation; EF, ejection fraction; LVOT VTI, left ventricular outflow tract velocity time integral.

Radiological Parameters

Radiological parameters such as X-ray chest, USG, and 2D echo are equally important in assessing the cannula position and looking for intrathoracic complications like pneumothorax, hemothorax, hemopericardium, etc.[18] Head ultrasound and CT brain help in assessing the neurological complications, especially the intracranial bleed that might occur during the course of illness (**Box 37.13**).

Once ECMO Is Initiated, Monitoring too Is Initiated

Once ECMO is initiated the metabolism of the patient undergoes major metabolic changes. Therefore, as a first step, soon after initiating ECMO get an arterial blood gas done to correct the electrolyte disturbances. If the patient shows some neurological deterioration then it is wise to withhold sedation and paralytic agents for some time. All evaluations are made on the patient's bedside in the ICU, as patients are very sick. A X-ray, ultrasound/echocardiography done at the bedside, crunches the diagnosis. If seizures are seen, then an EEG is done (**Table 37.5**).[19]

Conclusion

Monitoring during ECMO requires an understanding of the physiological basis for the monitor's validity. Many conventional forms of ICU hemodynamic monitoring lack validity in ECMO patients. Nevertheless, used appropriately, these tools are invaluable to the intensivist.

ECMO is not a causal therapy. Monitoring of patients under ECLS comprises time-consuming and staff-intensive

Table 37.5 Unstable patients

Stage	Steps to be performed
First few hours of ECMO initiation	ABG, lab parameters, X-ray, ultrasound, ECHO, POC test; ACT EEG
Semistable patients	• Daily team meeting • Start thinking of an alternative support or weaning from ECMO • Discuss with team on patient's progress • Update to the family are given from time to time
Bedside recovery of ECMO patients	• Larger pulse pressure (from previous flat one on ECMO) on arterial tracing is observed • Opening of aortic valve on Echo • Check ejection of blood to prevent thrombosis and pulmonary congestion • Addition of IABP or impella may be warranted • Atrial septostomy to unload the left ventricle may be needed from ECMO support • Appropriate intervention to be done judiciously, as ECMO is best for 7–14 d only

Abbreviations: ABG, arterial blood gas; ACT, activated clotting time; ECHO, echocardiography; ECMO, extracorporeal membrane oxygenation; EEG, electroencephalogram; POC, point of care.

management. Besides intensive care monitoring, special aspects of ECLS should be checked regularly and optimized. With regard to patient-side monitoring control of hemodynamics, gas exchange, anticoagulation status, leg perfusion as well as neurological monitoring is very important.[20]

Summary

Accuracy, adequacy, and safety are in general a key to success. To maintain this constantly one is required to have vigilant monitoring. Proper monitoring of the system functionality can prevent life-threatening complications. Thorough check of the ECMO system along with the vital parameter and laboratory value will lead to safe and successful ECMO. ECLS as a cardiopulmonary bypass is a cardiovascular and lung support system. However it is not a causal therapy. Monitoring of patients under ECLS comprises time-consuming and staff-intensive management. Besides intensive care monitoring, special aspects of ECLS should be checked regularly and optimized. With regard to patient-side monitoring control of hemodynamics, gas exchange, anticoagulation status, leg perfusion, as well as neurological monitoring is very important. In terms of device monitoring pump flow per minute, fresh gas flow, and inspiratory O_2-fraction have to be regularly documented. A multiprofessional and interdisciplinary team of caretakers and physicians well-skilled in use of ECLS system is indispensable in a qualitative and patient-safe ECLS setting.

References

1. Trummer G, Bein B, Buerke M, et al. Standardized terminology of mechanical heart, lung and circulatory assist devices: a recommendation of the Section "Heart and Circulation" of the German Interdisciplinary Association of Critical Care Medicine. Appl Cardiopulm Pathophysiol 2011;15:181–182
2. ELSO Guideline for Cardiopulmonary Extracorporeal Support Extracorporeal Life Support Organization Extracorporeal Life Support Organization. August 2017 (Version 1.4)
3. Abrams D, Garan AR, Abdelbary A, et al; International ECMO Network (ECMONet) and The Extracorporeal Life Support Organization (ELSO). Position paper for the organization of ECMO programs for cardiac failure in adults. Intensive Care Med 2018;44(6):717–729
4. Chung M, Shiloh AL, Carlese A. Monitoring of the adult patient on venoarterial extracorporeal membrane oxygenation. Scientific World J 2014;2014:393258
5. Taylor MA, Maldonado Y. Anesthetic management of patients on ECMO. In: Firstenberg M, ed. Extracorporeal membrane oxygenation—advances in therapy. InTech; 2016. doi: 10.5772/63309
6. Fox J, Troughton G. Blood conservation with a patient dedicated arterial blood gas analyser. September 2015, Sphere Medical White Paper. http://www.spheremedical. com/ content/ clinical-resources
7. Venkat G, Pranay O. Monitoring on extracorporeal membrane oxygenation. In: Kapoor PM, ed. Manual of Extracorporeal Membrane Oxygenation (ECMO) in the ICU. Jaypee Brothers Medical Publishers; 2014:76–80
8. Cook OJ. Neurologic effects of cardiopulmonary bypass. In: Davis RF, Stammers AH, Ungerleider RM, Gravlee GP, eds. Cardiopulmonary bypass: principles and practice. 3rd ed. Philadelphia, PA: Lippincott Williams and Wilkins; 2008
9. Nasr DM, Rabinstein AA. Neurologic complications of extracorporeal membrane oxygenation. J Clin Neurol 2015; 11(4):383–389
10. Maldonado Y, Singh S, Taylor MA. Cerebral near-infrared spectroscopy in perioperative management of left ventricular assist device and extracorporeal membrane oxygenation patients. Curr Opin Anaesthesiol 2014;27(1):81–88
12. Extracorporeal Life Support Organization. ELSO guidelines for cardiopulmonary extracorporeal life support. ELSO; 2013. https://www.elso.org/Portals/0/IGD/Archive/FileManager/92 9122ae88cusersshyerdocumentselsoguidelinesgeneral alleclsversion1.3.pdf
13. Annich G. ECMO: extracorporeal cardiopulmonary support in critical care. Extracorporeal Life Support Organization; 2012. https://www.elso.org/Publications/RedBook4thEdition.aspx
14. Zanella A, Mojoli F, Castagna L, et al. Respiratory monitoring of the ECMO patient. In: Sangalli F, Patroniti N, Pesenti A, eds. ECMO-extracorporeal life support in adults. Milano: Springer; 2014
15. Belliato M, Degani A, Buffa A, et al. A brief clinical case of monitoring of oxygenator performance and patient-machine interdependency during prolonged veno-venous extracorporeal membrane oxygenation. J Clin Monit Comput 2017;31(5):1027–1033
16. Smith A, Hardison D, Bridges B, Pietsch J. Red blood cell transfusion volume and mortality among patients receiving extracorporeal membrane oxygenation. Perfusion 2013;28(1): 54–60
17. Kilburn DJ, Shekar K, Fraser JF. The complex relationship of extracorporeal membrane oxygenation and acute kidney injury: causation or association? BioMed Res Int 2016;2016:1094296
18. Lee S, Chaturvedi A. Imaging adults on extracorporeal membrane oxygenation (ECMO). Insights Imaging 2014;5(6):731–742
19. Krishnan S, Schmidt GA. Hemodynamic monitoring in the extracorporeal membrane oxygenation patient. Curr Opin Crit Care 2019;25(3):285–291
20. Merkle J, Azizov F, Fatullayev J, et al. Monitoring of adult patient on venoarterial extracorporeal membrane oxygenation in intensive care medicine. J Thorac Dis. 2019;11(Suppl 6):S946–S956

38

Perfusion Perspectives for Integrated Venoarterial ECMO: AIIMS Experience

Poonam Malhotra Kapoor, Suruchi Hasija, Sukesan Subin, and Sandeep Chauhan

Introduction

Extracorporeal membrane oxygenation (ECMO) used for severe cardiac and respiratory failure is here to stay in every intensive care unit (ICU). Not only does it drain blood from the patient's body, it also removes the carbon dioxide, oxygenates the blood, and returns it to the patients. The return of oxygenated blood from the ECMO machine is into either the venous or the arterial circulation. This handling of the ECMO machine components entails an expert perfusionist with an in-depth knowledge of ECMO nuances. Optimization of the patients' blood and care during ECMO will be handled deftly by a perfusionist with the right ECMO circuitry and equipment for many days at a stretch. Unlike a cardiopulmonary bypass (CPB), which entails a few hours only, the resistance and expertise needed for prolonged ECMO duration is immense. Hence, the need for a teamwork for best results on ECMO.

Journey of AIIMS from ECMO to Integrated ECMO

In the past two decades AIIMS (All India Institute of Medical Sciences) has functioned in a judicious manner with ECMO. AIIMS has increasingly provided leadership in the area of public health; one such example is "Use of Integrated ECMO in Cardiac Surgery" in last 20 years with good results.

The ECMO components and circuitry in the modern era are sleeker, easier to run, and more compact. The same machine with different disposable items and sizes can be used in neonates, pediatric, and adult patients alike. The ECMO circuit is heparin coated and biocompatible; thus, it can be used for longer time periods with less numbers of changes and minimal complications of bleeding, thrombosis, and physiological derangement inherent to an ECMO circuit with article. We require immediate postoperative mechanical support with the early application of ECMO, which was initiated in AIIMS as Integrated ECMO Concept in an attempt to manage cases like primary arterial switch operation (ASO) in transposition of the great arteries (TGA) with intact ventricular septum (IVS) beyond 3 weeks of life (**Box 38.1**). *Patients who had severely regressed left ventricle were operated on integrated ECMO.*[1-3]

Description of Integrated CPB ECMO Circuit

The two parallel circuits of ECMO and CPB are integrated at the level of the membrane oxygenator (MO) and the heat exchanger. During surgery (on CPB), the "hard shell" noncollapsible cardiotomy reservoir is used; and after surgery (on ECMO), the collapsible soft reservoir "bladder" of the ECMO is used. The entire assembling is performed prior to the initiation of surgery.

ECMO is a last resort in managing a critical patient, when other conservative and radical measures fail. Multiple reports have shown that transporting high-risk patients on ECMO is beneficial if the risk of transporting them without extracorporeal support is life-threatening. Patients transported on mechanical circulatory support may have improved outcomes when a dedicated team travels to initiate support and stabilize the patient before transport. These unique integrated circuit designing has provided significant improvements over more traditional ECMO circuits, particularly when patient requires an immediate mechanical support postsurgery. Contraindications to ECMO should always be kept in mind too (**Boxes 38.2 and 38.3**).[5]

Box 38.1 Indications of integrated extracorporeal membrane oxygenation (ECMO) support

The indigenous redesign of the venoarterial ECMO is done in AIIMS for the following surgeries:
- Transposition of great arteries with intact ventricular septum, beyond 3 weeks, undergoing an arterial switch operation
- Obstructed total anomalous pulmonary venous connection (TAPVC)
- Anomalous left coronary artery from pulmonary artery (ALCAPA) for preoperative and postoperative support, including performance of surgery on the ECMO circuit
- Anticipated inabilities to wean from cardiopulmonary bypass (CPB) in a complex redo case
- Border line cases of late primary switch operation (<3 wk):
  ➢ dTGA and IVS, D-Shaped LV, abnormal coronary origin

Abbreviations: dTGA, dextro-transposition of the great arteries; IVS, intact ventricular septum; IVS, intact ventricular septum; LV, left ventricle.

Box 38.2 Criteria for ECMO specific to adults

- Cardiorespiratory failure >90% mortality
- Indications:
  ➢ Failure of conventional medical therapy
  ➢ Transpulmonary shunt >30% ($FiO_2 > 69\%$)
  ➢ Static compliance <0.5 mL/cmH$_2$O/kg
  ➢ Diffusely abnormal chest roentgenogram
  ➢ Cardiac failure or cardiac arrest
  ➢ Hypercapnia with pH >7.20
- Contraindications:
  ➢ Age >60 y (relative)
  ➢ Duration of ventilation >5–7 d
  ➢ Incurable condition
  ➢ Intracranial bleed or closed space bleed

Abbreviations: ECMO, extracorporeal membrane oxygenator; FiO$_2$, fraction of inspired oxygen.

Components of an ECMO Circuit

The ECMO circuit is made up of a number of components that have been customized at AIIMS in the form of integrated circuit with customized low-cost ECMO cart having battery backup to support patients with severe cardiac failure. In a conventional ECMO circuit, there is a blood pump, a gas exchanging device, and a heat exchange all of which are connected together by a circuit tubing. Other

components of an ECMO circuit include blood flow and pressure monitors, continuous oxy-hemoglobin saturation monitors, circuit access sites, and a bridge connecting the venous and arterial limbs of the ECMO circuit together taking the ECMO from a simple to an advanced cardiohelp type of format. Recent advancements in ECMO component (**Box 38.2**) and circuitry (**Figs. 38.1** and **38.2**) have provided inroads into safe ECMO procedures and outcomes today in 2022.

Box 38.3 Contraindications to neonatal ECLS

- Only absolute:
  - ➤ Do not resuscitate?
- Neurological impairment
- End stage, inoperable, irreversible disease
- Uncontrolled bleeding and DIC
- Inaccessible vessels on CPR
- No major cardiac malformation like coarctation of aorta
- Birth weight <2.0 kg—due to limitations of catheter size
- Gestational age <34 wk—due to risk of IVH (intraventricular hemorrhage)
- Lethal or untreatable nonpulmonary disease
- Grade II–IV intracranial hemorrhage—due to risk of extension of bleeding
- Relative contraindications:
  - ➤ Mechanical ventilation for >10 d (high risk of irreversible lung injury)
  - ➤ Grade I IVH
  - ➤ Uncontrolled bleeding or coagulopathy

Abbreviations: CPR, cardiopulmonary resuscitation; DIC, disseminated intravascular coagulation; ECLS, extracorporeal life support; IVH, intraventricular hemorrhage.

The AIIMS ECMO Circuit

To fulfil the need for a cardiac surgery in the postoperative period, ECMO is frequently required to continue supporting a weak functioning heart. Most often, since there is a delay in implementation of ECMO more mortality on ECMO is seen than survival. The AIIMS cardiac center, in 2010, circumvented this problem, with the implementation and formation of an integrated CPB venoarterial (VA) ECMO circuit, which has in the last 11 years proved beneficial in survival and better outcomes. It is used chiefly as outlined in **Box 38.1**, patient who may require CPB support post–cardiac surgery for a few more hours or days.

1. **Concept/design of the integrated CPB:** The first circuit design has two parallel circuits of both ECMO and CPB integrated together at the level of both the membrane oxygenator (MO) and the heat exchanger (HE). During the cardiac surgical procedure, the hardshell cardiotomy reservoir which is noncollapsible (as in CPB) is used. Post-CPB, ECMO is initiated automatically with prior circuitry arrangement, in which the reservoir is removed from the circuit and the "ECMO bladder" which is a soft collapsible reservoir is used.

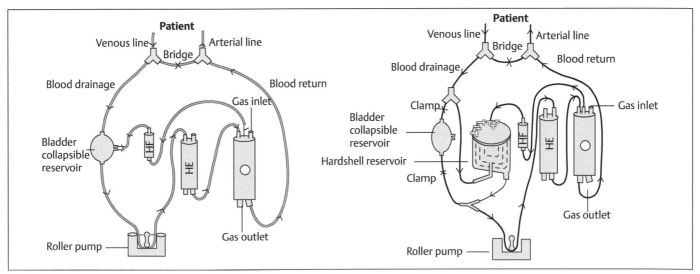

Fig. 38.1 Integrated extracorporeal membrane oxygenation (ECMO) circuit beginning. Abbreviations: HF, hemofilter; HE, heat exchanger; O, oxygenator.

2. **Circuit assembly:** During surgery on CPB (**Fig. 38.1**) blood superior vena cava (SVC) and inferior vena cava (IVC) cannulas are connected to a Y-piece and then into "hardshell" reservoir and then to the patient as explained in **Flowchart 38.1**.

Post–Cardiac Surgery Circuit While on ECMO

After surgery on ECMO, the circuit followed is blood to SVC and IVC cannulas and then to single right atrial (RA) cannula.

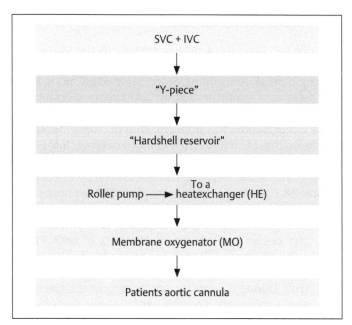

Flowchart 38.1 Flow of steps for integrated extracorporeal membrane oxygenation (ECMO) circuits and ECMO connections. Abbreviations: IVC, inferior vena cava; SVC, superior vena cava.

From RA it goes to the bladder, the roller pump/cone to the heat exchange. From this it goes to the MO and then to aortic cannula and to the patient. All this is depicted in **Fig. 38.2**.

Today, integrated CPB-ECMO circuit at AIIMS is followed routinely by all for all elected and most emergency pediatric congenital cases. It has many advantages, which are listed in **Box 38.4**.

The Oxygenator for Integrated ECMO

In a neonate coming for pediatric cardiac surgery, with the indications as cited for integrated ECMO-CPB circuit, a EUROSETS (EUROSETS A.L. ONE, ECMO Paediatric Oxygenator, Italy) oxygenator is used at AIIMS. An integrated ECMO-CPB circuit uses a Capiox SX (Terumo Corporation) reservoir with a bridge line to the arterial access. From the reservoir, it is joined by a BIOMEDICUS (Italy) pump, which leads to the oxygenator along with the heat exchanger incorporated together. All throughout the cardiac surgery, a hemoconcentrator is routinely incorporated into the circuit, as shown in **Fig. 38.3**.[5,6]

Various safety features incorporated in the ECMO circuit are listed in **Box 38.5** and are shown in **Fig. 38.4**.

Box 38.4   Advantages of the redesigning venoarterial integrated CPB-ECMO
• Incorporate cardiopulmonary bypass (CPB) circuit • Increase preparedness/availability of the ECMO circuit • Cut-down assembly time • Reduce possibility of cardiopulmonary resuscitation • Increase cost-effectiveness

Abbreviation: CPB-ECMO, cardiopulmonary bypass–extracorporeal membrane oxygenation.

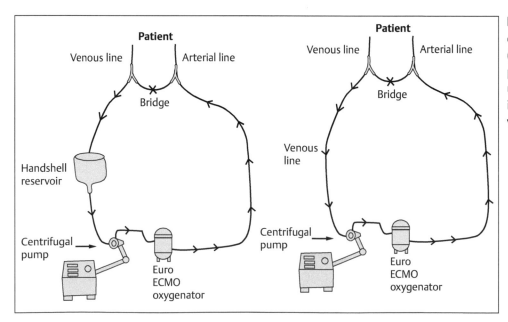

Fig. 38.2 Integrated extracorporeal membrane oxygenation (ECMO) circuit modified by AIIMS perfusionist and team at present use in 2023. Abbreviations: IVC, inferior vena cava; SVC, superior vena cava.

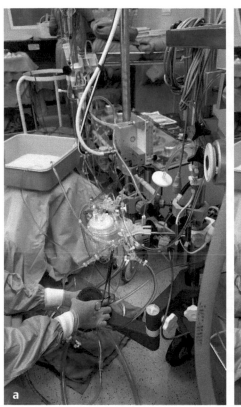
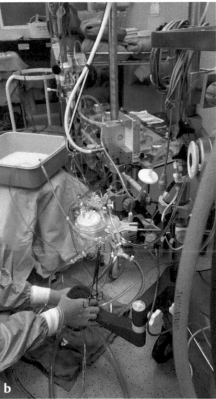
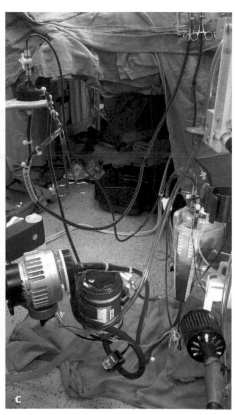

Fig. 38.3 The integrated cardiopulmonary bypass–extracorporeal membrane oxygenation (CPB-ECMO) circuit. **(a)** Preparation in the operating room with pump. **(b)** Reservoir oxygenation. **(c)** Hemofiltration.

> **Box 38.5 Different safety features incorporated in the ECMO circuit**
>
> - Venous bladder and pump controller
> - The ECMO Bridge (**Fig. 38.4**)
> - Mixed venous oxygen saturation monitor
> - Transonic flow meter—pressure alarm, battery backup, supplementary electrical supply on the ECMO trolley

Perfusion Details During Surgery and Postoperative on the ECMO Circuit

CPB is established by utilizing aortic cannula and venous cannula for both SVC and IVC. The heart is then arrested using either Delnido cardioplegia or St. Thomas cardioplegia and is given manually by the surgeon to the aortic root. After cooling the patients to 30 to 32°C, and maintaining a mean arterial pressure (MAP) between 50 and 60 mmHg, the topical temperature is maintained using a Bair Hugger machine.

A near-infrared spectroscopy (NIRS) is routinely used at AIIMS in all cardiac surgical cases. When the surgery is over, the surgeon excludes the CPB limb of the venous reservoir from the perfusion circuit. A straight venous cannula is used to drain blood from the RA appendage, maintaining an optimum drainage outflow. As the ECMO circuit begins,

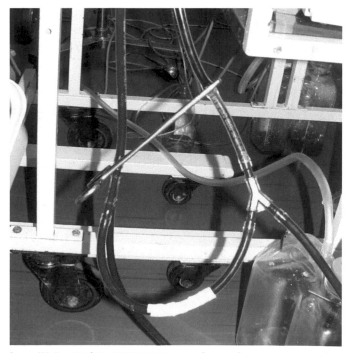

Fig. 38.4 Bridge in extracorporeal membrane oxygenation (ECMO) circuit. It provides bypass if patient requires isolation from the circuit and also ensures unclamping for brief periods to ensure patency of the line, so that no air is entrapped.

then with the use of the bridge (**Fig. 38.4**), the aortic circuit and cannula remaining the same, the patient is isolated from CPB into ECMO, skin is closed, encompassing both the cannula sites. On this ECMO support the patients is shifted to the ICU. Heparin infusion is continued at the rate of 10 U/kg/h to keep an optimal activated clotting time (ACT) of 180 to 220 seconds when the ECMO procedure is on. It is important at all times to maintain a hematocrit more than 40% and a platelet count greater than one lakh twenty thousand with use of the right components therapy (**Boxes 38.6** and **38.7**; **Tables 38.1** and **38.2**).

ECMO Management in ICU

In the ICU as heparin continues at the infusion rate of 8 to 10 U/kg/h and ACT, hematocrit, and platelet count are maintained (**Box 38.8**), an X-ray chest is done to confirm the tube position is in place, the ECMO ventilatory settings are put on "rest," lung protective mode of tidal volume. The tidal volume is kept between 4 to 5mL/kg with an FiO_2 of 21%. At all times, it is imperative to maintain the body temperature to near normothermia, around 36 to 37°C, using a conventional body warmer. On a four hourly basis by an intensivist and all throughout by a perfusionist and nurse the patient is monitored both clinically and biochemically. Central venous pressure/left atrial pressure (CVP/LAP), heart rate, central and peripheral venous oxygenation temperature, urine output, and MAP are maintained within normal limits all throughout the ECMO run.

Special attention is paid to the ECMO flows (high vs. low flows for optimal hemodynamics), cannula positioning, daily blood cultures for sepsis, and imaging. A transthoracic echocardiography is done once daily and so is a cranial ultrasound to rule out intracranial hemorrhage (**Fig. 38.5**).

Weaning is initiated when all parameters are satisfactory. A decrease in flow rates every 1 to 2 hours by 10% or more is done to maintain the flow at around 30 to 40 mL/kg/min.[13] A trial off for an hour is given without ECMO. It is then initiated by declamping the recirculation line or bridge and clamping simultaneously the arterial and venous cannulas. Decannulation is done when the child is passing adequate urine (at least 1 mL/kg/h) and the arterial blood gases show

---

Box 38.6 Sizes of venovenous cannula (Origin Biomedical Inc.)

For Integrated CPB-ECMO circuits, sizes of venovenous cannula are:
- 12 Fr for children 2–5 kg
- 15 Fr for children 4–8 kg
- 18 Fr for children 7–12 kg

Box 38.7 Integrated ECMO-CPB circuit complications

- Assist reservoir complication
- Inadequate return → Air embolism (Late sign)
- Hypovolemia
- Increased intrathoracic pressure
- Venous cannulas' occlusion pressure rising
- Capillary leak syndrome
- Drainage insufficiency due to clots or small drainage cannula size, leading to obstruction at the drainage cannula, inlet site

---

Table 38.1 Pump flows on integrated CPB-ECMO circuit

Age group	Heparin infusion
Neonates	150 mL/min × body weight
Pediatric up to 10 kg	100–150 mL/min × body weight
Pediatric >10 kg	2400 mL/m²/min × body surface area (BSA)
Adults	2400 mL/m²/min × body surface area (BSA)

Abbreviations: CPB, cardiopulmonary bypass; ECMO, extracorporeal membrane oxygenation.

Table 38.2 Merits and demerits of integrated ECMO-CPB circuit

Merits	Demerits
Less cumbersome (shifting circuit)	More cumbersome (circuit components increase)
Economical (if circuit is used)	Expensive (if unused)
Less time off CPB	More initial time to assemble circuit
Less hesitancy to take decision	Less familiar
Less risk (reduce possibility for cardiac massage)	

Abbreviations: CPB, cardiopulmonary bypass; ECMO, extracorporeal membrane oxygenation.

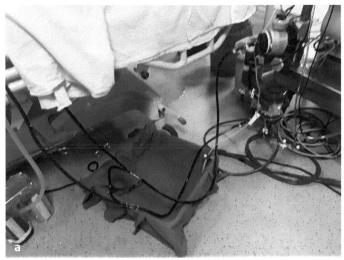
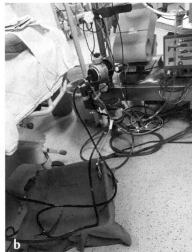
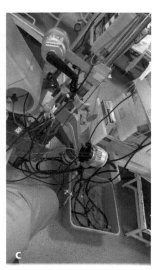

Fig. 38.5 **(a)** Disposable circuit tubings in trays; the extracorporeal membrane oxygenation (ECMO) trolley. **(b)** The membrane oxygenator (MO) and heat exchanger (HE) and monitors remain at the patient's bedside till weaned off. **(c)** Dedicated perfusionist, nurse, and intensivist monitor the ECMO in the intensive care unit (ICU) continuously, postweaning too.

minimal acidosis with optimal PaO_2 and $PaCO_2$. The sternum is closed the next day and child is subsequently extubated.

The advantages of integrated circuit ECMO at AIIMS are as follows:

- No time lag to initiate ECMO (even experienced personnel need 20–25 min to assemble and deair circuit).
- Enables left ventricle (LV) "retraining" under normoxemia and controlled loading.
- Early initiation prevents end-organ damage by reducing chances of cardiac arrest and prolonged low cardiac output.
- Surgical asepsis and cost-effective.
- Saves blood and blood products especially in cases where patients have rare blood group.

Complications of Integrated Circuit

Bleeding complications have not been observed at AIIMS because of intensive hemostasis, a good platelet count maintenance, strict ACT maintenance between 180 and 220 seconds, low threshold for packed RBCs and platelet transfusion, and performing point-of-care tests for right component therapy whenever feasible (**Box 38.8**).

In select cases, the use of ECMO may result in patients' neurologically intact survival; however, the question remains as to whether this benefit is consistently observed in comparison to conventional care in the variety of settings in which it is used. Currently, these strategies are not incorporated into comparative evaluations of ECMO, as there exists no validated prognostic approach for identifying appropriate patients at ECMO initiation (**Table 38.3**). Such entry criteria for ECMO have been described as a "moving target." Author's review therefore focuses on the current

---

Box 38.8 Flow rates, ACT, and ECHO parameters

- Maximal flow rates on ECMO (125–150 mL/kg)[4–6,13]
- Activated clotting time between 180–220 s and FIBTEM >10 mm[10–12]
- Weaning and recovery: echocardiographic parameters of possible recovery are:
  - ➤ LVEF >35–40%
  - ➤ LVED diameter <55 mm
  - ➤ Aortic velocity-time integral >10 cm
  - ➤ Aortic valve opening pattern
  - ➤ Absence of LV dilatation
  - ➤ Lactate clearance[14,15]

Abbreviations: ACT, activated clotting time; ECMO, extracorporeal membrane oxygenation; LV, left ventricle; LVED, left ventricular end-diastolic pressure; LVEF, left ventricular ejection fraction.

---

use of ECMO, differentiated by indication (**Tables 38.4** and **38.5**). In this way, they will be addressing the question of what patient populations, as defined by indication, might be best served by integrated ECMO treatment. Still the issue will be more careful delineation of those patient populations in which ECMO remains an exercise in futility, or a "bridge to nowhere." Although VA ECMO was developed to rescue patients with cardiogenic shock, the impact of ECMO on hemodynamics is often unpredictable and can lead to hemodynamic collapse, so ECMO initiation should be immediate without any hurdle. This has been made easier by integrated ECMO. Infection, renal failure, and intracranial hemorrhage were leading causes of mortality; however, mechanical complications have lowered down with time and experience.[7,8]

Table 38.3 Outcome by time of initiation and use of integrated ECMO-CPB circuit[13]

Time of intervention	Survived (%)	Died (%)
Integrated ECMO-CPB circuit	150 (76)	45 (23)
Failure to wean from CPB	30 (45)	36 (54)
Postoperative ECMO	9 (33)	18 (66)

Abbreviations: CPB, cardiopulmonary bypass; ECMO, extracorporeal membrane oxygenation.

Table 38.4 Outcome by diagnosis in the use of integrated ECMO-CPB circuit

Diagnosis	Survived (%)	Died (%)
TGA with IVS/TGA with VSD	177 (67)	84 (32)
VSD	2 (66)	1 (33)
TOF	2 (66)	1 (33)
ALCAPA	4 (66)	2 (33)
Truncus ateriosus	2 (66)	1 (33)
AVSD	2 (66)	1 (33)

Abbreviations: ALCAPA, anomalous left coronary artery from pulmonary artery; AVSD, atrioventricular septal defect; CPB, cardiopulmonary bypass; ECMO, extracorporeal membrane oxygenation; IVS, intact ventricular septum; TGA, transposition of the great arteries; TOF, tetralogy of Fallot; VSD, ventricular septal defect.

Table 38.5 Outcome by duration of ECMO run

Duration of ECMO run (h)	Survived (%)	Died (%)
24–48	108 (80)	27 (20)
48–72	69 (71)	27 (13)
>72	12 (25)	36 (75)

Abbreviation: ECMO, extracorporeal membrane oxygenation.

Conclusion

Management of pediatric patients requiring mechanical support after immediate surgery requires a well-coordinated multidisciplinary team of surgeon anesthetist, clinical perfusionist, nursing staff, and intensivist with pre-planned techniques like integrated ECMO which can lead to successful management of these scenarios.

The integrated circuit ECMO may be a useful tool in patients with high predictability of postoperative mechanical support. Not only does it save time, but also reduces the hesitancy to initiate ECMO, and hence, it cuts down the overall cost of surgery. In conclusion, ECMO support if used in the operating room, after assorting a completeness of surgical repair, thereby improves the surgical rates in all scenarios. Early institution of ECMO remains the key to survival. Today's integrated circuit is cost-effective with lesser exposure to blood, and circulating area is also reduced intraoperatively as well as postoperatively. Use of low-flow ECMO could enhance the ECMO outcomes, keeping in mind that low flows can be used easily without complications in the integrated ECMO circuit.[16] Integrated ECMO therapy can be used as destination for which patient's mortality chances are more than 90%.

Mendes et al, in experiments animals recently concluded that the use of ECMO support with consequent increase in venous oxygen pressure induced a significant drop in PAPm with no detectable effect on regional lung perfusion in different scenarios of ventilation/perfusion mismatch.[17]

References

1. Chauhan S, Subin S. Extracorporeal membrane oxygenation, an anesthesiologist's perspective: physiology and principles. Part 1. Ann Card Anaesth 2011;14(3):218–229
2. Chauhan S, Subin S. Extracorporeal membrane oxygenation: an anaesthesiologist's perspective—Part II: clinical and technical consideration. Ann Card Anaesth 2012;15(1):69–82
3. Kapoor PM, Malik V, Singh P, Chauhan S, Kiran U. Role of integrated extracorporeal membrane oxygenation in ALCAPA patients. Manual of extracorporeal membrane oxygenation (ECMO) 2013 in the ICU. Jaypee Publications 2013; Chapter 26: 160–164

4. Bisoi AK, Sharma P, Chauhan S, et al. Primary arterial switch operation in children presenting late with d-transposition of great arteries and intact ventricular septum. When is it too late for a primary arterial switch operation? Eur J Cardiothorac Surg 2010;38(6):707–713

5. Singh SP, Chauhan S, Bisoi AK, Sahoo M. Lactate clearance for initiating and weaning off extracorporeal membrane oxygenation in a child with regressed left ventricle after arterial switch operation. Ann Card Anaesth 2016;19(1):188–191

6. Chauhan S, Pal N, Bisoi AK, Chauhan Y, Venugopal P. Extending the boundaries of primary arterial switch operation: the integrated ECMO-CPB circuit. Anesthesiology 2007;107:A212

7. Singh P, Kapoor PM, Devagourou V, Bhuvana V, Kiran U. Use of integrated extracorporeal membrane oxygenator in anomalous left coronary artery to pulmonary artery: better survival benefit. Ann Card Anaesth 2011;14(3):240–242

8. Development of the AIIMS Integrated CPB–ECMO. Ann Pediatr Cardiol 2013;6(1):105 108

9. Pooboni S, Goyal V, Oza P, Kapoor PM. ECMO challenges and its future: Indian scenario. J Cardiac Critical Care TSS 2017;1(02):89–94

10. Kapoor PM, Karanjkar A, Bhardwaj V. Review article: evaluation of coagulopathy on veno-arterial ECMO (VA) extracorporeal membrane oxygenation using platelet aggregometry and standard tests: a narrative review. Egypt J Crit Care Med 2018;6(3):73–78

11. Bhardwaj V, Malhotra P, Hasija S, Chowdury UK, Pangasa N. Coagulopathies in cyanotic cardiac patients: an analysis with three point-of-care testing devices (thromboelastography, rotational thromboelastometry, and sonoclot analyzer). Ann Card Anaesth 2017;20(2):212–218

12. Bhardwaj V, Kapoor PM. Re-exploration can be deterred by point-of-care testing in cardiac surgery patient. J Card Crit Care TSS 2017;1:48–50

13. Airan R, Sharan S, Malhotra Kapoor P, Chowdhury U, Velayoudam D, John A. Low flow venoarterial ECMO support management in postcardiac surgery patient. J Card Crit Care 2021;5:103–107

14. Kapoor PM. Echocardiography in extracorporeal membrane oxygenation. Ann Card Anaesth 2017;20(Supplement):S1–S3

15. Ladha S, Kapoor PM, Singh SP, Kiran U, Chowdhury UK. The role of blood lactate clearance as a predictor of mortality in children undergoing surgery for tetralogy of Fallot. Ann Card Anaesth 2016;19(2):217–224

16. Airan R, Malhotra Kapoor P, Kumar Chowdhury U, Sharan S, Sehgal L. Low flows ECMO support management in post cardiac patient. J Card Crit Care TSS 2021;5(02):103–107

17. Mendes PV, Park M, de Azevedo LCP, et al. Lung perfusion during veno-venous extracorporeal membrane oxygenation in a model of hypoxemic respiratory failure. Intensive Care Med Exp. 2022;10(1):15

39

Nutrition in Extracorporeal Membrane Oxygenation Patients

Yatin Mehta, Anshu Joshi, Gaurav Kochhar, and Poonam Malhotra Kapoor

Introduction

Extracorporeal membrane oxygenation (ECMO) is a life-saving procedure used in neonates, children, and adults with severe, reversible, cardiopulmonary failure. ECMO uses a heart-lung machine with a membrane oxygenator in cardiorespiratory failure settings. Successful usage of ECMO in pediatric and adult patients has been done, and the most frequent indication has been neonatal respiratory failure in conditions such as congenital diaphragmatic hernia (CDH), persistent pulmonary hypertension, meconium aspiration, and congenital heart disease.[1] Metabolic/Nutritional burden in such pediatric patients is high. ECMO provides a cardiopulmonary rest, but the metabolic catabolism continues unabated in ECMO patients, especially in newly born babies who undergo extreme protein catabolism while on ECMO. Thus, to judiciously plan nutrition requirements during ECMO, it is essential to know the metabolic stores and the nutritional requirements which change minute to minute in these ECMO patients.[2-4]

Revelly et al, in 2001, showed clearly that patients post cardiopulmonary bypass, requiring high doses of vasopressors tolerate enteral nutrition (EN) well.[1-4]

Patients Receiving ECMO Are Critically Ill

Patients on venoarterial (VA) ECMO remain on high doses of inotropes and are critically ill. These patients usually receive high doses of vasoactive agents (especially in VA ECMO), sometimes steroids, and require long stay in critical care. Medications adversely affect the gastric emptying, impacting enteral feeding and subsequent caloric adequacy.

Most of these indisposed ill patients have limited nutrients as endogenous stores; thus, it is important to administer nutritional support as early as possible in these moribund patients. Patients have limited endogenous nutrient stores and relatively high nutritional requirements; therefore, early institution of nutritional support is important.[5,6] This, however, is delayed in the intensive care unit (ICU) setting. Enteral nutrition (EN) stimulates intestinal hormone secretion. As ECMO patients have limited nutritional reserves, and high nutritional requirements are essential in these sick patients, early feeding during ECMO is essentially needed.[7,8]

As EN is begun, multifold benefits appear; some of these are listed in **Box 39.1**.

VA ECMO patients undergo malnutrition and consumptive protein catabolism. Hence, their nutritional requirements are immense (**Box 39.2**).

Literature has shown over time that both nonocclusive bowel necrosis and mesenteric ischemia are seen in ECMO patients especially, if reporting is not adhered to by the intensivists themselves (**Table 39.1**). Most patients on ECMO

may have had earlier circulatory shock, and the timing of inserting an ECMO, in a phase of cardiogenic shock, till date remains debatable.

Research has concluded that when patients are on high inotrope doses in a case of ECMO then enteral nutrition can be resorted to with a very low incidence of both nonocclusive bowel necrosis and mesenteric ischemia.[9]

The ECMO run brings with it inflammation and oxidative stress.[10,11] The incidence of latter has decreased with the use of newer biocompatible materials such as polysulfone membranes and cellulose acetate membranes for protein oxidation.[10,11] The addition of renal replacement

---

Box 39.1 Benefits of enteral nutrition (EN)

- Prevents sepsis
- Stimulates structural functional changes in the gut through the release of intestinal hormones in the gut
- Is well tolerated and safe
- High vasopressor support can be started
- Post cardiopulmonary bypass (CPB) on high vasopressors, enteral nutrition (EN) is successful

---

Box 39.2 VA ECMO and nutrition-based clinical outcomes

- Protein soaking up in the body during ECMO process leads to malnourishment in the patients
- Administration of appropriate nutrition to these patients is difficult because of hemodynamic instability and multiorgan failure. The aim of this study was to evaluate the relationship between nutritional supply and clinical outcomes in patients undergoing VA ECMO
- If the daily requirement of proteins in the VA ECMO patients over 8 to 14 days is met with, then it reduces the 90-day mortality by 18%

Abbreviations: ECMO, extracorporeal membrane oxygenation; VA, venoarterial.

Table 39.1 Enteral nutrition on ECMO with prevalence as percentage of nonocclusive bowel necrosis and mesenteric ischemic

Authors	NOMI and NOBN in EN patients (n/N)
Scott et al[3]	0/26
Lucas et al[12]	0/45
Marvin et al[13]	0/7a
Shankat et al[14] Lawler et al[15]	3/30
Ohbe et al[16]	9/1769

Abbreviations: ECMO, extracorporeal membrane oxygenation; EN, enteral nutrition; NOMI, nonocclusive mesenteric ischemia; NOBN, nonocclusive bowel necrosis.

therapy (RRT) also aids in stress reduction during ECMO.[1] Continuous renal replacement therapy (CRRT) with ECMO induces a systematic inflammatory response with increase in multiorgan failure and mortality with the advent of new polymethyl pentene membrane of the ECMO oxygenators, diffusion of lipid emulsions, and heavy molecular-weight-based nutrients for patient benefit as EN therapy surmounts. An in-depth knowledge of the type of membrane and nutrient details is essential to circumvent these problematic issues. This progress observed in RRT can also improve the stress induced by ECMO. This technique increases whole body protein breakdown[1] and induces systemic inflammatory response syndrome, which can be associated with multiorgan failure and mortality.[17] As there was excessive use of intravenous lipid infusion, the older type of microporous ECMO oxygenators would get impaired.[18] However, such issues can be resolved with the new generation of diffusion (polymethylpentene) membrane oxygenators in use today in most modern ECMO machines. Understanding the metabolic changes during these techniques becomes important to prevent side effects due to the ECMO membrane lung.

In most of the studies shown in **Table 39.1**, it is apparent that:

1. Enteral nutrition is tolerated better with norepinephrine and dopamine and less with a vasopressin infusion.[13]
2. Also, if enteral nutrition was started within 6 hours of the surgery, there were improved results.[14]
3. NOBN occured more in those with nasojejunum feeding.[15]
4. More the vasopressors, greater the NOBN.[19]
5. Hepato sphlanchnic and cardiac index all increased; with increased, blood flow during ECMO. In patients on ECMO, who develop sepsis a low dose postpyloric enteral nutrition in the ICU, is beneficial.[20]

Nutrition Practices in Patients Supported with ECMO

Survey conducted by Thomas et al[21] found that there are a vast majority of extracorporeal life support (ECLS) among the various parameters at Extracorporeal Life Support Organization (ELSO) centers providing EN to neonatal and pediatric patients receiving ECLS. However, significant variability existed in the patient and clinical parameters while deciding initiation of EN (**Box 39.3**). The survey found that 55 and 71% of respondents provide EN "often" or "always" for VA and venovenous (VV) ECLS, respectively. EN was reported as given "often" or "always" by 24% with increased vasopressor support, 53% with "stable" vasopressor support, and 60% with weaning of vasopressor support. Patient's underlying diagnosis and vasopressor support were important factors influencing physician's decision to implement EN, and were the primary or secondary determinants of whether to provide EN 81 and 72% of the time, respectively. However, only 38% of ECLS centers reported an institutional feeding protocol for providing EN.

Uncertainty about nutrition in ECMO may be associated with concerns of involved paralysis and/or heavy sedation with neonatal ECMO, which may affect the gut function, in addition to the effect of VA ECMO itself, which may reduce perfusion of the gut.[22] Heavy seduction on ECMO may impair the gut function; VA ECMO may add to it by decreasing gut perfusion low cardiac output in a peripheral hospital before ECMO or pre-ECMO hypoxia may all hamper gut perfusion on VA ECMO, fluid overload with excessive intravenous fluids leads to generalized edema and anasarca with hampered gut motility. EN is safe in both VA and VV ECMO and can be well tolerated when patient is stable on ECMO shown in **Box 39.4**.[18]

However, the venous congestion of the bowel resolves with the reduction of airway pressure, subsequently improving feeding tolerance.

Nutritional Requirements in Adult Patients

Clinical guidelines are developed for the nutrition therapy of neonates undergoing ECMO. However, no such guidelines exist for adult patients.[23] EN is preferred in critical patients and this should be considered for adult population supported with ECMO. Timing to initiate and preferred route for EN should be similar to the recommendations of critical care nutrition guidelines.

Enteral nutrition guidelines for adults on ECMO (unlike those for neonates on ECMO) do not exist. The guidelines for a critically ill adult patient receiving ECMO in the ICU

Box 39.3 Important prognostic factors for decision-making before initiating EN

- Underlying patients diagnosis, for which ECMO was initiated
- Patients vasopressor requirements
- Sedation levels of the ECMO patients
- Low cardiac output
- Prolonged hypoxia

Abbreviations: ECMO, extracorporeal membrane oxygenation; EN, enteral nutrition.

Box 39.4 Factors lowering gut perfusion on ECMO

- Low cardiac output
- Hypoxia
- Heavy sedation
- Excessive intravenous fluids
- Increased airways pressures

Abbreviation: ECMO, extracorporeal membrane oxygenation.

for EN should be same as those that exist for critically ill adults in ICU, without an ECMO support. Indirect calorimetry is not successful in estimating energy requirements in ECMO patients. Weight-based predictive equations used for critically ill patients can be used in such patients also. As per the American Society for Parenteral and Enteral Nutrition (ASPEN) 2016 guidelines, 25 to 30 kcal/kg/d can be used for patients with BMI less than 30 units. Edema-free body weight needs to be used. Estimated energy for the obese patient (BMI > 30) can be estimated as 22 to 25 kcal/kg/d of ideal body weight.

Taking care of cardiac cachexia and wound healing, addressing adequate energy needs, and minimizing catabolism are necessary in an adult on ECMO. Daily protein administration range from 1.3 to 1.5 g/kg/d will help to increase protein synthesis and attenuate the loss of muscle mass. This range can be tailored to patient's underlying clinical conditions and protein requirements. Higher amounts are needed for patients with RRT. Carbohydrate intake should be tailored to meet energy requirements. However, hyperglycemia needs to be avoided. Sodium restriction will improve fluid balance, minimize fluid weight gain, and optimize diuretic therapy.

Reaching nutritional goals may also be affected by fluid status. In fact, patients with higher positive fluid balances have shown less achievement of nutritional target compared to patients with low or negative fluid balance.[22] Extra fluid balance restricts the intake of nutritional fluids. Hence, the choice of EN formula can be a concentrated one. For improving tolerance, the enteral formula can be initiated at a rate below the target.

EN often gets discontinued in patients presenting large gastric residual volumes. Using prokinetic medications such as metoclopramide or erythromycin may prevent unnecessary interruptions in feeding due to large gastric residuals (**Box 39.5**). EN often is done away while on ECMO with CRRT. **Box 39.4** reiterates the nutritional support adequacy needed in this valuable group, where frequent discontinuation of nutritional therapy is practiced in patients due to larger residual gastric volumes seen in these patients.

Nutritional Requirements in Neonates[24]

For providing neonatal ECMO support nutrition, ASPEN has postulated guidelines in 2010 which are used till date. As neonates are born with limited nutritional reserves, they require nutrition for adequate growth, expedited nutritional support is mandatory (Grade D) with protein requirement up to 3 g/kg/d grade D nonprotein nitrogen calories of greater than 60 kcal/kg/d, and a positive nitrogen balance of more than 240 mg/kg/d, and free fatty acids (FFAs) both medium and long chain are used clinically to provide efficient carbon substrate sources of ATP-generated energy consumption, during ECMO. Glutamate enrichment is needed for the same (**Box 39.6**).

Neonates on ECMO have enhanced catabolism; so their slower tolerance to EN has a nearly fourfold longer stay in the hospital, than those who are feeding early by 3-4 weeks while on ECMO.

Renal Replacement Therapy in Critically Ill Patients Receiving ECMO

Single-center studies using the RIFLE[25,26] (risk, injury, failure, loss, and end stage) definition in ECMO patients show the incidence of acute kidney injury (AKI) as: 71% of neonates with CDH,[27] 71% of children with a cardiac indication for ECMO,[28] 78% of adults with respiratory failure,[29] and 81% of postcardiotomy adult patients.[30]

RRT imitation requires adequate fluid load and nutritional support in the patient on ECMO.

Fluids

During RRT initiation, fluid accumulation in the body should be prevented. ECMO itself brings about rapid changes in hemodynamics of the patients with perturbations in renal blood flow and impending AKI (**Flowchart 39.1**).[31]

Box 39.5 CRRT adequate nutrition supplementation is needed
• Tailor carbohydrates
• Avoid hyperglycemia
• Restrict sodium
◆ Minimize fluid weight gain
◆ Optimize diverted therapy
◆ Improve fluid balance
• Higher amounts of proteins
• Prefer a negative or low fluid balance
• Prevent frequent interruptions in EN by using optokinetic medications

Abbreviations: CRRT, continuous renal replacement therapy; EN, enteral nutrition.

Box 39.6 Nutritional requirements on neonatal ECMO as per ASPEN guidelines
• Protein requirements up to 3 g/kg/d
• Nonprotein nitrogen calories greater than 60 kcal/kg/d
• Positive nitrogen balances more than 240 mg/kg/d
• Nitrogen intake >400 mg/kg/d
• Sodium requirements without diuretics is 4–7 mEq/kg/d
• Enteral feeding in neonates on ECMO should be initiated when the patients on ECMO have clinically stabilized
• Provision of adequate dietary proteins promotes a positive protein balance and promotes the anabolic effect of insulin

Abbreviations: ASPEN, American Society for Parenteral and Enteral Nutrition; ECMO, extracorporeal membrane oxygenation.

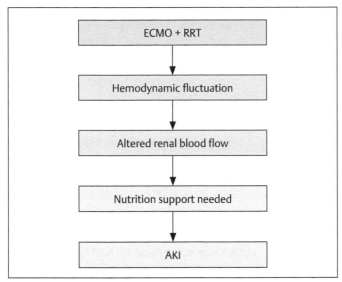

Flowchart 39.1 Algorithm depicting the progress to AKI. Abbreviations: AKI, acute kidney injury; ECMO, extracorporeal membrane oxygenation; RRT, renal replacement therapy.

RRT initiation requires nutrition support which takes care of protein losses, thiamine/folic acid losses, and other nutrient losses, which happen during the process.

Other Practical Issues

EN as suggested by Ridley et al was found to be the most common route of nutritional support on ECMO patients, with interruptions in 53% of the days citing residual gastric volumes and prolonged fasting for therapeutic and diagnostic procedures as main reasons for barriers for EN mode.[32]

Lukas et al in a retrospective study found that the change in nutritional support delivered in the ICU was found to be more after ECMO removal (in 71%) than during ECMO support (in 55%).[12] Thus, adequate nutritional support is mandatory and requires detailed and meticulous planning and execution. Nutritional support should be the aim in the care of these sick, moribund patients on ECMO and RRT, due to protein, thiamine, folic acid, and other nutrient losses.[2]

Nutrition support in ECMO patients should ensure that nutrition adequacy goals are maintained and interruptions are minimized by using optimum nutrition delivery mode.

What is New in Enteral Nutrition in Pediatric Patients on ECMO?

In January 2022, Gema Pierez et al,[33] from Spain, concluded that most pediatric patients on ECMO are undernourished, especially those who are less than two years of age. Most patients do receive enteral nutrition in some phase of ECMO. In the hundred odd children studied by them, they surmised, that if enteral nutrition is started within 48 hours of ECMO initiation, then both gastro-intestinal complications, as well as mortality is less. These authors found no association between enteral nutrition and mortality. Early enteral nutrition (EEN) is safe in ECMO is what has been recently concluded by them.[33]

Conclusion

No clinical guidelines exist for nutrition during ECMO in the adult population but exist for neonates; in both VV ECMO and VA ECMO, EN seems to be well accepted by most patients. The nutrition support clinician's expertise is essential in providing appropriate nutrition support for the patient undergoing ECMO support. It is apparent that the clinical practice guidelines for nutrition support in adult ECMO patients are well accepted for now. ASPEN 2010 guidelines can be referred to in case of neonates requiring ECMO support. In 2019 clinical guidelines for validating the body composition came up for assessment in clinical populations. The ASPEN clinical guidelines for 2019 reiterate and highlight the influence of acute and chronic inflammation in body composition and underscore the importance of inflammation for nutritional assessment. When methods for validating relevant body composition method for lean mass assessment in a variety of diseases were compared, the dual-energy X-ray absorptiometry (DXA) was found to be better than ultrasound or bioelectrical impedance analysis (BIA) methods.[31]

Current opinions and recommendations on nutrition strategies in patients receiving ECMO are mostly based on observational data with that have a low level of evidence and expert consensus. In general, MNT should be carefully adapted to each individual patient, considering enteral and GI tolerance, comorbidities, and phase of critical illness. This evidence-based guidance provides extensive recommendations for MNT in patients receiving ECMO.[34]

References

1. Keshen TH, Miller RG, Jahoor F, Jaksic T. Stable isotopic quantitation of protein metabolism and energy expenditure in neonates on- and post-extracorporeal life support. J Pediatr Surg 1997;32(7):958–962, discussion 962–963
2. Lukas G, Davies AR, Hilton AK, Pellegrino VA, Scheinkestel CD, Ridley E. Nutritional support in adult patients receiving extracorporeal membrane oxygenation. Crit Care Resusc 2010;12(4):230–234
3. Scott LK, Boudreaux K, Thaljeh F, Grier LR, Conrad SA. Early enteral feedings in adults receiving venovenous extracorporeal membrane oxygenation. JPEN J Parenter Enteral Nutr 2004;28(5):295–300
4. Revelly JP, Tappy L, Berger MM, Gersbach P, Cayeux C, Chiolero R. Metabolic, systemic and splanchnic hemodynamic responses to early enteral nutrition in postoperative patients treated for circulatory compromise. Intensive Care Med 2001;27:540–547
5. Brown RL, Wessel J, Warner BW. Nutrition considerations in the neonatal extracorporeal life support patient. Nutr Clin Pract 1994;9(1):22–27

6. Evans RA, Thureen P. Early feeding strategies in preterm and critically ill neonates. Neonatal Netw 2001;20(7):7–18

7. Heyland DK, Cook DJ, Guyatt GH. Enteral nutrition in the critically ill patient: a critical review of the evidence. Intensive Care Med 1993;19(8):435–442

8. Moore FA, Feliciano DV, Andrassy RJ, et al. Early enteral feeding, compared with parenteral, reduces postoperative septic complications. The results of a meta-analysis. Ann Surg 1992;216(2):172–183

9. Patel JJ, Rice T, Heyland DK. Safety and outcomes of enteral nutrition in circulatory shock. JPEN J Parenter Enteral Nutr 2020;44(5):779–784

10. Walker RJ, Sutherland WH, De Jong SA. Effect of changing from a cellulose acetate to a polysulphone dialysis membrane on protein oxidation and inflammation markers. Clin Nephrol 2004;61(3):198–206

11. Takouli L, Hadjiyannakos D, Metaxaki P, et al. Vitamin E-coated cellulose acetate dialysis membrane: long-term effect on inflammation and oxidative stress. Ren Fail 2010;32(3): 287–293

12. Lucas A, Bloom SR, Aynsley-Green A. Postnatal surges in plasma gut hormones in term and preterm infants. Biol Neonate 1982;41(1-2):63–67

13. Marvin RG, McKinley BA, McQuiggan M, Cocanour CS, Moore FA. Nonocclusive bowel necrosis occurring in critically ill trauma patients receiving enteral nutrition manifests no reliable clinical signs for early detection. Am J Surg. 2000;179(1):7-12

14. Shankar B, Daphnee DK, Ramakrishnan N, Venkataraman R. Feasibility, safety, and outcome of very early enteral nutrition in critically ill patients: results of an observational study. J Crit Care. 2015;30(3):473-475

15. Lawlor DK, Inculet RI, Malthaner RA. Small-bowel necrosis associated with jejunal tube feeding. Can J Surg. 1998;41(6): 459-462

16. Ohbe H, Jo T, Matsui H, Fushimi K, Yasunaga H. Differences in effect of early enteral nutrition on mortality among ventilated adults with shock requiring low-, medium-, and high-dose noradrenaline: a propensity-matched analysis [published online ahead of print February 15, 2019]. Clin Nutr. https://doi.org/10.1016/j.clnu.2019.02.020.

17. Kozik DJ, Tweddell JS. Characterizing the inflammatory response to cardiopulmonary bypass in children. Ann Thorac Surg 2006;81(6):S2347–S2354

18. Montoya JP, Shanley CJ, Merz SI, Bartlett RH. Plasma leakage through microporous membranes. Role of phospholipids. ASAIO J 1992;38(3):M399–M405

19. Mancl EE, Muzevich KM. Tolerability and safety of enteral nutrition in critically ill patients receiving intravenous vasopressor therapy. JPEN J Parenter Enteral Nutr. 2013;37(5): 641-651.

20. Rokyta R, Jr., Matejovic M, Krouzecky A, Senft V, Trefil L, Novak I. Post-pyloric enteral nutrition in septic patients: effects on hepatosplanchnic hemodynamics and energy status. Intensive Care Med. 2004;30(4):714-717.

21. Desmarais TJ, Yan Y, Keller MS, Vogel AM. Enteral nutrition in neonatal and pediatric extracorporeal life support: a survey of current practice. J Pediatr Surg 2015;50(1):60–63

22. Ferrie S, Herkes R, Forrest P. Nutrition support during extracorporeal membrane oxygenation (ECMO) in adults: a retrospective audit of 86 patients. Intensive Care Med 2013;39(11):1989–1994

23. Farías MM, Olivos C, Díaz R. Nutritional implications for the patient undergoing extracorporeal membrane oxygenation. Nutr Hosp 2015;31(6):2346–2351

24. Jaksic T, Hull MA, Modi BP, Ching YA, George D, Compher C; American Society for Parenteral and Enteral Nutrition (A.S.P.E.N.) Board of Directors. A.S.P.E.N. Clinical guidelines: nutrition support of neonates supported with extracorporeal membrane oxygenation. JPEN J Parenter Enteral Nutr 2010;34(3):247–253

25. Bellomo R, Ronco C, Kellum JA, Mehta RL, Palevsky P; Acute Dialysis Quality Initiative workgroup. Acute renal failure: definition, outcome measures, animal models, fluid therapy and information technology needs: the Second International Consensus Conference of the Acute Dialysis Quality Initiative (ADQI) Group. Crit Care 2004;8(4):R204–R212

26. Akcan-Arikan A, Zappitelli M, Loftis LL, Washburn KK, Jefferson LS, Goldstein SL. Modified RIFLE criteria in critically ill children with acute kidney injury. Kidney Int 2007;71(10):1028–1035

27. Gadepalli SK, Selewski DT, Drongowski RA, Mychaliska GB. Acute kidney injury in congenital diaphragmatic hernia requiring extracorporeal life support: an insidious problem. J Pediatr Surg 2011;46(4):630–635

28. Smith AH, Hardison DC, Worden CR, Fleming GM, Taylor MB. Acute renal failure during extracorporeal support in the pediatric cardiac patient. ASAIO J 2009;55(4):412–416

29. Lin CY, Chen YC, Tsai FC, et al. RIFLE classification is predictive of short-term prognosis in critically ill patients with acute renal failure supported by extracorporeal membrane oxygenation. Nephrol Dial Transplant 2006;21(10):2867–2873

30. Yan X, Jia S, Meng X, et al. Acute kidney injury in adult postcardiotomy patients with extracorporeal membrane oxygenation: evaluation of the RIFLE classification and the Acute Kidney Injury Network criteria. Eur J Cardiothorac Surg 2010;37(2):334–338

31. Keckler SJ, Laituri CA, Ostlie DJ, St Peter SD. A review of venovenous and venoarterial extracorporeal membrane oxygenation in neonates and children. Eur J Pediatr Surg 2010; 20(1):1–4

32. Ridley EJ, Davies AR, Robins EJ, Lukas G, Bailey MJ, Fraser JF; Australian and New Zealand Extracorporeal Membrane Oxygenation Nutrition Therapy. Nutrition therapy in adult patients receiving extracorporeal membrane oxygenation: a prospective, multicentre, observational study. Crit Care Resusc 2015;17(3):183–189

33. Gema Perez, Elena Gonzalez, Laura Zamora, Sarah N. Fernandez, Amelia Sanchez et al. Early Enteral Nutrition and Gastrointestinal Complications in Pediatric Patients on Extracorporeal Membrane Oxygenation. JPGN 2022;74: 110–115

34. Dresen E, Naidoo O, Hill A, et al. Medical nutrition therapy in patients receiving ECMO: Evidence-based guidance for clinical practice. JPEN J Parenter Enteral Nutr. 2022

40

Extracorporeal Cytokine Hemoadsorption Therapy in the Management of ICU Sepsis

Prachee Sathe and Prashant Sakhwalkar

Introduction

Sepsis has to be treated as a medical emergency. The word *Sepsis* describes the systemic immunological response by patient, when an insult like an infection or sometimes a noninfectious but severe inflammatory process affects the body. Sepsis has potential to harm various organs, causing mild-to-severe organ dysfunction or end-stage organ damage which may even lead to death. Though there are significant insights in understanding the pathophysiology of this dangerous clinical syndrome, along with the advances in hemodynamic monitoring tools and resuscitation measures, despite that sepsis remains one of the major causes of prolonged organ support in intensive care unit (ICU) and mortality in critically ill patients.[1] A rough estimate is that approximately more than 30 million patients get affected by sepsis every year worldwide, leading to 6 million deaths attributable to sepsis every year. The reported mortality rates vary between 20 and 41% (in Indian ICUs mortality rate is 36%, as per INDICAP study).[1]

Evolution of Definition and Understanding of Severe "Sepsis"

Research has helped in understanding the complex pathophysiology of sepsis better, leading to a more precise definition of sepsis. As the disease process is heterogenous, there are serious difficulties in recognizing the right time to treat the right patient as well as to study sepsis.[2] Roger Bone and his colleagues were the leaders to lay the foundation, during the SCCM-ACCP conference in 1991, the first consensus meeting to define "sepsis." Since then, regular revisions have happened, which reached the third version. We now have a better understanding of cell biology, biochemistry of intermediate sepsis molecules, immunobiology, as well as changes in endothelial function which lead to defects in circulation causing organ dysfunction. All this understanding has helped in reaching compact "Sepsis treatment bundles"[2] (SSC guideline 1,2,3).[3–6]

Current Definition, Sepsis 3 (Third International Consensus Definition of Sepsis and Septic Shock)

The working group for SEPSIS 3 tried to make a better definition of sepsis. Sepsis is portrayed as "life-threatening organ dysfunction caused by a dysregulated host response to infection" and septic shock is defined as lactate levels rising above 2 mmol/L with hypotension (in the absence of hypovolemia) and need for initiation of vasopressor treatment to keep mean arterial pressure above 65 mmHg. SOFA indicates Sequential Organ Failure assessment, which helps to identify organ dysfunction. If there is an acute change in total SOFA score ≥2 points consequent to the infection, then the score of ≥2 reflects an overall mortality risk of approximately 10%[6]. An increase of two points or more in quick SOFA (qSOFA) score corresponds to a 3- to 14-fold increase in hospital mortality.[7]

Sepsis is not only the process of infection but what happens inside the body in response to an infective insult. Hence the new definition accepts sepsis as "Dysregulated host response" to infective insult. This opens up the possibility of some therapeutic interventions, or at least the research and application of some promising new modalities to bring back the immune homeostasis and avoid self-harm (even though it may not be accepted in guidelines yet).[8–12]

Sepsis Care Bundles and Their Limitations in Affecting the Sepsis Outcomes

Surviving Sepsis Campaign guidelines (2008) suggested about how to use sepsis resuscitation bundles. There were two sets of bundle components recommended to be achieved in 6 hours and in 24 hours, respectively, to try and improve the outcomes when applied simultaneously. In 2012, learning with previous experience, the 6-hour resuscitation bundle was made more focused by further breaking it into two bundles: "the severe sepsis 3-hour resuscitation bundle" and "the 6-hour septic shock bundle," which contain all therapeutic goals to be completed, respectively.[9] It was then thought that we were missing the window of opportunity for successful treatment; hence, in 2018, the 3- and 6-hour bundles were combined into a single 1-hour bundle highlighting the urgency of treatment to be completed within window period.[13–18] Observational studies show that with 60% adherence to sepsis bundles, overall 14% improvement in mortality could be achieved. Some guidelines like early goal-directed therapy (EGDT) were removed from the bundles because it was a single-center study which could not be reproduced for the validity of the results, it added to the complexity of the management, and it had the potential risks of mandatory central line placement for measurement of central venous pressure (CVP) and central venous oxygen saturation (ScvO$_2$) monitoring.[19] Also some multicenter trials disproved certain elements in the bundles,[20] approving the pragmatic approach in management reaching to the current concepts seen in surviving sepsis guidelines.

Immunobiological Understanding of Sepsis and Its Therapeutic Implications

The research to understand the molecular basis of sepsis found the newer and complex interplay between the infective agent or insult, inflammatory process, and the response of the host, all of which are likely to produce the diverse manifestations of sepsis.

The host response to the pathogen starts with the activation of innate immune cells. The pathogen-associated molecular patterns (PAMPs) stimulate the basic cells for immune response, viz. macrophages, monocytes, neutrophils, and natural killer cells. PAMPS including bacterial endotoxins and fungal β-glucans bind to specific pattern recognition receptors. Then there are damage-associated molecular patterns (DAMPs). DAMPs are intracellular material or molecules released from dead or damaged host cells, such as adenosine triphosphate (ATP) and mitochondrial DNA and the release of proinflammatory cytokines like tumor necrosis factor-α (TNF-α), interleukin-1 (IL-1), and IL-6, and anti-inflammatory cytokines like IL-10, IL-1β, and IL-18. Various DAMPs can initiate what is called *programmed cell death*. Various effects of proinflammatory cytokines include the following: (1) activation and proliferation of leukocytes, (2) activation of the complement system, (3) upregulation of endothelial adhesion molecules, and (4) expression of chemokines. In addition, there is increased tissue factor production and induction of hepatic acute phase reactants. During the process of unregulated sepsis, the above immune response gets amplified, which may result in unintentional collateral damage. This can cause the death of host cells and tissues producing clinical syndrome of organ dysfunction.

Strangely, the initial proinflammatory state of sepsis may get followed by a prolonged state of immunosuppression/relative immunoparesis[21] which can cause repeated waves of secondary sepsis or chronic ICU syndromes (**Fig. 40.1**).

Need to Improve Treatment Pathways Based on Immunobiology in Sepsis

Just the antibiotics and source control with fluid resuscitation cannot save every septic patient. Looking at the complexity of the sepsis something more is needed; simple modulation of pro- and anti-inflammatory mediators would not translate into improved patient outcomes and may result in further dysregulation leading to worsening of outcomes in sepsis, by transition into a late anti-inflammatory phenotype referred to as sepsis-associated immunosuppression (SAI). Hence, research on more targeted therapies is required.

When trying to ascertain the correlation between mortality and elevated cytokine levels, several studies found high pro- as well as anti-inflammatory cytokine levels associated with higher mortality (**Fig. 40.2**).

IL-6 is found to have a relatively fast induction couple and a short half-life; these characteristics make it an ideal inflammatory marker, suitable for patient monitoring. Similarly, among anti-inflammatory cytokines, IL-10 is the most studied and has similar kinetics to IL-6.[22–25]

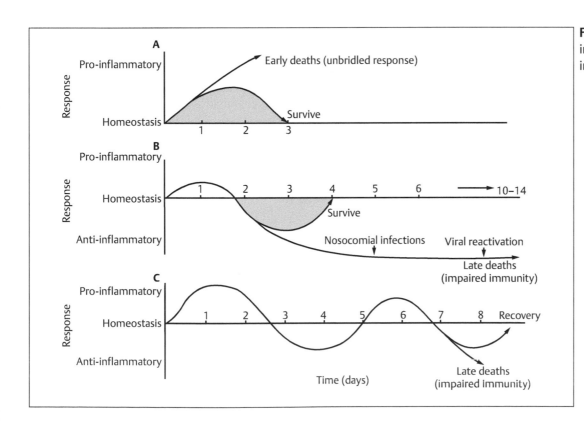

Fig. 40.1 Potential inflammatory responses in sepsis.

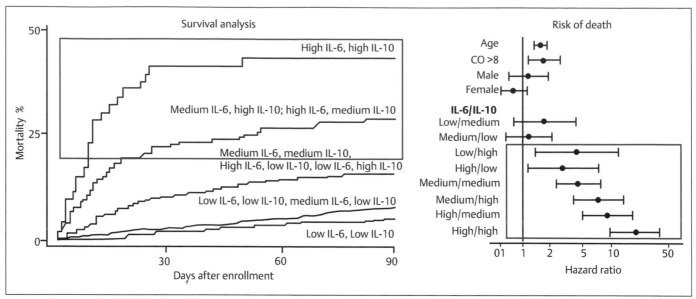

Fig. 40.2   Impact of IL-6 and IL-10 changes on mortality in sepsis patients (n = 1886) with community-acquired pneumonia.

Cytokine Storm in Progression of Sepsis Syndrome

As discussed in the immunobiological understanding of the sepsis, proinflammatory cytokines play an important role in the elimination of infection which is an integral part of sepsis.[23-26] But at the same time it is observed that, if produced excessively, they can cause tissue and organ damage. Increase in cytokines such as IL-6, IL-8, IL-10, IL-18, and TNF-α may have implications in diagnosis and treatment of sepsis. Initial phases of sepsis may be characterized by severe cytokine storm which if progresses unregulated with high pro- and anti-inflammatory cytokine levels can cause self-harm with organ dysfunction.

Consideration and Scope for Blood Purification in Cytokine Storm in Severe Sepsis

Basically, early treatment of severe sepsis in intensive care unit (ICU) includes monitoring and treatment bundles as per the recommendations of SSC-SEPSIS 3. Though bundle adherence has improved mortality, but it still remains high, highlighting the limitations of current treatment options. Hence, the idea is being considered for removal of excess damaging levels of pro- and anti-inflammatory cytokines.

Various methods including extracorporeal blood purification techniques (BPT) have also been tried. These techniques that have been tried over a period include: (1) hemofiltration, (2) hemoperfusion (HP), (3) intermittent or continuous high-volume hemofiltration (HVHF), (4) plasmapheresis, or (5) hemadsorption. One of the important extracorporeal organ support techniques is extracorporeal membrane

oxygenator (ECMO), mostly applied in venovenous mode. Acute kidney injury in septic patients is common; continuous renal replacement therapies (CRRTs) in mild-to-severe kidney dysfunction offer a significant support for solute and fluid control. Similarly extracorporeal supports are offered by left ventricular-assist devices in case of refractory heart failure or albumin dialysis and HP in case of liver dysfunction and hyperbilirubinemia offering some type of blood purification. Dysregulated cytokine production may propagate sepsis; hence, it follows that removal of these substances via specific extracorporeal BPTs may help attenuate the response particularly if used in the early phase of sepsis[28] when it is still in reversible stage.

Various postulates to explain the potential mechanisms responsible for potential benefit include cytotoxic theories, one of which is the **peak concentration hypothesis** (**Fig. 40.3**). It proposes that all the inflammatory mediators are removed at a certain rate, and the rate of clearance, depending upon the concentration gradient and the type of BPT used, will decide which of the filterable/adsorbable cytokines can be removed based on their molecular weight. Another hypothesis is **cytokinetic theory,** which proposes that because of the process of gradual cytokine removal, a cytokine gradient is created between the bloodstream and tissues allowing leucocyte-enhanced trafficking (**Fig. 40.4**). This helps to reduce the collateral damage caused by the cytokine "storm."[29] Similarly, cytokine levels have various actions as communicating messengers; when they communicate with cells, they initiate various actions on cells to recruit some, depress others, and reduce cell metabolism for some others.

The HVHF with higher flows has been tried for increased cytokine removal, but out of multiple multicenter trials and controlled studies hardly any could translate it in

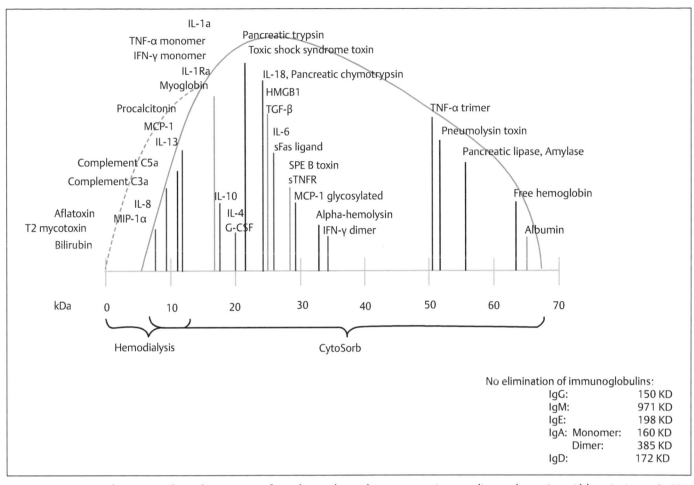

Fig. 40.3 CytoSorb removes broad spectrum of cytokines through concentration gradient adsorption. Abbreviations: G-CSF, granulocyte-macrophage colony-stimulating factor; HMGB1, high mobility group protein B1; IFN-γ, interferon gamma; IL, interleukin; MCP-1, monocyte chemotactic protein-1; MIP-1α, macrophage inflammatory protein-1 alpha; SPE B, streptococcal pyrogenic exotoxin B; sTNFR, soluble tumor necrosis factor receptors; TGF-β, transforming growth factor-β; TNF-α, tumor necrosis factor-alpha.

survival benefit (the cytotoxic threshold immune modulation hypothesis).[30]

Randomized controlled trials (RCTs) have not been conclusive for other extracorporeal blood purification therapies to demonstrate a reproducible survival benefit. When blood levels of the mediators are high, it implies that there has been saturation of the interstitial and cellular compartments. This is called **tip of the iceberg theory.**[31] This is what leads to overwhelming systemic inflammation. Other proposed factors for high levels of mediators in the blood include the intensity of production, the number of cell receptors, the clearance of such mediators, and the affinity of the receptors for such mediators. The endosomal DAMPs also play a key role in inducing cellular damage and apoptosis, and these DAMPs can be eliminated via the BPT. That is why the initial "positive" observational trials were observed with HVHF. Also an improvement is observed in the hemodynamic status, with or without lactate reduction during HVHF, may be as a result of dilutional effects of fluid

replacement therapy made with large volumes of crystalloids containing high buffer concentrations during HVHF. Improvement in hypotension[32] can be explained by rise in pH indirectly affecting the affinity of catecholamines to their receptors.

Cytokine Storm and Capillary Leak

Capillary leak is a prototype of early sepsis syndrome. This may represent the dysregulated, disproportionate, and unwanted movement of fluid and electrolytes with or without protein into the interstitial compartment of fluid. Because of this fluid movement, edema develops in sepsis, generalized as well as in end organs, leading to various organ dysfunction and/or failure. The global increased permeability syndrome (GIPS) can be defined as a positive cumulative fluid balance and new onset organ dysfunction/failure in patients with persistent systemic inflammation resulting in continuing transcapillary albumin leakage. GIPS or

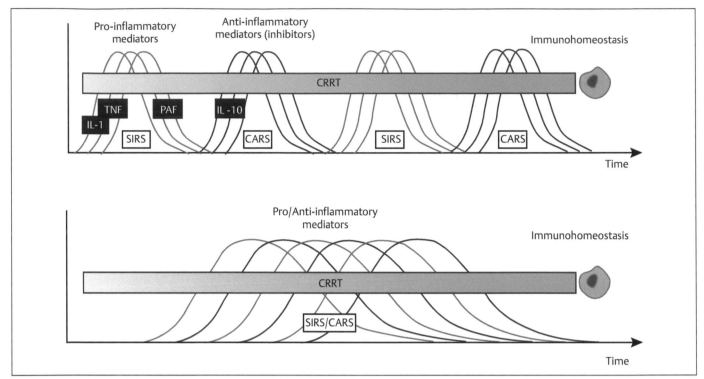

Fig. 40.4 Peak concentration hypothesis. Abbreviations: CARS, compensatory anti-inflammatory response syndrome; CRRT, continuous renal replacement therapy; IL-10, interleukin 10; PAF, platelet activating factor; SIRS, systemic inflammatory response syndrome; TNF, tumor necrosis factor.

third spacing as it is commonly known as may represent the third phase after the initial cytokine storm and ischemia–reperfusion injury. Clinically, this observation could be a potential indication to start blood purification therapy.[33]

Rationale for Extracorporeal Therapy and Cytokine Removal in Sepsis

We do not have any pharmacological treatment available for progressive organ dysfunction syndromes. Hence, we are left with only organ support, such as mechanical ventilation and hemodynamic support, renal replacement therapy (RRT), etc., as possible therapeutic strategies, knowing that the cytokine storm with excessive inflammatory response seen in septic shock leads to various organ failures leading to high death rates.[34] This fact correlates with high production of pro- and anti-inflammatory mediators rather than imbalance between pro- and anti-inflammatory mediators, giving us a window of opportunity to use BPT with the intention to decrease the harmful levels of the same.[35]

It is advisable to review available main BPTs objectively, such as (1) filtration, (2) dialysis (diffusion), and (3) adsorption. Continuous venovenous hemofiltration (CVVH) with dialysis or continuous hemodiafiltration (CHDF) are not considered as BPT because of the inability to remove middle molecular weight toxins raising the need for supplementary hemoadsorption therapy.[36] In this chapter, the

authors will review the evolution of currently available modalities.

Various studies investigated the use of increased filtration volumes by using HVHF with high cut-off membranes, and suggested that more multicenter RCTs are required before these therapies can be recommended for routine use.[37]

Researched and developed in Japan for gram-negative sepsis, direct hemoperfusion using a polymyxin B is one such modality. PMX filter uses an endotoxin-adsorbing column (PMX-DHP). It is marketed as Toraymyxin (Toray Industries, Tokyo, Japan). Technically it is a polycationic antibiotic column containing multiple polymyxin B-immobilized fibers, which have been shown to neutralize bacterial endotoxins.[38]

Other than this, a multitude of adsorption hemofilters are being studied and tried, such as (1) polymethyl-methacrylate (PMMA) membranes, (2) AN69 surface-treated (AN69ST) membranes, and (3) modified AN69ST membranes (oXiris).

The PMMA membrane is microporous hydrophobic, synthetic, polymeric membrane. In the past, PMMA hemofilters were used as an adjunct to maintenance hemodialysis and utilized PMMA for diffusion of small- and medium-size solutes across the membrane while extracting cytokines and larger solutes such as proteins (e.g., albumin, uremic toxins, and immunoglobulin light chains). Hence, PMMA membrane attracted attention as a supportive treatment for organ dysfunction in sepsis.[39]

The modified AN69ST membrane marketed as oXiris (Baxter, Meyzieu, France) is designed to increase endotoxin adsorption by increased polyethyleneimine in it. An additional attractive feature in oXiris is the immobilized heparin in it, which is useful to reduce thrombogenicity.[40] The oXiris membrane can help to adsorb both endotoxin and cytokines. However, there are limited clinical trials utilizing this device. Shum et al found that, after 48 hours, the SOFA score of patients undergoing concurrent oXiris therapy decreased by 38% compared to their admission score. It could not be proven to show significant difference in ICU and in-hospital mortality benefit.[41]

Among currently available devices, CytoSorb (CytoSorbents Corporation, Monmouth Junction, NJ, USA) is a latest available device for bedside use. This device incorporated in extracorporeal circuit helps to reduce serum level of both pro- and anti-inflammatory cytokines. The benefits are described to be the maximum with CytoSorb when treatment is started within 24 hours of diagnosed sepsis. To catch the time window of first 24 hours for the deserving patients requires training and strict protocol formation in the treating units. It is designed to reduce the systemic cytokine burden to a "normal" range ensuing hemodynamic and metabolic stabilization which is seen commonly after the highly unstable stage of cytokine storm.[42]

CytoSorb therapy has recently gained acceptance in Europe in the treatment of sepsis, burn injuries, trauma, and acute respiratory distress syndrome. It is the only specifically approved extracorporeal cytokine adsorber in the European Union. CytoSorb is approved for various clinical conditions in which increased levels of cytokines are found as a part of underlying cytokine storm. It has been approved in cytokine storm in COVID-19 as well (intended use).

On April 10, 2020 the US Food and Drug Administration (FDA) issued an Emergency Use Authorization (EUA) for using CytoSorb to treat COVID-19 patients 18 years of age or older admitted to the ICU with confirmed or imminent respiratory failure. On May 6, 2020, CytoSorb received DCGI approval for use in conditions where levels of cytokines and/or bilirubin and/or myoglobin are elevated. The device is also indicated for removal of P2Y12 inhibitor-ticagrelor intraoperatively during cardiopulmonary bypass. Till now, with the help of this device more than 2,300 COVID-19 patients have been treated worldwide.[42]

In their ninth interim analysis of hemoadsorption in the critically ill patients, CytoSorb International Registry found that, almost irrespective of the patient population in which it was applied, (a) the treatment was safe, (b) there was significantly improved cardiovascular and pulmonary function, (c) there was reduced levels of routinely measured inflammatory markers such as PCT and IL-6, (d) selected patient populations had potential benefit on survival, and finally (e) the majority of treating physicians found an overall improvement in their patients as far as SOFA score and the use of vasopressors were concerned, as an effect of the therapy.

The Blood Purifier Technology in CytoSorb

With the increasing usage of extra corporeal membrane oxygenator (ECMO) for various infective etiology related disease conditions, cytokine adsorption therapy may find its role in the selected patients. We need more robust data to support it further. The cartridge comes in the form of a single-use, disposable device to be used as a stand-alone therapy or as an add-on with CRRT, either pre- or postdialyzer. It can be incorporated in cardiopulmonary bypass machines or extracorporeal membrane oxygenation circuit too. It requires a large-bore intravenous access like hemodialysis cannula; the cartridge is attached in a series with a pump and a closed-loop circuit for the potential beneficiary (**Fig. 40.5**). For this type of BPT, the venous blood from the patient is passed through into the hemoadsorption cartridge and reinfused into the patient at the other end. It requires systemic anticoagulation mostly with heparin, to maintain activated partial thromboplastin time (aPTT) of 60 to 80 seconds. For this BPT with CytoSorb, blood flow rates can be maintained between 150 and 500 mL/min through the extracorporeal circuit, based on the tolerance as per patient's hemodynamic instability. Studies have shown significant reduction in serum levels of inflammatory markers and cytokines in patient's blood, after this therapy. The use of a single cartridge is recommended for up to 24 hours at a time, after which if extended support is still needed, a new cartridge can be replaced daily for the duration between 2 and 7 consecutive days.

There are many indications of CytoSorb therapy like severe sepsis with rapidly worsening SOFA score, refractory septic shock, and vasoplegic shock. Other indications with reported evidence are toxic shock syndrome, necrotizing fasciitis, meningococcal sepsis, pancreatitis, burns, trauma, liver failure, and rhabdomyolysis, among others. The procedure is reported to be safe.[43]

Current Evidence for Cytokine Adsorption Therapy

Collectively, many case reports and case series show improved clinical outcomes with various hemoadsorption devices (e.g., CYT-860-DHP membrane, AN69ST, modified AN69ST, PMMA, and CytoSorb). Arguably, the scientific value of these studies gets limited due to small sample sizes and, at best, they advocate for larger RCTs to evaluate any proven potential benefits in terms of reduced mortality in septic patients. The use of CYT-860-DHP membrane has been shown to effectively reduce cytokine levels and to improve general respiratory and circulatory status in patients with SOFA scores ≥5.[44]

Since its free availability in the EU, more and more clinical evidence have started building up on the use of CytoSorb. A case series of 16 patients undergoing cardiopulmonary bypass with CytoSorb therapy and CRRT demonstrated

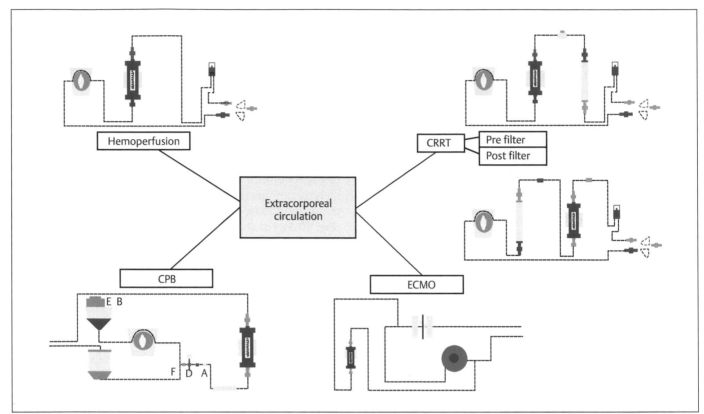

Fig. 40.5 Incorporation of blood purification cartridge (CytoSorb) in various extracorporeal circuits. Abbreviations: CPB, cardiopulmonary bypass; CRRT, continuous renal replacement therapy; ECMO, extracorporeal membrane oxygenation.

decreased serum levels of circulating cytokines, improved organ function, and improved hemodynamic stability. Kobe et al have reported a retrospective case series of 26 septic patients having two-system organ failure who were treated with CytoSorb therapy.[45] They observed increased hemodynamic stability, decreased serum lactic acid levels, and decreased vasopressor demands with this therapy. They recommended that the use of this therapy within 24 hours of diagnosis could lead to decreased mortality in both medical and postsurgical patients. The replicating findings of drop in serum lactate levels and falling vasopressor requirements were also confirmed in a single-center prospective cohort of 20 patients with refractory septic shock. The limitations of this study included the lack of a control group to compare clinical outcomes with. None of these case series reported any device-associated adverse effects. CytoSorb has been approved for use by the International Organization of Standardization (ISO, Geneva, Switzerland) since 2010. The large body of preclinical trials and case series is now starting to translate to randomized controlled human trials. Thus, there are two major accepted, clinical indications currently for CytoSorb therapy, viz. (1) severe sepsis with worsening SOFA scores and septic shock and (2) postcardiopulmonary bypass systemic inflammatory response syndrome.[46] Recently, the device has been approved by FDA and DCGI for use in cytokine storm in COVID-19 patients.

The Future of Cytokine Adsorption Therapy

Clinical studies in humans show that hemoadsorption devices effectively remove cytokines from the bloodstream when the levels are high. This needs to be conclusively proven by high-quality data to demonstrate improved clinical outcomes. The difficulties faced for this are (a) the broad and heterogenous clinical spectrum that gets included by a diagnosis of sepsis, (b) the difficulties in ascertaining the onset of sepsis to identify the time window and the correct timing of therapy, or (c) patient-to-patient variation in the innate immune response to infection. It is known that there are genetic factors which affect the course of sepsis, and single-nucleotide polymorphisms can greatly affect the serum levels of cytokines such as TNF-α in specific patients. The same factors, therefore, could be responsible for the variation in clinical outcomes between patients following hemoadsorption therapy. That may be the reason why 70 years of immunomodulation research in sepsis (dating way back for the use of corticosteroids in 1951) so far has no conclusive results.[47]

Hopefully, a better understanding of the immune dysregulation and cytokine storm in sepsis will help in enabling treatment to be more tailored to patient's needs. It holds true also for the specific use of different in vitro adsorption properties of oXiris, Toraymyxin, and CytoSorb. CytoSorb and other hemoadsorption devices work in a concentration-dependent manner; hence, patients with high serum cytokine loads are expected to benefit from these therapies. Early initiation of therapy (preferably within 24 h from the onset of worsening SOFA) also appears to be important in view of possible window of opportunity to reverse the syndrome, improve hemodynamic stability, and lower the predicted rate of mortality. But practically it has been that, due to the clinical heterogeneity of sepsis and hospital presentation of patients at different stages in the evolution of sepsis syndrome, many a times it is difficult to treat patients optimally early to derive significant benefit.[47]

One has to bear in mind that cytokines play various roles in the course of health and disease. They are necessary for the proper functioning of the localized and systemic host immune response. Removal of IL-6 and TNF-α may, for example, alter cell signaling and may attenuate the innate immune response to PAMPs and DAMPs. One must remember that the nature has created both pro- and anti-inflammatory cytokine responses during the evolution, as a part of "common responses" to infectious stimuli.[48,49]

The range of indications including nonspecific cytokine adsorption therapy seems to be broad. However, combined with the paucity of listed contraindications and randomized clinical trials, it should make clinicians wary of the risks of indiscriminate use of this technology. As of April 2018, the Food and Drug Administration approved the REFRESH II-AKI trial, the first randomized, controlled multicenter trial in the United States investigating the effect of CytoSorb during cardiac surgery on postoperative acute kidney injury, hospital length-of-stay, and mortality. The study has been completed on 18th January, 2022.[50]

The Center for Clinical Studies at the University of Jena, Germany constantly monitors the International CytoSorb Registry which collects and analyzes treatment data from all over the world. This helps in tracking patient mortality (primary end point) and secondary outcomes such as hospital and intensive care unit length of stay, vasopressor use, renal replacement therapy, and changes in end-organ function such as P/F ration for oxygenation. It is interesting to note the real-life experience, which showed multicenter data from 198 patients (68% of whom had sepsis with a mean APACHE II score of 33.1). This was analyzed in the registry's third interim analysis reported in 2017. Unequivocal findings include serum IL-6 levels following CytoSorb therapy were markedly decreased and the reported mortality with this therapy was 65% (compared to 78% predicted by their APACHE II score). None of the patients were affected by any device-associated side effects as per the investigators' observations.[51-55]

Conclusion

To date, there is a paucity of randomized controlled studies and data surrounding the use of hemoadsorption therapies in the treatment of cytokine storm states and septic shock. The registry and available published data show trend toward improvement of various parameters and primary end points in severe sepsis and septic shock patients, if this therapy is used early. As always only through well-conducted randomized controlled studies with appropriate patient selection criteria and end points of physiological relevance will we know whether the promise given by various hemoadsorption techniques as a future therapy for controlling dysregulated immune response in sepsis holds true. Till then, we still consider hemadsorption in sepsis/cytokine storm in ICU patient as a promising therapy worth trying, after all the current guidelines are exhausted.

CytoSorb© therapy is able to reduce inflammation and potentially improves survival in ARDS patients treated with V-V ECMO. Early initiation of CytoSorb© in conjunction with ECMO might offer a new approach to enhance lung rest and promote recovery in patients with severe ARDS.[56]

References

1. Kaukonen KM, Bailey M, Suzuki S, Pilcher D, Bellomo R. Mortality related to severe sepsis and septic shock among critically ill patients in Australia and New Zealand, 2000-2012. JAMA 2014;311(13):1308–1316
2. Gül F, Arslantaş MK, Cinel İ, Kumar A. Changing definitions of sepsis. Turk J Anaesthesiol Reanim 2017;45(3):129–138
3. Bone RC, Balk RA, Cerra FB, et al; The ACCP/SCCM Consensus Conference Committee. American College of Chest Physicians/ Society of Critical Care Medicine. Definitions for sepsis and organ failure and guidelines for the use of innovative therapies in sepsis. Chest 1992;101(6):1644–1655
4. Kaukonen KM, Bailey M, Pilcher D, Cooper DJ, Bellomo R. Systemic inflammatory response syndrome criteria in defining severe sepsis. N Engl J Med 2015;372(17):1629–1638 AQ14
5. Levy MM, Fink MP, Marshall JC, et al; SCCM/ESICM/ACCP/ATS/ SIS. 2001 SCCM/ESICM/ACCP/ATS/SIS International Sepsis Definitions Conference. Crit Care Med 2003;31(4):1250–1256AQ15
6. Singer M, Deutschman CS, Seymour CW, et al. The Third International Consensus Definitions for Sepsis and Septic Shock (Sepsis-3). JAMA 2016;315(8):801–810
7. Raith EP, Udy AA, Bailey M, et al; Australian and New Zealand Intensive Care Society (ANZICS) Centre for Outcomes and Resource Evaluation (CORE). Prognostic accuracy of the SOFA score, SIRS criteria, and qSOFA score for in-hospital mortality among adults with suspected infection admitted to the intensive care unit. JAMA 2017;317(3):290–300
8. Vincent JL, Moreno R, Takala J, et al. Working group on sepsis-related problems of the European society of intensive care medicine: the SOFA (Sepsis-related Organ Failure Assessment)

score to describe organ dysfunction/failure. Intensive Care Med 1996;22(7):707–710

9. van der Poll T, Opal SM. Host-pathogen interactions in sepsis. Lancet Infect Dis 2008;8(1):32–43

10. Esmon CT. The interactions between inflammation and coagulation. Br J Haematol 2005;131(4):417–430

11. Heagy W, Nieman K, Hansen C, Cohen M, Danielson D, West MA. Lower levels of whole blood LPS-stimulated cytokine release are associated with poorer clinical outcomes in surgical ICU patients. Surg Infect (Larchmt) 2003;4(2): 171–180

12. Vieillard-Baron A. Septic cardiomyopathy. Ann Intensive Care 2011;1(1):6

13. Gyawali B, Ramakrishna K, Dhamoon AS. Sepsis: the evolution in definition, pathophysiology, and management. SAGE Open Med 2019;7:2050312119835043

14. Nguyen HB, Jaehne AK, Jayaprakash N, et al. Early goal-directed therapy in severe sepsis and septic shock: insights and comparisons to ProCESS, ProMISe, and ARISE. Crit Care 2016; 20(1):160

15. Hayes MA, Timmins AC, Yau EH, Palazzo M, Hinds CJ, Watson D. Elevation of systemic oxygen delivery in the treatment of critically ill patients. N Engl J Med 1994;330(24): 1717–1722

16. Rivers E, Nguyen B, Havstad S, et al; Early Goal-Directed Therapy Collaborative Group. Early goal-directed therapy in the treatment of severe sepsis and septic shock. N Engl J Med 2001;345(19):1368–1377

17. Dellinger RP, Levy MM, Rhodes A, et al; Surviving Sepsis Campaign Guidelines Committee including the Pediatric Subgroup. Surviving sepsis campaign: international guidelines for management of severe sepsis and septic shock: 2012. Crit Care Med 2013;41(2):580–637

18. Yealy DM, Kellum JA, Huang DT, et al; ProCESS Investigators. A randomized trial of protocol-based care for early septic shock. N Engl J Med 2014;370(18):1683–1693

19. Park SK, Shin SR, Hur M, Kim WH, Oh EA, Lee SH. The effect of early goal-directed therapy for treatment of severe sepsis orseptic shock: a systemic review and meta-analysis. J Crit Care 2017;38:115–122

20. Levy MM, Evans LE, Rhodes A. The surviving sepsis campaign bundle: 2018 update. Intensive Care Med 2018;44(6):925–928

21. Pfortmueller CA, Meisel C, Fux M, Schefold JC. Assessment of immune organ dysfunction in critical illness: utility of innate immune response markers. Intensive Care Med Exp 2017;5(1):49

22. Venet F, Lukaszewicz AC, Payen D, Hotchkiss R, Monneret G. Monitoring the immune response in sepsis: a rational approach to administration of immunoadjuvant therapies. Curr Opin Immunol 2013;25(4):477–483

23. Coudroy R, Payen D, Launey Y, et al; ABDOMIX group. Modulation by polymyxin-B hemoperfusion of inflammatory response related to severe peritonitis. Shock 2017;47(1):93–99

24. Pachlopnik Schmid J, Ho CH, Chrétien F, et al. Neutralization of IFNgamma defeats haemophagocytosis in LCMV-infected perforin- and Rab27a-deficient mice. EMBO Mol Med 2009; 1(2):112–124

25. Tesi B, Sieni E, Neves C, et al. Hemophagocytic lympho-histiocytosis in 2 patients with underlying IFN-γ receptor deficiency. J Allergy Clin Immunol 2015;135(6):1638–1641

26. Vastert SJ, van Wijk R, D'Urbano LE, et al. Mutations in the perforin gene can be linked to macrophage activation

syndrome in patients with systemic onset juvenile idiopathic arthritis. Rheumatology (Oxford) 2010;49(3):441–449

27. Shimizu M, Nakagishi Y, Inoue N, et al. Interleukin-18 for predicting the development of macrophage activation syndrome in systemic juvenile idiopathic arthritis. Clin Immunol 2015;160(2):277–281

28. Ronco C, Tetta C, Mariano F, et al. Interpreting the mechanisms of continuous renal replacement therapy in sepsis: the peak concentration hypothesis. Artif Organs 2003;27(9):792–801

29. Grupp SA, Kalos M, Barrett D, et al. Chimeric antigen receptor-modified T cells for acute lymphoid leukemia. N Engl J Med 2013;368(16):1509–1518

30. van der Poll T, van de Veerdonk FL, Scicluna BP, Netea MG. The immunopathology of sepsis and potential therapeutic targets. Nat Rev Immunol 2017;17(7):407–420

31. Cavaillon JM, Munoz C, Fitting C, Misset B, Carlet J. Circulating cytokines: the tip of the iceberg? Circ Shock 1992;38(2): 145–152

32. Clark E, Molnar AO, Joannes-Boyau O, Honoré PM, Sikora L, Bagshaw SM. High-volume hemofiltration for septic acute kidney injury: a systematic review and meta-analysis. Crit Care 2014;18(1):R7

33. Malbrain MLNG, Van Regenmortel N, Saugel B, et al. Principles of fluid management and stewardship in septic shock: it is time to consider the four D's and the four phases of fluid therapy. Ann Intensive Care 2018;8(1):66

34. Ronco C, Ricci Z, Husain-Syed F. From multiple organ support therapy to extracorporeal organ support in critically ill patients. Blood Purif 2019;48(2):99–105

35. De Vriese AS, Colardyn FA, Philippé JJ, Vanholder RC, De Sutter JH, Lameire NH. Cytokine removal during continuous hemofiltration in septic patients. J Am Soc Nephrol 1999; 10(4):846–853

36. Ronco C. Sorbents: from bench to bedside. Can we combine membrane separation processes and adsorbent based solute removal? Int J Artif Organs 2006;29(9):819–822

37. Borthwick EM, Hill CJ, Rabindranath KS, Maxwell AP, McAuley DF, Blackwood B. High-volume haemofiltration for sepsis in adults. Cochrane Database Syst Rev 2017;1:CD008075

38. Payen DM, Guilhot J, Launey Y, et al; ABDOMIX Group. Early use of polymyxin B hemoperfusion in patients with septic shock due to peritonitis: a multicenter randomized control trial. Intensive Care Med 2015;41(6):975–984

39. Hattori N, Oda S. Cytokine-adsorbing hemofilter: old but new modality for septic acute kidney injury. Renal Replacement Therapy 2016;2:1–8

40. Nakada TA, Oda S, Matsuda K, et al. Continuous hemodiafiltration with PMMA Hemofilter in the treatment of patients with septic shock. Mol Med 2008;14(5-6):257–263

41. Shum HP, Chan KC, Kwan MC, Yan WW. Application of endotoxin and cytokine adsorption haemofilter in septic acute kidney injury due to Gram-negative bacterial infection. Hong Kong Med J 2013;19(6):491–497

42. Cytosorbents. CytoSorb—The Therapy, 2018. http://cytosorb-therapy.com/the-therapy/ (Last accessed July 5, 2018).

43. Gruda MC, Ruggeberg KG, O'Sullivan P, et al. Broad adsorption of sepsis-related PAMP and DAMP molecules, mycotoxins, and cytokines from whole blood using CytoSorb® sorbent porous polymer beads. PLoS One 2018;13(1):e0191676

44. Zhang J, Peng Z, Maberry D, et al. Effects of hemoadsorption with a novel adsorbent on sepsis: in vivo and in vitro study. Blood Purif 2015;39(1-3):239–245

45. Kobe Y, Oda S, Matsuda K, Nakamura M, Hirasawa H. Direct hemoperfusion with a cytokine-adsorbing device for the treatment of persistent or severe hypercytokinemia: a pilot study. Blood Purif 2007;25(5-6):446–453

46. Friesecke S, Stecher SS, Gross S, Felix SB, Nierhaus A. Extracorporeal cytokine elimination as rescue therapy in refractory septic shock: a prospective single-center study.J Artif Organs 2017;20(3):252–259

47. Chousterman BG, Swirski FK, Weber GF. Cytokine storm and sepsis disease pathogenesis. Semin Immunopathol 2017;39(5):517–528

48. Drutskaya MS, Efimov GA, Kruglov AA, Nedospasov SA. Can we design a better anti-cytokine therapy? J Leukoc Biol 2017;102(3):783–790

49. Multhoff G, Molls M, Radons J. Chronic inflammation in cancer development. Front Immunol 2012;2:98

50. Rauch S, Borgato A, Gruber E, Leggieri C, Bock M, Seraglio PME. Case Report: Prevention of Rhabdomyolysis-Associated Acute Kidney Injury by Extracorporeal Blood Purification With Cytosorb®. Front Pediatr. 2022 24;9:801807

51. Cytosorbents. Cytosorb registry. n.d. http://www.cytosorb-registry.org/?lang=en (Last accessed June 14, 2018)

52. Hawchar F, László I, Öveges N, Trásy D, Ondrik Z, Molnar Z. Extracorporeal cytokine adsorption in septic shock: A proof of concept randomized, controlled pilot study. J Crit Care 2019;49:172–178

53. Schädler D, Pausch C, Heise D, et al. The effect of a novel extracorporeal cytokine hemoadsorption device on IL-6 elimination in septic patients: a randomized controlled trial. PLoS One 2017;12(10):e0187015

54. Bellani G, Laffey JG, Pham T, et al; LUNG SAFE Investigators; ESICM Trials Group. Epidemiology, patterns of care, and mortality for patients with acute respiratory distress syndrome in intensive care units in 50 countries. JAMA 2016;315(8):788–800

55. Honore PM, Hoste E, Molnár Z, et al. Cytokine removal in human septic shock: Where are we and where are we going? Ann Intensive Care 2019;9(1):56

56. Akil A, Napp LC, Rao C, et al. Use of CytoSorb© Hemoadsorption in Patients on Veno-Venous ECMO Support for Severe Acute Respiratory Distress Syndrome: A Systematic Review. J. Clin. Med. 2022: 11, 5990

41

ECMO for Cardiodiabetes

Poonam Malhotra Kapoor, H. K. Chopra, and Mohit Prakash

Introduction

ECMO or "extracorporeal membrane oxygenation" traditionally is used in cases of respiratory failure (venovenous or VV ECMO) and severe cardiac failure (venoarterial or VA ECMO). In addition, ECMO is also used for providing postoperative support following cardiac surgery, short-term therapy in postcardiotomy syndrome, acute myocarditis, and refractory severe decompensated heart failure as a bridge to recovery or as a bridge to decision (heart transplant). The results have been encouraging in neonates and infants[1] but not so in adults.[1,2]

Options for managing heart failure in patients with refractory cardiogenic shock (CS) are limited. Given the circumstances, with dearth of randomized trials and lack of consensus for standard practices, survival has improved only slightly over the years. CS is still associated with high mortality in adults (50–60%)[1] despite revascularization and pharmacologic therapies.

With increasing technological advancements in designs of circuit, pumps, and oxygenators, recent years have witnessed an increasing use of ECMO as a bridge to definitive therapy in cases of CS from acute coronary syndromes and as a bridge to transplant with or without the use of other ventricular-assist devices (VADs). Use of ECMO following cardiac arrest is rapidly growing in popularity. Authors' basic focus in this chapter would mainly be use of ECMO in CS and heart failure.

Indications of ECMO in Cardiac Patients with Diabetes

People with cardiovascular disease have a higher incidence of development of diabetes, particularly when patients develop diabetic cardiomyopathy. The indications for using an ECMO in diabetic patients are listed in **Box 41.1**.

Risk Factors for Heart Failure and Diabetes

- Increasing age.
- Hypertension.
- Hyperlipidemia.
- Obesity.
- Atherosclerosis.
- Coronary artery disease.

Numerous clinical trials report increased correlation between occurrence of heart failure and diabetes but exact pathophysiology is still unknown.

ECMO in Heart Failure—Why the Need for ECMO?

Diabetic patients are more prone to develop acute heart failure (AHF). According to the European Society of Cardiology (ESC) guidelines,[7] AHF is rapid onset or worsening of symptoms and/or signs of heart failure requiring urgent evaluation and treatment. AHF may appear de novo or mostly as acute or chronic heart failure. It may be primarily because of cardiac dysfunction or precipitated by extrinsic factors in chronic heart failure. Acute myocardial dysfunction (ischemic, inflammatory, or toxic), acute valve insufficiency, or pericardial tamponade is among the most frequent acute primary cardiac causes of AHF. Decompensation of chronic HF can occur because of infection, uncontrolled hypertension, rhythm disturbances, or nonadherence with drugs/diet.

With advancement in cardiovascular sciences, challenges have grown in terms of the disease spectrum available for treatment. Various permutation and combinations can be seen such as chronic systolic dysfunction and acute decompensated heart failure, high-risk multivessel disease requiring percutaneous coronary intervention (PCI) or other procedures, patients having coexisting cardiac dysfunction after myocardial infarction (MI) despite successful reperfusion, and so on. The prognosis is grave if associated with diseases like diabetes. Such patients who are not stabilized with medical therapy alone can be supported using mechanical circulatory devices. These serve to unload the failing ventricle and maintain end-organ perfusion. Biventricular-assist devices, extracorporeal life support (ECLS),[8] and intra-aortic balloon pump (IABP) are usually used. According to 2011 American College of Cardiology/American Heart Association/Society for Cardiovascular Angiography and Interventions (ACC/AHA/SCAI) guidelines[9] for PCI, percutaneous mechanical circulatory support is recommended in two clinical settings: high-risk PCI (Class IIb) and CS with ST-elevation MI (Class Ib).

Box 41.1 Indications for ECMO in cardiodiabetes

- Bridge to decision for transplant or LVAD/BiVAD
- Support post cardiac surgery, in low output
- Cardiogenic shock
- Fulminant myocarditis
- Pulmonary hypertension and right heart failure
- Pulmonary embolus with hemodynamic compromise
- Cardiac arrest
- Drug overdose
- Nonischemic cardiomyopathy including sepsis-induced cardiomyopathy
- Heart failure and diabetes
- STEMI
- ECPR for diabetes
- ECMO in infants with diabetes

Abbreviations: ECMO, extracorporeal membrane oxygenation; ECPR, extracorporeal cardiopulmonary resuscitation; LVAD, left ventricular assist device; BiVAD, biventricular assist device; STEMI, ST-elevation myocardial infarction.

High-risk PCI is characterized as in the following patient categories.

- *Patient-specific variables:*
  - ➢ Increased age.
  - ➢ Symptoms of heart failure.
  - ➢ Diabetes mellitus.
  - ➢ Chronic kidney disease.
  - ➢ Prior MI.
  - ➢ Multivessel or left main disease.
  - ➢ Peripheral arterial disease.
- *Lesion-specific variables:*
  - ➢ Left main stenosis.
  - ➢ Bifurcation disease.
  - ➢ Saphenous vein graft.
  - ➢ Ostial stenosis.
  - ➢ Heavy calcified lesions.
  - ➢ Chronic total occlusions.
  - ➢ Dissection or occlusion during PCI.
- *Left ventricular (LV) dysfunction especially acute decompensated heart failure with difficult lesions.*

ECMO in Diabetics with Heart Failure

Diastolic dysfunction is more common in elderly persons, partly because of increased collagen cross-linking, increased smooth muscle content, and loss of elastic fibers (**Flowchart 41.1**). These changes tend to decrease ventricular compliance, making more susceptible to the adverse effects of hypertension, tachycardia, and atrial fibrillation. It worsens in diabetes, leading to acute decompensated heart failure and patient may be required to be put on a mechanical device such as ECMO for a short while.

Pathophysiology of Diabetes and Heart Failure

Framingham Heart Study reports higher incidence of heart failure in diabetics compared to controls (men: two times more; women: five times more).[10] Idiopathic cardiomyopathy also has increased incidence of diabetes (22%) compared to normal population (11%).[11,12] Increasing age, duration of disease,[13] extent of metabolic disturbances, and requirement of drug therapy (regardless of drug used) are strongly correlated with development of increased risk of heart failure in diabetic patient.[14] Since diabetes is associated with silent MI and sudden cardiac death, it is important to periodically screen diabetic patients for development of heart failure so that appropriate therapy may be initiated at the earliest (**Flowchart 41.1**).

Management is same as for other heart failure patients with special attention to the following:

- Strict glycemic control.
- Monitoring of renal dysfunction and need for renal replacement therapy.
- Atherosclerosis in peripheral and central arteries may affect the decision in case mechanical support is required in advanced cases.

- Autonomic dysfunction may affect hemodynamic management.

Initiation of ECMO

Since cardiac dysfunction is primary pathology in heart failure and CS, VA ECMO is invariably used. Usually VA ECMO initiated peripherally is adequate for majority of cases of CS (**Fig. 41.1**).

It, however, requires frequent echocardiographic monitoring for progressive ventricular dilatation because ECMO does not allow for venting of left ventricle. If ventricular dilatation occurs then either configuration of ECMO circuit can be changed or a percutaneous atrial septostomy can be performed.

Another pitfall associated with the use of peripheral ECMO stems from the fact that native cardiac output generated from the dysfunctional heart theoretically may mechanically oppose the cardiac output generated by the ECMO in the femoral aortic cannula. This may lead to increased LV stress. If an added respiratory insult ensues, there is inadequate oxygenation with deterioration in the medical condition of the patient despite optimal ECMO flows.

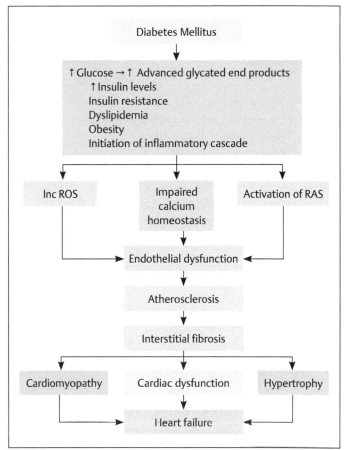

Flowchart 41.1 Pathophysiology of heart failure in diabetic patients. Abbreviations: RAS, renin-angiotensin system; ROS, reactive oxygen species.

Types of ECMO

ECMO was first used successfully for life-threatening respiratory failure in an adult in 1971 and in a neonate with meconium aspiration in 1975.

There are two types of ECMO:

- **VA ECMO:** It allows gas exchange and hemodynamic support while blood is pumped from the venous to the arterial side (**Fig. 41.2a**).
- **VV ECMO:** It facilitates gas exchange; blood is removed from the venous side and then pumped back into it, but does not provide hemodynamic support (**Fig. 41.2b**).

The circuit setup for VA or VV is almost identical. Blood movement is facilitated by an external pump that then pushes the blood through a membrane allowing gas exchange (oxygenation and CO_2 removal), before returning the blood to the patient's circulation via a warmer. Due to its configuration,

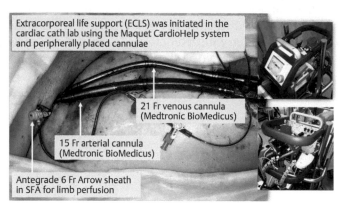

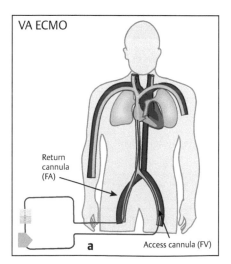

Fig. 41.1 Extracorporeal membrane oxygenation (ECMO) cannula placement: femoral approach with antegrade sheath. Adapted with permission from Chopra HK, Kapoor PM. Role of Extracorporeal Membrane Oxygenation for Acute Decompensated Heart Failure. In: Kapoor PM, ed. Manual Of Extracorporeal Membrane Oxygenation (ECMO) In The ICU, 1 ed. India: Jaypee Publication; 2014.

VA-ECMO bypasses the patient's heart and lung and part or all of the blood flow is diverted through the ECMO circuit (**Fig. 41.3**). In contrast, VV-ECMO returns the blood before it enters the pulmonary circulation. So, VA-ECMO is ideal for ST-elevation myocardial infarction (STEMI) patients. In fact, in a study done by Rajsic et al,[15] patients included for ECMO support (>85% of the total) were those with profound CS undergoing cardiopulmonary cerebral resuscitation (CPCR) and in whom a prompt ECMO was instituted.

ECMO timing for initiation and weaning has always been crucial and controversial. For patients with advanced heart failure, Interagency Registry for Mechanical Assisted Circulatory Support (INTERMACS)[7] has defined seven clinical profiles (**Table 41.1**).

Interagency Registry for Mechanically Assisted Circulatory Support (INTERMACS)

Out of seven levels, patients at one and two levels are considered for mechanical circulatory support. Availability of advanced mechanical support systems has resulted in improvements in survival and quality of life in patients with advanced cardiac failure.[16]

Although human studies demonstrating benefits of ECMO for myocardial protection are limited, increase in use is based on the hypothesis that ventricular support may provide myocardial preservation during periods of acute ischemic insult. It serves to improve hemodynamic condition with reduction in infarct size.

Beneficial Hemodynamic Effects of ECMO

Whether it is VV ECMO or VA ECMO, the overall benefits, accrued from ECMO use, are:

- Decreases LV volume, wall stress, and oxygen consumption.

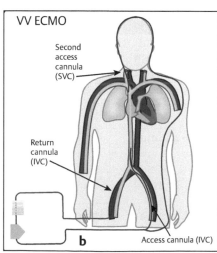

Fig. 41.2 (a) Venoarterial extracorporeal membrane oxygenation (VA ECMO). **(b)** Venovenous (VV) ECMO. Abbreviations: FA, femoral artery; FV, femoral vein; IVC, inferior vena cava; SVC, superior vena cava.

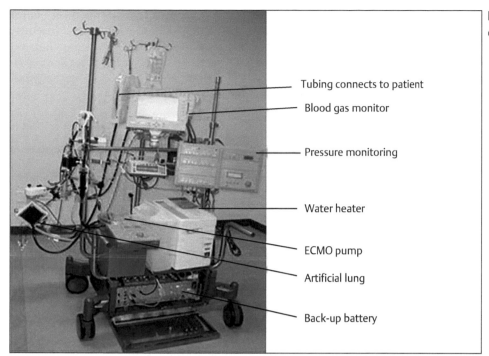

Fig. 41.3 Extracorporeal membrane oxygenation (ECMO) circuit machine.

Tubing connects to patient

Blood gas monitor

Pressure monitoring

Water heater

ECMO pump

Artificial lung

Back-up battery

Table 41.1 Interagency registry for mechanical assisted circulatory support (INTERMACS) stages for classifying patients with advanced heart failure

INTERMACS	NYHA Class	Description	Device	Ly survival with LVAD therapy
Cardiogenic shock "Crash and run"	IV	Hemodynamic instability in spite of increased doses of catecholamines and/or mechanical circulatory support with critical hypoperfusion of target organs	ECLS, ECMO, percutaneous support devices	52.6 ± 5.6%
Progressive decline despite inotropic support "Sliding on inotropes"	IV	Intravenous inotropic support with acceptable blood pressure but rapid deterioration of renal function, nutritional state, or signs of congestion	ECLS, ECMO, LVAD	63.1 ± 3.1%
Stable but inotrope dependent "Dependent stability"	IV	Hemodynamic stability with low or intermediate doses of inotropic but necessary due to hypotension, worsening of symptoms, or progressive renal failure	LVAD	78.4 ± 2.5%
Resting symptoms "Frequent flyer"	IV Ambulatory	Temporary cessation of inotropic treatment is possible but patient presents with frequent symptom recurrences and typically with fluid overload	LVAD	78.7 ± 3.0%
Exertion intolerant "Housebound"	IV Ambulatory	Complete cessation of physical activity, stable at rest, but frequently with moderate fluid retention and some level of renal dysfunction	LVAD	93.0 ± 3.9%
Exertion limited "Walking wounded"	III	Minor limitation on physical activity and absence of congestion while at rest Easily fatigued by light activity	LVAD/Discuss LVAD as option	–
"Placeholder"	III	Patient in NYHA Class III with no current or recent unstable fluid balance	Discuss LVAD as option	–

Abbreviations: ECLS, extracorporeal life support; ECMO, extracorporeal membrane oxygenation; LVAD, left-ventricular-assist devices; NHYA, New York Heart Association.

- Limits the infarct size.
- Improves coronary perfusion.
- Maintains perfusion to other vital organs.
- Decreases cardiac filling pressures.

Contraindications for Initiation of VA ECMO in Cardiac Failure

- Irreversible disease (malignancy, cardiac dysfunction).
- Chronic multiorgan dysfunction (chronic obstructive pulmonary disease [COPD], renal dysfunction, hepatic dysfunction).
- Prolonged cardiopulmonary resuscitation (CPR) without adequate tissue perfusion or unwitnessed cardiac arrest.
- Compliance limitation (financial, cognitive, psychiatric, social).
- Bleeding diathesis.
- Central nervous system (CNS) injury (intracranial bleed, encephalitis, persistent vegetative state, hypoxic ischemic encephalopathy, intractable seizures).

ECMO in CS associated with sepsis is controversial due to concerns about bacteremia, inflammation, and bleeding following disseminated intravascular coagulopathy. VA ECMO might be considered for mixed cardiogenic and septic shock, provided benefits outweigh the risks of bleeding and thrombosis.[17]

ECMO in Cardiogenic Shock

In diabetics, CS is present when systemic tissue hypoperfusion occurs due to inadequate cardiac output. In such patients circulatory blood volume and LV filling pressures are, however, adequate.[18] Diagnostic criteria include: a systolic blood pressure <90 mmHg for 30 min; a drop in mean arterial blood pressure >30 mmHg below baseline, with a cardiac index (CI) <1.8 L/min/m² without hemodynamic support or </= 2.2 L/min/m² with support; and a pulmonary capillary wedge pressure >15 mmHg. It most commonly occurs after acute MI due to myocardial dysfunction or is the result of mechanical complications such as acute ventricular septal defect, cardiac rupture, papillary muscle rupture, and cardiac tamponade. Consequently, inability to maintain

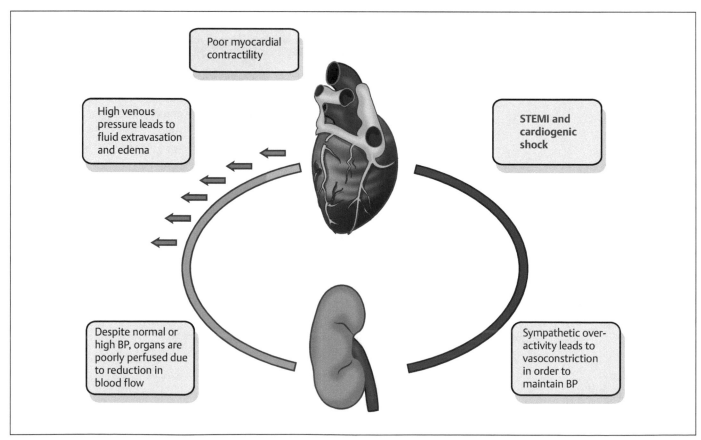

Fig. 41.4 Sequence of events leading to cardiogenic shock in ST-elevation myocardial infarction (STEMI). Adapted with permission from Chopra HK, Kapoor PM. Role of Extracorporeal Membrane Oxygenation for Acute Decompensated Heart Failure. In: Kapoor PM, ed. Manual Of Extracorporeal Membrane Oxygenation (ECMO) In The ICU, 1 ed. India: Jaypee Publication; 2014.

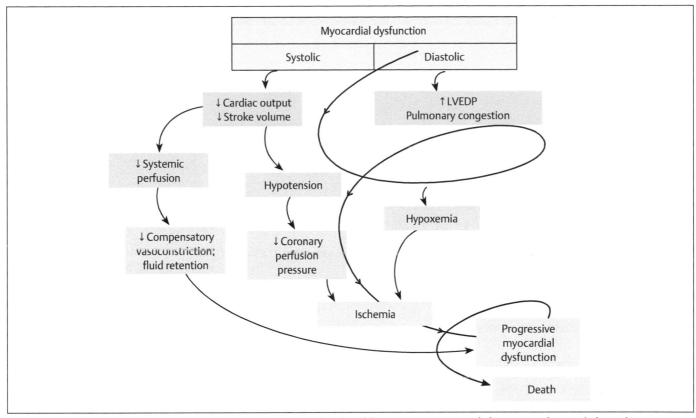

Flowchart 41.2 The downward spiral in cardiogenic shock. Abbreviation: LVEDP, left ventricular end-diastolic pressure. Adapted with permission from Chopra HK, Kapoor PM. Role of Extracorporeal Membrane Oxygenation for Acute Decompensated Heart Failure. In: Kapoor PM, ed. Manual Of Extracorporeal Membrane Oxygenation (ECMO) In The ICU, 1 ed. India: Jaypee Publication; 2014.

tissue perfusion and oxygenation is associated with poor prognosis[19] (**Fig. 41.4** and **Flowchart 41.2**).

Treatment consists of initial medical stabilization with oxygen, aspirin, morphine, fluids, inotropes, vasopressors, diuretics in pulmonary edema and vasodilators according to patient's hemodynamic status. Supportive measures include mechanical support (IABP, VADs, ECLS), reperfusion therapy (fibrinolytics, PCI), and surgery (coronary artery bypass grafting).

Use of IABP in refractory cases of CS is controversial as it is not effective when CI is less than 1.2 L/min/m²[20,21] Other partial support therapies like VADs have also been used.[22] However VADs have not shown to improve mortality in severe cases.[23]

Significant limitations of IABP and VAD include availability, cost, and time delay during initiation and need for personnel trained in providing specialized support according to the degree of hemodynamic compromise. The situation is further complicated with the development of respiratory compromise following hypoxemia, hypercarbia, and consequent pulmonary edema. ECMO emerges as a rescue therapy in such a scenario.

ECMO has been used in acute CS with left or biventricular failure for initial short-term assistance till the time cardiac and other organ functions have recovered and more definitive therapy can be planned. Time duration is usually restricted from few days to weeks. Percutaneous cardiopulmonary bypass can also be used to provide support.[24]

The ESC guidelines for the diagnosis and treatment of acute and chronic heart failure recommend short-term mechanical circulatory support (as a "bridge to recovery") in patients remaining severely hypoperfused despite inotropic therapy and with a potentially reversible cause (e.g., viral myocarditis) or a potentially surgically correctable cause (e.g., acute interventricular septal rupture)[16] (**Box 41.2**).

ECMO and STEMI

Patients who present with STEMI complicated by CS that suffer a cardiac arrest have high mortality rates. Little data exist on using ECMO as a rescue device during CPR in the CS patient.

Box 41.2 ESC guidelines for the diagnosis and management of heart failure

Indications for ECMO in heart failure
- Cardiogenic shock secondary to acute coronary syndrome
- Viral myocarditis
- Cardiogenic shock with acute severe mitral regurgitation and aortic regurgitation
- Postcardiotomy cardiogenic shock
- Failure to wean off from cardiopulmonary bypass
- Poisoning: beta blocker, calcium channel blocker, aluminum phosphide
- Patient waiting for left-ventricular-assist device
- Patient is waiting for cardiac transplant

Criteria for initiation of ECMO
Presence of any two criteria mentioned below observed over a period of 4–6 h after maximum medical resuscitation:
- Refractory arrhythmias
- Cardiogenic shock with high inotropic requirements
- Lactate level >5 mmol/L or rising titer or $ScvO_2$ <65% with maximum medical management
- Signs of poor tissue perfusion

Contraindications for ECMO in heart failure
- Irreversible disease (e.g., malignancy)
- Dilated cardiomyopathy except for waiting for final destination therapy or transplant
- Age >75 y
- Patient on ventilator from 15 d
- Intracranial bleed
- Active bleeding from noncompressible site
- Patient of gross multiorgan failure
- Severe CNS injury including encephalitis, persistent vegetative state, hypoxic ischemic encephalopathy, intractable seizures
- Unwitnessed arrest or arrest >30 min

Echocardiography criteria for contraindications to ECMO
- Severe aortic regurgitation (AR)
- Severe aortic stenosis (AS)
- Coarctation of aorta
- Aortic dissection

Essential targets to be reached on ECMO in cardiogenic shock

- $ScvO_2$ >70%
- MAP >60 mmHg (in case of full support with nonpulsatile flow)
- MAP >70 mmHg (in case of partial support with pulsatile flow)
- Avoid full flow and give partial flow about two-thirds through ECMO
- Maintain oxygen saturation of 90% or PaO_2 of >50 mmHg (in young patient) and >60 (in elderly and with CAD or CVA)
- Maintain coronary saturation of >70%

Abbreviations: CAD, coronary artery disease; CNS, central nervous system; CVA, cerebro-vascular accidents; ECMO, extracorporeal membrane oxygenation; ESC, European Society of Cardiology; MAP, mean arterial pressure; PaO_2, partial pressure of oxygen; $ScvO_2$, central venous saturation.

ECMO and Hypothermia as Rescue Therapy

ECMO can be a lifesaving rescue technique when instituted by an experienced shock team in the CV lab for refractory pulseless electrical activity (PEA) arrest occurring in the CV lab. Lucas CPR was a valuable adjunct. Striking recovery of LV function can also occur in several days. The combination of ECMO and therapeutic hypothermia was associated with excellent neurologic outcomes as well. ECMO may have a role in selected PCI centers with advanced specialized teams.

The use of ECMO, accompanied by mechanical CPR, in patients with massive MIs can lead to unexpected survival. ECMO is an advanced technology that functions as a replacement for a critically ill patient's heart and lungs.

"For many patients who present with a severe heart attack, or ST-elevation myocardial infarction (STEMI), complicated by cardiogenic shock that progresses to cardiac standstill, the result is almost uniformly fatal," says Michael R. Mooney, MD, a research cardiologist at the Minneapolis Heart Institute Foundation (MHIF) and a physician at the Minneapolis Heart Institute at Abbott Northwestern Hospital in Minneapolis. "This aggressive approach despite its complexity extends our ability to salvage the most devastating complication of acute MI."

Early ECMO-assisted primary PCI improved 30-day outcomes in STEMI patients complicated with profound CS.

Extracorporeal CPR (E-CPR)

ECMO can also be initiated percutaneously with ongoing cardiopulmonary resuscitation, that is, extracorporeal CPR (E-CPR). It aims to restore circulation during cardiac arrest in conjunction with ongoing advanced life support strategies. E-CPR has resulted in improved in-hospital survival free from major neurologic impairment.[25,26] Surgical assistance is not always necessary. Financial implications are difficult to determine due to the complexity of the intervention.

Disadvantages of Intra-Aortic Balloon Pump (IABP) and Ventricular-Assist Devices (VADs)

ECMO bypasses all the disadvantages of IABP and VAD. In ECMO, optimal gas exchange is possible as lungs are bypassed. It can provide up to 7 L/min of flow if required. With increasing use of peripheral cannulation techniques, availability of integrated portable pump systems and development of management guidelines have drastically reduced the time required for initiation of ECMO and can be performed bedside. In fact, the time for initiating ECMO is comparable to that required for percutaneous/catheter-directed therapies performed in cardiac catheterization laboratory or hybrid operating rooms.[27,28]

A nonrandomized study by Abrams et al et al depict survival advantage when mechanical support, including ECMO, is initiated early in acute MI with CS, as an initial therapy for cardiopulmonary stabilization (in-hospital mortality: 33%; 5-y survival: 81%) compared to early PCI or coronary artery bypass graft alone (in-hospital mortality: 81%; 5-y survival: 6.2%).[29] Selection bias, nonrandomization, and variable management protocols were major drawbacks in this study. This study clearly demonstrates that ECMO can improve outcomes if used early in carefully selected suitable candidates before the onset of a reversible shock and organ failure. Early identification and resuscitation are the keys for

improving outcomes.[30,31] Studies have also demonstrated the beneficial role of ECLS for high-risk PCI, particularly in cases of acute CS.[32]

VA ECMO in acute MI with CS has shown improved in-hospital survival and reduced 30-day mortality in conjunction with revascularization.[20,33] Careful selection of candidates for early initiation of VA ECMO at the first sign of CS provides the greatest chance for survival before development of irreversible multiple end-organ failure.[34,35] This allows for hemodynamic stabilization and optimization of reperfusion via PCI or surgery.

CS may also occur as part of nonischemic process in the form of fulminant myocarditis and sepsis-associated cardiomyopathy. Patients with fulminant myocarditis stabilized with VA ECMO have similar outcomes as myocarditis patients without shock.[36]

Survival after Venoarterial ECMO (SAVE)

The SAVE score can help in predicting the survival rate of patients receiving ECMO for refractory CS.[30] It should be used in conjunction with clinical assessment and not solely for decision-making related to use of ECMO (**Fig. 41.5**). SAVE score like the platelet, lactate levels pulmonary hypertension (PH) and Sequential Organ Failure Assessment (SOFA) scores are good prognostic markers for predicting survival in VA ECMO heart failure patients, depending on the days on ECMO.

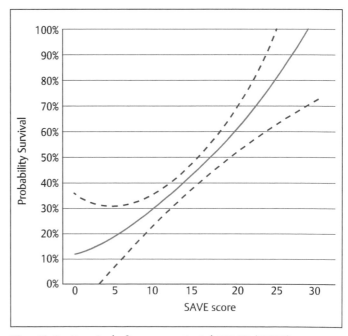

Fig. 41.5 Survival after venoarterial ECMO (SAVE) score.

Complications of ECMO

- Bleeding (30–60%): With newer pumps and circuitry, comparatively low levels of anticoagulation may suffice in reducing the incidence of bleeding.
- Neurological complications: These either result from intracranial bleed or emboli in the circuit (clot/air bubble). Overall incidence of stroke is 3 to 12%.

Box 41.3 Maquet CardioHelp extracorporeal life support (ECLS)

Smallest commercially available pump and integrated oxygenator (all in one heart-lung support system) with the following features:
- Biocompatible surface coatings for optimum protection
- Extracorporeal mechanical circulatory support
- Partial or complete cardiac output
- Support for CO_2 removal and oxygenation
- 10 kg (22 lb)
- 14 × 10 × 17 in
- Optional sprinter cart for in-hospital mobility

Source: Adapted with permission from Chopra HK, Kapoor PM. Role of ECMO and ADHF. In: Kapoor PM, ed. Manual of ECMO in ICU, 1 ed. India: Jaypee Publication; 2014.

- Nosocomial infection: 50 to 60%.
- Mechanical complications due to device failure.
- Multiorgan dysfunction: 33%.
- Others: Limb ischemia, hepatic dysfunction, renal dysfunction, hemolysis, and anemia.

Newer Developments in ECMO

Maquet CardioHelp system, a portable version, has revolutionized the ECMO era. The ease of insertion and increased mobility of patients may permit its use in cardiac catheterization laboratories in future (**Fig. 41.6**; **Box 41.3**).

Conclusion

The availability of ECMO has increased the horizon of therapeutic options available for patients requiring high level of hemodynamic support. Early initiation of ECMO in cases of impaired oxygenation in acute decompensated heart failure or large acute MI requiring revascularization may reduce mortality and morbidity. More randomized controlled trials for testing the efficacy of routine use of ECMO for salvaging the myocardium are needed. Introduction of portable ECMO devices may play an important role in future.[37] Patients with

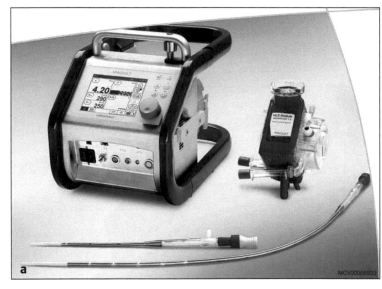

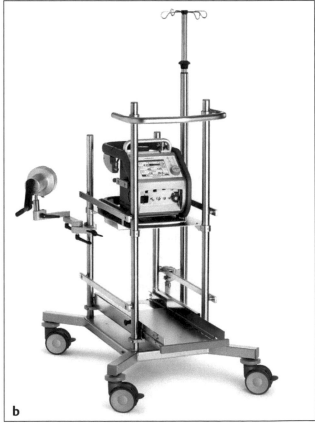

Fig. 41.6 **(a, b)** CardioHelp from Maquet. Adapted with permission from Kapoor PM. ECMO in STEMI management. In: Chopra HK, ed. STEMI: A Cardiology Update, 1 ed. India: Jaypee Publication; 2014.

refractory hypoxemia or hypercarbia as well as patients with right ventricular failure resulting from hypercarbia, acidemia, or hypoxic pulmonary vasoconstriction may benefit from ECLS through VV ECMO. Failure to wean from VA ECMO is due to a ECMO gap due to maltiorgan failure, thus detailed and prevention of contributing factors to MOF are warranted ventricle arrhythmias, dyssynchronopathy etc. maintaining sinus rhythm on ECMO is key to success.[38]

ECMO can be considered for patients whose cause of cardiac arrest is potentially reversible.[39] When DKA patients develop fatal dysrhythmia or even cardiac arrest induced by severe hypokalemia, ECMO could maintain circulation and provide time to correct electrolyte imbalances, while continuous renal replacement therapy (CRRT) could be used to restore homeostasis.[40]

References

1. Lowry AW, Morales DL, Graves DE, et al. Characterization of extracorporeal membrane oxygenation for pediatric cardiac arrest in the United States: analysis of the kids' inpatient database. Pediatr Cardiol 2013;34(6):1422–1430

2. Smedira NG, Moazami N, Golding CM, et al. Clinical experience with 202 adults receiving extracorporeal membrane oxygenation for cardiac failure: survival at five years. J Thorac Cardiovasc Surg 2001;122(1):92–102

3. Killip T III, Kimball JT. Treatment of myocardial infarction in a coronary care unit. A two year experience with 250 patients. Am J Cardiol 1967;20(4):457–464

4. Goldberg RJ, Gore JM, Alpert JS, et al. Cardiogenic shock after acute myocardial infarction. Incidence and mortality from a community-wide perspective, 1975 to 1988. N Engl J Med 1991;325(16):1117–1122

5. Tipoo FA, Quraishi AR, Najaf SM, et al. Outcome of cardiogenic shock complicating acute myocardial infarction. J Coll Physicians Surg Pak 2004;14(1):6–9

6. Hochman JS, Boland J, Sleeper LA, et al. Current spectrum of cardiogenic shock and effect of early revascularisation on mortality. Results of an international registry. SHOCK registry investigators. Circulation 1995;91:873–881

7. Ponikowski P, Voors AA, Anker SD, et al; ESC Scientific Document Group. 2016 ESC Guidelines for the diagnosis and treatment of acute and chronic heart failure: the Task Force for the diagnosis and treatment of acute and chronic heart failure of the European Society of Cardiology (ESC) developed with the special contribution of the Heart Failure Association (HFA) of the ESC. Eur Heart J 2016;37(27):2129–2200

8. Bartlett RH, Roloff DW, Custer JR, Younger JG, Hirschl RB. Extracorporeal life support: the University of Michigan experience. JAMA 2000;283(7):904–908

9. American College of Cardiology/American Heart Association/ Society for Cardiovascular Angiography and Interventions (ACC/AHA/SCAI) guidelines for percutaneous coronary intervention. ACC/AHA/SCAI 2011

10. Kannel WB, McGee DL. Diabetes and cardiovascular disease. The Framingham study. JAMA 1979;241(19):2035–2038

11. Bertoni AG, Tsai A, Kasper EK, Brancati FL. Diabetes and idiopathic cardiomyopathy: a nationwide case-control study. Diabetes Care 2003;26(10):2791–2795

12. Hamby RI, Zoneraich S, Sherman L. Diabetic cardiomyopathy. JAMA 1974;229(13):1749–1754

13. Lind M, Bounias I, Olsson M, Gudbjörnsdottir S, Svensson AM, Rosengren A. Glycaemic control and incidence of heart failure in 20,985 patients with type 1 diabetes: an observational study. Lancet 2011;378(9786):140–146

14. Kasznicki J, Drzewoski J. Heart failure in the diabetic population: pathophysiology, diagnosis and management. Arch Med Sci 2014;10(3):546–556

15. Rajsic S, Breitkopf R, Jadzic D, Popovic Krneta M, Tauber H, Treml B. Anticoagulation Strategies during Extracorporeal Membrane Oxygenation: A Narrative Review. J Clin Med. 2022 Aug 31;11(17):5147

16. Rose EA, Gelijns AC, Moskowitz AJ, et al; Randomized Evaluation of Mechanical Assistance for the Treatment of Congestive Heart Failure (REMATCH) Study Group. Long-term use of a left ventricular assist device for end-stage heart failure. N Engl J Med 2001;345(20):1435–1443

17. Bréchot N, Luyt CE, Schmidt M, et al. Venoarterial extracorporeal membrane oxygenation support for refractory cardiovascular dysfunction during severe bacterial septic shock. Crit Care Med 2013;41(7):1616–1626

18. E2015 SCAI/ACC/HFSA/STS Clinical Expert Consensus Statement on the Use of Percutaneous Mechanical Circulatory Support Devices in Cardiovascular Care. Endorsed by the American Heart Association, the Cardiological Society of India, and Sociedad Latino Americana de Cardiologia Intervencion; Affirmation of Value by the Canadian Association of Interventional Cardiology-Association Canadienne de Cardiologie d'interventionVOL. 65, NO. 19, 2015. http://dx.doi.org/10.1016/j.jacc.2015.03.036

19. Menees DS, Peterson ED, Wang Y, et al. Door-to-balloon time and mortality among patients undergoing primary PCI. N Engl J Med 2013;369(10):901–909

20. Thiele H, Zeymer U, Neumann F-J, et al; IABP-SHOCK II Trial Investigators. Intraaortic balloon support for myocardial infarction with cardiogenic shock. N Engl J Med 2012;367(14): 1287–1296

21. Thiele H, Zeymer U, Neumann F-J, et al; Intraaortic Balloon Pump in cardiogenic shock II (IABP-SHOCK II) trial investigators. Intra-aortic balloon counterpulsation in acute myocardial infarction complicated by cardiogenic shock (IABP-SHOCK II): final 12 month results of a randomised, open-label trial. Lancet 2013;382(9905):1638–1645

22. Norman JC, Cooley DA, Igo SR, et al. Prognostic indices for survival during postcardiotomy intra-aortic balloon pumping. Methods of scoring and classification, with implications for left ventricular assist device utilization. J Thorac Cardiovasc Surg 1977;74(5):709–720

23. Myat A, Patel N, Tehrani S, Banning AP, Redwood SR, Bhatt DL. Percutaneous circulatory assist devices for high-risk coronary intervention. JACC Cardiovasc Interv 2015;8(2):229–244

24. Vogel RA, Shawl F, Tommaso C, et al. Initial report of the National registry of elective cardiopulmonary bypass supported coronary angioplasty. J Am Coll Cardiol 1990;15(1):23–29

25. Shin TG, Jo IJ, Sim MS, et al. Two-year survival and neurological outcome of in-hospital cardiac arrest patients rescued by extracorporeal cardiopulmonary resuscitation. Int J Cardiol 2013;168(4):3424–3430

26. Maekawa K, Tanno K, Hase M, Mori K, Asai Y. Extracorporeal cardiopulmonary resuscitation for patients with out-of-

hospital cardiac arrest of cardiac origin: a propensity-matched study and predictor analysis. Crit Care Med 2013;41(5): 1186–1196

27. Brodie D, Bacchetta M. Extracorporeal membrane oxygenation for ARDS in adults. N Engl J Med 2011;365(20):1905–1914

28. Arlt M, Philipp A, Voelkel S, et al. Early experiences with miniaturized extracorporeal life-support in the catheterization laboratory. Eur J Cardiothorac Surg 2012;42(5):858–863

29. Tayara W, Starling RC, Yamani MH, Wazni O, Jubran F, Smedira N. Improved survival after acute myocardial infarction complicated by cardiogenic shock with circulatory support and transplantation: comparing aggressive intervention with conservative treatment. J Heart Lung Transplant 2006; 25(5):504–509

30. Rihal CS, Naidu SS, Givertz MM, et al; Society for Cardiovascular Angiography and Interventions (SCAI); Heart Failure Society of America (HFSA); Society of Thoracic Surgeons (STS); American Heart Association (AHA), and American College of Cardiology (ACC). 2015 SCAI/ACC/HFSA/STS clinical expert consensus statement on the use of percutaneous mechanical circulatory support devices in cardiovascular care: endorsed by the American Heart Association, the Cardiological Society of India, and Sociedad Latino Americana de Cardiologia Intervencion; Affirmation of Value by the Canadian Association of Interventional Cardiology-Association Canadienne de Cardiologie d'intervention. J Am Coll Cardiol 2015;65(19): e7–e26

31. Abrams D, Combes A, Brodie D. Extracorporeal membrane oxygenation in cardiopulmonary disease in adults. J Am Coll Cardiol 2014;63(25 Pt A):2769–2778

32. Spina R, Forrest AP, Adams MR, Wilson MK, Ng MK, Vallely MP. Veno-arterial extracorporeal membrane oxygenation for high-risk cardiac catheterisation procedures. Heart Lung Circ 2010;19(12):736–741

33. Hochman JS, Sleeper LA, Webb JG, et al. Early revascularization in acute myocardial infarction complicated by cardiogenic shock. SHOCK Investigators. Should we emergently revascularize occluded coronaries for cardiogenic shock? N Engl J Med 1999;341(9):625–634

34. Takayama H, Truby L, Koekort M, et al. Clinical outcome of mechanical circulatory support for refractory cardiogenic shock in the current era. J Heart Lung Transplant 2013;32(1):106–111

35. Rastan AJ, Dege A, Mohr M, et al. Early and late outcomes of 517 consecutive adult patients treated with extracorporeal membrane oxygenation for refractory postcardiotomy cardiogenic shock. J Thorac Cardiovasc Surg 2010;139(2): 302–311, 311.e1

36. Asaumi Y, Yasuda S, Morii I, et al. Favourable clinical outcome in patients with cardiogenic shock due to fulminant myocarditis supported by percutaneous extracorporeal membrane oxygenation. Eur Heart J 2005;26(20):2185–2192

37. Joshua Krieger MD, Jenelle Badulak MD. The use of ECMO in patients with cardiopulmonary failure due to COVID-19. American College of Cardiology. 2020. https://www.acc.org/latest-in-cardiology/articles/2020/08/03/12/44/the-use-of-ecmo-in-patients-with-cardiopulmonary-failure-due-to-covid-19

38. Meuwese, CL, Brodie D, Donker DW. The ABCDE approach to difficult weaning from venoarterial extracorporeal membrane oxygenation. Crit Care 2022;26:216

39. Li Y, Xu R, Cao CS, Huang L. The successful use of extracorporeal membrane oxygenation combined with continuous renal replacement therapy for a cardiac arrest patient with refractory hypokalemia and diabetic ketoacidosis. World J Emerg Med. 2022;13(4):337–340

40. Kato Y, Kuriyama A, Hata R, Ikegami T. Extracorporeal membrane oxygenation for hypokalemia and refractory ventricular fibrillation associated with caffeine intoxication. J Emerg Med. 2019 S0736–S4679(19)30806–6

42

Utility of ECMO in Accidental Poisoning and Intoxication

Vivek Gupta, Rajiv Gupta, and Gurpreet Singh Wander

Introduction

As a result of severe poisoning there may be cardiac intoxication, dysfunction leading to cardiac arrest, arrhythmias, or cardiogenic shock. In the western world, the common intoxicants used for self-poisoning are analgesics, tricyclic antidepressants, antipsychotics, and cardiotoxic drugs. In the developing world, however, the main intoxicants used as suicide/homicide poisons are household pesticides and toxins, rat poisons, or alum. So poisons and their contents vary globally. Majority of the self-poisoning patients are young and inherently healthy. Extracorporeal membrane oxygenation (ECMO) today is used along with renal replacement therapy (RRT) and transplant as salvage therapy or as a bridge to antidote. So, ECMO is used as a bridge to transplant, a bridge to recovery, and now as a bridge to antidote. Despite conventional supportive therapy, when patient continues to remain in refractory hypoxemia or cardiogenic shock, then ECMO is very useful. ECMO facilitates removal of toxins by redistributing them from the central cannulation, facilitates their metabolism, and hastens their removal. Evidence in literature has shown the beneficial effects of ECMO in enhancing contractility and oxygenation in poisoned patients, yet ECMO remains an underutilized entity even in developing countries. Literature reiterates initiating ECMO early for best results, but prognostication, time to initiation, and criteria to initiate ECMO remain largely unanswered. Future studies and extracorporeal life support organization (ELSO) contribution in developing global data for poisoned patients will help in answering these questions in the near future and thus provide the above answer.

ECMO When Conventional Therapy Fails

A common observation in the emergency department is mild-to-severe form of cardiac OR respiratory failure following the ingestion of chemical, drugs, or other pharmaceutical substances.[1] Though conventional therapy and specific antidotes exist for most toxic substances but these may not be enough to sustain life when cardiorespiratory arrest happens. In children, particularly, any inadvertent accidents or mishaps come to notice immediately, whereas in adults the toxic substance ingestion is deliberate and not accidental, with intent to suicide. Thus, emergency presentation of patients with toxic ingestion is either accidental or suicidal in nature.[2]

The number of patients presenting to the emergency department of a hospital due to self-ingestion of poison has increased over the years. Inadvertent or accidental poisoning is an important cause of mortality, is usually more common in the younger age group, and far exceeds the road traffic accidents. The nature of poisons varies across different continents.[3,4]

ECMO Use in Adults and Pediatric Population is on the Rise

ECMO use in patients in the past four decades has increased by leaps and bounds. The increase in adult followed the success of the HINI influenza.[5] Today in COVID pandemic, ECMO use in adults and children is similar.[6] ECMO provides time and acts as a bridge to the failing heart and lungs, when all other conventional therapy fails.[7] So, ECMO is a temporary measure till definitive therapy is available. A good example is a patient with pulmonary embolus resulting in right ventricular (RV) failures—such a patient can undergo pulmonary thrombectomy on ECMO for a short period of time.

ECMO with Adjuvant Mechanical Support is the Norm

Poisoning and intoxication can lead to mortality due to failure of essential organs. Sedation-induced respiratory failure markedly improves with mechanical ventilation. RRT helps to remove toxins causing acute renal failure. However, the use of ECMO in cardiac failure due to acute poisoning has been a controversial issue.[8,9] ECMO helps in providing both perfusion and oxygenation in an acutely poisoned patient till the toxin levels are completely eliminated. Similarly, continuous renal replacement therapy (CRRT) may be added to aid ECMO for complete toxin elimination (**Flowchart 42.1**).

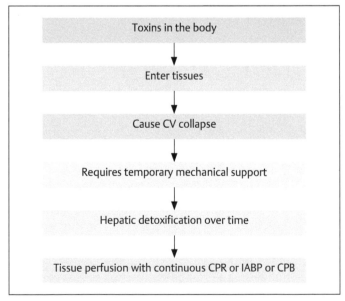

Flowchart 42.1 ECMO use with toxins ingestion. Abbreviations: CPB, cardiopulmonary bypass; CPR, cardiopulmonary resuscitation; CV, cardiovascular; ECMO, extracorporeal membrane oxygenation; IABP, intra-aortic balloon pump.

In a patient with increased amlodipine intoxication, Schmidt et al used venoarterial ECMO for hemodynamic support and added to it a high cut-off dialyzers called CytoSorb adsorbed, in two different sessions, for complete amlodipine elimination. ECMO alone, without CytoSorb use could not have eliminated the drug, the authors concluded.

The new ECMO circuit with its miniaturization, heparin-coated circuits, and better oxygenation has made treatment of intoxication safe in the hands of the ECMO intensivists (**Flowchart 42.1**).[10–12] There are many new developments related to specific strategies for treating patients post poisoning exposures, but the simplest treatment remains symptomatic and supportive care.[13]

COVID-19 and VV ECMO

Shimoyama et al[14,15] treated COVID-19-induced thrombosis and bleeding by relating the cause of bleeding in COVID-19 patients to increased fragility of capillary vessels. These patients may need massive transfusions and venovenous (VV) ECMO with meticulous monitoring of anticoagulation with free heparin intervals. Thus, intensivists should explore, in greater depth, the realms of ECMO in toxic patients. As yet, even ELSO has not declared ECMO as rescue modality in acute intoxication with cardiac arrest. This chapter gives a brief outline of existing literature on this subject.

It is the miniaturization of the ECMO circuit, along with sleeker circuitry of the ECMO components and advanced ECMO component technology, which has paved the way for intensivists to promote the use of ECMO in the ICU. ECMO with or without an intra-aortic balloon pump (IABP) or CRRT for detoxication is today a well-known rescue therapy, but it has not been included in any guidelines or textbook chapter. This chapter deals with intoxicants across the globe, their clinical epidemiology, acute cardiotoxic intoxicants, extracorporeal life support (ECLS) practices across the globe, and ECMO as a bridge to antidote.[16]

Types of Common Intoxications

Three types of poisonous substances exist in nature. The first group is that of chemicals used for industrial, agricultural, medical, and healthcare products. The second is a group of biological poisons used as plant and animal toxins. The third group is that of chemicals used for intentional or unintentional poisoning. The clinical symptoms of poisoning may range from mild to severe and life-endangering cardiovascular collapse. The types of poisoning too may range from suicides, homicides, intentional or unintentional, or lead or occupational as in mica mining.[17] The clinical effects of poisoning may range from minor effects of atropine poisoning, not requiring intensive treatment, to intentional poisoning requiring much and more than acute active treatment.

Pesticide poisoning is on the rise globally, accounting for nearly 2.5 million deaths,[18] in a country like India and other developing South Asian countries. It is agricultural poisoning which is a major menace. Around four lakh victims die due to both accidental and unintentional chemical poisoning in India, each year, thus contributing nearly 6.3% of them to chemical cardiotoxic substances.[17] The highest mortality is with pesticide intoxication, most commonly in the western world. Mortality is due to biological substances of abuse and illegal drugs and some culprit drugs such as tricyclic antidepressants, analgesics, most of the cardiac drugs, as well as many antipsychotics and sedatives.[17,19] It is the younger population which is more afflicted with poisoning (**Box 42.1** and **Table 42.1**).

Box 42.1   Resuscitation protocol for managing poisoning
• Prompt assessment and maintenance of compromised airway
• Support breathing
• Optimize the circulations[9]
• Provide short-term ventilator support in case of difficulty in breathing following ingestion, till the poisonous substance is eliminated or metabolized[20]
• Optimize blood pressure
• Give intravenous fluid boluses continuously till hemodynamic is stable
• Administer specific antidote at the earliest
• Use vasopressor and inotropes, if hypotension persists despite fluids[19]
• Use antiarrhythmic drugs to combat the tachycardia and arrhythmias that may occur
• Correct the acidosis, hypokalemia, hypomagnesaemia, and hypoxia at the earliest to reduce the arrhythmias[21]
• Bedside hemodynamic monitoring, improved treatment of cardiovascular shock, and intensive fastidious therapy are the backbone of all success[21,22]
• CV collapse due to poisoning is as high as 17%, as seen in sudden collapse in the young[23]
• Severity and toxic efficacy of the poison determines "the severity of the symptom"[24]

Abbreviation: CV, cardiovascular.

Table 42.1 List of toxic substances with immense cardiotoxic potential

Toxic substances and conditions	Examples
Medical conditions	Hypoxia, hypokalemia, hypovolemia, systemic vasodilatation, decreased myocardial function, arrhythmias
Acute toxic cardiac failure	Reduced myocardial contractility[25]
Membrane-stabilizing drugs	**Class I antiarrhythmic drugs (Vaughan-Williams class I)** • β-Blocker • Bupropion • Phenytoin and carbamazepine • Tricyclic antidepressants • Cocaine • Amphetamines • Dextropropoxyphene like opioids
Other drugs	• Colchicine • Digoxin • Calcium channel blockers • Meprobamate
Pesticides, herbicides, and rodenticides	• Organophosphorus • Parquet • Alum • Yellow phosphide • Zinc phosphide
Plant toxins	• Aconite taxus
Carbon monoxide inhalation Cyanide poisoning	

Poisoning leads to respiratory and cardiac collapse, as shown in **Flowchart 42.2**, and its consequences are disastrous.[20–24]

ECMO use in acute heart or lung failure, despite supraoptimal medical therapy, warrants letting the patient relatives know of the high risk of mortality. As in other indications for ECMO, so also in these sick patients of poisoning, ECMO should be considered based on the factors listed in **Box 42.2**.

The indications for ECMO whether VV ECMO (respiratory) or venoarterial (VA) ECMO (cardiorespiratory failure) may vary in poisoning patients. Whenever there are situations of cardiac dysfunction or ventilator and oxygenation problems, which do not improve with standard ventilation, then ECMO is very useful.[27] Examples of such cases may include organic substances (e.g., hydrocarbon-containing thinners and paint removers), which bring about good results if initiated at an early stage for a reversible cause. As no guidelines on ECMO for toxicology exist, on clinical judgment alone, for initiating ECMO, in a patient without irreversible effects, some intensivists may depend on a scoring system such as the Murray score, but these scores aid in identifying the grade 3 and 4 patients. This scoring system for classifying a poisoned patient has its own limitations due to its subjective nature; however, it may help in identifying the most severe form of patients.[28]

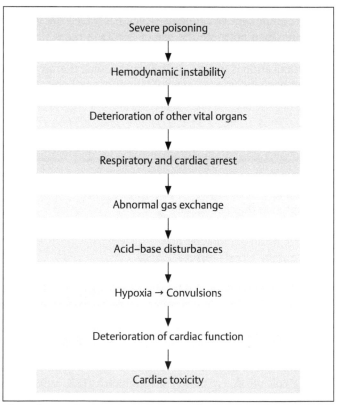

Flowchart 42.2 Consequences of cardiac and respiratory poisoning.

ECMO Types in Toxicity

NO recovery is seen in a toxicity patient with conventional therapy, especially when no antidote for the poison is ingested. It is in this case that a VA ECMO can help revive the biventricular cardiac dysfunction, give the lung a "Rest-period," revive a cardiac collapse/shock, and ensure recovery of the cardiorespiratory function. Factors on which the time period of ECMO is dependent are enumerated in **Box 42.3**. VA ECMO here acts as "bridge to recovery" as it not only enhances the cardiac and respiratory function but also reduces the requirement of oxygen consumption. VV ECMO can be initiated in those patients who upon ingestion of the toxin develop acute respiratory distress syndrome (ARDS) and who is unresponsive to non-ECMO management. VV ECMO takes care of the ventilator support to the patient, by providing "lung rest." Patient in cardiogenic shock, due to poisoning with unknown multiple drugs, can benefit from the VV ECMO. It also helps in the management of malignant arrhythmias. The elimination of poisonous metabolic is proportional to the duration of ECMO support.[29-31]

ECMO, as described above, aids recovery and is a temporary procedure. It can act as a bridge for many situations as listed in **Box 42.4** and **Table 42.2**.

How Extracorporeal Therapies Benefit Poisoning

RRT may be useful in acute severe intoxication in several ways: it not only helps in removing certain toxins but also helps in optimizing hemodynamics by metabolic acidosis correction. This improved hemodynamics further helps in redistribution, and enhances metabolism and elimination of toxic substance.

The modalities employed for treating acute intoxication may be divided into two groups as listed in **Table 42.3**. For example, in acute poisoning of methanol, which may sometimes land up in a mass casualty of methanol poisoning,

RRT may be given either in an intermittent or a continuous manner, as shown in **Box 42.5**. We are all aware that the blood of the patient and the dialysate move in a countercurrent mechanism. Toxin removal depends on a few factors as enumerated in **Box 42.6**. Surface area and pore size of the artificial kidney are the most important factors.

Some substances which have a low molecular weight, less than 500 Daltons such as salicylates, and lithium which has low lipid solubility are most easily dialyzable. These substances have a rather small volume of distribution and poor protein binding as well. Based on the principle of convection therapy, we can use the hemofiltration therapy for substances with a higher molecular weight (>30,000 Da) such as vancomycin, parquet, procainamide, hirudin, thallium, lithium, and methotrexate.[29-36] Generally, we look at the protein binding and the sieving coefficient of higher molecular weight substances for successful hemofiltration and toxin elimination.[37-41]

Whenever, a patient of ECMO develops a Acute Kidney Injury or has a hemodynamic compromise, continuous renal replacement therapy (CRRT) is the treatment of choice.[42-45] Lactate production due to shock alters both intracellular and extracellular pH.[46] Patients having severe acidosis are relatively resistant to the action of vasopressors.[47] Moreover, an initial response with vasopressors decreases and requires higher doses with the development of metabolic acidosis. The correction of acidosis has shown the improvement of cardiac function and hemodynamics.[48] The main principle for acidosis correction is correction of underlying cause; however, in some severely hypotensive patients RRT helps in correcting metabolic acidosis and improving the hemodynamics as bridge till the underlying cause is addressed.[49] Continuous therapies are preferred for correction of pH and more effective clearance of lactate and prevention of rebound. Furthermore, patients with severe metabolic acidosis can be effectively managed with CRRT in correcting the acid–base disturbances.[50] Lactate clearance

Table 42.2 ECMO as a bridge in poisoning

ECMO in intoxicated patient	Description
Bridge to antidote	FAB fragments for dioxin toxicity till they are available; ECMO takes care of the cardiogenic shock and the malignant arrhythmias[34,35]
Bridge to toxin elimination	Dialysis, RRT, and ECMO are well-known methods to remove many poisons. The modality is dependent upon the protein-binding types, the molecular weight of the toxin, and the volume of distribution of the toxin (**Box 42.5**).[36,37] RRT is known to remove substances only in plasma, so toxins with a large volume of distribution will be removed from the body using RRT alone, very slowly. That is why ECMO and RRT can be used together for synergistic effects.[38] If on VV ECMO hemodynamic instability persists, then a VA ECMO may be initiated to optimize the hemodynamic. The mechanism of hemofiltration and hemeadsorption is different. But they all eliminate the toxin well, either alone or in combination. Author uses plasmapheresis for acute poisoning, wherein the toxins are highly protein bound. During ECMO, prefer to do a continuous renal replacement therapy (CRRT) or a slow low efficiency dialysis (SLED) over intermittent dialysis[39,40]
Bridge to transplant	VV ECMO can be used in pulmonary fibrosis, before and during a lung transplant. During the interim period before a lung transplant VV ECMO acts as a bridge to transplant[41]

Abbreviations: ECMO, extracorporeal membrane oxygenation; RRT, renal replacement therapy; VA, venoarterial; VV, venovenous.

Table 42.3 Essential therapies for acute intoxication

Continuous therapy	Intermittent therapy
• Continuous renal replacement therapy (CRRT) • Peritoneal dialysis (PD)	• Sustained low-efficiency dialysis • Hemodialysis

Box 42.5 Methods used for toxin elimination

• Dialysis
• Hemoperfusion and hemadsorption
• Hemofiltration
• RRT
• ECMO VV or VA
• Plasmapheresis

Box 42.6 Factors on which toxin removal depends[39]

• Surface area of artificial kidney
• Pore size of artificial kidney membrane
• Blood flow rate
• Type and total amount of dialysate

Abbreviations: ECMO, extracorporeal membrane oxygenation; RRT, renal replacement therapy; VA, venoarterial; VV, venovenous.

with CRRT may be <3% as compared to normal kidney but improvement in hemodynamics with metabolic acidosis correction may improve the lactate clearance.[51] CRRT uses both diffusive and corrective principle for solute removal depending on the chosen therapy. The advantages of CRRT include not only the institution of therapy in hemodynamically unstable, acutely intoxicated patients, but also prevention of rebound phenomenon in certain toxins due to large volume of distribution and slow redistribution among the various body compartments.[52]

Does ECMO in Poisoning Show Substantial Medical Evidence?

Weiner et al, in 2019,[53] reiterated VA ECMO for cardiac drug overdose toxicity and concluded that VA ECMO improved the hemodynamics as the metabolic parameters in patients with drug-induced cardiogenic shock, despite a few randomized control studies only having sporadic case reports and literature reviews on the literature shows sporadic case reports and review articles on the use of any form of ECMO for drug induced toxicity. No guidelines exist on the same and for ARDS and ECMO as well.[53] So, caution should be warranted in all poison cases before starting and maintaining an ECMO. Also, the duration of ECMO use in most animal studies has been recorded for drugs such as lidocaine, desipramine, or amitriptyline. But, animal studies show positivity in ECMO use for refractory cardiogenic shock, if ECMO is started in these sick and toxic patients immediately and patients are closely monitored during the ECMO support. In a cohort of 17 patients receiving ECMO for refractory cardiac arrest, 14 patients were stable on VA ECMO. Between the refractory cardiac arrest and the drug poisoning group, the survival was better in the latter.[54] In another French study on a smaller population, care should be monitored for the above cases. Also in cases of overdose of propafenone tricyclic antidepressants, chloroquine diuretics, and sclerosing agents, the patients benefit with the use of VA ECMO. Cardiogenic shock due to drug poisoning responds well to

VA ECMO than the refractory cardiogenic shock. The survival rate was 86% in ECMO versus 48% in conventional therapy for cardiogenic shock in a retrospective French study.[55] The number of cases studied were far too small in all trials so far. Case reports on ECMO use for drugs, as listed in **Box 42.7**, exist in literature but these drugs in both adult and pediatric patients are all on VA ECMO.

In cases of drug poisoning the time of ECMO initiation and ECMO duration were different. As per case reports intensivist should use ECMO early for less mortality, even though these case reports have a degree of bias in them. The use of VA ECMO for poisoning with membrane-stabilizing drugs reported 90% success.[56] Patients were weaned off easily from emergency cardiopulmonary bypass (ECPB) when it was first started in these patients. Bleeding, ischemia, hemorrhage, and thrombosis were witnessed in almost all cases of cardiogenic shock on VA ECMO for drug toxicity. RRT was also started in some patients along with ECMO.[38] The authors concluded that ECPB is a safe method for managing severely poisoned patients due to drug overdose, who are in cardiogenic shock and require VA ECMO.

ECMO has been used successfully for many years for the drugs listed in **Box 42.7**. Drug poisoning with pesticides, plant toxins, cyanides, and carbon monoxide is common in developing world and ECMO is not so commonly used in such cases. So, only a few sporadic case reports exist. Baran et al, in October 2020,[57] successfully reported the use of VV ECMO, in a 10-year-old child with carbon monoxide poisoning, who looked "PINK," was in altered sensorial, and whose carboxyhemoglobin was 18%. Using the right internal jugular vein (IJV) in the catheterized laboratory and the carboxyhemoglobin levels soon decreased. VV ECMO was weaned off the next day. Yu et al[58] also have shown good result of ECMO use for acute toxic intoxications. Both VV and VA ECMO[56] may be used successfully to manage the tissue hypoxia, seen in carbon monoxide poisoning and other toxic inhalational pesticides (**Box 42.8**). Another poison is aluminum phosphide, which is used as poison for suicide/homicide purposes in the northern and north-western parts of India. Patients poisoned with aluminum phosphide show good results on a VA ECMO, especially improvement in left baseline left ventricular (LV) ejection fraction. A longer delay in hospital presentation was found to be mortality predictors in an Indian study. Taxus is a plant toxin which heralds the onset of cardiogenic shock with severe ventricular arrhythmias. These patients too have been successfully managed on a VA ECMO.[59] VV ECMO is good in treating phosphorus poisoning of organs and patients with pulmonary fibrosis post poisoning as VV ECMO efficiently improves gas exchange.[60]

Conclusion

ECMO is getting a good pedestal over conventional therapy in acutely poisoned patient with refractory cardiogenic shock. It is not easily available, is expensive, needs

---

Box 42.7   Drugs implicated for cardiogenic shock and requiring ECMO therapy
• Flecainide • β-Blocker • Calcium channel blockers • Digoxin • Tricyclic antidepressants • Bupropion • Methamphetamine • Mepivacaine

Box 42.8   Indications for the use of VV and VA ECMO in intoxication
VA ECMO • Persistent/progressive hypotension despite high inotropic support • Persistent severe metabolic and/or lactic acidosis • Refractory arrhythmias • Cardiac arrest **VV ECMO** • Acute reversible lung injury with inhalational toxins • Severe hypoxemia ($PaO_2/FiO_2 < 80$) • Uncompensated hypercapnia (pH < 7.2)

Abbreviations: ECMO, extracorporeal membrane oxygenation; PaO_2, partial pressure of oxygen; VA, venoarterial; VV, venovenous.

a team of experts to run it successfully, and because of these constraints, it remains a rarely used modality. Acute toxic poisons of all kinds get eliminated by an antidote or extracorporeal therapies like ECMO, CRRT, hemoperfusion, hemodialysis, hemadsorption, or slow low-efficiency dialysis (SLED). The life-threatening complications of ECMO also hinder its active use. The use of VA ECMO or VV ECMO in an acute intoxication depends on the type of poison and the damaged end organ. The ELSO data registry is also working on collecting data globally in order to create ECMO guidelines on acute intoxications. ECMO should not be used in cases of irreversible organ damage. There should be no hesitancy, to institute ECMO with CRRT in cases of hemodynamic compromise. ECMO provides both hemodynamic and respiratory support, in cases of toxic ingestion by patients. ECMO specially helps in cases of patients in refractory shock, cardiac arrest or respiratory failure.[61] (BOX 12) As observed in literature patients generally report more with incidence of intentional poisoning VA ECMO use has been shown to be cost-effective in life-years consistent use of CRRT, hemodialysis, hemoperfusion, apheresis with ECMO, should be considered with the multi-speciality ECMO team. Early treatment by a medical toxicologist and ECMO intensivist is crucial for survival, as has been observed recently, by C ward et al, in a patient with yew tree berries poisoning, wherein the patient's cardiogenic shock condition was treated with prompt institution of ECMO.[62]

It should be noted that ECMO is a bridge to recovery, to a more durable bridge, to a definitive treatment, or to a better clinical decision, and is a powerful tool that should be used judiciously.[63]

References

1. Kapur N, House A, Creed F, Feldman E, Friedman T, Guthrie E. Management of deliberate self-poisoning in adults in four teaching hospitals: descriptive study. BMJ 1998;316(7134): 831–832

2. Office for National Statistics. Numbers of deaths from drug-related poisoning by underlying cause, England and Wales, 1998–2002. In: Census UK 2001.London: Office for National Statistics; 2001

3. 49th edition of the Report of National Crime Records Bureau. Accidental Deaths & Suicides in India–2015. http://ncrb.gov.in

4. Mowry JB, Spyker DA, Brooks DE, et al. 2015 Annual Report of the American Association of Poison Control Centers' National Poison Data System (NPDS): 33rd Annual Report. Clin Toxicol 2016;54(10):924–1109

5. Domínguez-Cherit G, Lapinsky SE, Macias AE, et al. Critically Ill patients with 2009 influenza A (H1N1) in Mexico. JAMA 2009;302(17):1880–1887

6. Sauer CM, Yuh DD, Bonde P. Extracorporeal membrane oxygenation use has increased by 433% in adults in the United States from 2006 to 2011. ASAIO J 2015;61(1):31–36

7. MacLaren G, Combes A, Bartlett RH. Contemporary extra-corporeal membrane oxygenation for adult respiratory failure: life support in the new era. Intensive Care Med 2012;38(2): 210–220

8. Albertson TE, Dawson A, de Latorre F, et al; American Heart Association; International Liaison Committee on Resuscitation. TOX-ACLS: toxicologic-oriented advanced cardiac life support. Ann Emerg Med 2001;37(4, Suppl):S78–S90

9. Holzer M, Sterz F, Schoerkhuber W, et al. Successful resuscitation of a verapamil-intoxicated patient with percutaneous cardio-pulmonary bypass. Crit Care Med 1999;27(12):2818–2823

10. Schmidt JJ, Busch M, David S, et al. Life-threatening amlodipine over dose requiring ECMO support treated by high-cut-off dialysis and Cytosorb. J Clin Toxicol 2021;11(3):1000479

11. Orr DA, Bramble MG. Tricyclic antidepressant poisoning and prolonged external cardiac massage during asystole. Br Med J (Clin Res Ed) 1981;283(6299):1107–1108

12. Jeyaratnam J. Acute pesticide poisoning: a major global health problem. World Health Stat Q 1990;43(3):139–144

13. Eddleston M. Patterns and problems of deliberate self-poisoning in the developing world. QJM 2000;93(11):715–731

14. Abrams D, Lorusso R, Vincent JL, Brodie D. ECMO during the COVID-19 pandemic: when is it unjustified? Crit Care 2020; 24(1):507

15. Shimoyama K, Azuma K, Oda J. A patient with COVID-19 and bleeding complications due to neurofibromatosis type 1 during VV-ECMO: a case report. Medicine (Baltimore) 2021; 100(51):e28094

16. Gupta V, Gupta R, Wander GS. Role of ECMO in life threatening intoxication. Egyptian J Crit Care Med 2018;6(3):103–109

17. Kishi M, Ladou J. International pesticide use. Introduction. Int J Occup Environ Health 2001;7(4):259–265

18. Santana VS, Moura MC, Ferreira e Nogueira F. [Occupational pesticide poisoning mortality, 2000-2009, Brazil]. Rev Saude Publica 2013;47(3):598–606

19. Jones AL, Dargan PI. Churchill's pocket book of toxicology. London: Churchill Livingstone; 2001

20. Mokhlesi B, Leikin JB, Murray P, Corbridge TC. Adult toxicology in critical care: Part II: specific poisonings. Chest 2003;123(3):897–922

21. Riou B, Barriot P, Rimailho A, Baud FJ. Treatment of severe chloroquine poisoning. N Engl J Med 1988;318(1):1–6

22. Clemessy JL, Taboulet P, Hoffman JR, et al. Treatment of acute chloroquine poisoning: a 5-year experience. Crit Care Med 1996;24(7):1189–1195

23. Manini AF, Nelson LS, Stimmel B, Vlahov D, Hoffman RS. Incidence of adverse cardiovascular events in adults following drug overdose. Acad Emerg Med 2012;19(7):843–849

24. Huikuri HV, Castellanos A, Myerburg RJ. Sudden death due to cardiac arrhythmias. N Engl J Med 2001;345(20):1473–1482

25. Kolecki PF, Curry SC. Poisoning by sodium channel blocking agents. Crit Care Clin 1997;13(4):829–848

26. ELSO guidelines for cardiopulmonary extracorporeal life support. Extracorporeal Life Support Organization, Version 1.4 August 2017 Ann Arbor, MI USA. www.elso.org

27. Mielck F, Quintel M. Extracorporeal membrane oxygenation. Curr Opin Crit Care 2005;11(1):87–93

28. Persson HE, Sjöberg GK, Haines JA, Pronczuk de Garbino J. Poisoning severity score. Grading of acute poisoning. J Toxicol Clin Toxicol 1998;36(3):205–213

29. Chung M, Shiloh AL, Carlese A. Monitoring of the adult patient on venoarterial extracorporeal membrane oxygenation. ScientWorld J 2014;2014:393258

30. Mohamed YA, Akram AA, Mohamed MK. Veno-venous extracorporeal membrane oxygenation in a case of organo-phosphorus poisoning. Egyptian J Crit Care Med 2016;4:43–46

31. Roberto R, Barbara C, Roberto M, et al. Extra-corporeal life support for near-fatal multi-drug intoxication: a case report. J Med Case Reports 2011;5:231

32. Lee J-H, Kim H-S, Park J-H, et al. Incidence and clinical course of left ventricular systolic dysfunction in patients with carbon monoxide poisoning. Korean Circ J 2016;46(5):665–671

33. Hassanian-Moghaddam H, Zamani N, Rahimi M, Hajesmaeili M, Taherkhani M, Sadeghi R. Successful treatment of alu-minium phosphide poisoning by extracorporeal membrane oxygenation. Basic Clin Pharmacol Toxicol 2016;118(3): 243–246

34. Idialisoa R, Jouffroy R, Lamhaut L, et al. Extra corporeal life support in life-threatening digoxin overdose: a bridge to antidote Austin. Emerg Med 2016;2(5):1029

35. Chan BS, Buckley NA. Digoxin-specific antibody fragments in the treatment of digoxin toxicity. Clin Toxicol (Phila) 2014;52(8):824–836

36. Doolan PD, Walsh WP, Wishinsky H. Acetylsalicylic acid intoxication; a proposed method of treatment. J Am Med Assoc 1951;146(2):105–106

37. Holubek WJ, Hoffman RS, Goldfarb DS, Nelson LS. Use of hemodialysis and hemoperfusion in poisoned patients. Kidney Int 2008;74(10):1327–1334

38. Daubin C, Lehoux P, Ivascau C, et al. Extracorporeal life support in severe drug intoxication: a retrospective cohort study of seventeen cases. Crit Care 2009;13(4):R138

39. Winchester JF. Dialysis and hemoperfusion in poisoning. Adv Ren Replace Ther 2002;9(1):26–30

40. Amir AR, Winchester JF. Hemodialysis and hemoperfusion in the management of drug intoxication. In: Massry SG, Glassock RJ, eds. Massry & Glassock's textbook of nephrology, 4th ed. Philadelphia: Lippincott Williams and Wilkins; 2001: 1729–35

41. Tang X, Sun B, He H, et al. Successful extracorporeal membrane oxygenation therapy as a bridge to sequential bilateral lung transplantation for a patient after severe paraquat poisoning. Clin Toxicol (Phila) 2015;53(9):908–913

42. Kraut JA, Kurtz I. Use of base in the treatment of acute severe organic acidosis by nephrologists and critical care physicians: results of an online survey. Clin Exp Nephrol 2006;10(2): 111–117

43. Lutz PL, Lapennas GN. Effects of pH, CO2 and organic phosphates on oxygen affinity of sea turtle hemoglobins. Respir Physiol 1982;48(1):75–87

44. Berger DS, Fellner SK, Robinson KA, Vlasica K, Godoy IE, Shroff SG. Disparate effects of three types of extracellular acidosis on left ventricular function. Am J Physiol 1999;276(2):H582–H594

45. Otter D, Austin C. Simultaneous monitoring of vascular contractility, intracellular pH and intracellular calcium in isolated rat mesenteric arteries; effects of weak bases. Exp Physiol 2000;85(3):349–351

46. Levy B, Collin S, Sennoun N, et al. Vascular hyporesponsiveness to vasopressors in septic shock: from bench to bedside. Intensive Care Med 2010;36(12):2019–2029

47. Teplinsky K, O'Toole M, Olman M, Walley KR, Wood LD. Effect of lactic acidosis on canine hemodynamics and left ventricular function. Am J Physiol 1990;258(4 Pt 2):H1193–H1199

48. Weil MH, Houle DB, Brown EB Jr, Campbell GS, Heath C. Vasopressor agents; influence of acidosis on cardiac and vascular responsiveness. Calif Med 1958;88(6):437–440

49. Peters N, Jay N, Barraud D, et al. Metformin-associated lactic acidosis in an intensive care unit. Crit Care 2008;12(6):R149

50. Hilton PJ, Taylor J, Forni LG, Treacher DF. Bicarbonate-based haemofiltration in the management of acute renal failure with lactic acidosis. QJM 1998;91(4):279–283

51. Levraut J, Ciebiera J-P, Jambou P, Ichai C, Labib Y, Grimaud D. Effect of continuous venovenous hemofiltration with dialysis on lactate clearance in critically ill patients. Crit Care Med 1997;25(1):58–62

52. Leblanc M, Raymond M, Bonnardeaux A, et al. Lithium poisoning treated by high-performance continuous arterio-venous and venovenous hemodiafiltration. Am J Kidney Dis 1996;27(3):365–372

53. Weiner L, Perroud N, Weibel S. Attention Deficit Hyperactivity Disorder And Borderline Personality Disorder In Adults: A Review Of Their Links And Risks. Neuropsychiatr Dis Treat. 2019 Nov 8;15:3115–3129

54. Mégarbane B, Leprince P, Deye N, et al. Emergency feasibility in medical intensive care unit of extracorporeal life support for refractory cardiac arrest. Intensive Care Med 2007;33(5): 758–764

55. Masson R, Colas V, Parienti JJ, et al. A comparison of survival with and without extracorporeal life support treatment for severe poisoning due to drug intoxication. Resuscitation 2012;83(11):1413–1417

56. Shenoi AN, Gertz SJ, Mikkilineni S, Kalyanaraman M. Refractory hypotension from massive bupropion overdose successfully treated with extracorporeal membrane oxygenation. Pediatr Emerg Care 2011;27(1):43–45

57. Baran DA, Stelling K, McQueen D, Pearson M, Shah V. Pediatric veno-veno extracorporeal membrane oxygenation rescue from carbon monoxide poisoning. Pediatr Emerg Care 2020; 36(10):e592–e594

58. Yu D, Xiaolin Z, Lei P, Feng L, Lin Z, Jie S. Extracorporeal membrane oxygenation for acute toxic inhalations: case reports and literature review. Front Med (Lausanne) 2021;8:745555

59. Mohan B, Singh B, Gupta V, et al. Outcome of patients supported by extracorporeal membrane oxygenation for aluminum phosphide poisoning: an observational study. Indian Heart J 2016;68(3):295–301

60. Vardon Bounes F, Tardif E, Ruiz S, Gallart JC, Conil JM, Delmas C. Suicide attempt with self-made Taxus baccata leaf capsules: survival following the application of extracorporeal membrane oxygenation for ventricular arrhythmia and refractory cardio-genic shock. Clin Toxicol (Phila) 2017;55(8):925–928

61. Upchurch C, Blumenberg A, Brodie D, MacLaren G, Zakhary B, Hendrickson RG. Extracorporeal membrane oxygenation use in poisoning: a narrative review with clinical recommendations. Clin Toxicol (Phila). 2021 Oct;59(10):877-887.

62. Ward C, Meeks D, Trimlett R, Alçada J. Taxine alkaloid poisoning successfully supported with venoarterial extracorporeal membrane oxygenation: a case report. Eur Heart J Case Rep. 2022;6(2):ytac039.

63. Yu D, Xiaolin Z, Lei P, Feng L, Lin Z, Jie S. Extracorporeal Membrane Oxygenation for Acute Toxic Inhalations: Case Reports and Literature Review. Front Med (Lausanne). 2021;8:745555

43

Intervention Lung Assist: Pumpless Extracorporeal and Paracorporeal Technology for Refractory Respiratory Failure

Poonam Malhotra Kapoor, P. Praveen, S. Rajmohan, Ritu Airan, and Rajiv Gupta

➢ Introduction

➢ The Novalung ILA

- Device Implantation and Operation
- Technique for Implantation of NovaLung ILA

➢ Indications for Therapy

➢ Complications and Adverse Effects of ECLA Devices

➢ Installation of Other Artificial Lung Devices

➢ Conclusion

Introduction

Acute respiratory distress syndrome (ARDS) is a life-threatening condition which is multifactorial in etiology. Breathing dysfunction occurs secondary to severe lung inflammation due to damage to underlying alveolar epithelium and surrounding capillaries, affecting their ability to exchange oxygen and carbon dioxide.[1,2] Fluid leak occurs across once-damaged alveolocapillary membrane. There is limitation of the lungs to have proper gas exchange as the alveolar spaces fill with extravasated fluids instead of air. Treatment of ARDS thus primarily involves provision of sufficient oxygen and removal of carbon dioxide from the blood. This has traditionally been achieved with the use of mechanical ventilation, antibiotics, analgesics, sedatives, and diuretics. The most effective and widely accepted intervention to reduce mortality due to ARDS has been mechanical ventilation[1] with reduction in tidal volumes (TVs)[2] and application of an adequate positive end-expiratory pressure (PEEP).

A mechanical ventilation of 8 to 10 mL/kg weight has adverse effects; thus, in most ARDS patients who have respiratory failure with acidosis and hypoxia, it is advisable to use protective ventilation strategies of low TVs (4–6 mL/kg body weight). An extracorporeal device to provide oxygen and remove carbon dioxide from such a patient may also become necessary in some extreme cases, so that gas exchange may be optimal.[3] Extracorporeal lung-assist (ECLA) devices are invasive alternatives that work by establishing a venovenous or venoarterial shunt, which bypass the failing heart and/or lungs and provide a reliable gas exchange.

They comprise a roller or centrifugal pump, a membrane for gaseous exchange, and a heat exchanger to maintain blood temperature (**Fig. 43.1**).

Extracorporeal technology complications, such as bleeding, inflammation, and surgical side effects, limit its use to advanced, specialized extracorporeal membrane oxygenation (ECMO) trained centers only. The significant blood trauma caused by ECLA devices can cause hemolysis and various coagulation disorders. Besides, the ECLA technique requires extensive knowledge and understanding of the complex equipment used. Dedicated paramedical staff which is well-trained in the technique is required and this is an expensive proposition.

The Novalung ILA

The NovaLung Interventional Lung-Assist (ILA; NovaLung GmbH, Hechingen, Germany) device is a membrane ventilator that allows the process of oxygen and carbon dioxide gas exchange to occur by simple diffusion[4,5] (**Figs. 43.2** and **43.3**). It is a low-resistance lung-assist device designed to be driven by the pulsatile blood flow of the patient, independent of any extracorporeal pump assistance. It consists of a plastic gas exchange module with diffusion membranes made from polymethylpentene (PMP) fibers woven into a complex configuration of hollow fibers. Blood flows over the exterior surface of the device's fibers and the ventilating gas flows inside these fibers, allowing gas exchange to take place without direct contact with blood. While being used

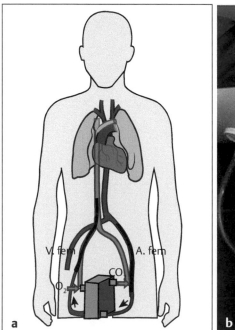
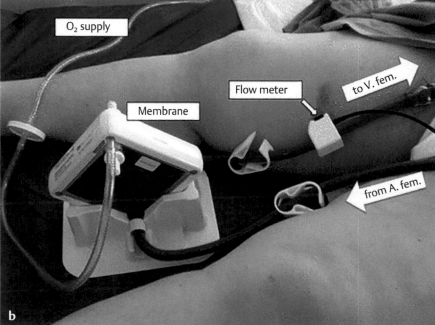

Fig. 43.1 **(a, b)** The circuit and components of the extracorporeal lung assist device (ECLA) for optimal gas exchange.

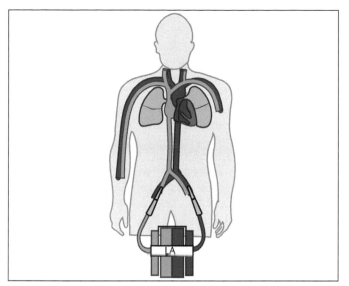

Fig. 43.2 Principles of gas exchange across a membrane lung.

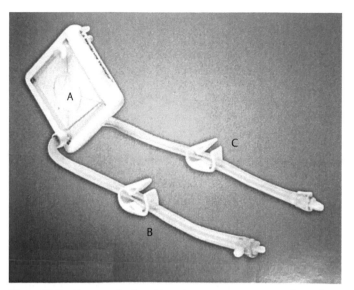

Fig. 43.3 Parts of the Novalung extracorporeal carbon dioxide removal device. A represents membrane lung; B and C represent connections to cannulas placed in femoral vein and femoral artery respectively.

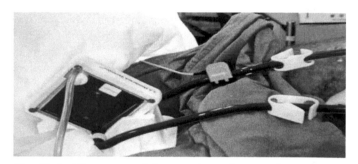

Fig. 43.4 Placement of the Novalung device in between the patient's lower limbs.

as an adjunct to mechanical ventilation, it allows for the use of lung-protective ventilation strategies, with the objective of giving the lungs time to heal while attempting to minimize ventilation-induced lung injury.[6,7] This causes reduced inflammation-induced endothelium disruption, and therefore less bleeding.

Device Implantation and Operation

ILA (**Fig. 43.2**) is attached to the systemic circulation and receives a part of the left ventricular output for extracorporeal gas exchange.[8,9] The venous and arterial cannulas are usually inserted percutaneously by Seldinger technique and application of serial dilatators. In case of presence of atherosclerotic plaques or small caliber of vessels, an open surgical wound exposure is preferable (**Fig. 43.4**).

Technique for Implantation of NovaLung ILA

For the purpose of cannulation, a single bolus of heparin (100 units/kg) is often recommended. The system usually operates on a heparin-coated system that obviates any need for systemic anticoagulation. The postoperative period, however, warrants the maintenance of the ideal activated clotting time (ACT) between 130 and 150 seconds and activated partial thromboplastin time (aPTT) between 40 and 50 seconds. The entire device with all its accessories, tubing, etc., is deaired with normal saline and oxygen through a simple gas diffusion process. These are the basic principles on which effective gaseous exchange across a membrane lung occurs in the device called NovaLung ILA (**Figs. 43.2** and **43.3**). The blood flow offers resistance to a plastic gas exchange module which encases membranes made from polymethyl pentive (PMP) fibers, which are woven into a complex array of hollow fibers. Once the tubing is connected

to the cannulas, the vascular clamps are removed allowing blood flow through the arterial line into the device and return of oxygenated blood back into the patient through the venous cannula. A flow probe is connected to the tubing line to monitor the circulating blood volume through the device. Since it is a low-gradient device designed to operate without the help of an external pump, an adequate mean arterial blood pressure (70–90 mmHg) ensures an optimal driving force.

Removal of carbon dioxide depends on the sweep gas flow rate, and oxygenation depends on shunt, arterial oxygenation saturation, and other variables. The sweep gas flow (O_2) for the gas exchange module is set at 6 to 12 L/min. The device is routinely placed in a stable position in-between patient's lower limbs for proper functioning (**Fig. 43.4**). Lower extremities are frequently examined in all patients clinically and with the use of Doppler ultrasonography to ensure adequate blood supply to the lower limbs and for prevention of limb ischemia. Once implanted, the entire system can handily be placed in between the legs.

Indications for Therapy

1. Ventilation-resistant severe hypercapnia and respiratory acidosis secondary to trauma, lung infection, and ARDS.
2. Bridge to lung transplant in patients with end-stage pulmonary failure.
3. Posttransplantation complications, such as severe acute rejection and acute graft failure.

Complications and Adverse Effects of ECLA Devices

The shunt flow is dependent on the patient's heart rate. Thus, the use of this pumpless device is of no use in patients with low cardiac output, on high and low ejection fraction. It has limited oxygenation capacity and is ideal for hypercapnic conditions. Those patients with oxygenation problems may not benefit much from ILA. As the ILA therapy involves securing large-bore vascular accesses, a 5 to 10% incidence of complications associated with establishment of vascular access and limb ischemia has been reported, which can be prevented from happening by direct central cannulation. Loss of core body temperature through the extracorporeal circulation of the ILA can be a clinically significant problem in the intensive care unit (ICU) and active interventions to prevent heat loss should be undertaken.

Installation of Other Artificial Lung Devices

As enumerated in **Table 43.1**, patients with good cardiac reserve can be supported with low-resistance artificial lungs (ALs). With an arterial drainage and venous perfusion the AL can be installed using the patient's own cardiac output. Those patients who suffer from CO_2 retention (hypercapnia) can undergo extracorporeal CO_2 removal using low-resistance ALs without a centrifugal pump, because CO_2 exchange requires less blood flow than O_2 exchange. In patients who chronically retain carbon dioxide both pumpless (NovaLung ILA) and with the centrifugal pump in the circuit (Hemolung reticular activating system (RAS)) can be carried out successfully (**Fig. 43.5**).[10-12]

There are three types of ALs. An extracorporeal AL is placed outside of the patient's body. A paracorporeal AL is placed on the patient's body. An implantable AL is placed in the patient's body.

In patients with pulmonary artery hypertension, the circuits placed in series should be avoided as it enhances the risk of right-sided heart failure. In latter cases, an AL with circuit in parallel is preferable as it decreases the right ventricular afterload especially in patients with pulmonary arterial hypertension (PAH), thus increasing coronary perfusion.

Although the coatings of ALs (**Table 43.2**) decrease the thrombogenicity of the devices, the design of many ALs is primarily square, which causes stagnation and clot formation in the corners. The clot formation then causes increased resistance in the oxygenator and decreased capacity for gas exchange. The same device, cannot be used for more than 4 weeks as clots form, and there is decrease in gaseous exchange and increase in afterload. As it is a foreign surface, it will require more anticoagulation, with increased risk of bleeding.[13-15] The AL causes damage to blood cells by shear stress. Thus, there will be increased hemolysis with loss in important blood factors like Von Willebrand factor and factor XIII leading to acquired Von Willebrand disease with ventricular-assist device (VAD) due to related VAD shear wear and tear.[16,17]

Conclusion

The ILA system is a gas exchange device that provides pulmonary support for patients suffering from ventilation-refractory severe hypercapnia and respiratory acidosis. The device is easy to handle, does not require continuous technical/perfusionist support, and is conveniently managed at bedside with routine nursing care. The costs associated with the use of the ILA are much less than the pump-driven ECLA because it does not need a pump, blood warming device, or external power source, and can be used for a longer period of time. ILA could serve as an extracorporeal assist to support mechanical ventilation by enabling low TV and a reduced inspiratory plateau pressure.[19]

Table 43.1 Extracorporeal CO_2-related complications with extracorporeal life support (ECLS) devices[18]

Type	Complications
Patient complications	• Anticoagulation-related bleeding • Hemolysis • Heparin-induced thrombocytopenia • Acquired coagulopathy • Recirculation
Catheter-related complications	• Catheter-site bleeding • Catheter malposition, dislodgement, or kinking • Catheter infection • Vascular occlusion • Thrombosis • Hematoma, aneurysm, pseudoaneurysm formation
Device-related complications	• Pump failure • Oxygenator failure • Heat exchanger malfunction • Clot formation • Air embolism

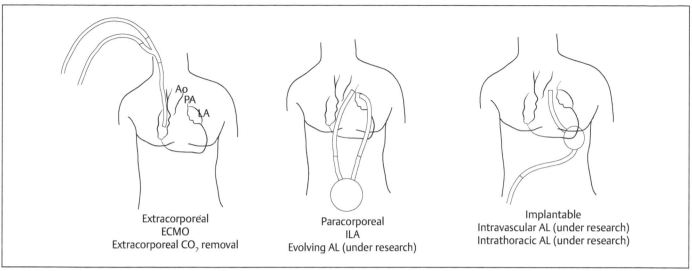

Fig. 43.5   Types of artificial lungs. Abbreviations: AL, artificial lung; Ao, aorta; ECMO, extracorporeal membrane oxygenation; ILA, interventional lung-assist device; LA, left atrium; PA, pulmonary artery.

Table 43.2   Characteristics of commercially available artificial lungs

Device	Manufacturer	Usage	Pump-in system	Priming volume (mL)	Pressure drop	Heparin coating or not
QUADROX-i	Maquet, Rastatt, Germany	Extracorporeal membrane oxygenation (ECMO)	No	215	50 mmHg at 5.0 L/min	Yes
Affinity NT	Medtronic, Eden Praire, Minnesota	ECMO	No	270	50 mmHg at 5.0 L/min	Yes
NovaLung	Xenios AG, Heilbronn, Germany	Extracorporeal CO_2 removal Paracorporeal	No	175	11 mmHg at 2.5 L/min	Yes
Hemolung	ALung Technologies, Pittsburgh, Pennsylvania	Extracorporeal CO_2 removal Paracorporeal	Yes	260	10 mmHg at 2.0 L/min	Yes

Despite a significant reduction in the mechanical power, ultra-lung-protective ventilation during 48 h did not reduce biotrauma in patients with vv-ECMO-supported ARDS. The impact of this ventilation strategy on clinical outcomes warrants further investigation.[20]

References

1. Boyle AJ, Sklar MC, McNamee JJ, et al; International ECMO Network (ECMONet). Extracorporeal carbon dioxide removal for lowering the risk of mechanical ventilation: research questions and clinical potential for the future. Lancet Respir Med 2018;6(11):874–884
2. MacLaren G, Combes A, Bartlett RH. Contemporary extracorporeal membrane oxygenation for adult respiratory failure: life support in the new era. Intensive Care Med 2012;38(2):210–220
3. Zapol WM, Snider MT, Hill JD, et al. Extracorporeal membrane oxygenation in severe acute respiratory failure. A randomized prospective study. JAMA 1979;242(20):2193–2196
4. Matheis G. New technologies for respiratory assist. Perfusion 2003;18(4):245–251
5. Liebold A, Philipp A, Kaiser M, Merk J, Schmid FX, Birnbaum DE. Pumpless extracorporeal lung assist using an arteriovenous shunt. Applications and limitations. Minerva Anestesiol 2002;68(5):387–391
6. Zwischenberger JB, Alpard SK. Artificial lungs: a new inspiration. Perfusion 2002;17(4):253–268
7. Tao W, Brunston RL Jr, Bidani A, et al. Significant reduction in minute ventilation and peak inspiratory pressures with arteriovenous CO2 removal during severe respiratory failure. Crit Care Med 1997;25(4):689–695
8. Reng M, Philipp A, Kaiser M, Pfeifer M, Gruene S, Schoelmerich J. Pumpless extracorporeal lung assist and adult respiratory distress syndrome. Lancet 2000;356(9225):219–220
9. Liebold A, Reng CM, Philipp A, Pfeifer M, Birnbaum DE. Pumpless extracorporeal lung assist - experience with the first 20 cases. Eur J Cardiothorac Surg 2000;17(5):608–613
10. Zwischenberger JB, Conrad SA, Alpard SK, Grier LR, Bidani A. Percutaneous extracorporeal arteriovenous CO2 removal for severe respiratory failure. Ann Thorac Surg 1999;68(1):181–187
11. Lick SD, Zwischenberger JB, Alpard SK, Witt SA, Deyo DM, Merz SI. Development of an ambulatory artificial lung in an ovine survival model. ASAIO J 2001;47(5):486–491

12. Schmid C, Philipp A, Hilker M, et al. Bridge to lung transplantation through a pulmonary artery to left atrial oxygenator circuit. Ann Thorac Surg 2008;85(4):1202–1205

13. Mazzeffi M, Greenwood J, Tanaka K, et al. Bleeding, transfusion, and mortality on extracorporeal life support: ECLS Working Group on Thrombosis and Hemostasis. Ann Thorac Surg 2016; 101(2):682–689

14. Dalton HJ, Garcia-Filion P, Holubkov R, et al; Eunice Kennedy Shriver National Institute of Child Health and Human Development Collaborative Pediatric Critical Care Research Network. Association of bleeding and thrombosis with outcome in extracorporeal life support. Pediatr Crit Care Med 2015;16(2):167–174

15. Kawahito S, Maeda T, Yoshikawa M, et al. Blood trauma induced by clinically accepted oxygenators. ASAIO J 2001;47(5):492–495

16. Hendrix RHJ, Ganushchak YM, Weerwind PW. Contemporary oxygenator design: shear stressrelated oxygen and carbon dioxide transfer. Artif Organs 2018;42(6):611–619

17. Crow S, Chen D, Milano C, et al. Acquired von Willebrand syndrome in continuous-flow ventricular assist device recipients. Ann Thorac Surg 2010;90(4):1263–1269, discussion 1269

18. Morales-Quinteros L, Del Sorbo L, Artigas A. Extracorporeal carbon dioxide removal for acute hypercapnic respiratory failure. Ann Intensive Care 2019;9(1):79

19. Zimmermann M, Bein T, Arlt M, et al. Pumpless extracorporeal interventional lung assist in patients with acute respiratory distress syndrome: a prospective pilot study. Crit Care 2009;13(1):R10 10.1186/cc7703

20. Guervilly C, Fournier T, Chommeloux J, et al. Ultra-lung-protective ventilation and biotrauma in severe ARDS patients on veno-venous extracorporeal membrane oxygenation: a randomized controlled study. Crit Care. 2022;26(1):383

44

Utility of Extracorporeal Cardiopulmonary Resuscitation in Extracorporeal Cardiopulmonary Resuscitation

Jumana Yusuf Haji, Poonam Malhotra Kapoor, Anju Grewal, Kanwal Preet Sodhi, and Gunjan Chanchlani

Introduction

Cardiogenic shock and acute cardiac arrest both carry a poor prognosis, despite advanced cardiac life support (ACLS) initiated early. In this scenario, if extracorporeal cardiopulmonary resuscitation (ECPR), which utilizes extracorporeal life support (ECLS) to revive[1] vital organs, is initiated early as part of ACLS, the cardiac arrest patient may be revived. This was introduced by Kennedy in 1996, but it became popular in 2009, with the HINI pandemic and widespread use of ECLS in COVID-19 pandemic (2020–22). Venoarterial extracorporeal membrane oxygenation (VA-ECMO) is implanted in patients who experience a sudden and unexpected pulseless condition attributable to cessation of cardiac mechanical activity. The main aim of ECPR is to provide perfusion-associated mechanical support to reverse the end-organ damage in a falling heart/lung. ECPR requires high-end machinery and equipment along with a highly motivated, trained multidisciplinary team of experts. The latter is generally limited to larger tertiary care centers. In the last 10 years, the Extracorporeal Life Support Organization (ELSO) registry has recorded a 10-fold increase in ECPR procedures. ECPR is feasible in both in-hospital and out-of-hospital cardiac arrest cases (**Flowchart 44.1**).

There should be no uncertainty in the multidisciplinary team as to when to initiate ECMO. At all times, this team should be armed to reach out and provide during a cardiac arrest, not just with continuous cardiac compressions but also expedite emergency help to initiate ECMO within minutes of the cardiac arrest. For a successful ECPR outcome, the following criteria should be ideally fulfilled:
- A well-established running ECPR program within the institute or within reach in a reasonable time period.
- Preserved functional reserve of the patient before cardiac arrest.

Factors Influencing the Outcomes of ECPR

- The quality of conventional CPR.
- Nature of the ECMO device used.
- Expertise of the center performing ECPR.
- Availability of resources.
- Condition of the patient.
- Outcome measures used.

Ideally, a no-flow interval (i.e., time from cardiac arrest to initiation of CPR) should be less than 10 minutes. Application of ECMO during ECPR does not reverse the cardiac arrest. Therefore, this technique must always be combined with a diagnostic work-up to identify the cause of cardiac arrest (5Hs [Hypoxia, Hypovolemia, Hydrogen ions (acidosis), Hyper/Hypokalemia, Hypothermia] and 5Ts [Tension pneumothorax, Tamponade-cardiac, Toxins, Thrombosis-coronary (MI), Thrombosis-pulmonary (PE)])

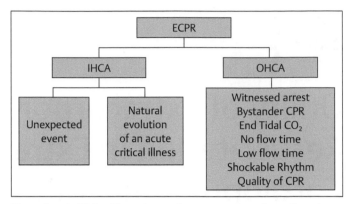

Flowchart 44.1 Flowchart of extracorporeal cardiopulmonary resuscitation (ECPR) in both in-hospital (IHCA) and out-of-hospital cardiac arrest (OHCA).

and interventions to treat the underlying pathology. For an effective in- and out-of-hospital ECPR program, system preparedness, capacity, training of personnel involved, and logistics for ECPR should be in place.

Indications of ECPR

ECPR can be applied for supporting a patient on cerebral cardiopulmonary resuscitation (cerebral-CPR) in the following ways:
- "Bridge-to-recovery": by giving time to initiate procedures and therapies such as ventricular-assist device (VAD) if needed.
- "Bridge-to-organ transplantation" as a means to consider initiating organ transplantation during the arrest period.
- "Bridge-to-decision" to continue or stop advanced cardiopulmonary support, or as a bridge to palliative care plan.

ECPR being a highly invasive, resource-intensive, and expensive technique needs careful selection of patient population.[2] ECPR is usually carried out in patients who continue to be in cardiac arrest despite conventional CPR (CCPR) (i.e., refractory cardiac arrest). EC PR is also indicated in patients:
- Witnessing cardiac arrest.
- Undergoing continuous CPR.
- Not responding to CCPR.
- Having reversible cause of cardiac arrest.

Timing of ECPR

Most of the guidelines recommend that ECPR should be implemented within 60 minutes of collapse. For this, a program should be built according to local resources knowing that the optimal team will require pre-established specific roles with personnel dedicated to conventional resuscitation and others to make preparation for ECPR.[3]

Contraindications

All contraindications to routine ECMO use apply to ECPR patients also. Poor candidates for ECPR are:
- Gestational age < 34 weeks.[4]
- Those weighing 1.5 kg or less.
- Severe congenital abnormality.
- Concomitant major trauma.
- End-stage terminal illness or significant medical comorbidities, such as cachexia, obesity, or preexisting renal failure.
- Uncontrolled hemorrhage.

A large number of authors have been researching on ECPR, in recent times. Some of them are enlisted in **Table 44.1**.

Boxes 44.1 and **44.2** indicate which cases would benefit from ECPR.

In-Hospital Cardiac Arrest

Among the many causes of use of ECPR in in-hospital cardiac arrest patients, the etiology for the cardiac arrest MUST BE REVERSIBLE—this is the basic premise for ECPR. Thus in conditions like intractable VTVF (ventricular tachycardia [VT] and ventricular fibrillation [VF]) due to metabolic or ischemic changes not responding to conventional resuscitation or any disease where there is likelihood of reversibility of the condition, with an artificial heart and lung machine like ECMO, for some period of rest, ECPR adds value to life with hope (**Box 44.3**).[12]

Complications of ECPR include the following: (1) those due to the extracorporeal circuit; (2) any vascular injury

Box 44.1   ECPR with good prognosis
- ECPR is initiated in a cardiac arrest
- Is a witnessed cardiac arrest
- Cardiac arrest is of a basic cardiac or respiratory etiology
- Cardiac arrest is of less than 60 minutes duration before ECPR is initiated
- Patient is hypothermic (32° C)
- Cardiac arrest is due to vasoactive poisoning
- Reversible etiology of cardiac arrest exists
- Patient is devoid of multiple comorbidities
- CCPR was begun within 10 minutes
- Age of patients is between 12 and 70 years

Abbreviations: CCPR, conventional cardiopulmonary resuscitation; ECPR, extracorporeal cardiopulmonary resuscitation.

Box 44.2   When is ECPR contraindicated?
ECPR should be withheld if one of the following conditions coexist:
- Cardiac arrest time is more than 60 minutes
- Advanced age of the patient
- Trained staff not available
- No reversible cardiac or respiratory physiology is observed
- CCPR initiated late (later than 10 minutes after cardiac arrest)
- Patient is in septic shock due to hemorrhage
- Cardiac arrest follows a stroke, dementia, or traumatic brain injury
- No trained or expert staff for ECPR is available

Abbreviations: CCPR, conventional cardiopulmonary resuscitation; ECPR, extracorporeal cardiopulmonary resuscitation.

Table 44.1   Work done on CPR in recent times

Authors	Work done on ECPR
Holmberg et al 2018[5]	In their review they concluded that there is no evidence to either support or refute the use of ECPR in IHCA and OHCA (LOE)
Richardson et al 2017[6]	Out of 176 ECPR patients 29% saw out of hospital discharge and 3 patients in their study group needed advanced ECMO technology
CHEER trial 2015[7]	Survival rate of 45% in OHCA and 60% in IHCA following ECPR with good neurological outcome
Siao et al 2015[8]	Comparing ECPR to CCPR recovery it was 35% vs 18.3% with a longer duration in the ECPR group which also had sustained recovery with better neurological outcomes
Matsuoka et al 2019[9]	Reported a better sustained outcome in the ECPR group compared to the CCPR group (22.9% vs 8.5%)
Dalia et al 2020[10]	In a single center experience with a hospital survival of 33.8% in their 71 patients who had CRRT with ECPR initiated, the mortality was the highest with a hospital survival of only 5.3%
MacLaren et al 2020[11]	ECPR with CPR alone survival of OHCA versus IHCA was 8% vs 33% but with ECPR it ranged from 19% to 60% with good neurological outcomes

Abbreviations: CPR, cardiopulmonary resuscitation; CCPR, conventional cardiopulmonary resuscitation; ECMO, extracorporeal membrane oxygenation; ECPR, extracorporeal cardiopulmonary resuscitation; IHCA, in-hospital cardiac arrest; LOE, level of evidence; OHCA, out-of-hospital cardiac arrest.

occurring during ECPR cannulation; (3) aberrant or unsuccessful placement of the ECPR cannula; (4) bleeding and/or thrombosis; (5) pneumonia; (6) sepsis; (7) transient ischemic attack (TIA) or stroke.[13]

Thus in postresuscitation care the end targets like target mean arterial pressure (MAP), target CO_2, and target hypothermia transport are all easier to achieve.

Need for an Interdisciplinary Team to Provide ECPR

Intensivists, cardiac anesthesiologists, physicians, and cardiothoracic surgeons take on the mantle of ECMO specialists. ECPR requires a multidisciplinary team working in unison for initiation and maintenance of ECMO resuscitation in patients with cardiac arrest. An ECMO cart for ECPR should be prepared in the ICU with preassembled provision of ECMO circuit, serial dilators, clamps, cannulas of different sizes, antiseptic solutions, surgical drapes and aprons, disposable gloves, surgical tray with blades, suture material of different types, and an ECMO consent form. This team takes instructions for coordinated work. ECPR kit with all essential equipment listed above for rapid ECPR initiation is made available for easy wheeling in at the site of cardiac arrest (**Box 44.4**).[14]

A simulation drill is conducted in most centers so that every team member learns to run each step of the ECMO meticulously. Code blue for ECMO alert its activation pathway should be created for all specialists in the ECPR team to be alert and on vigil for receiving the ECPR patient and initiate the ECPR the system (**Fig. 44.1**).[14]

The ECMO continuous renal replacement therapy (CRRT) cart should be made available at appropriate location for easy, ready use and for effective time usage (**Box 44.4**).

Maintenance

- In ECPR, cerebral CPR remains the central target. For this, meticulous attention and coordinated action of each team member is essential. At all times, cerebral perfusion should be maintained. The ECMO team should discuss beforehand the patients ECMO flow, perfusion pressures, cannula sizes, which will differ according to the patient's age and diagnosis. From minute to minute, the circuit blood flow need to be increased to maintain target perfusion pressures. Gas flows need to be titrated time to time by expert perfusionists so that both hypocapnia and hypercapnia are avoided. The latter is essential to maintain secondary brain ischemia.
- Neuroprotection during and after CPR is critical and therapies known to improve survival and neurological outcomes after CPR such as hypothermia should be included in the ECPR program also.

- Postresuscitation, neurological examination by a neurologist should be a standard protocol after discontinuation of neuromuscular blocking agents and once hemodynamic stability is achieved.

Weaning Off ECPR

ECPR duration varies in different institutions. ECPR should be weaned off as per institution protocol, once there is return of spontaneous circulation (ROSC). The confusion arises when the decision as to how and when to withdraw/wean ECPR has to be taken. The treating physician decides

---

Box 44.3 Complications of low cardiac output state where ECPR adds hope

Cardiac stunning and ECPR support:
- Imbalance in calcium homeostasis
- Ineffective I/V calcium, vasodilators, cardiac pacing, and LV decompression measures

Neurological support with ECPR:
- Decrease in cerebral oxygen delivery
- After good oxygenation, a reperfusion injury occurs
- Serum enolase biomarker after 48 hours of cardiac arrest aids in detecting cerebral hypoxia

Abbreviations: ECPR, extracorporeal cardiopulmonary resuscitation; LV, left ventricular.

Box 44.4 Where should the ECMO CRRT cart be located?

ECPR to be initiated within:
- Emergency room
- Intensive care unit of the hospital
- Main operating room area
- Coronary care unit
- Main hospital emergency unit

Abbreviations: CRRT, continuous renal replacement therapy; ECMO, extracorporeal membrane oxygenation; ECPR, extracorporeal cardiopulmonary resuscitation.

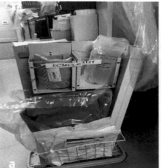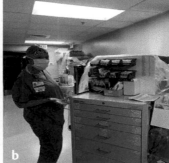

Fig. 44.1 (a, b) Extracorporeal membrane oxygenation (ECMO) continuous renal replacement therapy (CRRT) can be combined in many scenarios when acute kidney injury (AKI) is present with ECMO.

according to the patient's condition, but it is the patient's family that takes the final decision as to when ECPR should be finally terminated.

An essential part of the ECPR program is providing this final guidance to the patient's family.

Ethical Considerations

ECPR was initially a rescue therapy for cardiac arrests in the hospitals.[15] However, studies and reviews since the late 1980s have increasingly suggested ECPR as a feasible option for out-of-hospital cardiac arrest (OHCA) adult patients as well.[16] The main ethical issue is to choose between continuing CCPR with uninterrupted, effective compressions or to move patients and expose them to the avoidable risk involving transportation and placing on ECMO and increasing circulatory downtime.[14] On the other hand, in truly refractory VF/VT, the chances of survival may reduce substantially with only CCPR. Randomized controlled trials (RCTs) suggesting criteria for appropriate patient selection for early and judicious use of ECPR are needed.[17] Due to the time sensitivity involved with initiation of ECPR, the decision-making for the same is seldom shared with the next of kin and is usually medically driven. The next of kin is often involved later in the process after ECMO has been initiated and at times late enough to consent to withdrawal of life supporting system when ECMO is more of a "bridge to nowhere."[18]

Cost-Effectiveness

ECPR is highly resource demanding and has a huge cost burden. To determine a threshold value to assess the cost-effectiveness of a therapy is highly challenging. Also, the survival rate, quality of life following ECPR, contributes to the analysis. A recent retrospective analysis of ECPR for 6 years from 2012 to 2018 at Chicago Medical Center found the therapy cost-effective at their institution.[19] Similarly, another recent study conducted by the Sydney ECMO research interest group found ECPR to be a cost-effective technique for refractory cardiac arrests.[20] It also reported that the higher costs involved with ECPR in in-hospital cardiac arrest (IHCA) patients compared to OHCA patients were offset by the higher survival rate and increased mean quality-adjusted life year (QALY) in these set of patients. They also found a similar cost-effectiveness ratio between ECPR and CCPR. It is estimated that cost-effectiveness will be better with ECPR, when the higher neurological favorable survival is proven with the use of ECPR.

ECPR versus CCPR

In order to improve CPR quality and survival in OHCA, the approach used by emergency medical service (EMS) providers favored "stay-and-play" in order to decrease circulatory downtime,[21] whereas ECPR demands an approach of "load-and-go" for OHCA patients. It involves early recognition of refractory cardiac arrest. A predominant cause of cardiac arrest is coronary artery disease. If ECPR is initiated too early, there is a possibility that the patients who may have possibly recovered with CCPR would be exposed to the risks of ECMO. On the other hand, delaying the initiation increases the possibility of anoxic brain damage. The cut-off time for initiation of ECPR to have good neurological outcomes is yet to be defined.

Conclusion

ECMO providers in India are often called upon for instituting ECMO with impending failure window. There is a requirement for standard operating procedures (SOPs) conducive to the available resources for rapid institution of ECMO. It is essential to educate and instill the concept of ECPR in future CPR guidelines. Training manpower from relevant specialties to have a round-the-clock multidisciplinary team is need of the hour. Future brain death testing guidelines should take cognizance of patients on ECMO as potential brain dead donors. ECMO specialists should be trained to deal with financial, legal, ethical issues that arise while counseling in high pressure clinical scenarios convincingly.

When there is a patient with respiratory/cardiac failure there is an urgent need for an ECMO provider. In India, we need to initiate, maintain, and wean-off from ECPR. There is very little evidence-based literature in favor of this modality for saving an arrest patient. Going through review articles on current ECPR protocols as done by Jeong et al, it is clear that ECPR brings about good neurological outcomes in up to 21.3% of patients, if the time to ECPR is early.[22] A major contributing factor for the same was defining recent cardiac arrest (RCA) as >10 minutes, which contributed to a good neurological survival of 26.7%. The second factor contributing to good neurological outcomes for ECPR protocols was defining the ECPR access route. It is seen by most that combining percutaneous cannulation technique (Seldinger method) with a good imaging of ultrasound or fluoroscopy to guide cannulation had good cannulation time and less complication rates.

Cannulation complications in ECPR led to worst outcomes.[23] As recent studies on ECPR taught us, to implement a successful ECPR program, it is imperative to have an optimized chain of survival with early bystander-initiated CPR, rapid EMS response time, high-performance CPR on-scene, mechanical CPR devices for transport of patients in refractory arrest with ongoing chest compressions, availability of high-volume cardiac arrest center (CAC) for immediate ECPR, rigorous postarrest care, and careful selection of patients to undergo this expensive yet effective treatment.[24,25]

To conclude, ECPR is a feasible method and therapeutically a treatment for refractory cardiac arrest that, if available, should be considered to enhance the survival rate in critically ill cardiac arrest patients.[26] Most ECPR circuits of ECPR can deliver more than 4 L/min blood flow with a single cannula with a 15 Fr arterial return cannula. The access cannula position should be confirmed with fluoroscopy or echocardiography prior to cannula securing and dressing. The tip of the drainage cannula should be positioned in the right atrium. Both cannulas should be secured once an acceptable position is achieved.[7]

There is strong support amongst clinicians for further research into the optimal use of ECMO and ECPR and provides a framework for prioritizing future clinical trials and research agendas.[27]

References

1. Abrams D, MacLaren G, Lorusso R, et al. Extracorporeal cardiopulmonary resuscitation in adults: evidence and implications. Intensive Care Med 2022;48(1):1–15

2. Gottula AL, Neumar RW, Hsu CH. Extracorporeal cardiopulmonary resuscitation for out-of-hospital cardiac arrest: who, when, and where? Curr Opin Crit Care 2022;28(3):276–283

3. Hutin A, Abu-Habsa M, Burns B, et al. Early ECPR for out-of-hospital cardiac arrest: best practice in 2018. Resuscitation 2018;130:44–48

4. Napp LC, Sanchez Martinez C, Akin M, et al. Use of extracorporeal membrane oxygenation for eCPR in the emergency room in patients with refractory out-of-hospital cardiac arrest. PLoS One 2020;15(9):e0239777

5. Holmberg MJ, Geri G, Wiberg S, et al; International Liaison Committee on Resuscitation's (ILCOR) Advanced Life Support and Pediatric Task Forces. Extracorporeal cardiopulmonary resuscitation for cardiac arrest: a systematic review. Resuscitation 2018;131:91–100

6. Richardson AS, Schmidt M, Bailey M, Pellegrino VA, Rycus PT, Pilcher DV. ECMO Cardio-Pulmonary Resuscitation (ECPR), trends in survival from an international multicentre cohort study over 12-years. Resuscitation 2017;112:34–40

7. Stub D, Bernard S, Pellegrino V, Smith K, Walker T, Sheldrake J, Hockings L, Shaw J, Duffy SJ, Burrell A, Cameron P, Smit de V, Kaye DM. Refractory cardiac arrest treated with mechanical CPR, hypothermia, ECMO and early reperfusion (the CHEER trial). Resuscitation. 2015 Jan;86:88–94

8. Siao FY, Chiu CC, Chiu CW, et al. Managing cardiac arrest with refractory ventricular fibrillation in the emergency department: conventional cardiopulmonary resuscitation versus extracorporeal cardiopulmonary resuscitation. Resuscitation 2015;92:70–76

9. Matsuoka Y, Ikenoue T, Hata N, et al. Hospitals' extracorporeal cardiopulmonary resuscitation capabilities and outcomes in out-of-hospital cardiac arrest: a population-based study. Resuscitation 2019;136:85–92

10. Dalia AA, Lu SY, Villavicencio M, et al. Extracorporeal cardiopulmonary resuscitation: outcomes and complications at a quaternary referral center. J Cardiothorac Vasc Anesth 2020; 34(5):1191–1194

11. MacLaren G, Masoumi A, Brodie D. ECPR for out-of-hospital cardiac arrest: more evidence is needed. Crit Care 2020;24(1):7

12. Shanmugasundaram M, Lotun K. Refractory out of hospital cardiac arrest. Curr Cardiol Rev 2018;14(2):109–114

13. Kumar KM. ECPR-extracorporeal cardiopulmonary resuscitation. Indian J Thorac Cardiovasc Surg 2021;37(Suppl 2): 294–302

14. Monaco F, Belletti A, Bove T, Landoni G, Zangrillo A. Extracorporeal membrane oxygenation: beyond cardiac surgery and intensive care unit: unconventional uses and future perspectives. J Cardiothorac Vasc Anesth 2018;32(4): 1955–1970

15. Cardiopulmonary resuscitation. JAMA 1966;198(4):372–379

16. Ortega-Deballon I, Hornby L, Shemie SD, Bhanji F, Guadagno E. Extracorporeal resuscitation for refractory out-of-hospital cardiac arrest in adults: a systematic review of international practices and outcomes. Resuscitation 2016;101:12–20

17. Yannopoulos D, Bartos JA, Martin C, et al. Minnesota Resuscitation Consortium's advanced perfusion and reperfusion cardiac life support strategy for out-of-hospital refractory ventricular fibrillation. J Am Heart Assoc 2016;5(6):10

18. Henry B, Verbeek PR, Cheskes S. Extracorporeal cardiopulmonary resuscitation in out-of-hospital cardiac arrest: ethical considerations. Resuscitation 2019;137:1–6

19. Bharmal MI, Venturini JM, Chua RFM, et al. Cost-utility of extracorporeal cardiopulmonary resuscitation in patients with cardiac arrest. Resuscitation 2019;136:126–130

20. Dennis M, Zmudzki F, Burns B, et al; Sydney ECMO Research Interest Group. Cost effectiveness and quality of life analysis of extracorporeal cardiopulmonary resuscitation (ECPR) for refractory cardiac arrest. Resuscitation 2019;139:49–56

21. Smith RM, Conn AK. Prehospital care: scoop and run or stay and play? Injury 2009;40(Suppl 4):S23–S26

22. Ryu JA, Cho YH, Sung K, Choi SH, Yang JH, Choi JH, Lee DS, Yang JH. Predictors of neurological outcomes after successful extracorporeal cardiopulmonary resuscitation. BMC Anesthesiol. 2015 Mar 8;15:26

23. Olasveengen TM, Wik L, Steen PA. Quality of cardiopulmonary resuscitation before and during transport in out-of-hospital cardiac arrest. Resuscitation 2008;76(2):185–190

24. Dennis M, Lal S, Forrest P, et al. In-depth extracorporeal cardiopulmonary resuscitation in adult out-of-hospital cardiac arrest. J Am Heart Assoc 2020;9(10):e016521

25. Hu L, Peng K, Huang X, et al. A novel strategy sequentially linking mechanical cardiopulmonary resuscitation with extracorporeal cardiopulmonary resuscitation optimizes prognosis of refractory cardiac arrest: an illustrative case series. Eur J Med Res 2022;27(1):77

26. Richardson ASC, Tonna JE, Nanjayya V, et al; Interim Guideline Consensus Statement from the Extracorporeal Life Support Organization. Extracorporeal cardiopulmonary resuscitation in adults. ASAIO J 2021;67(3):221–228

27. Dennis M, Southwood TJ, Oliver M, Nichol A, Burrell A, Hodgson C. Extracorporeal membrane oxygenation and Extracorporeal Membrane Oxygenation Cardiopulmonary Resuscation (ECPR) research priorities in Australia: A clinician survey. Aust Crit Care. 2023:S1036-7314(22)00242-9

45

Importance of Mechanical-Assist Devices in Acute Decompensated Heart Failure

H. K. Chopra, Poonam Malhotra Kapoor, Navin C. Nanda, and Kul Aggarwal

Introduction

Acute decompensated heart failure (ADHF) is one of the highest risk situations encountered by a critical care specialist. The ensuing mortality with ADHF is often very high—to a tune of more than 50%. Drug therapy, oral or even systemic medical treatment, is generally ineffective, and even harmful in most cases. Post-risk stratification with biomarkers, genetic typing, and newer medications are used for heart failure. Mechanical device therapy is a rapidly evolving modality today. It is the definitive treatment when all else fails in ADHF patients.[1] Timely institution of a left ventricular assist device (LVAD) is life-saving in patients with end-stage cardiac disease. In early stages, intra-aortic balloon pump (IABP) may be sufficient, but in more advanced cases an Impella device or a tandem heart or even an extracorporeal membrane oxygenation (ECMO) device (temporary bypass) may be required. The key to success lies in proper selection of the assist device at an appropriate time.

Etiology of Decompensated Heart Failure (DHF)

The reason for poor outcomes without treatment in case of DHF is perhaps related to the etiology of acute heart failure, which encompasses both hemodynamic compromise and ischemic damage (**Box 45.1** and **Flowchart 45.1**). Acute myocardial infarction (AMI) and high-risk percutaneous coronary intervention (PCI) in patients with cardiogenic shock contribute more to ischemic damage. It is mainly pathologies like myocardial ischemia and hemodynamic changes that bring about hemodynamic compromise in situations such as cardiogenic shock.[1,2] It then becomes a phasic double-edged sword situation, wherein one condition causes another (**Fig. 45.1**) leading to maximum decompensation.

It is essential to diagnose the myocardial infraction, as the appropriate therapy is dependent upon the stage of diagnosis. AMI or hemodynamic compromise is the most important contributor to diseases with predominantly myocardial damage like myocarditis or aluminum phosphide poisoning. In cardiogenic shock, the two mechanics involved are acute myocardial infarction and hemodynammic disturbances.

Device Therapy for Acute Decompensated Heart Failure (ADHF)

Mechanical-assist device may be considered in those cases of ADHF which are not amenable to drugs alone. IABP assists in adequate unloading of the heart and so does ECMO and VADs such as the tandem heart.[3-5] So, it is imperative to learn the plus and minus of all three types of devices with immense team work among all concerned too.[5]

> **Box 45.1** Causes of acute decompensated heart failure (ADHF)
>
> - High-risk percutaneous coronary intervention (PCI)
> - Acute myocardial infarction
> - Other causes (myocarditis, tricuspid stenosis, hypertensive emergency, aluminum phosphide poisoning)
> - Cardiogenic shock (CAD)

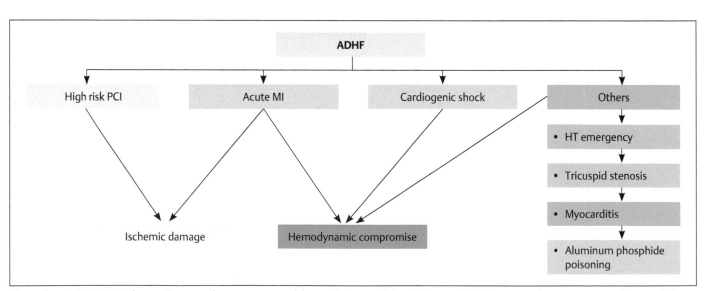

Flowchart 45.1 Etiology of acute decompensated heart failure. Abbreviations: ADHF, acute decompensated heart failure; HT, hypertensive; MI, myocardial infarction; PCI, percutaneous coronary intervention.

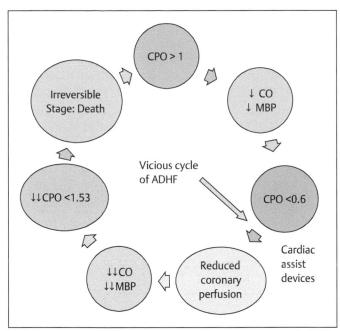

Fig. 45.1 Course of hemodynamic compromise. Abbreviations: CO, cardiac output; MBP, mean blood pressure; CPO, cardiac power output.

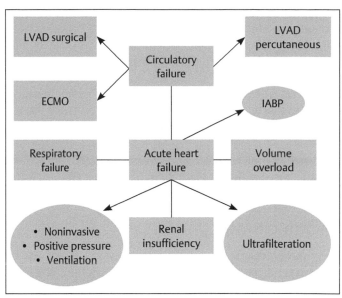

Flowchart 45.2 Algorithm depicting a brief overview of the devices available for managing acute heart failure during shock, as it moves the pressure-volume curve to the left as seen with tandem heart. Abbreviations: ECMO, extracorporeal membrane oxygenation; IABP, itra-aortic balloon pump; LVAD, left ventricular assist device.

Table 45.1 Pros and cons of IABP for acute heart failure

Pros	Cons
Increases coronary perfusion	Increases cardiac output less than ECMO/VAD
Decreases preload and afterload	No high support level
Modestly increases cardiac output	No cardiac unloading
Mature technology	Essential to have cardiac reserve
Easy to transport patients	Requires a stable rhythm
Patients can be awake	Seen with a lot of side-effects, for example, bleeding, embolism/thrombosis, thrombocytopenia, limb ischemia, aortic dissection, infection/sepsis
Nurse managed	
Relatively inexpensive	

Abbreviations: ECMO, extracorporeal membrane oxygenation; IABP, intra-aortic balloon pump; VAD, ventricular assist device.

Cardiac-Assist Devices

Several cardiac-assist devices are currently available, but they have to be carefully chosen based on implantation procedure (concept, technique of implantation, indication for device—whether destination or bridging therapy, ease/timing of implantation), mechanism of action, expected magnitude of benefit, risk of complication, and other issues. Most VADs today decrease the work of pump function (**Flowchart 45.2**). Hemodynamic and ischemic support by most cardiac arrest patients has to be upgraded once decompensation sets in.

Intra-Aortic Balloon Pump (IABP)

A lot of pros and cons exist when we consider IABP as the only therapy for a failing heart (**Table 45.1**).

For IABP the concept involves indirect LV unloading and augmentation of stroke volume (SV) and mean arterial pressure (MAP). The implantation technique is simple, requires single arterial puncture and 8 Fr sheath in adults, and can be easily implanted within 5 minutes (if done by a trained person). The mechanism of action involves hemodynamic internal mammary artery perforator (IMAP), total stroke volume (TSV) (cardiac power output [CPO] improves by 10%), but predominantly ischemic-LV unloading shifts pressure-volume area (PVA) slightly to the left. Thus, IABP is ideally suited to early stages of high-risk PCI preferably prophylactically.[6]

The magnitude of benefit of IABP is modest, and its institution may transiently stabilize if adequate pressure head is present. The complications involve limb ischemia and stroke, and its use is contraindicated in aortic incompetence, aortic disease, uncontrolled sepsis, and coagulopathy. An important issue with IABP is that it requires stable rhythm and some pressure head.

Both ECMO and IABP inserted in the catheterization laboratory act as a bridge to LVAD/RVAD as destination therapy.

Mechanical-Assist Devices

Temporary mechanical circulatory support (MCS) as a bridge to transplant, recovery/destination therapy, has nowhere been found to be a definitive and therapeutic treatment in shock states. More literature, clinical guidelines, and expertise are needed for its global acceptability. To better the outcomes of different types of circulatory support, the individual advantages and disadvantages of each type must be found from recent ongoing trials.[7]

IABP, ECMO, and VAD in Peripartum Cardiomyopathy with Decompensated Heart Failure (DHF)

According to Gevaert et al,[8] as shown in **Flowchart 45.3**, there is a tendency to use ECMO as a temporary mechanical support in all cases of ADHF. A patient presenting with advanced heart failure requires a more robust treatment in the form of the destination therapy or a bridge to transplant to correct the biventricular or LV/RV failure. A permanent (HeartMate II and III) or a temporary Impella serves as an LV-assist device, whereas CentriMag is a good temporary RV-assist device (**Flowcharts 45.3** and **45.4**). LVAD implantation, in those patients where cost is of no concern, is on the rise (**Fig. 45.2a, b**). HeartWare ventricular-assist device (HVAD), which has a centrifugal pump, is at par with HeartMate II[9] in terms of clinical outcomes, but had a high incidence of cerebrovascular incidents.[10] The Heart Ware II, with a miniaturized access in minimally invasive cardiac surgery and reduce surgical complications. HeartMate II also showed good clinical outcomes.[11] It is used as a destination therapy and a bridge to transplant. With all modalities, survival rates have improved to nearly 78%. HeartMate III is a fully, magnetically levitated centrifugal flow pump, but it has several complications such as bleeding, infection, stroke, right heart failure, and arrhythmias.[12] SynCardia, the sole Total Artificial Heart (TAH) with US FDA approval, could be the final answer for patients with biventricular failure and small surface area.[13]

Tandem Heart

Here the communication is from left artery (LA) to common innominate artery (CIA) and thus involves LA unloading and thus indirect LV unloading. However, implantation of the tandem heart is a 30-minute procedure, where the process

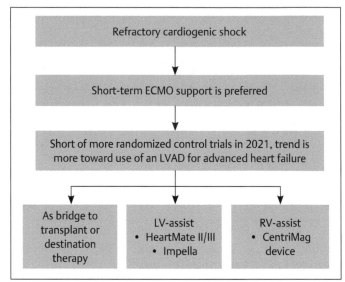

Flowchart 45.3 Uses of ventricular assist device. Abbreviations: ECMO, extracorporeal membrane oxygenation; LVAD, left ventricular assist device; LV, left ventricle; RV, right ventricle.

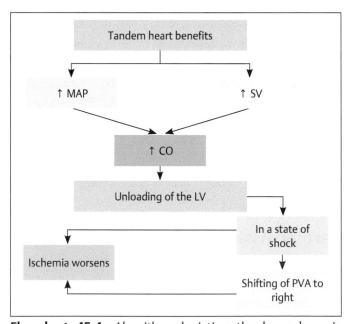

Flowchart 45.4 Algorithm depicting the hemodynamic benefits of tandem heart. The tandem heart is a left atrial to femoral artery bypass system that includes a transseptal cannula, arterial cannulae and a centrifugal pump. Abbreviations: CO, cardiac output; LV, left ventricle; MAP; mean arterial pressure; PVA, pressure volume area; SV, stroke volume.

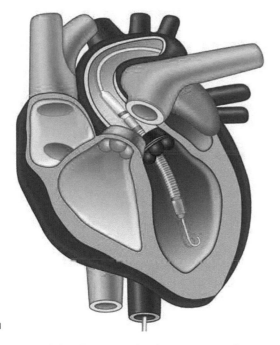

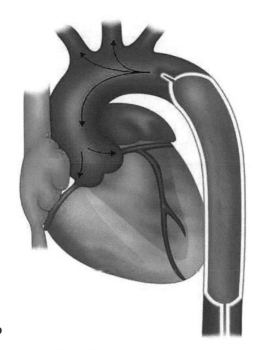

a

b

Fig. 45.2 **(a)** Left ventricular device across the aortic valve and axial pump. **(b)** Left ventricle in diastole with an intra-aortic balloon pump (IABP) in site.

entails a transeptal puncture with a venous (21 Fr for LA) and arterial (15 Fr) cannula, in a double fashion. The mechanism of beneficial action is predominantly hemodynamic: ↑MAP, ↑SV (4 L/min) (CPO improves by 80%). The ischemic benefit involves indirect LV unloading, but during shock it paradoxically worsens ischemia by shifting PVA to the right. Tandem heart system can offer innovative and superior options for ECMO delivery to heart failure patients.

The hemodynamic benefits of tandem heart are well enumerated in **Flowchart 45.4**. In this procedure, the cardiac output (CO) increases by nearly 50 percent. Thus, the basic issue with this procedure is technical: large arterial access and need for trans-septal. An additional concern is that in very sick patients it may paradoxically worsen ischemic damage (**Box 45.2**).[14]

Impella Device

In an Impella device, the communication is always between the left ventricle and the ascending aorta, which will lead to unloading of the left ventricle. It requires a single puncture in the artery with a 13 Fr cannula (in Impella 5; **Fig. 45.3**). In a percutaneous, easy-to-perform procedure, the time taken in expert hands is about 10 to 15 minutes. Like the tandem heart it provides hemodynamics increase in the CO by increasing the MAP (Increase MAP) and the SV by 4 L/min causing a nearly hundred percent with the use of Impella 5. For ischemic benefits (**Box 45.3**), it shifts the LV-unloading PVA curve to the left, during shock; thus, benefits of both hemodynamics and ischemia are provided by Impella 5

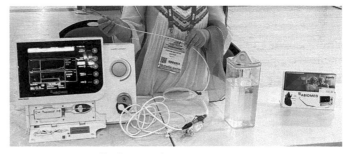

Fig. 45.3 Impella device placement.

Box 45.2 Complications of tandem heart
• Complications of aortic puncture
• Limb ischemia
• Bleeding risk
• Transfusion requirement
• Residual atrial septal defect (ASD) risk
• Need for trans-septal large access

device. Minimal complications do exist with the Impella device, which are listed in **Box 45.4**.

The mechanism of action is obtained by providing hemodynamic support: ↑MAP, ↑SV (4 L/min) (CPO improves by 50% in Impella 2.5 and 100% in Impella 5) but there is ischemic benefit as well by direct LV unloading which shifts PVA curve to the left even during shock. Thus, overall it provides good hemodynamic benefit (Impella 2.5 < Tandem heart < Impella 5) which is coupled with a good ischemic

Box 45.3   Benefits of Impella left ventricular-assist device (LVAD)

- Increase in mean arterial pressure (MAP)
- Increase in stroke volume (SV)
- Increase in cardiac output (CO)
  - ➤ 50% by Impella 2.5
  - ➤ 100% by Impella 5.0
- Left ventricle (LV) unloading with both the types 2.5 and 5.0
- Ischemia benefit also in cardiogenic shock

Box 45.4   Complications with the Impella left ventricular-assist device (LVAD)

- Moderate risk of limb ischemia
- Minimal risk of bleeding
- Minimal need for blood transfusion
- Cardiac ischemia (C/I) of Impella is in following conditions:
  - ➤ Left ventricle (LV) thrombus
  - ➤ Ventricular septal defect (VSD)
  - ➤ Severe aortic stenosis (AS)
  - ➤ Right ventricle (RV) failure
- Requires a large vascular access

benefit as well. The implantation carries a moderate risk of limb ischemia but a minimal risk of bleeding and requirement of transfusion. Its use is contraindicated in the presence of LV thrombus, ventricular septal defect (VSD), severe atrial stenosis (AS), and RV failure. The only problem with this device is requirement of relatively large arterial access.[15,16]

The sequence provided for both benefits in the three types of LVADs is: Impella 2.5 < Tandem Heart < Impella 5.0.

Extracorporeal Membrane Oxygenation (ECMO): In Decompensated Heart Failure (DHF)

ECMO, which is a partial cardiopulmonary bypass (CPB), provides good LV uploading and is a good choice in patients with low CO.

Venovenous/Venoarterial Extracorporeal Membrane Oxygenation

There are many indications of venovenous (VV) ECMO in the cardiac patient requiring increase in CO. These can primarily be summarized as cardiogenic shock, pulmonary support, postcardiotomy, and post-heart/lung transplant.

In the 1970s and 1980s, the ECMO machine was big, bulky with multiple lines. An ECMO circuit looked complex (**Fig. 45.4**), but over the years, it has become miniaturized, sleek, and portable (**Fig. 45.5**).

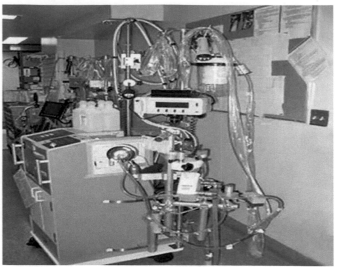

Fig. 45.4 Figure shows extracorporeal membrane oxygenation used in the 1970s and 1980s.

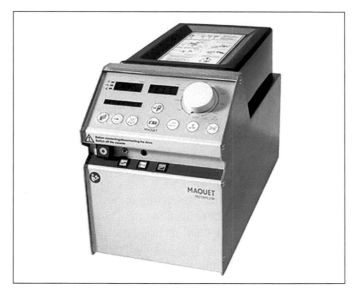

Fig. 45.5 The modern Maquet portable Rotaflow Pump along with the cardiohelp which is very useful for extracorporeal membrane oxygenation (ECMO) cardiopulmonary resuscitation.

VV/VA Extracorporeal Membrane Oxygenation in 2020

It is portable, can be inserted in a cath lab, requires 17 to 21 Fr cannulas, and can be used along with IABP to reduce afterload (can continue with ECMO). The Maquet centrifugal pump with 2 to 4 L/min flow rate is used as a bridge to surgical VAD, transplant, or recovery.

The Process of ECMO

Close monitoring of the coagulation parameters is needed, and it is, therefore, labor-intensive. Patients on ECMO are treated with ultrafiltrate heparin to obtain an activated clotting time (ACT) of 170 to 200 seconds. Antithrombin III (ATIII) levels are analyzed daily.

ATIII concentrate is given if the ATIII activity drops below 70 percent. It is advisable to perform beyond ACT and antithrombin II levels, a routine aPTT (activated partial thromboplastin time with kaolin), and serum fibrinogen levels as well. Point-of-care viscoelastic tests such as ROTEM/TEG (rotational thromboelastometry/thromboelastography) or Sonoclot can be done if bleeding persists. These tests provide prompt action as they have shorter turnaround time.[17] Patients on arteriovenous ECMO are ventilated with conventional settings, with a FiO_2 to achieve an acceptable PaO_2 (at least 60 mmHg). Inotropic support can be slowly weaned off but a more potent inodilator which has strong vasodilator effects at the tissue level like milrinone can be continued. Fluid management is aimed at preserving renal function and ensuring a stable circulation (**Fig. 32.3**).

Role of Echocardiography in ECMO

For successful outcomes, echocardiography becomes essential. From selecting the right patient and the time when ECMO has to be initiated to discerning the type of ECMO, echocardiography is required. ECHO aids in the placement of cannulas and their migrations, monitoring biventricular function, LV distension, aortic valve opening, pressure of pericardial effusion/tamponade, cardiac thrombus/casts around cannulas, and also decide whether patient is ready for ECMO weaning and trial off. This is essential, as ECMO is flow dependent. ECMO is flow dependent; therefore, an ECHO can help decide the hemodynamics and SV when ECMO flow is being decreased before weaning off.

Selection of the Right Mechanical Device for a Failing Heart for ECMO Induced CPR (E-CPR)

Postpartum cardiomyopathy has an acutely decompensated failing heart. Timely intervention starting from an IABP and going on to the VAD can salvage life[18,19] in these postpartum mothers with acute LV dysfunction.

The ECMO can be inserted at the bedside. It is relatively cheap (as compared to the implantable LVAD) and gives the treating physicians some time to wait for recovery or a more stable condition. Cannula malpositioning and migration during an ECMO run can be well visualized on echocardiography.

The Surgical Concerns in Mechanical Circulatory Support Placement

Mechanical-assist devices are more reliable today than ever before. The European Association for Cardio-Thoracic Surgery (EACTS) expert opinion on the use of long-term (LT) MCS[20] has reiterated that there is an increased demand of MCS implants, especially of the continuous-flow LVADs (CF-LVADS) in end-stage, DHF patients. With a paucity in the availability of a donor heart, the number of patients on LT-MCS will grow further. Thus, optimization of its management becomes imperative. Optimization of all body organs (liver, lungs, coagulation nutrition, etc.) is important as is their anesthetic management, monitoring, and postoperative concerns. An ECHO monitoring to rule out an intracavitary thrombus or a patient foramen ovale or intracardiac shunts, right ventricular assessment, and positioning of inflow and outflow cannulas are all very important.[7] The level of evidence recommended for off-pump implantation of an LT-MCS is IC.[21] The placement of the inflow cannula parallel to the septum is recommended (Level of evidence IB) by performing the outflow graft anastomosis on the ascending aorta which is again recommended as level of evidence IC. Liberal deairing via the outflow graft is recommended with on-pump surgery (IC).[22]

Postoperative Concerns in Long-term Mechanical Circulatory Support (LT-MCS) Placement

According to Potapov et al in postoperative patients with MCS, continuous electrocardiography, pulse oximetry, central venous pressure, and invasive arterial blood pressure monitoring are all recommended (LOE IC). Miniaturized transesophageal echocardiographic probes that can be maintained in the esophagus in site for up to 72 hours may be considered to assist in the management of fluid resuscitation and to look for complications. Transpulmonary thermodilution and pulse contour–derived measurement are inadequate in case of both CF-VADs and biventricular devices. Thus, according to the EACTS expert opinion in 2019, these are not recommended. However, a pulmonary artery catheter is good for managing fluids and looking out for any complications (LOE II ac).[23]

Daily monitoring postoperatively of plasma-free hemoglobin and lactate dehydrogenase levels are recommended today (LOE IC). Echocardiography is temporary right ventricular support (LOE IB).[24] It is imperative to use postoperative mechanical ventilation in such a way that hypercarbia is avoided at all times as it leads to rise in pulmonary artery pressure and right ventricular afterload (LOE IC). If intraoperative extracorporeal life support or off-pump implantation is done, then a low-dose heparin is needed. The international normalized ratio target should be between 2.0 and 3.0 (LOE IC) and the use of low-molecular-weight heparin and acetyl/salicylic acid is recommended (LOE IC). For any major bleeding event, discontinue the anticoagulant being used, and use of judicious blood components and Vitamin K-dependent coagulation factors is recommended (LOE IC).

Conclusion

Cardiac-assist devices can be a useful safety technique in ADHF. It is very important to use right device at right time; thus, it may be of value to use IABP early, even prophylactically rather than waiting for patient to get sick and then institute as a rescue therapy. Broadly, in nonischemic situations, devices improving hemodynamic status are more useful but in ischemic settings like high-risk PCI ischemic protection is better than mere hemodynamic support. However, once patient destabilizes, additional hemodynamic support is of paramount importance. Impella device gives best combination of ischemic protection, hemodynamic support, ease of insertion, and safety. As the number of heart failure patients in the United States itself rises to 8 million by 2030 and interventional heart failure therapies,[25] for improving the quality of life. ECMO has a major position to occupy in these patients. As the unloading and hemodynamic support levels with a left ventricular assist device (LVAD) are limited, VA-VA ECMO has both strong hemodynamic supportive effect if ECMO trained staff exists in that centre.[25,26] ECMO is good for bridging strategies, post-operative outcomes in acute decompensated heart failure-related cardiogenic shock patients undergoing heart transplantation or durable left ventricular assist device implantation or as a bridge to LVAD.[27]

New technologies can be challenging from the beginning because the precise indication for use and the success and failure criteria are not completely defined. Only a pragmatic trial with clinically relevant endpoints will bring tangible benefits to patients, without adding costs and unnecessary interventions.[28]

References

1. Choi H-M, Park M-S, Youn J-C. Update on heart failure management and future directions. Korean J Intern Med (Korean Assoc Intern Med) 2019;34(1):11–43
2. Burkhoff D, Cohen H, Brunckhorst C, O'Neill WW; Tandem Heart Investigators Group. A randomized multicenter clinical study to evaluate the safety and efficacy of the Tandem Heart percutaneous ventricular assist device versus conventional therapy with intraaortic balloon pumping for treatment of cardiogenic shock. Am Heart J 2006;152(3):469.e1–469.e8
3. Chandra D, Kar B, Idelchik G, et al. Usefulness of percutaneous left ventricular assist device as a bridge to recovery from myocarditis. Am J Cardiol 2007;99(12):1755–1756
4. Lietz K, Long JW, Kfoury AG, et al. Outcomes of left ventricular assist device implantation as destination therapy in the post-REMATCH era: implications for patient selection. Circulation 2007;116(5):497–505
5. Costanzo MR, Guglin ME, Saltzberg MT, et al; UNLOAD Trial Investigators. Ultrafiltration versus intravenous diuretics for patients hospitalized for acute decompensated heart failure. J Am Coll Cardiol 2007;49(6):675–683
6. Firstenberg MS, Orsinelli DA. ECMO and ECHO: the evolving role of quantitative echocardiography in the management of patients requiring extracorporeal membrane oxygenation. J Am Soc Echocardiogr 2012;25(6):641–643
7. Kapoor PM. Echocardiography in extracorporeal membrane oxygenation. Ann Card Anaesth 2017;20(Supplement):S1–S3
8. Gevaert S, Van Belleghem Y, Bouchez S, et al. Acute and critically ill peripartum cardiomyopathy and "bridge to" therapeutic options: a single center experience with intra-aortic balloon pump, extra corporeal membrane oxygenation and continuous-flow left ventricular assist devices. Crit Care 2011;15(2):R93
9. Rogers JG, Pagani FD, Tatooles AJ, et al. Intrapericardial left ventricular assist device for advanced heart failure. N Engl J Med 2017;376(5):451–460
10. Chatterjee A, Feldmann C, Dogan G, et al. Clinical overview of the HVAD: a centrifugal continuous-flow ventricular assist device with magnetic and hydrodynamic bearings including lateral implantation strategies. J Thorac Dis 2018;10(Suppl 15):S1785–S1789
11. Miller LW, Pagani FD, Russell SD, et al; HeartMate II Clinical Investigators. Use of a continuous-flow device in patients awaiting heart transplantation. N Engl J Med 2007;357(9): 885–896
12. Mehra MR, Goldstein DJ, Uriel N, et al; MOMENTUM 3 Investigators. Two-year outcomes with a magnetically levitated cardiac pump in heart failure. N Engl J Med 2018;378(15):1386–1395
13. Wells D, Villa CR, Simón Morales DL. The 50/50 cc total artificial heart trial: extending the benefits of the total artificial heart to underserved populations. Semin Thorac Cardiovasc Surg Pediatr Card Surg Annu 2017;20:16–19
14. Hajjar LA, Teboul JL. Mechanical circulatory support devices for cardiogenic shock: state of the art. Crit Care 2019;23(1):76
15. Dixon SR, Henriques JP, Mauri L, et al. A prospective feasibility trial investigating the use of the Impella 2.5 system in patients undergoing high-risk percutaneous coronary intervention (the PROTECT I trial): initial U.S. experience. JACC Cardiovasc Interv 2009;2(2):91–96
16. O'Neill WW, Kleiman NS, Moses J, et al. A prospective, randomized clinical trial of hemodynamic support with Impella 2.5 versus intra-aortic balloon pump in patients undergoing high-risk percutaneous coronary intervention: the PROTECT II study. Circulation 2012;126(14):1717–1727
17. Malhotra Kapoor P, Karanjkar A, Bhardwaj V. Evaluation of coagulopathy on veno-arterial ECMO (VA) extracorporeal membrane oxygenation using platelet aggregometry and standard tests: a narrative review. Egyptian J Crit Care Med 2018;6(3):73-78
18. Nichol G, Karmy-Jones R, Salerno C, Cantore L, Becker L. Systematic review of percutaneous cardiopulmonary bypass for cardiac arrest or cardiogenic shock states. Resuscitation 2006;70:381–394
19. Jaski BE, Ortiz B, Alla KR, et al. A 20-year experience with urgent percutaneous cardiopulmonary bypass for salvage of potential survivors of refractory cardiovascular collapse. J Thorac Cardiovasc Surg 2010;139(3):753–7.e1, 2
20. Potapov E, Antonides C, Crespo-Leiro MG, et al. 2019 EACTS Expert Consensus on long-term mechanical circulatory support. Eur J Cardiothorac Surg 2019;56(2):230–270

21. Windecker S, Stortecky S, Meier B. Paradoxical embolism. J Am Coll Cardiol 2014;64(4):403–415

22. Neumann FJ, Sousa-Uva M, Ahlsson A, et al; ESC Scientific Document Group. 2018 ESC/EACTS Guidelines on myocardial revascularization. Eur Heart J 2019;40(2):87–165

23. Burns PB, Rohrich RJ, Chung KC. The levels of evidence and their role in evidence-based medicine. Plast Reconstr Surg 2011;128(1):305–310

24. Arora S, Singh PM, Goudra BG, Sinha AC. Changing trends of hemodynamic monitoring in ICU—from invasive to non-invasive methods: are we there yet? Int J Crit Illn Inj Sci 2014;4(2):168–177

25. Saku K, Yokota S, Nishikawa T, Kinugawa K. Interventional heart failure therapy: a new concept fighting against heart failure. J Cardiol 2022;80(2):101–109

26. Thiele H, Jobs A, Ouweneel DM, et al. Percutaneous short-term active mechanical support devices in cardiogenic shock: a systematic review and collaborative meta-analysis of randomized trials. Eur Heart J 2017;38(47):3523–3531

27. Varshney AS, Berg DD, Zhou G, et al. Temporary mechanical circulatory support bridging strategies and post-operative outcomes in acute decompensated heart failure-related cardiogenic shock patients undergoing heart transplantation or durable left ventricular assist device implantation: a Society of Thoracic Surgeons Database analysis. J Card Fail 2022;28(5):S52–S53

28. de Oliveira Cardoso C, Elgalad A, Li K, Perin EC. Device-based therapy for decompensated heart failure: An updated review of devices in development based on the DRI2P2S classification. Front Cardiovasc Med. 2022;9:962839

46

Echocardiography in ECMO

*Poonam Malhotra Kapoor, Muralidhar Kanchi, Kanwal Kapur,
Naman Shastri, and Navin C. Nanda*

Definition

Extracorporeal membrane oxygenation (ECMO) is a complex critical care therapy used to provide cardiac and/or respiratory support in severely ill patients in whom maximum conventional medical management has failed. It can provide prolonged cardiac and/or pulmonary support for days, weeks, and even months.

Using echocardiography on an ECMO patient is a synergistically, life-saving procedure in a supplementary manner. Echocardiography helps in selecting patients for ECMO, monitoring, maintaining, and weaning off ECMO. ECHO provides great information in each phase of ECMO implementation, but its use is limited due to either unavailability of the Echo machine at the ECMO site or because echo may, in a transthoracic mode, give a poor acoustic window. The latter may be overcome by using either transesophageal echocardiography (TEE) or a contrast echocardiography. The use of many other imaging modalities that may require use of radio-opaque contrast media or ionizing radiations should be completely avoided. Contrast-enhanced echocardiography can give good insights into ECMO implantation and detecting its complications. The best use of ECHO on ECMO is its safety potential as ECHO is noninvasive and inert with no radiations.

Role of Echocardiography in ECMO

Although transthoracic echocardiography[1,2] (TTE) has been in existence for more than 50 years (Edler and Hertz, 1954) and ECMO has been in use for the last 40 years (Hill, 1971), there is a paucity of data on the use of echocardiogram during ECMO support. The potential for use of echocardiogram during ECMO support is immense. Echocardiography provides high-resolution images of the heart and blood vessels. It is easily available, is cost-effective, and can be performed in the emergency room, ICUs, catheterization laboratories, and operating rooms. The utility of echocardiogram in critically ill patients in the ICU is well known. Recently, echocardiogram has been widely used in the hemodynamic evaluation of critically ill patients and has, to a large extent, replaced invasive monitoring in this setting. However, despite its obvious potential advantages, there are several limitations to the use of echocardiogram in the critically ill patients. Poor acoustic window is compounded by the restricted access in the ICU setting owing to several cannulas, tubing, and the use of several monitoring and therapeutic devices. With the advent of TEE it has been possible to overcome many of these limitations. The judicious use of both TTE and TEE provides accurate and comprehensive evaluation of critically ill patients requiring ECMO support. Echocardiography provides crucial information during the entire period of the ECMO support, beginning from the assessment of patients likely to benefit from ECMO, identifying contraindications to the commencement

of ECMO support and observing complications, and deciding on timing of weaning and trial-off while on ECMO support (**Boxes 46.1–46.3**).

Box 46.1 Echocardiography and ECMO

- Echocardiography is the side-kick of ECMO
- Its use is of key importance during:
  - ➤ Assessment of ECMO indications and contraindications
  - ➤ Cannulation and guidance of ECMO initiation
  - ➤ Follow-up, monitoring, and detecting complications during ECMO
  - ➤ Weaning from ECMO

Abbreviation: ECMO, extracorporeal membrane oxygenation.

Box 46.2 Assessment of ECMO indications and contraindications

- Even in situations of severe hemodynamic compromise (E-CPR), go for a focused and goal-oriented echocardiography
  - ➤ Refractory cardiac arrest because of tamponade does not need to be treated with ECMO
- Choice between respiratory and cardiac ECMO is not always easy; ECHO can help
  - ➤ Up to 35% with ARDS have severe RV dysfunction; VV ECMO will often resolve the problem, but sometimes switching to (Venoarterial-Venous) VAV ECMO is needed
- Prognostication and treatment plan
  - ➤ Preexisting RV dysfunction is a predictor of outcome in patients treated with ECMO after cardiac surgery
  - ➤ Cardiogenic shock after myocardial infarction is not always due to severe LV dysfunction; look for mechanical complications
- Contraindications
  - ➤ Look for aortic dissection and aortic regurgitation

Abbreviations: ARDS, acute respiratory distress syndrome; ECHO, echocardiography; ECMO, extracorporeal membrane oxygenation; E-CPR, ECMO cardiopulmonary resuscitation; LV, left ventricle; RV, right ventricle; VV, venovenous.

Box 46.3 Cannulation and guidance of ECMO initiation

The essential ECHO views are:
- Ultrasound is beneficial in gaining vascular access
- Identification of severe atheromatous disease with artery stenosis at access site
- Combined echocardiography and fluoroscopy is in authors' point of view ideal for guidewire and cannula placement
- For specific situations (Avalon dual lumen cannula), combining TEE and TTE can be beneficial
- Subcostal (TTE) and bicaval (TEE) views are the most important views for procedure guidance and cannula positioning in an ECMO circuit (**Fig. 46.1**)

Abbreviations: ECMO cardiopulmonary resuscitation; TEE, transesophageal echocardiography; TTE, transthoracic echocardiography.

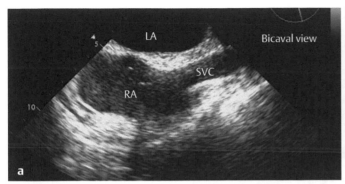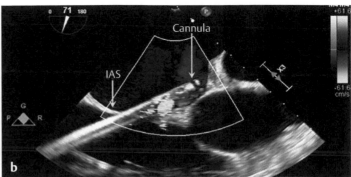

Fig. 46.1   (a, b) Bicaval view is showing the cannula from SVC into the RA cavity on TEE. **(b)** The draining ECMO cannula in the ECHO; descending thoracic aorta view showing dilated cardiomyopathy and return cannula in the descending thoracic aorta cardiomyopathy. Abbreviations: ECHO, echocardiography; ECMO, extracorporeal membrane oxygenation; IAS, interatrial septum; LA, left atrium; RA, right atrium; SVC, superior vena cava; TEE, transesophageal echocardiography.

Cannula and Guidance of ECMO Initiation

Extra attention is needed when implanting an Avalon elite dual-lumen cannula, avoiding cannulation of a hepatic vein. Paying attention that the tip of the cannula cannot clearly be identified with the guidewire in place. In femoral VV ECMO, the tip of a femoral drainage cannula should be placed at IVC/RA junction. Placement of a drainage cannula too deep in RA, might lead to damage to cardiac structures and to problems of recirculation. Girand et al, in their case report of a 56-year-old in refractory cardiogenic shock, reiterated that echocardiography should be essential in ECMO venous cannula placement. They found that the tip of the venous cannula was lying in the left atrium, instead of the right atrium, in the midesophageal four chamber view.

Echocardiography for Follow-up, Monitoring, and Detecting Complications during ECMO

In a VA ECMO follow-up: it is important to do the evaluation of aortic valve opening with TEE. In peripheral VA ECMO, afterload of retrograde aortic flow will interfere with left ventricular (LV) ejection of stroke volume. This will lead to LV distention with secondary problems of increased wall stress, thrombus formation, and pulmonary edema. The need for LV decompression may arise with LV distention (intra-aortic balloon pump [IABP], Impella, percutaneous or surgical vent).

To appreciate the role of echocardiography during ECMO support, it is important to understand the types of ECMO supports available, the ECMO circuit, as well as the indications and the contraindications for ECMO.

Types of ECMO (Venovenous and Venoarterial)

Venovenous (VV ECMO) is used for gas exchange in patients with isolated refractory respiratory failure but adequate cardiac function. The oxygenated blood from the ECMO circuit is returned to the right heart where it mixes with the blood without passing through the circuit and then is pumped into the lungs and then to the left heart and systemic circulation. Of crucial importance is the fact that the right heart function, pulmonary vascular resistance, and left heart function should be adequate (**Fig. 46.2a, b**).

Venoarterial (VA ECMO) is used in the cardiac patient who is sick due to cardiogenic shock, heart failure, myocarditis, or low cardiac output. In **Fig. 46.2a** the venous cannula is seen in the femoral vein or in the right atrium (the drainage cannula) and the arterial cannula is placed in the femoral artery or ascending aorta (**Fig. 46.2b**). The venous blood thus enters the ECMO circuit and the oxygenated blood from the ECMO circuit flows via the return cannula into the patient's arterial tree (**Figs. 46.3** and **46.4**).

TEE ME descending thoracic aorta views show the drainage cannula in the inferior vena cava (IVC) and return cannula in the descending thoracic aorta, as shown in **Fig. 46.1(b)**. This is dilated cardio awaiting a heart transplant. A daily ECHO surveillance should be done on all ECMO patients in both types of ECMO—VV and VA. What parameters to look for while selecting the patient and monitoring and weaning from ECMO are well enlisted in **Table 46.1**.

Echocardiography and Monitoring ECMO Response

During ECMO, a large number of hemodynamic perturbations take place. Following a peripheral VA ECMO, there is a decrease in pulmonary blood flow which leads to decrease in preload, but a simultaneous increase in LV afterload. The latter is seen because the blood in the ECMO return cannula is under pressure. The ECMO cannula location and the type of ECMO become the decisive factors for maintaining the hemodynamic on ECMO. In case of severe LV dysfunction with an associated mitral regurgitation, the LV becomes even more dilated, with greater LV dysfunction and reduced

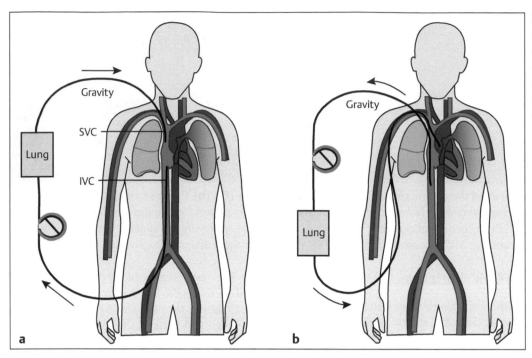

Fig. 46.2 (a, b) Cannulation sites in a venoarterial (VA) extracorporeal membrane oxygenation (ECMO). Abbreviations: IVC, inferior vena cava; SVC, superior vena cava.

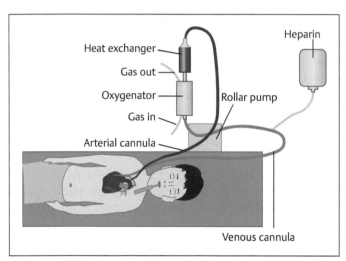

Fig. 46.3 Venoarterial extracorporeal membrane oxygenation (ECMO) showing the arterial circulation in a neonate.

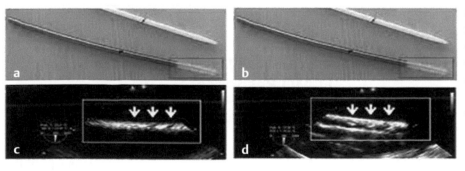

Fig. 46.4 (a) The drainage and return single cannula. **(b–d)** Transesophageal echocardiography (TEE). ME (midesophageal) descending thoracic aorta views showing the drainage cannula in the inferior vena cava (IVC) and return cannula in the descending thoracic aorta.

cardiac output. Because of latter changes, the aortic valve may not open at all. This may cause stagnation of blood in the LV cavity and the ascending and the pulmonary veins. Venting of the LV blood stasis is undertaken in such cases, as enumerated in **Table 46.2**. TEE is a procedure to be carried out for guiding the balloon atrial septostomy (BAS) procedure (**Fig. 46.5**).

Table 46.1 Echo parameters and views for VA and VV ECMO[2-5]

ECMO phase	ECHO views	ECMO types	
		Venovenous ECMO	**Venoarterial ECMO**
Patient selection	**TEE** • ME 4 chamber view • ME bicaval • HE view **TTE** • Apical • Subcostal • Parasternal long- and short-axis view	• IVC and SVC entering into the RA • IVC collapse • Flow reversal in hepatic veins during atrial systole • Anomalies such as AR, Chiari network, and PFO as these will obstruct • ECMO cannula placement and flow • Visualize both right and left SVC	• RV and LV function assessment • Systolic and diastolic function assessment • TAPSE • Pulmonary artery acceleration time • E/A • E/e' • Strain and strain rate • S1 • Rule out any AR
Monitoring on ECMO	• Add DEEP transgastric view for gradient • ME RV inflow-outflow view • ME long-axis view	• LV and RV size • LA and RA size • LA and RA volume • Any preexisting cardiac pathology • Position of cannulas • Any cardiac tamponade • Pericardial effusion • IVC size and collapsibility • ECMO flows and oxygenation	• LV and RV size • Reversible pathology for which ECMO is inserted • Opening of the aortic valve • RA and LA size and volume • Any spontaneous ECHO contrast • Presence of intra-cardiac thrombus in any of the four chambers • Migration of cannulas • Presence of ECMO flows and oxygenation
Weaning from ECMO	• ME 4 chamber view • ME 2 chamber view • ME SAX view • ME LAX view • ME bicaval view • TG–view • TG–SAX view to rule out hypovolemia	• Concerns here are more for recovery of lung function. The ECHO data should be on ECMO weaning with a decrease in PAP from the TR jet • Rule out R–L shunt across the IAS or IVS • Look for normal interventricular septum motion • TAPSE >11.5 mm • PAAT >110 ms	• ECHO for stable mics • LV global recovery • LVEF >20–25% or >35–40% • LVOT or VTI >10 cm • Absence of LV dilatation • No cardiac tamponade • A lateral mitral annulus peak systolic velocity of >6 cm/s

Abbreviations: AR, aortic regurgitation; E/A, early to late diastolic transmitral flow velocity; E/e', ratio between early mitral inflow velocity and mitral annular early diastolic velocity; ECHO, echocardiography; ECMO, extracorporeal membranous oxygenation; HE, hepato-esophageal view; IAS, interatrial septum; IVC, inferior vena cava; IVS, interventricular septum; LA, left atrium; LAX, long-axis echocardiographic imaging; LV, left ventricle; LVEF, left ventricular ejection fraction; LVOT, left ventricular outflow tract; ME, midesophageal; PAAT, pulmonary artery acceleration time; PAP, pulmonary arterial pressure; PFO, patent foramen ovale; RA, right atrium; RV, right ventricle; SAX, short-axis echocardiographic imaging; SVC, superior vena cava; TAPSE, tricuspid annular plane systolic excursion; TEE, transesophageal echocardiography; TG, transgastric; TR, tricuspid regurgitation; TTE, transthoracic echocardiography; VA, venoarterial ECMO; VTI, velocity time integral; VV, venovenous ECMO.

Echocardiography in Detection of ECMO Complications

ECMO support gives rise over a period of time to some pertinent complications, which can be salvaged with the use of echocardiography. Some complications such as thrombosis in any cardiac chamber, cardiac tamponade, or migration of ECMO cannulas from one chamber of the heart to the other usually arise. TTE has limited window of resolution. TEE is the ECHO of choice to detect most ECMO complications. TEE is most useful for all cannula-related problems, for example, positioning of ECMO cannulas, cardiac filling, tamponade-induced chamber compression and biventricular cardiac function, cardiac tamponade detection. and chamber thrombosis, and any collection or pericardial effusion goes unobserved in an ECMO generally, as it is a state of partial cardiopulmonary bypass (CPB).

Complications

ECMO is an adaptive form of conventional CPB. Patient selected for ECMO needs to have a pathology requiring ECMO which is reversible. ECMO physiology does not entail a cure, but putting a patient on short-term ECMO provides a supportive aid to the reversible pathology (e.g., ECMO acts

Table 46.2 Methods of LV venting on ECMO

A PCWP elevate, LV hypocontractile and distended	
Medical management	• Inotropes, vasopressors, diuretics, CVVH carefully titrated to decompress the LV on ECMO • Lowest ECMO flows possible to be given

Mechanical management	• BAS (balloon atrial septostomy)
	• IABP (intra-aortic balloon pump)
	• ECPELLA
	• VAD (ventricular-assist device):
	  ➢ Percutaneous left-atrial vents
	  ➢ Tandem heart
	  ➢ Impella

Surgical management	• Open surgical placement of LV vent • Minimally invasive LV venting with centrimag LVAD and ECMO

Abbreviations: CVVH, continuous venovenous hemofiltration; ECMO, extracorporeal membrane oxygenation; ECPELLA, ECMO and concomitant Impella support; LV, left ventricle; LVAD, left ventricular-assist device; PCWP, pulmonary capillary wedge pressure.

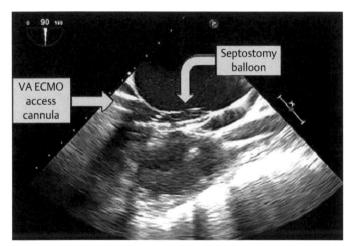

Fig. 46.5 Septostomy balloon. Abbreviation: VA ECMO, venoarterial extracorporeal membrane oxygenation.

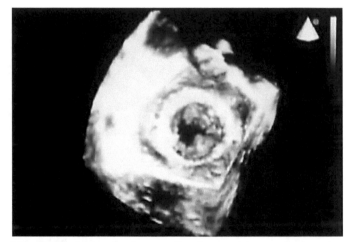

Fig. 46.6 Thrombotic complication on bioprosthetic valve due to heparin-induced thrombocytopenia.

as a bridge to recovery or a bridge to transplant). ECMO is used over a wide range of patients from the neonates to adults (**Figs. 46.6–46.12**).

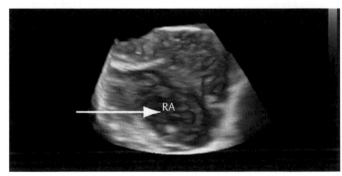

Fig. 46.7 3D transesophageal echocardiography (TEE) detects a right atrium (RA) thrombus post cannula insertion.

Echocardiography Weaning and Recovery from ECMO

As we decrease ECMO support and ECMO blood flow, there is generally a reduction in LV afterload and an increase in LV preload. Conventional ECHO recovery parameters, as described in **Box 46.4**, are dependent on loading conditions (**Figs. 46.8, 46.9,** and **Box 46.5**).[6] Kim et al[7] provided a framework for guiding VA ECMO weaning in cardiogenic shock, based on TEE parameters. As listed in **Box 46.5**, they proposed that as most ECHO parameters are affected by loading conditions, it is LV diastolic recovery (E1) and RV systolic recovery (S1) that are responsible in helping VA ECMO weaning. E1 helps in aiding the diastolic lusitropic function

of the LV and the improved S1 tells us about the remodeled RV systolic function of the patient. These parameters were found to be better than the LV and RV ejection fractions, despite the fact that weaning from VA ECMO is a biventricular reloading procedure involving biventricular functions.[8]

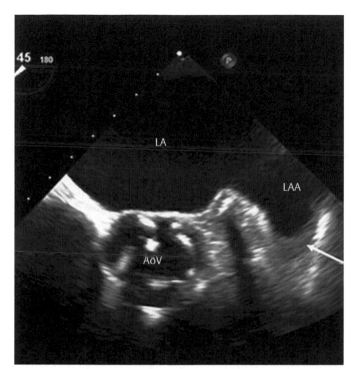

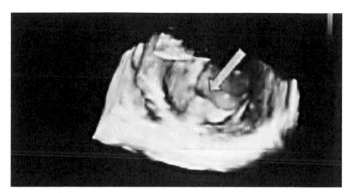

Fig. 46.10 Bleeding tamponade (*arrow*) seen with stasis and effusion on transesophageal echocardiography (TEE).

Fig. 46.8 Transthoracic echocardiography showing an extensive LA thrombus (*arrow*). Abbreviations: AoV, aortic valve; LA, left atrium; LAA, left atrial appendage.

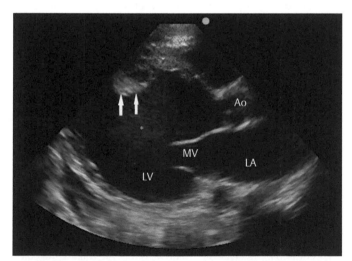

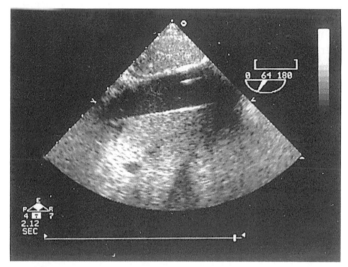

Fig. 46.11 Flow obstruction in lower esophageal view on transesophageal echocardiography (TEE).

Fig. 46.9 Transthoracic echocardiography showing severely dilated LV with spontaneous contrast and mural thrombus (*arrows*). Abbreviations: Ao, ascending aorta; LA, left atrium; LV, left ventricle; MV, mitral valve. *Spontaneous contrast; *arrows* pointing to mural thrombus.[6]

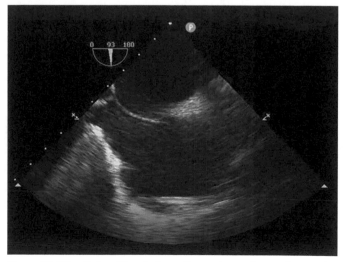

Fig. 46.12 Suboptimal transthoracic echocardiography (TTE) imaging in a patient on extracorporeal membrane oxygenation (ECMO) unlike what is seen on transesophageal echocardiography (TEE) wherein resolution is higher.

Conclusion

Quantitative assessment of both LV and RV by echocardiography is important for ECMO weaning. Patients with better LVEF and lower RV Tei index may have a better chance of successful weaning from ECMO.[9] The recovery of right ventricular systolic function is also an important echocardiographic indication that cannot be ignored in ECMO weaning.[10]

Summary

Echocardiography is a fundamental procedure that is performed in all of ECMO procedures: selecting the right patient for ECMO, verifying correct position of cannula, during daily surveillance, monitoring heart recovery, and evaluating daily recovery. At the time of cannula insertion, look out for complications such as pericardial effusion, tamponade, and intracardiac clotting.

Echocardiography should be performed on patients on mechanical assistance and on ECMO at least once daily. It is of great utility when choosing a patient for ECMO cannulation, monitoring the ECMO process, decannulating, and evaluating TEE findings along with clinical and functional status of the patient. Interpretation of ECHO observations should be handled by experts. When the transvalvular gradients are high, the aortic valve will remain closed, both in systolic and diastolic. The latter leads to stasis of blood in the aortic root with impending thrombus formation, especially

in peripheral VA ECMO patient.[11,12] The importance of ECHO for LV venting cannot be overlooked. ECHO for ECMO is a must for safe ECMO outcomes.[13]

References

1. Giraud R, Banfi C, Bendjelid K. Echocardiography should be mandatory in ECMO venous cannula placement. Eur Heart J Cardiovasc Imaging 2018;19(12):1429–1430
2. Aissaoui N, Guerot E, Combes A, et al. Two-dimensional strain rate and Doppler tissue myocardial velocities: analysis by echocardiography of hemodynamic and functional changes of the failed left ventricle during different degrees of extracorporeal life support. J Am Soc Echocardiogr 2012;25(6):632–640
3. Meani P, Gelsomino S, Natour E, et al. Modalities and effects of left ventricle unloading on extracorporeal life support: a review of the current literature. Eur J Heart Fail 2017;19(Suppl 2):84–91
4. Aissaoui N, El-Banayosy A, Combes A. How to wean a patient from veno-arterial extracorporeal membrane oxygenation. Intensive Care Med 2015;41(5):902–905
5. Ranasinghe AM, Peek GJ, Roberts N, et al. The use of transesophageal echocardiography to demonstrate obstruction of venous drainage cannula during ECMO. ASAIO J 2004;50(6):619–620
6. Bautista-Rodriguez C, Sanchez-de-Toledo J, Da Cruz EM. The role of echocardiography in neonates and pediatric patients on extracorporeal membrane oxygenation. Front Pediatr 2018;6:297
7. Kim D, Jang WJ, Park TK, et al. Echocardiographic predictors of successful extracorporeal membrane oxygenation weaning after refractory cardiogenic shock. J Am Soc Echocardiogr 2021;34(4):414–422.e4
8. Essandoh M, Graul T, Awad H. Venoarterial extracorporeal membrane oxygenation weaning in refractory cardiogenic shock: echocardiographic guidance may improve success. J Am Soc Echocardiogr 2022;35(1):134–135
9. Ye F, Yang Y, Liang Y, Liu J. Quantitative evaluation of hemodynamic parameters by echocardiography in patients with post-cardiotomy cardiac shock supported by extracorporeal membrane oxygenation. J Cardiothorac Surg. 2023;18(1):1
10. Huang KC, Lin LY, Chen YS, et al. Three-dimensional echocardiography-derivedright ventricular ejection fraction correlates with success of decannulation and prognosis in patients stabilized by venoarterial extracorporeal life support. J Am Soc Echocardiogr. 2018;31(2):169–179
11. Cevasco M, Takayama H, Ando M, Garan AR, Naka Y, Takeda K. Left ventricular distension and venting strategies for patients on venoarterial extracorporeal membrane oxygenation. J Thorac Dis 2019;11(4):1676–1683
12. Dickstein ML. The Starling relationship and veno-arterial ECMO: ventricular distension explained. ASAIO J 2018;64(4):497–501. 10.1097
13. O'Connor TA, Downing GJ, Ewing LL, Gowdamarajan R. Echocardiographically guided balloon atrial septostomy during extracorporeal membrane oxygenation (ECMO). Pediatr Cardiol 1993;14(3):167–168

Box 46.4 Echocardiography parameters of possible recovery

- TAPSE >11.5 mm
- PAAT >110 ms
- E/e¹ <15 (left free wall)
- E1—LV diastolic recovery
- S1—RV systolic recovery

Abbreviations: E/e', ratio between early mitral inflow velocity and mitral annular early diastolic velocity; LV, left ventricular; PAAT, pulmonary artery acceleration time; RV, right ventricular; TAPSE, tricuspid annular plane systolic excursion.

Box 46.5 Weaning and recovery: correct timing on a mechanical device

- Bridge to recovery, bridge to bridge VAD, bridge to transplant, and a bridge here to now
- No definitive weaning guidelines exist for ECMO; it is used as a bridge in most situations, so weaning gets dependent on the procedure

Abbreviations: ECMO, extracorporeal membrane oxygenation; VAD, ventricular assist device.

47

Role of Transesophageal Echocardiography Examination for Aortic Pathology

Kathirvel Subramaniam

Introduction

Transesophageal echocardiography (TEE) has advantages over transthoracic echocardiography (TTE) in the management of aortic disease because of the enhanced resolution with an unobstructed window, multiple examining planes, and the use of higher frequency transducers. TTE can be difficult in patients with thick chest wall and lung disease. However, it is a useful screening test and can be used to follow up aortic diameters in Marfan disease. Anatomically, aorta is divided into aortic root, ascending aorta, arch of aorta, and descending aorta. Aortic root includes aortic annulus, sinus of Valsalva, and sinotubular junction. Echocardiographically, aorta is indicated by six zones. Distal ascending (zone 3—site of cross clamping) and proximal arch (zone 4—site of aortic cannulation) cannot be visualized satisfactorily by TEE because of the intervening trachea and proximal bronchus. Epiaortic echocardiography with the probe placed directly on trachea is useful in evaluation of these zones for pathology.

There are certain safety considerations with TEE in aortic disease. Hypertensive response induced by TEE insertion or manipulations can cause rupture of aorta which is already dissected or enlarged. Anticipate probe insertion difficulties in patients with compression symptoms of enlarged aorta (dysphagia, dyspnea, and Horner syndrome). Patients with aortic disease also have coexisting cardiac disease. A comprehensive echocardiographic examination is recommended in such patients.

Typical TEE views for aortic examination include midesophageal aortic long axis, midesophageal aortic short axis, midesophageal aortic valve long and short axis, descending aortic short and long axis at multiple levels, upper esophageal aortic arch long and short axis, transgastric long axis. Imaging of right and left coronary arteries should also be done.

Artifacts such as reverberation artifact, side lobes, and shadowing can be frequent problems with aorta, and experience is required to avoid misdiagnosis of these artifacts as dissection. Random irregular movement of the dissection pathology should differentiate these fixed artifacts. Pericardial effusion can mimic dissection in the aortic arch.

Aortic diameter should be measured at various levels and care should be taken to avoid measuring in oblique axis as this will result in falsely high or low diameters.

Aortic Aneurysms

Aneurysms are defined as dilatation above two standard deviation from normal diameter after correction for body habitus. Thirty-three percent of aneurysms are thoracic, 65% abdominal, and 2% thoracoabdominal. Among thoracic aneurysm, more than 50% occur in ascending aorta. Ascending aortic aneurysms are caused by cystic medial necrosis and the descending aortic aneurysms are commonly associated with atherosclerosis. Hypertension is commonly associated with both. True aneurysms (contains all the layers of aorta) should be differentiated by echocardiography from pseudoaneurysms which are caused by rupture of the aortic wall and contained in the adventitial layer. Aneurysms are also classified according to shape as fusiform or saccular. Threshold for surgery in unruptured aorta is usually at the aortic diameter of 50 mm or more. Surgeons should be notified if the aortic diameter exceeds 40 mm and this was an accidental finding on perioperative echocardiography for another surgical procedure. Decision-making can be based on the etiology. If the dilatation is poststenotic from aortic stenosis, then aortic valve replacement may cure the problem. If the patient has Marfan syndrome, the dilatation is usually progressive and unrelated to aortic valve pathology. Marfan disease can present in three forms: Type 1 with cystic medial necrosis and ascending aneurysm, Type 2 with dissection of aorta, and Type 3 with mitral regurgitation and no aortic pathology. Sinus of Valsalva aneurysm can be congenital or traumatic. Usually it involves the right coronary cusp and protrudes into right atrium. Rupture into right atrium can cause sudden hemodynamic compromise.

Bicuspid aortic valve deserves special mention because of its association with dissections (6%), ascending aneurysms, coarctation of aorta, bicuspid pulmonary valve, and pulmonary artery dilatation.

Atherosclerosis

Aortic atheromas are the common reason for macroembolization and postoperative neurologic dysfunction. They also predict widespread peripheral vascular disease including coronary and carotid artery disease.

Aortic atheromas are graded as:
- *Grade 1:* Normal.
- *Grade 2:* Intimal thickening.
- *Grade 3:* Atheromas less than 5 mm.
- *Grade 4:* Atheromas more than 5 mm.
- *Grade 5:* Mobile atheromas.

Grades 4 and 5 are associated with 25% risk of postoperative stroke.

Atherosclerosis of aorta is diagnosed preoperatively by chest roentgenography, aortography, computed tomography (CT) and magnetic resonance imaging (MRI) scanning, and echocardiography. Intraoperative echocardiography is more readily available and is a sensitive method of diagnosing aortic atheromas.[1] Epiaortic can pick up more atheromas than TEE of ascending aorta. TEE is more sensitive to descending aortic atheromas. A combination of TEE and epiaortic imaging is recommended if significant disease is detected by TEE in the descending aorta.[2]

Epiaortic Scanning

Epiaortic scanning is superior to surgical palpation in the detection of aortic atheromas. Epiaortic scanning–directed surgical management decreased the postoperative neurological dysfunction. Current level of evidence for epiaortic scanning is class 2b.

Five different views are obtained by epiaortic scanning:
- Three short-axis views: proximal, mid, and distal ascending aortic short-axis view.
- Ascending aortic long axis.
- Proximal arch long axis including arch vessels.

Epiaortic scanning should be done by an echocardiographer or surgeon directed by the echocardiographer. Indications for epiaortic echocardiography included TEE-detected atheromas, mitral annular calcification, calcific aortic valve disease, age more than 60 years, calcified aortic knob on chest X-ray, palpable calcification in the ascending aorta, and patients with history of transient ischemic disease, cerebrovascular accidents, and peripheral vascular disease. Intravascular ultrasound with high-frequency probe is another modality which can be useful in detecting atheromatous disease of aorta.

Acute Aortic Syndromes

The term "acute aortic syndrome" includes acute dissection, intramural hematoma (IMH), and penetrating ulcers of the aorta. **Table 47.1** lists the terminologies used in differentiating between the true lumen and false lumen of aortic dissection.[3,4]

Dissection of Aorta

Dissection is splitting of aortic media between inner two-third and outer one-third creating a false channel within media. Stanford classified dissections into type A (all involving ascending aorta) and type B (dissection of descending aorta). Intimal flap is an undulating membrane 2 to 4 mm thick containing intima and one-third of media. Five percent of the dissections have no flap, and those will be missed by all noninvasive modalities. Presence of true and false lumen and intimal flap are characteristic of dissection. True and false lumens can be differentiated by the following. Other features such as entry tear, exit point, and re-entry tears can be recognized. Typical dissection begins on the anterior and right side of ascending aorta, courses over the superior surface of arch, and goes down on the left side of descending aorta. Therefore, it involves left intercostals, left renal vessels, left iliac vessels, and right coronary artery.[1]

TEE is very sensitive (97–100%) and specific (77–100%) and comparable to other modalities such as MRI and CT scanning. TEE requires no contrast, is minimally invasive, allows real-time assessment of cardiovascular system, and can be performed at bedside in short time in unstable patients.

The drawbacks of TEE include the artifacts seen which require experience and to differentiate between true dissection, learning curve, and blind spot where TEE may not be able to very nicely discern the landmarks of true versus false lines.[2]

Intraoperative Uses of TEE in Dissection

TEE answers the following questions in dissection of aorta:
- Is ascending aorta involved? Does the dissection involve intrapericardial portion of ascending aorta?
- Is the aortic valve involved in dissection?
- What is the mechanism of aortic insufficiency if present?
- Are the coronary arteries involved?
- Does the intimal flap originate in the arch? Are the neck vessels involved? Do the neck vessels originate in true or false?
- Is there any intimal invagination, intussusception, or compression by false lumen?
- Is there a dissecting aneurysm?
- Is the dissection ruptured or leaking?

Apart from answering these diagnostic questions, TEE is useful for the following intraoperatively:
- TEE-guided true lumen aortic cannulation.
- Cardiopulmonary bypass (CPB) related arterial flows in aorta can be assessed to rule out false lumen cannulation.
- Neck vessel perfusion can be assessed through surface echocardiography.

Table 47.1   Differentiation between true and false lumen in aortic dissection

S. no.	Characteristics	True lumen	False lumen
1.	Size	Small	Large
2.	Movement in systole	Expand with systole	Flap moves toward during systole
3.	Velocity flow	High velocity flow	Low velocity
4.	On ECHO	None (no pathology)	Thrombus/spontaneous echo contrast
5.	Contrast flow	Contrast flow faster	Contrast washout slower

- Aortic valve evaluation in valve-sparing surgery.
- Coronary artery flows if reimplanted.
- Ventricular function assessment post bypass period.
- False lumen flows after coming off cardiopulmonary bypass.
- Graft leak.

Descending thoracic aortic lesions are usually managed conservatively. Surgical indications include organ malperfusion, hemodynamic instability, ongoing or impending rupture, Marfan disease, and wide-open false lumen communicating to true lumen with chances of progression.

Intramural Hematoma

Intramural hematoma (IMH) is defined as the hemorrhage in the medial wall in the absence of intimal tear. It comprises 15 to 30% of acute aortic syndromes. Clinical presentation is similar to dissection and the management is similar.

Features

- Localized aortic wall thickness >7 mm in a circular or crescentic fashion.
- No intimal tear/dissection/smooth intimal surface.
- Aortic dilatation/dissection (localized)/rupture are sequelae to look for in TEE.
- Aortic thickness >11 mm and aortic diameter >60 mm are poor prognostic factors.[3]
- Treatment is surgical in ascending aorta and management is medical in descending aorta.[4]

Penetrating Aortic Ulcer

Develops in severe atherosclerotic aorta, commonly encountered in mid to distal descending aorta. The ulcer penetrates through media to produce subadventitial hematoma/pseudoaneurysm. Dissection is rare. Rupture through adventitia has been reported. Treatment is both surgical and medical.

Aortic Trauma

Severe deceleration injuries are associated with aortic injury with involvement of aortic isthmus in 90% of cases. TEE diagnosed these patients with 91% sensitivity and 100% specificity.[5]

Three types are recognized: intimal tears, subadventitial aortic disruption, and mediastinal hematoma. Subadventitial aortic disruption commonly involves isthmus, and flap contains media and intima, which runs vertically and is highly mobile. Aortic contour is deformed and asymmetric with preserved diameter. Re-entry and exit tears are absent. Mediastinal hematoma is present. Blood flow velocity is similar on either side of the flap and thrombus formation is absent.

Conclusion

In aortic disease though CT is the most used imaging technique in the diagnosis of its pathology, it is echocardiography which has a major role to play and is complimented to CT to complete a diagnosis of aortic disease. Echo thus plays a major role in the diagnosis. So best is to combine CT with contrast to TTE with contrast.[5] Before surgical procedures, it is wise to perform a TEE in the operative room, to know the extent of aortic disease, before and after surgical correction. Advantages of echocardiography in aortic disease examination are more than its limitations.[6,7]

Trans-esophageal echocardiography has been proven to be a simple, inexpensive, and easily reproducible way to measure the flow and peak systolic velocity in the celiac artery. Using TEE as an intraoperative monitoring during Aortic resections may be useful to evaluate the success of the surgical procedure, allowing the surgeon to obtain an intraoperative confirmation of the outcome of the resection, without the need to wait for postoperative follow-up evaluation.[8]

References

1. Feigenbaum H, Armstrong WF, Ryan T, eds. Diseases of aorta: Feigenbaum's echocardiography. 6th ed. New York: Lippincott Williams & Wilkins; 2005
2. Glas KE, Swaminathan M, Reeves ST, et al; Council for Intraoperative Echocardiography of the American Society of Echocardiography; Society of Cardiovascular Anesthesiologists. Guidelines for the performance of a comprehensive intraoperative epiaortic ultrasonographic examination: recommendations of the American Society of Echocardiography and the Society of Cardiovascular Anesthesiologists; endorsed by the Society of Thoracic Surgeons. J Am Soc Echocardiogr 2007; 20(11):1227–1235
3. Konstadt S, Kanchuger M. Assessment of surgery of the aorta. Robert Savage & Solomon Aronson: intraoperative transesophageal echocardiography. 1st ed. New York: Lippincott Williams & Wilkins; 2005
4. Willens HJ, Kessler KM. Transesophageal echocardiography in the diagnosis of diseases of the thoracic aorta: part 1. Aortic dissection, aortic intramural hematoma, and penetrating atherosclerotic ulcer of the aorta. Chest 1999;116(6):1772–1779
5. Evangelista A, Maldonado G, Gruosso D, et al. The current role of echocardiography in acute aortic syndrome. Echo Res Pract 2019;6(2):R53–R63
6. Erbel R, Aboyans V, Boileau C, et al; ESC Committee for Practice Guidelines; The Task Force for the Diagnosis and Treatment of Aortic Diseases of the European Society of Cardiology (ESC). 2014 ESC Guidelines on the diagnosis and treatment of aortic diseases: document covering acute and chronic aortic diseases of the thoracic and abdominal aorta of the adult. Eur Heart J 2014;35(41):2873–2926
7. Nienaber CA, Clough RE, Sakalihasan N, et al. Aortic dissection. Nat Rev Dis Primers 2016;2:16071
8. Lubian M, Nisi F, Giustiniano E, et al. Trans-Esophageal Echocardiography of the Descending Aorta and Celiac Trunk as an Intraoperative Monitoring for Median Arcuate Ligament Syndrome (MALS) Treatment: Technique Proposal and Two Case Reports. Surgeries 2023, 4, 17–25

48

Echocardiography for Left Ventricular Assist Device Management

Poonam Malhotra Kapoor, Priya Menon, Chirojit Mukherjee, Joerg Ender, and Minati Choudhury

Introduction

Patients with end-stage heart failure respond best to a cardiac transplant only. There exists a paucity of donors for all such patients to receive a heart transplant. Many patients thus remain on long-term or short-term mechanical circulatory support devices called left ventricular assist devices (LVADs), which provide all support to the ventricles and act as "Bridge" (to transplant/candidacy/recovery/destination therapy). The ideal tool to guide the placement, evaluation, management, and follow-up of patients with an LVAD in situ is expert echocardiography, which is the most essential.[1]

Ventricular assist devices (VADs) as they are popularly called are electromechanical pumps, which are applied to the patient's circulation in parallel and not in series. A typical VAD comprises of four parts (**Box 48.1**, **Fig. 48.1**).

The types of LVAD pumps widely range from the original roller pumps (e.g, Stockert) to the pulsatile pumps like Thoratec and HeartMate I. The axial flow devices like HeartMate II and Jarvik 2000 are the most recent ones, whereas BioMedicus and Tandem heart devices are centrifugal pump devices. These are well depicted in **Table 48.1**.

The HeartMate II LVAD, taken as a prototype, has the following positioning of its components. The rotor pump is first, followed by the inflow and, lastly, the outflow cannula. At the left ventricular (LV) apex lies the inflow cannula, whereas we find the outflow cannula attached to the right anterior aspect of the ascending aorta. The whole LVAD is housed within the peritoneal cavity. It is spinning of the rotor which suck in the blood from the inflow cannula through cardiac cycle into the ascending aorta (**Fig. 48.2** and **Box 48.2**).

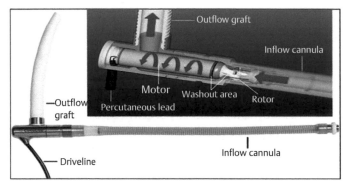

Fig. 48.1 Components of a left ventricular assist device (LVAD): Inflow cannula, outflow cannula, driveline motor, and pump pointing to the inner LVAD components.

> **Box 48.1** Components of a left ventricular assist device (LVAD)
>
> - **Inflow cannula.** This carries blood from the patient's heart into the LVAD
> - **Pump:** It pushes the blood forward into the body
> - **Outflow cannula:** This returns from the LVAD back into the patient
> - **Controller console:** This console accumulates and processes and returns all information and is most essential for LVAD pump function
>
> Abbreviation: LVAD, left ventricular assist device.

> **Box 48.2** Parts of a HeartMate II
>
> - It is an LVAD that provides short- or long-term circulatory support for intermediate to advanced heart failure patients
> - This small advice has only one moving part and provides same blood flow as that of a healthy heart
>
> Abbreviation: LVAD, left ventricular assist device.

Table 48.1 Types of left ventricular assist device (LVAD) pump devices

Types of LVAD pumps	Example
Traditional roller pumps	Stockist
Pulsatile LVAD pumps	• HeartMate I • Thoratec
Centrifugal pumps	• BioMedicus • Tandem Heart
Continuous axial flow devices with propeller and pump	• HeartMate II • Jarvik
Continuous flow third generation with a miniaturized centrifugal pump with bearing less magnetically levitated motor with active magnetic mounting	Heartware (HVAD) or HeartMate III
Component parts float rather than rub together	Can create an artificial pulse
Contactless and frictionless rotor	Makes it more durable
Microaxial continuous flow pump	Impella
Full Maglev flow technology with a centrifugal pump, a motor, a control console, a flow probe, tubing, and cannulae Pump priming volume is 31 mL	CentriMag with a maximum blood flow of 10 L/min

Abbreviation: HVAD, HeartWare ventricular-assist device; LVAD, left ventricular assist device.

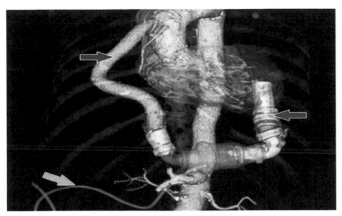

Fig. 48.2 HeartMate II displaying the inflow and outflow cannula.

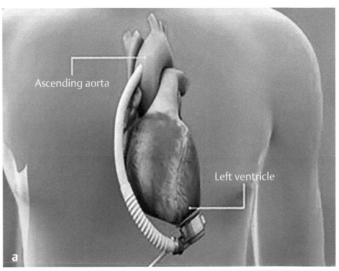

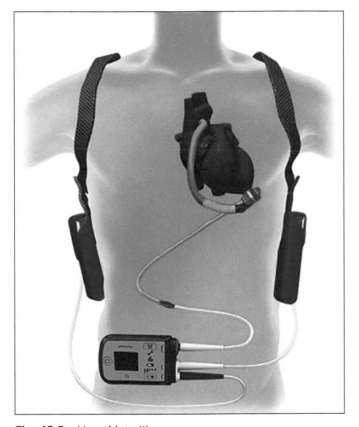

Fig. 48.3 HeartMate III.

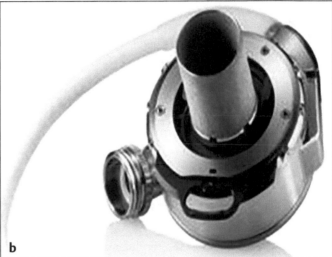

Fig. 48.4 **(a)** HeartMate III. **(b)** HeartMate III left ventricle assist system.

Difference Between HeartMate II and HeartMate III LVADs

The main difference between HeartMate II and HeartMate III is that the HeartMate III device is a pulsatile flow system without mechanical bearings, as against the HeartMate II device which is a continuous flow system with mechanical bearings.

The HeartMate II and Echocardiography

Echocardiography needs to be performed in four major areas for successful LVAD placement:

- Preoperative assessment of the patient.
- Echocardiography guidance during LVAD placement.
- To detect postoperative complications.
- Monitoring the cardiac parameters post LVAD.

The HeartMate III Device

As shown in **Figs. 48.3** and **48.4**, HeartMate III has a driveline through the skin into the abdomen which is made of titanium. It is virtually a silent machine, pumping blood into the patient's body like the native heart. The pump cable and the modular cable, in this LVAD, is attached at the base of the heart at base of LV with a small electric motor, which pumps blood. The pump and modular cables act as inflow and outflow cables. The modular cable is attached to the console (**Fig. 48.5**).

Strategies for Mechanical Circulatory Devices (MCDs)

As shown in **Box 48.3**, all MCDs like the LVAD, right ventricular assist device (RVAD), or BIVA (**Fig. 48.6**) can be used as either as a bridge to transplant, decision, candidacy, recovery, or destination therapy.

Who Needs Mechanical Circulatory Support (MCS)? Indications for LVAD

These are used by those patients with refractory heart failure. For a typical patient with a refractory heart failure, echocardiography is essential in all four phases from LVAD insertion to LVAD maintenance as stated below.

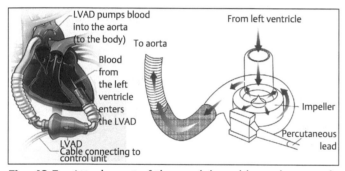

Fig. 48.5 Attachment of the modular cable to the console in HeartMate III device. Abbreviation: LVAD, left ventricular assist device.

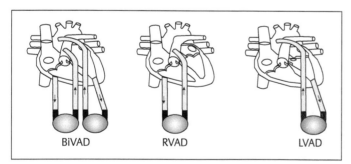

Fig. 48.6 Biventricular assist device (BiVAD), right ventricular assist device (RVAD), and left ventricular assist device (LVAD) with their connections.

Box 48.3 Strategies for mechanical circulatory support (MCS)
• Bridge to transplantation • Bridge to therapy • Bridge to candidacy • Bridge to decision • Bridge to recovery

Echocardiography for LVAD

Echocardiography in LVAD is most essential in four areas:
- Patient selection and preoperative assessment.
- Aiding VAD insertion.
- Detection of complications with LVAD in situ.
- Monitoring cardiac recovery while on LVAD.

Patient Selection

Echocardiography aids in two major ways:
- Is the patient suitable for an LVAD insertion? Making decision on whether or not to place the LVAD.
- To identify, preoperatively and postoperatively, cardiac abnormalities with different echocardiography views so that postoperative complications can be overcome. For this, it is important to assess each one of the following on echocardiography before LVAD placement:
  ➢ Left ventricle function.
  ➢ Right ventricle function.
  ➢ Ascending aorta, arch, and descending aorta.
  ➢ Valvular heart function (valvular regurgitation or stenosis).
  ➢ Assessment of prosthetic valve function.
  ➢ Rule out any ventricular scar or fibrosis.

Left Ventricular Assessment on Echocardiography

Depending on the etiology of heart failure, the LV function will be depressed with LV being dilated or of normal diameter. The left ventricular ejection fraction (LVEF) for requiring LVAD would also be only around 25 to 30%. The diastolic function too is restrictive in nature. This is generally picked up on pulsed wave Doppler of the pulmonary veins or on a tissue Doppler when the LV diastolic dysfunction is restrictive. It implies there is a high risk of apical thrombus formation. An apical thrombus is most commonly observed near the cannula insertion site. Whenever we find a restrictive LV diastolic function, we must cautiously rule out an apical thrombus formation. Use of an echocardiographic contrast injection can help in delineating with a high sensitivity the presence of an LV apical thrombus (**Flowchart 48.1**).[2]

Pre VAD Insertion: Assessment of Patients

It is imperative to perform a detailed preoperative echocardiography assessment of a patient selected for VAD insertion for guiding during VAD, and also postoperatively for detecting complications after VAD insertion. Monitoring the cardiac recovery on echocardiography is equally important, once the VAD is activated.

Pre VAD Insertion: Echocardiography Assessment

A detailed echocardiogram is required for two reasons: first, in the preoperative period to have a detailed knowledge of the suitability of the patient for LVAD insertion or not and second, postoperatively to learn the complications that may cause bad outcomes by preventing optimal efficiency of VAD.

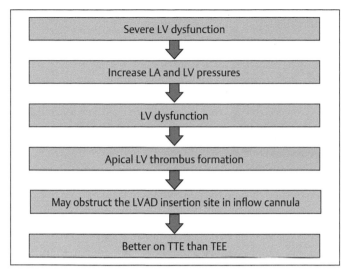

Flowchart 48.1 LV apical contrast injection helps delineate ventricular dysfunction and LVAD cannula obstruction. Abbreviations: LA, left atrium; LV, left ventricle; LVAD, left ventricular assist device; TEE, transesophageal echocardiography; TTE, transthoracic echocardiography.

The following need to be assessed in detail. Preoperatively on echocardiography it is important to rule out presence of intra-cardiac shunts, patient foramen ovalis (PFO), and certain other structural issues that may be surgically corrected at the time of LVAD insertion. Atheromas and dilatation in the ascending aorta (**Box 48.4**) or a pericardial effusion or the presence of an left atrium (LA), left ventricle (LV), or any cardiac chamber thrombus clot should be ruled out.

Preoperative RV Assessment on Echocardiography for LVAD Placement

It is well known that the output of the native right ventricle (RV) determines the preload of the LVAD. This implies that when there is a decrease in RV function the LVAD output too would decrease. Thus, RV dysfunction develops far too commonly in LVAD recipient patients. Postoperative RV dysfunction has a multifactorial etiology, but a complete RV assessment pre LVAD placement immensely aids in selecting the right patient for an LVAD or a BiVAD placement wherein low cardiac output period due to RV dysfunction has been preoperatively ruled out. **Box 48.5** shows how LVAD placement can influence the RV function.[3]

Preoperative RV Assessment on Echocardiography for Detecting RV Failure

LVAD recipients' most dreaded complication is the development of RV failure. This is because the output of the native RV determines the preload of the LVAD. A decrease in RV function will automatically decrease the LV function as well.

Transesophageal Echocardiography (TEE) Views to Detect RV Dysfunction

- Midesophageal (ME) RV inflow–outflow view.

Box 48.4 Pericardial effusion before LVAD insertion

- With or without cardiac tamponade including RV compression
- **Tamponade:** respire [phasic flow changes; poor RVOT SV, LV failure secondary to partial LV unloading (by serial exam comparison)
- **2D/3D:** increasing LV size by linear or volume measurements, increased AV opening duration, increased left atrial volume
- **Doppler:** increased mitral inflow peak E-wave diastolic velocity, increased E/A and E/e' ratio, decreased deceleration time of mitral E velocity, worsening fuctional MR and elevated pulmonary artery systolic pressure

Abbreviations: AV, atrioventricular; E/A, early to late diastolic transmitral flow velocity; E/e', ratio between early mitral inflow velocity and mitral annular early diastolic velocity; LVAD, left ventricular assist device; LV, left ventricle; MR, mitral regurgitation; RV, right ventricle; RVOT, right ventricular outflow tract; SV, sinus venosus.

Box 48.5 LVAD placement and its effect on RV function

- LVAD benefits RV function by reducing the afterload
- LVAD can further harm the RV by increasing preload to an already compromised RV
- LVAD can be more detrimental to the RV by reducing its contractility as it shifts the septum leftward during VAD support
- LVAD implantation predisposes a preoperatively dilated RV with increased RV preload and afterload to RV dysfunction

Abbreviations: LVAD, left ventricular assist device; RV, right ventricle; VAD, ventricular-assist devices.

- ME 4 chamber view.
- Transgastric long-axis view.
- Transgastric short-axis view.

Observations for RV Dysfunction

- RV dilatation and RV function measurement.
- RV base (tricuspid valve [TV] annulus) to apex motion and free-wall motion.
- Quantitative analysis of RV function and dilatation.
- The maximum derivative of the RV pressure (dP/dt max) have been used to quantify systolic function.

Global RV fractional area change (FAC): The global RV FAC is most often used in patients undergoing LVAD implantation. Normal global FAC is 20 to 60%. A value of FAC <20% infers right ventricular failure (RVF) on LVAD insertion.

Echocardiography Assessment for LVAD Implantation to Rule Out RV Diastolic Dysfunction

Before LVAD implantation, it is important to rule out the following lesions so that they may be corrected preoperatively or at the time of LVAD implantation, as shown in **Box 48.6** and **Fig. 48.7**.

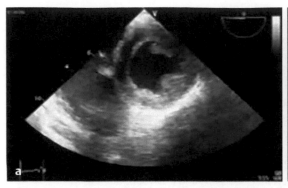
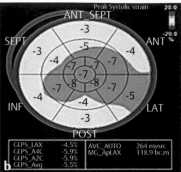

Fig. 48.7 (a) Preoperative right ventricular diastolic function and strain imaging. **(b)** Transthoracic strain echocardiography displaying a diffuse abnormal strain pattern in a 65-year-old man with ischemic cardiomyopathy. Global longitudinal peak systolic strain (GLPS) measure is –5.5%.

Box 48.6 Preoperative right ventricular diastolic function and strain imaging

- Global:
  - ➤ RV ejection fraction
  - ➤ RV fractional area change %
  - ➤ Dp/dt
  - ➤ Myocardial performance index
  - ➤ 2D straim
- Regional:
  - ➤ Tricuspid annular plane systolic excursion
  - ➤ S' (Doppler myocardial velocity in systole)

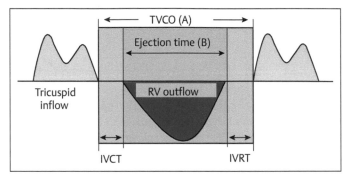

Fig. 48.8 Tei index. Abbreviations: IVCT, isovolumetric contraction time; IVRT, isovolumetric relaxation time; RV, right ventricular; TVCO, tricuspid valve cardiac output.

2D strain rate has limitations with regards to: Reflecting both systolic and diastolic abnormalities, possibility of reflecting heterogeneous myocardial abnormalities, ability to detect subclinical rejection, and angle dependent and frame rate limitations. Thus, 4D strain came up and is in current use.

A more quantitative evaluation of RV myocardial performance is the Tei index (**Fig. 48.8**). The Tei index is reproducible, independent of ventricular geometry, and not significantly impacted by heart rate or blood pressure. Ventricular loading conditions do not appear to affect the index. The calculation for the Tei index using the TV annular velocity is shown in **Fig. 48.8**.

Other RV Function Indices for RV Dysfunction

High specificity for an RV dysfunction:
- A TAPSE cut-off value of 17 mm yields abnormal from normal systolic function.
- Functional tricuspid regurgitation (TR).
- The mechanism of TR is extremely important to define and moderate or greater may require surgical correction at the time of LVAD implantation.
- Significant TV annular dilation.
- Absence of TR does not imply that the TV orifice is free from abnormality.
- Meticulous examination of RV size and function and TV pre-LVAD implantation.

Assessment of the Ascending Aorta

- The outflow cannula of an LVAD device is usually attached to the ascending aorta in an end-to-side anastomosis.
- The two main abnormalities that impact LVAD insertion are aneurysmal dilatation of the ascending aorta and atherosclerotic disease (**Fig. 48.9**).
- If there is significant dilatation of the ascending aorta (>45 mm) detected at the time of LVAD insertion, the ascending aorta is usually replaced with a Dacron graft and the LVAD cannula attached in an end-to-side manner to the graft.

Uncorrected Aortic Regurgitation (AR)

If left without correction, there is a negative impact on the forward flow of the LVAD as the VAD flow regurgitates back into the LV cavity. It is thus essential to first correct the moderate and severe AR before LVAD implantation. Aortic stenosis with LVAD does not have such negative side effects as AR, but in continuous flow device, with the set configurations aortic regurgitation too may limit forward flow and may require first surgical correction of as before LVAD implantation. TR is the commonest valve scenario observed in heart failure patients due to elevated pulmonary artery pressures. TR with >40 cm tricuspid annular dilatation may need correction as it causes much morbidity and mortality.[3]

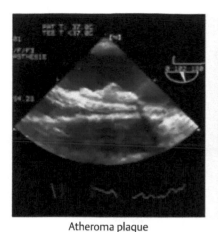
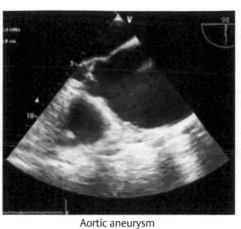
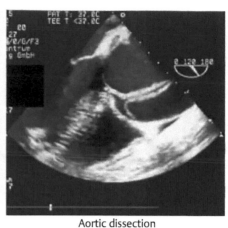

| Atheroma plaque | Aortic aneurysm | Aortic dissection |

Fig. 48.9 Aortic diseases, such as an atheromatous plaque or aortic aneurysm or aortic dissection, should be ruled out prior to implantation.

Pulmonary insufficiency and pressure right to left shunting (atrial and with a ventricular scar, especially at the cannulation site) may require an RVAD instead of an LVAD.

Prosthetic valve in situ patients represent a complex group for LVAD placements as an LVAD-induced low flow state increases risk of valve thrombosis.[4] Risk of thrombosis is there in both biological and mechanical valves. However, if a mechanical valve is in site at the time of valve implantation, it is wise to change it to a biological valve before LVAD implantation.[5]

Patients with incite prosthetic valves requiring LVAD represent a complex patients category as they are more prone to develop prosthetic valve thrombosis.[6]

Rule out moderate to severe aortic insufficiency (**Fig. 48.10**) as enumerated by Cowger et al.[7]

According to Kukucka et al, a tricuspid annular diameter greater than 43 mm is an independent predictor of survival after LVAD has been implanted. So this needs to be interrogated before LVAD on a detailed echocardiography examination as well.[8]

The following should be ruled out on echocardiography:
- Both mitral valve stenosis and mitral regurgitation using three-dimensional en-face view (**Fig. 48.11**). For this, the echocardiographic parameters to quantify mitral leaflet configurations are (**Fig. 48.12**):
  - ➢ Tethering area.
  - ➢ Mitral annulus size.
  - ➢ Papillary muscle distance.
  - ➢ LV end diastolic distance.

LV Assessment Pre LVAD Insertion on Echocardiography

Left ventricle (LV) function before LVAD insertion shows in most patients a depressed LV with a normal or dilated LV size due to heart failure, cardiomyopathy, etc before an LVAD implantation, the left ventricle LV has depressed contractility due to diseases like heart failure, cardiomyopathy etc. The LVEF also is less around 25-30% on Echo. It shows as a diastolic dysfunction, seen well on pulsed wave Echo with

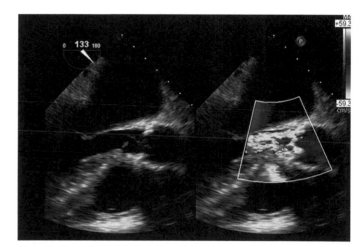

Fig. 48.10 Aortic valve insufficiency.

pulsed wave Doppler of the pulmonary veins and Doppler across the transmitral velocity. The restrictive LV diastolic functions implies there is increased LV and LA pressures, which mandates an LVAD insertion. This severe LV failure is also a high risk for thrombus formation or regional wall abnormalities development. For the latter a global, longitudinal strain, basal preoperative value is very helpful assist LV dimensions (LVAD) so that postoperative LV dilation or the strain becoming more negative is a poor outcome predictor. It can be overcome by optimizing the pump speed and RPM.

Tissue Doppler Imaging and Speckle Tracking Echocardiography

Strain rate analysis has a potential to detect even mild rejection. Kato et al[9] reported that the attenuation of LV longitudinal strain and the diastolic strain rate derived from TDI were associated with conventional International Society for Heart and Lung Transplantation (ISHLT) grade 1b or higher rejection without hemodynamic alterations (**Fig. 48.13**).[9]

Two-dimensional speckle-tracking echocardiography (2D-STE) was developed as an angle-independent

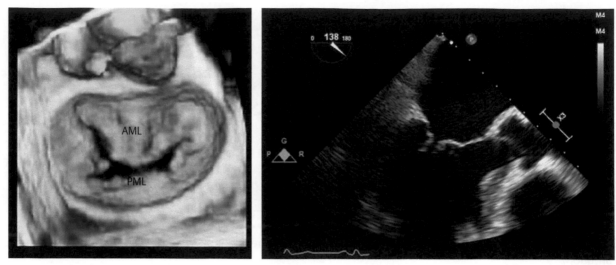

Fig. 48.11 Mitral valve stenosis/regurgitation using three-dimensional en-face view. Abbreviations: AML, anterior mitral leaflet; PML, posterior mitral leaflet.

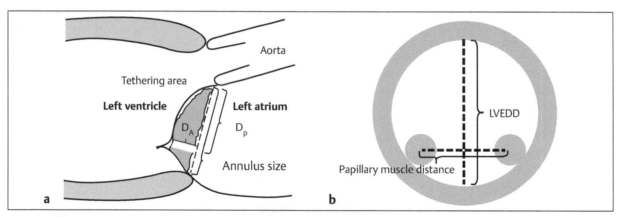

Fig. 48.12 (a, b) Preoperative assessment of echocardiography parameters. The tethering area (a) and LVEDD are good parameters to measure post LVAD implantation. Abbreviation: LVEDD, left ventricular end-diastolic diameter.

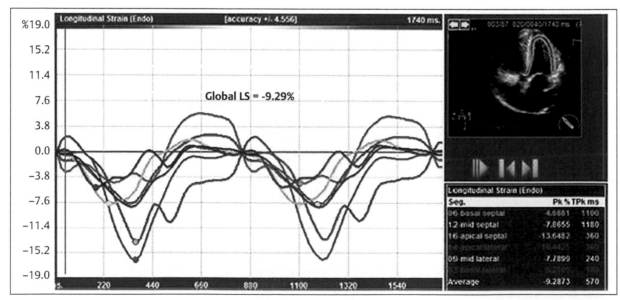

Fig. 48.13 Patient with grade 3A rejection has a GLS of -9.29% which is abnormal. GLS is a good predictor of successful outcomes, post LVAD implantation. Abbreviations: GLS, global longitudinal strain; LVAD, left ventricular assist device.

echocardiographic modality to evaluate cardiac mechanical function. The 2D-STE–derived parameters associated with rejection. The association between LV torsional deformation and rejection in transplant recipients has been reported since the 1980s. Sato et al reported that 2D-STE–derived LV torsion values are decreased in patients with rejection, and the serial assessments of an intra-patients comparison showed that a cut-off value of a 25% reduction of LV torsion from the baseline is associated with ISHLT grade 2 or higher rejection, which returns to the baseline after adequate rejection treatment.[10]

Echocardiography parameters needed in a stepwise approach are enumerated in **Box 48.7** and **Fig. 48.14**.

It was predicted that LVAD with LV dysfunction would not do well post implantation. So authors gave RVF score point (**Figs. 48.15–48.17**).

The wall thickness of LV and the LV mass index without rejection (left) were 9 mm and 88 g/m², respectively. The same parameters associated with rejection (right) were 13 mm and 112 g/m². The arrow in the right lower panel indicates a pericardial effusion (**Fig. 48.18a, b**).

Risk Factors for RV Dysfunction Post LVAD

RV dysfunction should be ruled out before LVAD insertion. RV failure when it sets in brings with it low cardiac output. An LVAD or MCD here reduces the afterload by (i) increasing the preload to compromise RV and (ii) it impairs the RV contractility through leftward septal shift during LVAD support.

A preoperative RV with raised preload, increased afterload, and RV dilatation predisposes to RV dysfunction after LVAD implantation.

> **Box 48.7** Echocardiography parameters for assessment of left ventricle (LV) diastolic function
>
> - M-mode
> - Mitral inflow
> - Pulmonary venous flow
> - PA systolic pressure
> - Flow propagation velocity (Vp)
> - Mitral annulus velocities by tissue Doppler (strain, strain rate)
> - 2D speckle imaging/VVI: strain, strain rate, rotation and twist
> - 3D speckle imaging: strain, strain rate, rotation, twist and torsion
> - Left ventricular hypertrophy
> - Left atrial volume index

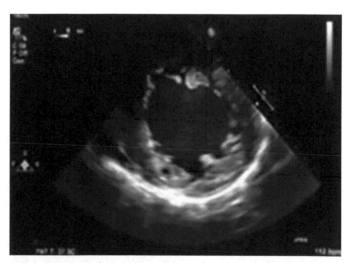

Fig. 48.14 Echocardiography showing left ventricular diastolic function.

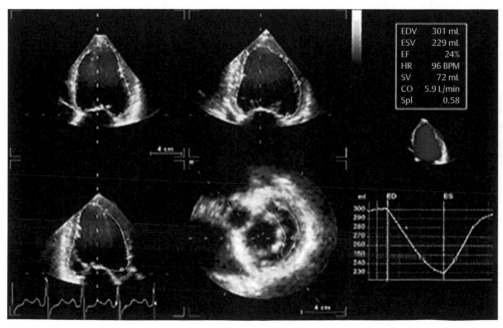

EDV	301 mL
ESV	229 mL
EF	24%
HR	96 BPM
SV	72 mL
CO	5.9 L/min
Spl	0.58

Fig. 48.15 Preimplantation left ventricular assist device evaluation using three-dimensional echocardiography to assess left ventricular end-diastolic (EDV) and end-systolic volume (ESV) and ejection fraction (EF). In this, if EDV is approximately 300 mL and ESV is 200 mL, then EF is around 32%.

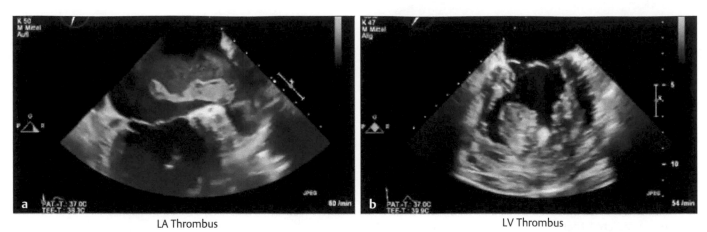

LA Thrombus

LV Thrombus

Fig. 48.16 **(a, b)** Preimplantation assessment of left atrium (LA) thrombus or left ventricular (LV) thrombus needs a detailed echocardiography in experienced hands.

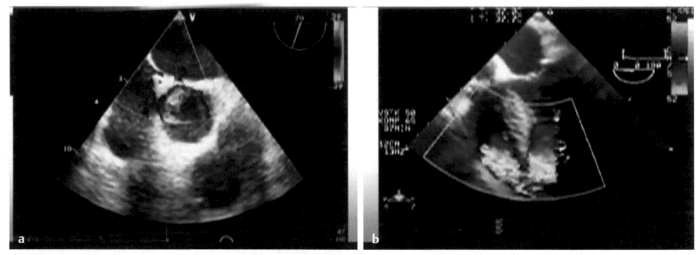

Fig. 48.17 **(a, b)** Check for shunts across the left atrium (LA), left ventricle (LV), right atrium (RA), and right ventricle (RV). Echo showing LA–LV stunts in **(a)**.

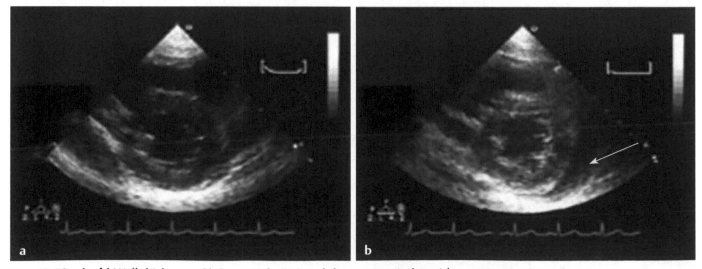

Fig. 48.18 **(a, b)** Wall thickness of left ventricle (LV) and the LV mass index without rejection (*arrow*).

Valvular Function Before LVAD

Assessment of Native Cardiac Valves

- In mitral insufficiency, there are chances of patient going into end-stage heart failure. The LVAD unloads the left ventricle following which there is often improvement in the severity of mitral regurgitation.
- Aortic insufficiency if left uncorrected has a negative impact on forward flow of the LVAD as the VAD flow regurgitation back into the LV cavity.
- Aortic stenosis is usually not of such clinical significance compared to aortic regurgitation.
- Tricuspid regurgitation is a relatively common condition in patients being assessed for mechanical support.
  - ➤ Assessment of prosthetic cardiac valves is important to rule out any of the following:
- Atrial and ventricular shunting especially R → L.
- Presence of pulmonary insufficiency, especially for an RVAD.
- Any scar, especially at cannulation site (**Fig. 48.19**).

It is important to note the inflow cannula positioning on two to three major transthoracic parasternal and apical views, and the inflow cannula positioning with LV apex palpation and LV apex needle placement (**Figs. 48.20** and **48.21**).

Detailed echocardiography for LVAD and RV function monitoring are shown in **Fig. 48.22**. It is essential to note the LV in totality especially as interavenous (IV) septum shifts rightwards and causes inadequate LV unloading (inadequate LVAD speed, suboptimal LVAD function, inflow-cannula obstruction) (**Fig. 48.23**).

Post activation of LVAD, a detailed echocardiography is essential to monitor the LV and RV function and position of both the interatrial septum (IAS) and interventricular septum (IVS) along with ejection fraction and functional area change (**Fig. 48.24**).

Guidance During VAD Insertion

- *Cannula flow pattern:* Both in LVAD, on echo, the color flow Doppler, the continuous wave Doppler, the pulsed wave Doppler, is essential to monitor. Also, to observe on ECHO adequate chamber decompression and presence of air within the circuit.

The apical inflow cannula can be confirmed with four-chamber (evaluate deviation toward the IVS) (**Fig. 48.25**) and two-chamber views (to evaluate anteroposterior direction) (**Figs. 48.26** and **48.27**).

The route taken by the flow of blood into an LVAD is depicted well in **Flowchart 48.2**.

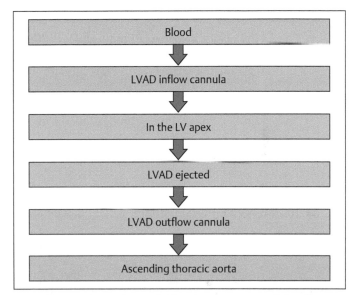

Flowchart 48.2 Flow of blood in LVAD and finally into the ascending thoracic aorta from the inflow cannula. Abbreviations: LV, left ventricle; LVAD, left ventricular assist device.

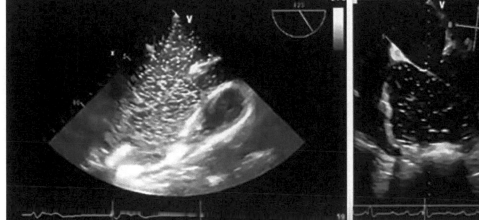
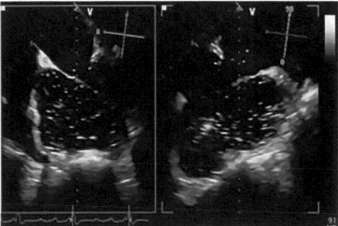

Fig. 48.19 De-airing on echocardiography helps to solve the problem of massive air seen in all four chambers during and after implantation.

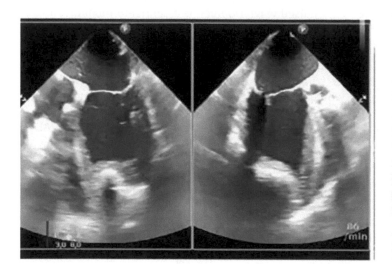

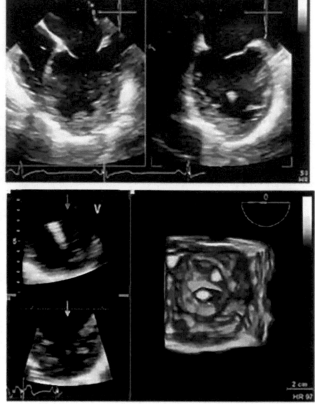

Fig. 48.20 Intraoperative monitoring during implantation.

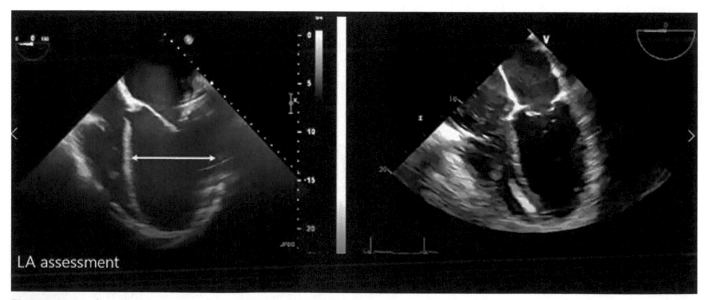

LA assessment

Fig. 48.21 Left atrium (LA) assessment and increase in left ventricular (LV) internal diameter are to be noted as well during implantation.

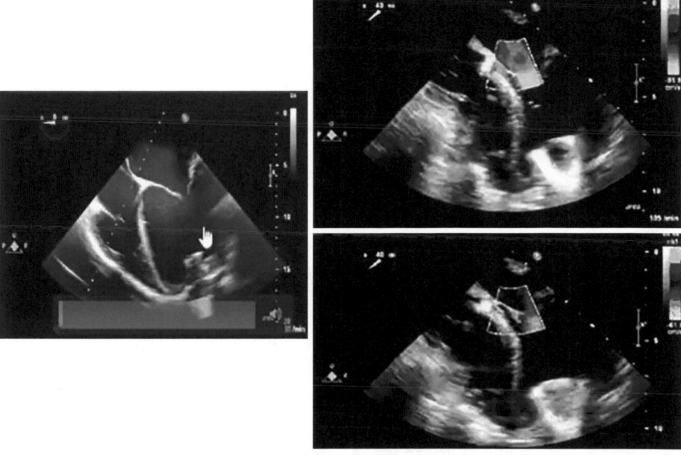

Fig. 48.22 Detailed echocardiography for left ventricular assist device (LVAD) and right ventricle (RV).

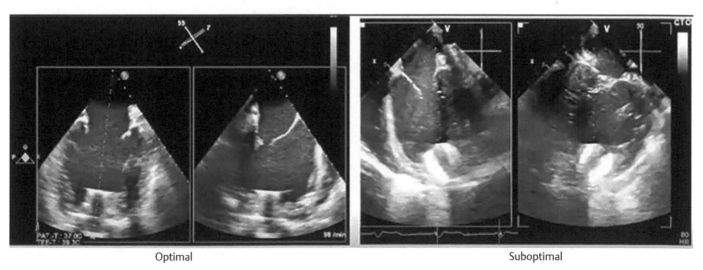

Optimal   Suboptimal

Fig. 48.23 The final position of cannula is to be noted before the left ventricular assist device (LVAD) is activated.

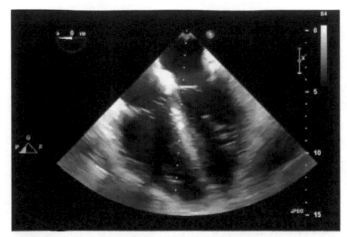

Fig. 48.24 Post activation of left ventricular assist device (LVAD).

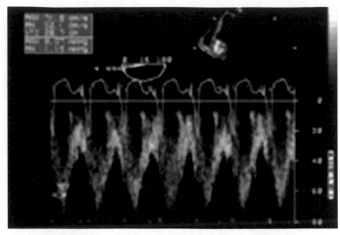

Fig. 48.25 Inflow cannula Doppler profile (normal).

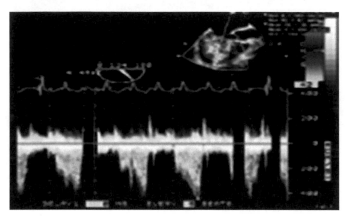

Fig. 48.26 Doppler flow turbulence—inflow cannula obstruction.

The alignment of the inflow cannula should be confirmed always by echocardiography. It should at all times be perpendicular to the plane of the mitral annulus and toward the P2 segment of the mitral valve. Its angulation should be directed toward the interventricular septum or the lateral wall of the LV.[11]

Assessment of the Outflow Cannula

Flow through the LVAD is generally unidirectional and pulsatile. For monitoring outflow cannula dynamics, it is important to monitor the same with a PWD sample volume cursor placed 1 cm proximal to the aortic anastomosis, so that good flow pattern can be observed. A normal outflow peak velocity ranges from 1 to 2 m/s with a specular pattern on Doppler evaluation. It is important to rule out kinking of the cannula if the LVAD outflow cannula flows are obstructed.

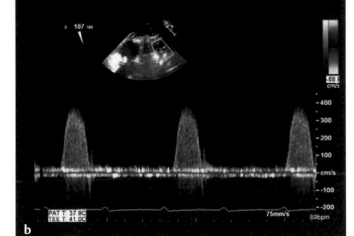

Fig. 48.27 (a, b) Left ventricular assist device outflow anastomosis in ascending aorta (ME Asc aorta long-axis color Doppler). Abbreviation: ME, midesophageal.

In latter scenarios, it is important to observe native valvular structure on echocardiography to evaluate valve function and its complications (e.g., aortic dissection).

Low LVAD Flows on Echocardiography

Low LVAD flows are seen if one of the following is seen to be existing:
- Inlet cannula obstruction.
- Reduced preload (hypovolemia).
- Severe TR.
- RV dysfunction with collapsed LV.
- Ventricular tachycardia.
- Cardiac tamponade.
- Detailed assessment of the outflow cannula.

In case of cardiac tamponade is seen, then on echocardiography it important is to observe low cardiac output and any big clot compressing any of the four cardiac chambers. Echocardiography features of interventricular dependence and cardiac tamponade may not be coexisting in an LVAD patient.

LVAD High Pump Flows

In an LVAD concept of de novo, aortic regurgitation should coexist, whenever we observed that if the pump flow is high then the cardiac output remains low. If there is LV dilation or/severe functional MR or regular opening of aortic valve secondary to inappropriate LV unloading or there is regurgitate flow through both inflows and outflow cannulas with an increase in systolic to diastolic velocity ratio, then there exists a pump thrombosis.

Weaning from LVAD

Echocardiography also plays an important role in weaning from LVAD as when we decrease the LVAD support reducing speed, the following changes are seen:
- The preload increases and left ventricular end-diastolic diameter (LVEDD) can decrease or increase suggesting recovery or failed weaning, respectively (**Table 48.2**).
- Dobutamine stress echocardiography testing in this setting has some evidence for assessing the degree of recovery with the LVAD weaned off.

Importance of Aortic Valve Opening

In an LVAD it is essential to observe aortic valve opening at all times, it:
- Prevents healing and chronic closure.
- Prevents thrombosis.
- In the event of LVAD dysfunction, allows LV ejection.

Post LVAD Assessment

Assessment of postoperative LVAD is depicted in **Flowchart 48.3**.

Valvular Insufficiency/Stenosis

Once LVAD is activated, the aortic leaflets are subjected to high pressure that might cause a worsening of the

Table 48.2 Different clinical situations and LVAD

	Hypovolemia	PAH	RVFD	AR
LVEDD	Decrease	Increase	Decrease	Same
RVEDD	±	Same	Increase	Same
Interventricular dependence	No change	No change	Shifts to the left	No change
MR	±	Increase	±	±
Pulsatility Index	Decrease	Increase	Decrease	Same
LVAD power	Remains the same	Same	Same	Same
LVAD power	Pump thrombosis	Cardiac tamponade		
LVAD power	Increase	Decrease		
LVAD power	Same	Decrease		
LVAD power	No change	No change		
LVAD power	Increase	Same		
LVAD power	Decrease	Decrease		
LVAD power	Increase	Same		

Abbreviations: AR, aortic regurgitation; LVAD, left ventricular assist device; LVEDD, left ventricular end-diastolic diameter; MR, mitral regurgitation; PAH, pulmonary arterial hypertension; RVEDD, right ventricular end-diastolic diameter; RVFD, right ventricular flow device.

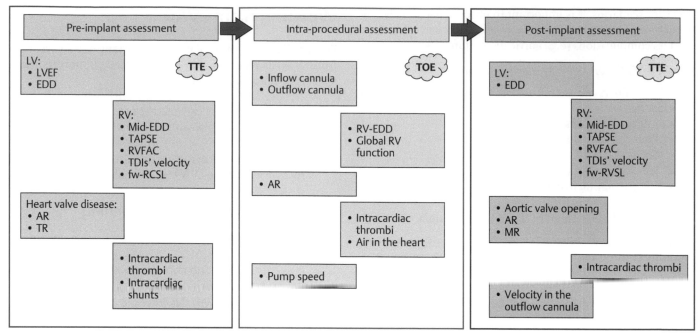

Flowchart 48.3 Assessment of postoperative LVAD. Abbreviations: AR, aortic regurgitation; EDD, end diastolic diameter; RVSL, right ventricular segment length; LV, left ventricle; LVAD, left ventricular-assist device; LVEF, left ventricular ejection fraction; MR, mitral regurgitation; RV, right ventricle; RV-EDD, right ventricular end diastolic diameter; RVFAC, right ventricular fractional area change; TAPSE, tricuspid annular plane systolic excursion; TDI, tissue Doppler imaging; TOE, transesophageal echocardiography; TEE, transesophageal echocardiography; TR, tricuspid regurgitation; TTE, transthoracic echocardiography.

regurgitation. Thus, in the presence of more than moderate aortic regurgitation, a surgical repair along with LVAD implant should be considered. Heart failure patients for heart transplantation showed good correlation with RV stroke work index (RVSWI), and it was the best predictor of RV failure after LVAD implantation. As a consequence, mitral regurgitation is generally not recommended to be corrected before LVAD implant since it is not a strong predictor of outcome after LVAD in contrast to tricuspid regurgitation (TR).

Device Specifications

- *Pulsatile devices:*
  - ➤ Continuous closure of the aortic valve.
  - ➤ Pulsatile flow velocities in device cannulas.
- *Axial flow devices:*
  - ➤ Intermittent opening of the aortic valve.
  - ➤ Pulsatile flow velocities in device cannulas superimposed on continuous velocity.
  - ➤ Left ventricular unloading, right ventricular function, and tricuspid regurgitation according to flow settings.

Hemodynamic Instability in Early Postoperative Days

- *Hypovolemia:* Should be considered when the RV and LV cavities are small.

- Acute RV dysfunction.
- Cardiac tamponade.
- Pulmonary embolism.
- *Suction cascade:* Most typical expression of acute RV dysfunction.
- *Echocardiography findings:* Dilated and hypo-contractile RV, significant functional tricuspid regurgitation, small left ventricle, and an intermittent inflow cannula obstruction by the collapsed LV wall.
- LVAD dysfunction or thrombosis (**Flowchart 48.4**) should be suspected when clinical (cardiogenic shock, low LVAD output), echocardiographic (rightward deviation of the interventricular and interatrial septum, significant functional mitral regurgitation, aortic valve opens in every cardiac cycle and the diastolic aortic pressure exceeds the LV diastolic pressure, resulting in a reverse flow from the ascending aorta through the outflow and inflow cannulas), and laboratory clues (intravascular hemolysis) are detected.[3]

Future of VADS on the Horizon

CentriMag for Heart Failure

CentriMag is an external blood pump connected to a surgically inserted cannula. It is designed for short-term cardiopulmonary support (up to 30 days) in adults and children with end-stage or acute heart failure. It can be used to

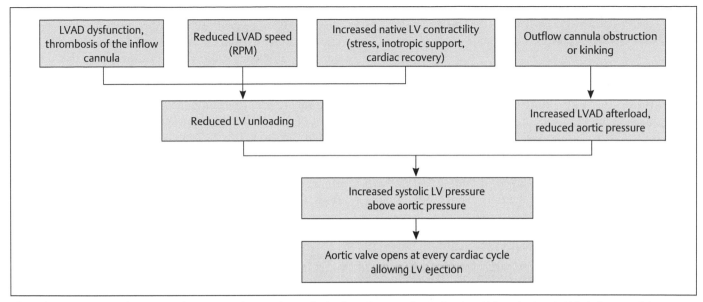

Flowchart 48.4 Left ventricular assist device (LVAD) dysfunction or thrombosis. Abbreviations: LV, left ventricle; RPM, revolutions per minute.

support patients until they recover (bridge to recovery), until they have a heart transplant (bridge to transplant), or while a decision is being made about suitable longer-term treatments (bridge to decision). The device can provide total circulatory support (acting as a biventricular assist device, or BiVAD) or individual left or right ventricular support (LVAD or RVAD). It can also be used as a part of an extracorporeal membrane oxygenation (ECMO) circuit, but this use is beyond the scope of this chapter (**Table 48.3** and **Fig. 48.28**).

Impella

Refer to **Fig. 8.7**.
Advantages of Impella:
- Small rotary pump.
- Can be placed percutaneously from femoral artery across aortic valve without need of trans-septal puncture or venous access.
- Can be easily removed.

Disadvantages of Impella:
- Hemolysis—although not felt to be clinically relevant.
- Provides partial cardiac output support of up to 2.5 L/minute in percutaneous model and up to 4 to 5 L/minute with model 5.0.
- Difficult to place in the setting of severe peripheral vascular disease.

Tandem Heart

Refer to **Fig. 8.8**.
Advantages of Tandem heart.
- Can be placed easily in the catheterization laboratory.
- Can supply up to 5 L/minute flow.
- Can be easily removed.

Table 48.3 Changes in hemodynamic parameters following Impella implantation

Index	Pre-Impella	Post-Impella
MAP (mmHg)	47	66
CVP (mmHg)	14	22
CI (L/min/m$_2$)	2.9	4.0
SVR (dyn-s-cm^{-5})	600	300

Abbreviations: CI, cardiac Index; CVP, central venous pressure; MAP, mean arterial pressure; SVR, systemic vascular resistance.

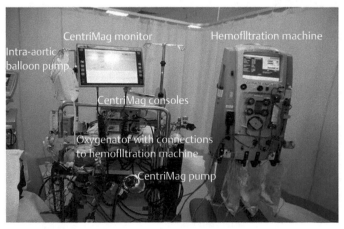

Fig. 48.28 Outcome of CentriMag™ extracorporeal mechanical circulatory support used in critical cardiogenic shock (INTERMACS 1) patients.[12]

Post LVAD Insertion on Echocardiography

On echocardiography, after LVAD insertion, it is important to look out for the *factors increasing TR such as:*

- Leftward shift of the IVS.
- Decreased RV function post LVAD implant.
- LVAD function increasing RV preload to an already dysfunctional RV.

Patients with elevated LVAD flow will demonstrate an IVS shift culminating in a spiral "suction event." This finding mandates decreasing the pump speed with a resultant reduction of TR, improved RV function, tamponade following chest closure, ascending and descending aortic dissection, aortic insufficiency, inflow and outflow valve dysfunction, and left ventricular unloading.

The interplay between an LVAD and the right ventricle is complex. The insertion of an LVAD can result in improvement of RV systolic function but may also result in reduction of the same. It is extremely difficult to foresee prior to insertion how an LVAD will influence RV systolic function. Significant right-to-left shunting can be visualized with TEE clinically as severe hypoxemia upon activation of the LVAD[13] (**Figs. 48.29–48.31**).

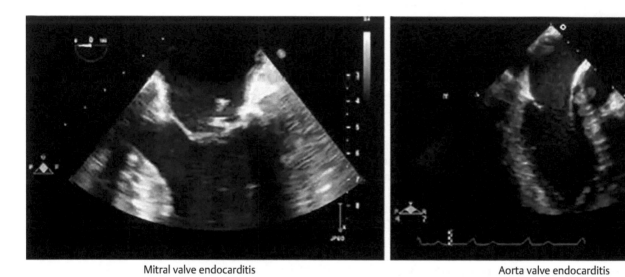

Mitral valve endocarditis   Aorta valve endocarditis

Fig. 48.29 Rule out endocarditis in postoperative echocardiography for left ventricular assist device (LVAD).

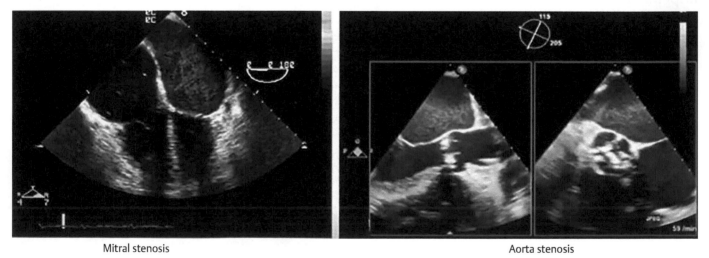

Mitral stenosis   Aorta stenosis

Fig. 48.30 Valve pathologies seen in postoperative echocardiography for left ventricular assist device (LVAD).

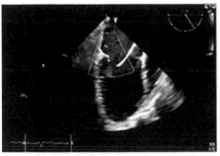
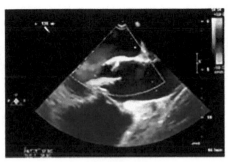
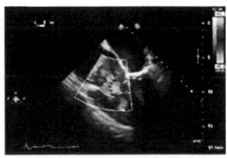

| Mitral regurgitation | Aortic regurgitation | Tricuspid regurgitation |

Fig. 48.31 Valve pathologies like mitral regurgitation, aortic regurgitation, and tricuspid regurgitation post left ventricular assist device (LVAD) placement also need to be ruled out before calling it a successful LVAD implantation.

Conclusion

Devices may become an important component in the management of acute heart failure. Although devices improve hemodynamic and metabolic parameters, there is currently no proven mortality benefits. Echocardiography should be considered an indispensable tool in the evaluation of patients with an LVAD. In fact, as outlined in this chapter, it provides useful and readily available information that could be crucial for the patient's survival. In the preoperative assessment, it is important to detect through echocardiography conditions and parameters that could hint to development of postoperative complications in order to treat them before LVAD implant or to consider the patient ineligible to this advanced treatment. Postoperatively, it rules out thrombosis and LVAD malfunction. During the implant, echocardiography provides information on whether the device is functioning correctly.

Particular attention should be paid to the importance of ECHO for detection and evaluation of ventricular reverse remodeling associated with improvement of contractile function during VAD support, as well as for weaning decision-making in patients with reversal of ventricular dilation and evidence of relevant and stable functional improvement.[15]

References

1. Westerdahl DE, Kobashigawa JA. Heart transplantation for advanced heart failure. Cardiac Intensive Care 2019;504–524
2. Gregoric ID, Poredos P, Jezovnik MK, et al. Use of transthoracic echocardiogram to detect left ventricular thrombi. Ann Thorac Surg 2021;111(2):556–560
3. Hayek S, Sims DB, Markham DW, Butler J, Kalogeropoulos AP. Assessment of right ventricular function in left ventricular assist device candidates. Circ Cardiovasc Imaging 2014;7(2):379–389
4. Cowger J, Rao V, Massey T, et al. Comprehensive review and suggested strategies for the detection and management of aortic insufficiency in patients with a continuous-flow left ventricular assist device. J Heart Lung Transplant 2015;34(2):149–157
5. Kukucka M, Stepanenko A, Potapov E, et al. Right-to-left ventricular end-diastolic diameter ratio and prediction of right ventricular failure with continuous-flow left ventricular assist devices. J Heart Lung Transplant 2011;30(1):64–69
6. Kato TS, Farr M, Schulze PC, et al. Usefulness of two-dimensional echocardiographic parameters of the left side of the heart to predict right ventricular failure after left ventricular assist device implantation. Am J Cardiol 2012;109(2):246–251
7. Cowger JA, Naka Y, Aaronson KD, et al; MOMENTUM 3 Investigators. Quality of life and functional capacity outcomes in the MOMENTUM 3 trial at 6 months: a call for new metrics for left ventricular assist device patients. J Heart Lung Transplant 2018;37(1):15–24
8. Kukucka M, Stepanenko A, Potapov E, Krabatsch T, Kuppe H, Habazettl H. Impact of tricuspid valve annulus dilation on mid-term survival after implantation of a left ventricular assist device. J Heart Lung Transplant 2012;31(9):967–971
9. Kato TS, Oda N, Hashimura K, et al. Strain rate imaging would predict sub-clinical acute rejection in heart transplant recipients. Eur J Cardiothorac Surg 2010;37(5):1104–1110
10. Sato T, Kato TS, Komamura K, et al. Utility of left ventricular systolic torsion derived from 2-dimensional speckle-tracking echocardiography in monitoring acute cellular rejection in heart transplant recipients. J Heart Lung Transplant 2011;30(5):536–543
11. Sciaccaluga C, Soliman-Aboumarie H, Sisti N, et al. Echocardiography for left ventricular assist device implantation and evaluation: an indispensable tool. Heart Fail Rev 2022;27(3):891–902
12. Hayek S, Sims DB, Markham DW, Butler J, Kalogeropoulos AP. Assessment of right ventricular function in left ventricular assist device candidates. Circ Cardiovasc Imaging. 2014 Mar;7(2):379–89
13. Mehta V, Venkateswaran RV. Outcome of CentriMag™ extracorporeal mechanical circulatory support use in critical cardiogenic shock (INTERMACS 1) patients. Indian J Thorac Cardiovasc Surg 2020;36(Suppl 2):265–274
14. Kapoor PM. ECMO and Ventricular Assist Devices as a Bridge to Transplant. Journal of Cardiac Critical Care TSS 2022; 06(03): 185–189
15. Michael D. Role of Echocardiography in the Management of Patients with Advanced (Stage D) Heart Failure Related to Nonischemic Cardiomyopathy. Rev. Cardiovasc. Med. 2022, 23(6), 214

49

Sonoanatomy for the Critical Care Physician

Sanchita Garg

Overview

The reach, availability, and acceptance of ultrasonography (USG) is growing every day. USG is operator dependent and this leads to interobserver variability. However, the facts that it is inexpensive, noninvasive, and easy to learn, and can be used at the bedside increase its popularity manifold. It allows for rapid and more accurate diagnosis of unstable critically ill patients at the bedside, thereby avoiding the risk of transporting such patients. It also makes it possible to avoid ionizing radiation. Its use has the potential to reduce time from presentation to diagnosis, expedite initiation of appropriate treatment, allow for better patient outcomes,[1] decreased complication rates in ultrasound (US)-guided procedures, reduced length of stay, and decreased cost of therapy.[2]

Today USG is becoming an essential tool in the armamentarium of not only the emergency department (ED) physicians and intensivists but also used perioperatively by anesthetists for vascular access and regional anesthesia. It is also important for assisting physicians in managing trauma, shock, dyspnea, and even cardiac arrest. US-guided protocols such as rapid ultrasound for shock and hypotension (RUSH)[3] and focused assessment using sonography for trauma (FAST)[4] have been established for delivering care in several of the above situations. The diagnosis of pulmonary pathologies such as pleural effusion and pneumothorax using point-of-care ultrasound (POCUS) is far superior to conventional radiography.[1] The POCUS is now also emerging as means for increasing patient safety by reducing complications in US-guided procedures such as thoracocentesis and paracentesis.[2] Therefore, it is vital for critical care physicians to have a hands-on knowledge about the basics of US. In this chapter, author will be exploring the basic sonoanatomy relevant for a critical care physician at the bedside.

USG Probes

Choosing the right probe for your area of interest is the most important first step in procuring a clear and meaningful image.[5] Some of the factors that go into determining which probe to be used are frequency, depth of penetration and footprint of the transducer, and location of the area of interest. Few particulars of the three most commonly used probes are described in **Table 49.1**. Portable USG machine used in our operating room (OR) and intensive care unit (ICU) is shown in **Fig. 49.1**.

Linear Probe

The linear probe, shown in **Fig. 49.2**, is a high-frequency transducer (5–15 MHz) that exchanges good resolution for a lower level penetration allowing us to see only superficial structures, to a depth of about 8 cm. It provides a rectangular field of view which corresponds with its linear footprint. It is commonly known as the vascular probe.

Curvilinear Ultrasound Probe

The curvilinear probe, shown in **Fig. 49.3**, is a low-frequency probe (2–5 MHz) and has a large/wide footprint. It is used to visualize deeper structures and allows for better lateral resolution (as compared to the phased-array probe). As it is most often used for scanning abdominal structures, it is commonly known as the abdominal probe, and is the probe used for the FAST and extended FAST exams.

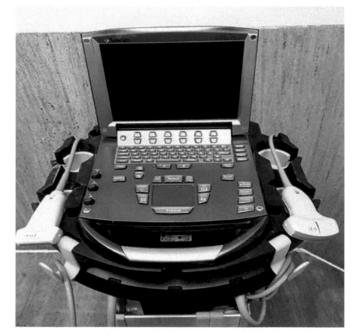

Fig. 49.1 Portable ultrasound machine.

Table 49.1 Characteristics of different transducers

Transducer type	Frequency range	Imaging depth	Applications in critical care
Linear (vascular)	5–15 MHz	8–9 cm	Visualization of arteries, veins, pleura, eyes, nerves, airway, line insertions
Curvilinear (abdominal)	2–5 MHz	30 cm	Gallbladder, liver, kidney, spleen, bladder, abdominal aorta, abdominal free fluid, uterus/ovaries, tapping
Phased array (cardiac)	1–5 MHz	35 cm	Heart, inferior vena cava, lungs, pleura, abdomen, transcranial Doppler, pericardiocentesis

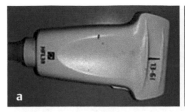

Fig. 49.2   (a, b) Linear probe with rectangular footprint.

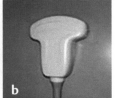

Fig. 49.3   (a, b) Curvilinear probe with wide footprint.

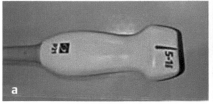

Fig. 49.4   (a, b) Phased-array probe with small and flat footprint.

Phased Array/Sector Probe

The phased array (or sector array), shown in **Fig. 49.4**, is a low-frequency probe (1–5 MHz) and has a smaller and flat footprint. The advantage of this probe is that its piezoelectric crystals are layered and packed in the center of the probe, making it easier to get in-between small spaces such as the ribs. It is commonly known and used as the cardiac probe. However, it can perform all of the applications of a curvilinear probe but with less lateral resolution.

Sonoanatomy: Imaging Windows and Views

Thomas Jefferson rightly said, "No knowledge can be more satisfactory to a man than that of his own frame, its parts, their functions, and actions."

Similarly, it is essential for a critical care physician in the current era who wishes to be well-versed in POCUS to have adequate knowledge of relevant human anatomy as viewed by an ultrasound probe. This section delineates the basic US anatomy that makes use of US in the critical care unit easy and meaningful.

Heart

There are four basic US views of the heart, namely, parasternal long axis (PLAX), parasternal short axis (PSAX), apical four-chamber, and subxiphoid (subcostal). They will be described briefly in this chapter. **Fig. 49.5** shows the ideal probe positions on the patient's torso.

Parasternal Long-Axis (PLAX) View

It is conventionally the first cardiac ultrasound view to be obtained. It is obtained by placing the probe at the fourth

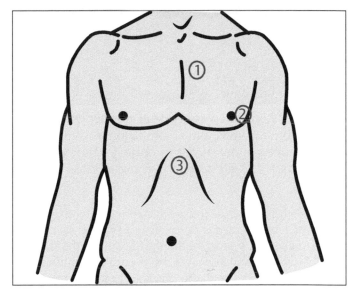

Fig. 49.5   Probe positions: 1: parasternal long-axis (PLAX) view (pointer toward right shoulder). 1: PSAX (pointer toward left shoulder), 2: apical view, 3: subcostal and inferior vena cava (IVC).

intercostal space and pointing the probe indicator/pointer toward the patient's right shoulder. The following structures are visualized, lying almost parallel to each other, and each occupies approximately one-third of the screen. Starting at the top (anteriorly), we see the right ventricle (RV), left-ventricular outflow tract (LVOT)-aorta in the middle, and the left artery (LA) posteriorly. Enlargement of any one of these structures directs toward the possible site of the pathology. For example, finding a dilated aortic root in case of Stanford type A aortic dissection. Structures visualized on the PLAX view are shown in **Fig. 49.6**. PLAX is used primarily to assess left ventricle (LV) size and function, left atrial (LA) size, aortic valve (AV), and mitral valve (MV). Circumferential pericardial effusions can also be detected.

Pro tip: If a collection lies anterior to the descending aorta then it is a pericardial effusion. A pleural effusion will be located posterior to the descending aorta.[6]

Parasternal Short-Axis (PSAX) View

To obtain the PSAX view, the transducer is simply rotated 90 degrees clockwise to point the transducer orientation marker toward the patient's left shoulder. Five different imaging planes can be achieved in the PSAX view by tilting

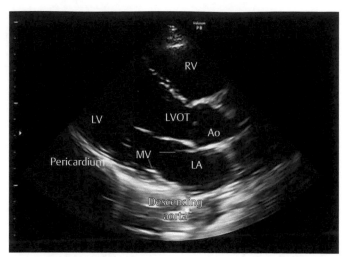

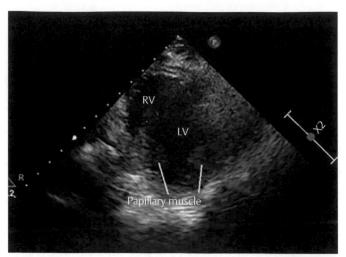

Fig. 49.6 Structures visualized on the parasternal long-axis (PLAX) view. Abbreviations: Ao, aorta; AV, aortic valve; DA, descending aorta; LV, left ventricle; LVOT, left ventricle outflow tract; LA, left atrium; MV, mitral valve; RV, right ventricle.

Fig. 49.7 Structures visualized on the parasternal short-axis (PSAX) view (midpapillary). Abbreviations: LV, left ventricle; RV, right ventricle.

the probe from the base toward the apex (pulmonary artery level, AV level/Mercedes Benz view, MV level/fish mouth view, midpapillary level, and apical level). In the midventricular or midpapillary level, both papillary muscles are symmetrically seen and the cross-sectional image of the LV cavity should appear circular, as shown in **Fig. 49.7**. This view is often favored by POCUS providers for its reliable portrayal of global LV systolic function and segmental LV wall motion, and estimation of LV filling. This view also helps in assessing the relative interventricular dependence and the shape and function of the interventricular septum (IVS), and helps in identifying patients having RV dilatation and dysfunction. Large- or moderate-sized circumferential pericardial effusions can also be well visualized. In the classical "D-sign" an acute increase in RV pressure (secondary to RV pressure overload as seen in pulmonary thromboembolism [PTE]) causes flattening of the IVS and causes the LV cavity to look like the letter D.

Apical Window

Apical view is the most difficult to master out of all the four views. Ideally, patients should be placed in left lateral position. However, in critically ill patients this is not always feasible. A compromise is reached upon by using supine position with some leftward tilt, although this results in some reduction in image quality. In obese or mechanically ventilated patients, obtaining good quality images may not always be possible. As shown in **Fig. 49.8**, all four chambers can be visualized along with MV and TV. Apical view gives excellent opportunity to document the signs of acute PTE[7] on cardiac US such as enlargement of the RV, RV strain, McConnell sign (mid-RV free-fall hypokinesia) can be easily detected by using the apical four-chamber view. The MV and TV can be assessed for detection of any stenosis or regurgitant flow.

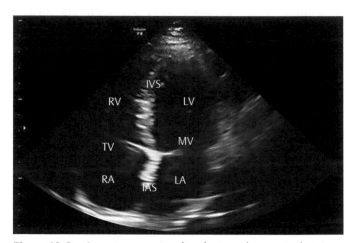

Fig. 49.8 Structures visualized in the apical view. Abbreviations: RV, right ventricle; IAS, inter-atrial septum; IVS, inter-ventricular septum; LA, left atrium; LV, left ventricle; MV, mitral valve; RA, right atrium; TV, tricuspid valve.

Any pericardial collection can also be detected. Signs of pericardial tamponade[8] (large pericardial effusion, systolic RA collapse, diastolic RV collapse, plethoric inferior vena cava [IVC]) can also be seen.

Subcostal Window

Subcostal view is obtained by keeping the probe in subcostal or subxiphoid location with the pointer cephalad and slightly to the left. All four chambers and the pericardial sac are well seen, as shown in **Fig. 49.9**. In a shocked patient undergoing cardiopulmonary resuscitation (CPR) or a crashed trauma patient, the subcostal view offers several advantages. Probe position is easy to identify with surface landmarks. It offers minimal interference to performance of

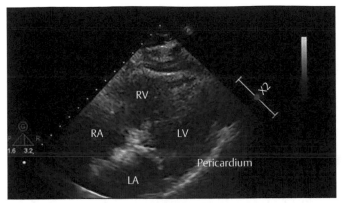

Fig. 49.9 Structures visualized in the subcostal view. Abbreviations: LA, left atrium; LV, left ventricle; RA, right atrium; RV, right ventricle.

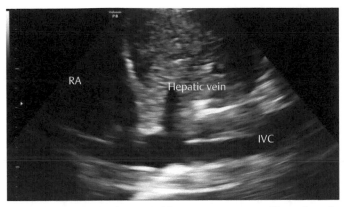

Fig. 49.10 IVC and its neighboring structures. Hepatic vein emptying into the IVC, along with the IVC itself draining into the RA. Abbreviations: RA, right atrium; IVC, inferior vena cava.

high-quality CPR. As compared to the other cardiac views, in patients on mechanical ventilation or having overdistended diseased lungs, the downward displacement of the heart may in fact lead to better quality images. Massive PTE and pericardial tamponade are two potentially life-threatening conditions that can be effectively diagnosed from this window by assessing the RV systolic function and the RV free wall. US from subxiphoid approach is also used to guide urgent intervention in the form of pericardiocentesis in patients of pericardial tamponade.

Inferior Vena Cava (IVC)

The IVC is best visualized using the subcostal approach. An alternative approach, the right lateral abdominal approach, exists as a rescue in patients with dressings or sutures in subcostal region and is hence also known as the rescue approach.[9] The IVC and aorta lie in close proximity. Several characteristics can help to distinguish the IVC from the aorta. The aorta has a thicker wall and is pulsatile (can be confirmed by Doppler). Most importantly, by tracing the hepatic veins draining into the IVC and furthermore the IVC draining into the RA. The IVC can be distinguished from the aorta, which arises from the left ventricle and open into the RA. Measurements of the IVC diameter and calculations of collapsibility are to be obtained 0.5 to 4 cm caudal to the IVC–right atrium junction. A plethoric IVC is seen in fluid overload, heart failure, massive PTE, and cardiac tamponade. A collapsible IVC essentially rules out the possibility of a tamponade physiology (**Fig. 49.10**).

It is essential to ensure that the ultrasound beam is centered in the center of the IVC. If the probe is toward the walls, when viewing the long axis of the IVC, it can underestimate the IVC diameter. Also if the probe is tilted and not perpendicular, when viewing the short axis of the IVC, it can over estimate the IVC diameter. Similarly, when using M-mode to measure the IVC diameter it is imperative to ensure that the beam is perpendicular to the walls of the IVC (**Fig. 49.11**).

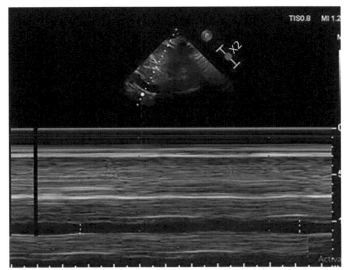

Fig. 49.11 Inferior vena cava (IVC) with M-mode to demonstrate IVC collapsibility.

Prediction of and correlation with CVP or fluid responsiveness is best at the extremes of measurement. A small collapsing IVC indicates need for fluids whereas a large non-collapsing IVC suggests its best to avoid fluids with possible need for diuretics.[10]

Abdominal Scan

US is primarily used to rule out any massive hemoperitoneum as the cause for shock and hypotension. Focused abdominal US is a rapid screening tool and can reliably detect intraperitoneal free fluid at the bedside. Evidence shows that US-guided abdominal paracentesis has better success rates and fewer procedural complications. The views and probe positions used are the same as that of a FAST exam, namely, the right upper quadrant (RUQ), the left upper quadrant (LUQ), the pelvic, and the subcostal views. These are also known as the four Ps: pericardial, perihepatic,

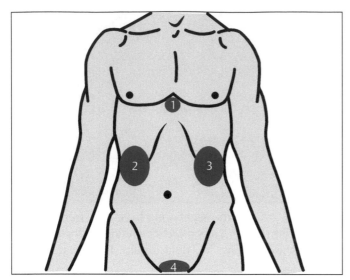

Fig. 49.12 Diagram showing probe positions for focused abdominal ultrasound (US). Probe positions: 1, subcostal; 2, right upper quadrant; 3, left upper quadrant; 4, pelvic.

perisplenic, and pelvic. **Fig. 49.12** depicts probe positions for focused abdominal US.

Cause of free fluid in the peritoneum can be either atraumatic (e.g., ruptured ectopic pregnancy, ruptured hollow viscus, and chronic ascites) or traumatic (unless proven otherwise, can be assumed to be due to solid organ injury, likely spleen or liver). USG cannot differentiate between different types of peritoneal free fluid. However, clear fluids such as ascites, blood, bile, lymph, and urine appear black, or anechoic, while fluid containing clotted blood, pus, fecal material, or debris appears more echogenic.[6]

Using a curvilinear probe, with marker-oriented cephalad, lateral to the rectus abdominis, paracentesis is done at the largest pocket of free fluid, avoiding nearby organs especially intestines.

Right Upper Quadrant (RUQ)

A curvilinear probe is placed at the level of the ninth to eleventh intercostal spaces posterior to the midaxillary line with the pointer cephalad. The three potential spaces where free fluid is most likely to accumulate in the RUQ are the right subdiaphragmatic space, hepatorenal space or "Morison pouch," and the inferior renal pole. Structures seen in the RUQ view are right lung, diaphragm, liver, and right kidney along with hepatorenal space or "Morison pouch," and suprahepatic space or right subdiaphragmatic space as shown in **Fig. 49.13**.

Left Upper Quadrant (LUQ)

A curvilinear probe is placed at the level of the sixth to ninth intercostal spaces posterior to the midaxillary line with the pointer cephalad. The three potential spaces where free fluid is most likely to accumulate in the LUQ are perisplenic space (left subdiaphragmatic space), the lienorenal recess, and the

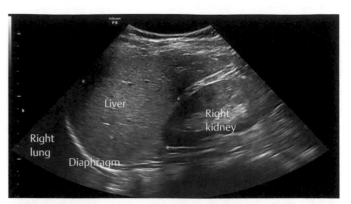

Fig. 49.13 Structures to identify in the right upper quadrant view are right lung, diaphragm, liver, and right kidney. * represents hepatorenal space or "Morison pouch," lower renal pole, and suprahepatic space.

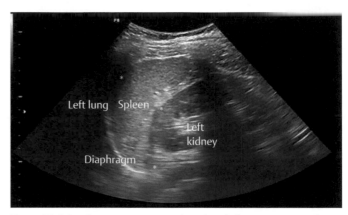

Fig. 49.14 Structures seen in the left upper quadrant (LUQ) view are left lung, diaphragm, spleen, and left kidney. * represents the perisplenic space (left subdiaphragmatic space), the lienorenal recess, and the inferior renal pole.

inferior renal pole. Structures seen in the LUQ view are left lung, diaphragm, spleen, and left kidney along with the perisplenic space (left subdiaphragmatic space), the lienorenal recess, and the inferior renal pole as shown in **Fig. 49.14**.

Pelvic and Subcostal View

A curvilinear probe is placed over the pubic symphysis with the pointer toward the patient's right. Collections of free fluid in the pelvis are found in the rectouterine space, or pouch of Douglas in women, and the rectovesicular space in men. In the pelvic area, collection is due to bleeding from the bladder injury, fractures of the pelvis, or large solid organ injury. Findings that can be significant in the subcostal view have been described above.

Aorta

When the curvilinear probe is placed just below the costal margin and scanning is done in downward direction, the aorta is identified anterior to the spine and to the left of the midline, as shown in **Fig. 49.15**. There are two catastrophic situations that can be detected by imaging the "PIPE" or the aorta. Early detection with help of US and timely intervention can drastically improve outcomes. The first is the abdominal aortic aneurysm (AAA) which is seen as a focal, abnormal dilation of the aorta. AAA may be surrounded by para-aortic fluid collection or free fluid in the abdomen (hemoperitoneum). An impending rupture should be feared in case of aneurysm sizes greater than 5 to 6 cm in diameter. POCUS has demonstrated high sensitivity (97.5–100%) and specificity (94.1–100%) for detection of AAA.[11] The second entity is an aortic dissection (AD). AD can arise from AV/aortic root or the descending aorta. An abdominal US might reveal an intimal flap if the descending aorta is involved. Abdominal US-guidance also allows for better placement of (ECMO) cannulas, resuscitative endovascular balloon occlusion of the aorta (REBOA) catheters, or intra-aortic balloon pumps.[6]

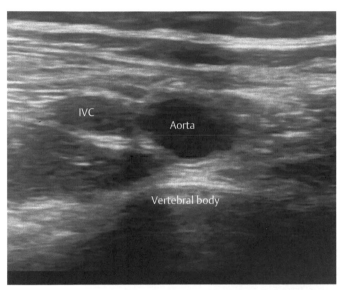

Fig. 49.15 Aorta lies anterior to the vertebral body to the left of the midline. Abbreviation: IVC, inferior vena cava.

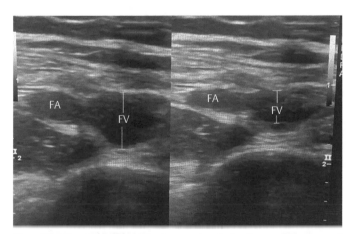

Fig. 49.16 Compressible femoral vein indicates absence of venous thromboembolic (VTE) disease. Abbreviations: FA, femoral artery; FV, femoral vein.

Lower Extremity Veins

Lower extremity veins are best visualized using a linear/vascular probe. Arteries are pulsatile and rounder as compared to their neighboring veins. Normally, veins are completely compressible even with slight pressure of the probe as shown in **Fig. 49.16**. By using two-dimensional (2D) imaging along with compression with/without the use of color Doppler US, we can diagnose lower limb venous thromboembolic (VTE) disease with more than 95% accuracy,[12] especially in proximal lower extremity veins. This establishes the role of POCUS, the diagnostic algorithm for massive PTE.[13]

Lung

The lung ultrasound (LUS) is performed by placing either the linear or the curvilinear probe perpendicular to the ribs. The characteristic Batwing sign is seen with two rib shadows seen with white pleural line on either side, shown in **Fig. 49.17**. When the patient breathes normally, the visceral and parietal pleura slide over one another, thus producing the lung sliding sign. Reverberation artifacts due to repeated reflection between the pleural line and the transducer produce A-lines. Their presence indicates that other pathologies (e.g., consolidation or pleural effusion) are absent. Upon placing M-mode over the pleural line in a normal lung we can see the seashore sign or sandy beach appearance (**Fig. 49.18**). This finding rules out the presence of a pneumothorax in the underlying lung. However, the absence of lung sliding does not always imply the presence of a pneumothorax. It can further be evaluated using M-mode which shows whether the patient has a normal seashore sign. Any reason that causes a separation of the parietal and visceral pleura or decreased movement thereof will lead to a reduced or absent lung sliding, for example, when they become separated by air (pneumothorax) or fluid (pleural effusion), or reduced movement due

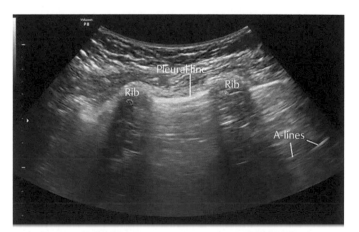

Fig. 49.17 Normal lung with Batwing sign, pleural line, and A-lines.

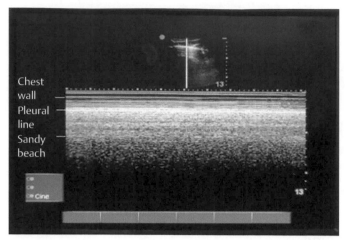

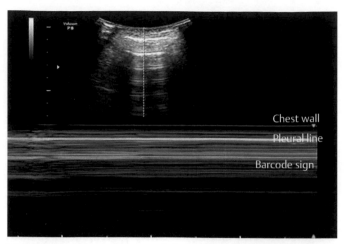

Fig. 49.18 Lung ultrasound showing the seashore sign or sandy beach appearance. Obtained by placing M-mode over the pleural line in a normal lung.

Fig. 49.19 Lung ultrasound showing the stratosphere sign. Obtained by placing M-mode over the pleural line in a lung with absent lung sliding.

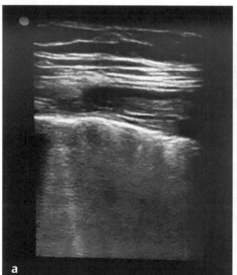

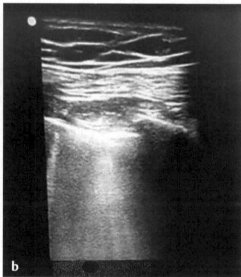

Fig. 49.20 Lung ultrasound. **(a)** Occasional B-lines. **(b)** Confluent multiple B-lines.

to severe consolidation, chemical pleurodesis, fibrotic lung diseases, acute respiratory distress syndrome, or mainstem intubation. The absence of lung sliding can also be demonstrated using M-mode, where lack of movement of air particles beneath the parietal pleura is seen as multiple straight lines (stratosphere sign and barcode sign; **Fig. 49.19**). The transition point between normal lung sliding (normal lung) and the absence of lung sliding (collapsed lung) is called the lung point. The presence of lung point is definitive proof of a pneumothorax. The lung point sign also allows you to quantify the size of the pneumothorax.

Build-up of fluid in the interlobular septa is demonstrated as B-lines (hyperechoic rocket-like artifacts arising from the pleural line that move with respiration). A few (1–3 per field)

may be present in a normal lung. In case of fluid overload, as lung tissue thickens or fills with fluid, B-lines converge (>3–5 per field) or coalesce and can create an appearance of "Confluent B-lines" (**Fig. 49.20**).

POCUS is an excellent modality for detection[14] and management[1] (thoracocentesis) of pleural effusions. Sensitivity and specificity for the detection of pleural effusions is higher than that of chest radiography.[14] It is important to scan behind the posterior axillary line as pleural fluid tends to accumulate in the dependent areas. The partially collapsed lung can be seen floating in the pleural fluid, the so-called "lung flapping" sign.[6] It is most important to rule pleural effusions in two situations: traumatic hemothorax or as evidence of fluid overload.

Conclusion

While point-of-care lung sonography may not necessarily replace other diagnostic modalities, it is becoming an important and indispensable tool for improving the care and outcomes of critically ill patients.[15]

Summary

- POCUS is rapidly gaining popularity because it is faster, cheaper, noninvasive, easy to use, and is readily available at the bedside.
- POCUS has become an essential tool that is utilized in several locations in a hospital to provide timely diagnosis in emergency situations while at the same time reducing exposure to ionizing radiation.
- US-guidance reduces errors, costs of treatment, and length of stay due to decrease in complications of common ICU procedures, including central-line insertions, paracentesis, and thoracentesis.
- Mastering POCUS is an essential skill in today's evidence-based era.
- Knowledge of relevant sonoanatomy and its practical application improves outcomes for patients and makes us better and safer physicians.

References

1. Chan KK, Joo DA, McRae AD, et al. Chest ultrasonography versus supine chest radiography for diagnosis of pneumothorax in trauma patients in the emergency department. Cochrane Database Syst Rev 2020;7(7):CD013031
2. Mercaldi CJ, Lanes SF. Ultrasound guidance decreases complications and improves the cost of care among patients undergoing thoracentesis and paracentesis. Chest 2013;143(2): 532–538
3. Weingart Scott D, Duque D, Nelson B. The rush exam; rapid ultrasound for shock and hypotension. Accessed: https://emcrit.org//rushexam
4. Scalea TM, Rodriguez A, Chiu WC, et al. Focused assessment with sonography for trauma (FAST): results from an international consensus conference. J Trauma 1999;46(3):466–472
5. Sargsyan AE, Blaivas M, Lumb P, Karakitsos D. Fundamentals: essential technology, concepts, and capability. In: Lumb P, Karakitsos D, eds. Critical care ultrasound: expert consult. Elsevier Health Sciences; 2015:2–15
6. Soni NJ, Arntfield R, Kory PD, eds. Point-of-care ultrasound: expert consult—online and print. 2nd ed. W.B. Saunders Company; 2014:111–125
7. Kurnicka K, Lichodziejewska B, Goliszek S, et al. Echocardiographic pattern of acute pulmonary embolism: analysis of 511 consecutive patients. J Am Soc Echocardiogr 2016;29(9):907–913
8. Goldstein JA. Introduction to pericardial disease. In: Kern MJ, Lim MJ, Goldstein JA, eds. Hemodynamic rounds: interpretation of cardiac pathophysiology from pressure waveform analysis. 4th ed. John Wiley & Sons Ltd.; 2018:197–218
9. Finnerty NM, Panchal AR, Boulger C, et al. Inferior vena cava measurement with ultrasound: what is the best view and best mode? West J Emerg Med 2017;18(3):496–501
10. Tan HL, Wijeweera O, Onigkeit J. Inferior vena cava guided fluid resuscitation: fact or fiction? Tren Anaesth Crit Care [Internet] 2015;5(2–3):70–75
11. Costantino TG, Bruno EC, Handly N, Dean AJ. Accuracy of emergency medicine ultrasound in the evaluation of abdominal aortic aneurysm. J Emerg Med 2005;29(4):455–460
12. Pomero F, Dentali F, Borretta V, et al. Accuracy of emergency physician-performed ultrasonography in the diagnosis of deep-vein thrombosis: a systematic review and meta-analysis. Thromb Haemost 2013;109(1):137–145
13. Konstantinides SV, Meyer G, Becattini C, et al; ESC Scientific Document Group. 2019 ESC Guidelines for the diagnosis and management of acute pulmonary embolism developed in collaboration with the European Respiratory Society (ERS). Eur Heart J 2020;41(4):543–603
14. Grimberg A, Shigueoka DC, Atallah AN, Ajzen S, Iared W. Diagnostic accuracy of sonography for pleural effusion: systematic review. Sao Paulo Med J 2010;128(2):90–95
15. Breitkopf R, Treml B, Rajsic S. Lung Sonography in Critical Care Medicine. Diagnostics 2022; 12, 1405

50

Ultrasound-Guided Vascular Access

Sanchita Garg

History

The practice of placing central venous catheters (CVCs) began in the 1950s with the first description of using ultrasound to access the internal jugular vein (IJV) by Ullman and Stoelting in 1978.[1] Yonei et al described the first use of real-time ultrasound guidance for IJV cannulation in 1986.[2] The 1990s saw an increase in ultrasound-guided central venous cannulation with the Agency for Healthcare Research and Quality recommending ultrasound use in 2001. The CDC in 2011 recommended ultrasound to be used for placement of all CVCs to decrease complications and number of attempts. In 2012 the ASA Task Force recommended the use of real-time ultrasonography for IJV cannulation and static ultrasound for femoral and subclavian cannulation.

Benefits of Ultrasound

Ultrasound-guided cannulation not only decrease the risk of an accidental arterial puncture of the IJV, but also reiterates, with its resolution, good imaging of the vessel. Since the 1996 study by Troianos et al[3] which showed that over half of the patients scanned had the IJV overlie the carotid artery by at least 75% of its diameter, use of ultrasound was implemented to decrease this risk. In 2003, Hind et al showed via a meta-analysis that while there was likely no increase in speed of central venous cannula placement, it did result in a 57% decrease in complications from cannulation of the IJV. Hind et al's meta-analysis also showed that there was a 41% improvement in first time cannulation as well as 86% decrease in failed IJV central venous cannula placement.[4] However, Gualtieri et al described this technique of ultrasound guidance as most beneficial in those who have minimal experience.[5] Recent studies have shown that a minimum of 10 to 20 ultrasound-guided CVC placements are needed in order to demonstrate competency. In IJV cannulation, ultrasound use has also shown that there is a decreased risk of pneumothorax. Ultrasound use also allows for improved confirmation of correct placement. It can be used to either confirm the wire is in the correct location in both the long axis and short axis or to confirm the cannula remains in the correct position. There have even been descriptions of using ultrasound to confirm the correct placement of the venous cannula into the superior vena cava in children. It is also useful in cases when placing CVCs is difficult such as when in prone position, kyphotic patients, or dehydrated patients. [6-8]

Probe and Equipment Selection

- The definitive mode of ultrasound-guided jugular vein cannulation is 2D ultrasound and not 3D ultrasound.[9] The role of 3D remains unclear for ICU at present in

2022. Both color Doppler and pulsed-wave Doppler are emerging technologies for differentiating arterial and venous vasculature.[10-13]

- As ultrasound usage becomes a part and parcel of routine care, its documentation on paper has both legal and patient care inferences.[5] All patient care data with images must be saved, documented on paper, and be available in an accessible part of sterility. Also it should be marinated with the use of good quality gel and a sterile cover. The type of probe used for ultrasound guidance should be in accordance to specific guidelines as described by the ASA transfusion (**Box 50.1**).[14]
- The machine should be with a high resolution to distinguish the vessels and their collapsibility from the adjoining vessels and also the ideal time imprint of the needle should be seen.

For IJV following guidelines must be followed:
1. *Adequate penetration*: Important to remember that SVC (superior vena cava) lies at a depth of 4 cm beneath the skin. IJV and PV (pulmonary vein) lie at a depth of 1 to 4 cm beneath the skin.[3]
2. *Adequate resolution and adjustable focal point*: It is important to have a probe with good resolution and an adjustable focal point.[4]

Technique

The two techniques to utilize ultrasound for central venous cannulation are either static or real time. The use of ultrasound in the static method helps to confirm the presence of a vessel when using the traditional anatomic landmark approach. Real-time ultrasonography allows for observation of the needle entering into the target vessel, and then confirmation of both the wire and central venous cannula inside the target vessel. Specific sites in which ultrasonography is useful include the IJV, subclavian vein (SCV), and femoral vein (**Table 50.1**).[7]

While the patient is in the correct position and properly prepped, a full body drape is used and the ultrasound transducer is draped in a sterile sheath. It is imperative to have a sterile sheath around the probe. This is done after a full body drape is performed. The transducer can be used in either the longitudinal or cross-sectional view. The advantage of the longitudinal view is that the needle is advanced in-plane while the disadvantage is that it is difficult to view the carotid at the same time. The advantage of the cross-sectional view

Box 50.1	Characteristics of ultrasound-guided probe

- Small footprint
- Probe should be between 20 and 40 mm in size and easily visible
- Able to visualize vessels in both short- and long-axis view
- Probe and needle should both be near the skin

Table 50.1 Machine and operator tray location for central line placement with ultrasound

Site	Machine location	Operating tray location
Right IJV	On right side toward patient's liver	Left side of the patient away from the u/s machine. Some practitioners prefer all equipment (u/s, operating tray) on the right side of the patient
Left IJV	On left side toward patient's spleen	Right side of the patient across from u/s machine. Some practitioners prefer all equipment (u/s, operating tray) on the left side of the patient
Right SCV	Left side of the patient at the level of the spleen	Right side of the patient across from the u/s machine
Left SCV	Right side of the patient at the level of the liver	Left side of the patient across from the u/s machine
Right femoral	Left side of the patient at the level of the pelvis	Left side of the patient next to the u/s machine and over the patient's legs
Left femoral	Right side of the patient at the level of the pelvis	Right side of the patient next to the u/s machine and over the patient's legs

Abbreviations: IJV, internal jugular vein; SCV, subclavian vein; u/s, ultrasound.

is that the carotid remains in real-time view; however, the needle is advanced out of plane, thus making it difficult to visualize the exact tip of the needle entering the target vessel. Regardless of the approach you decide to take with the needle, after the wire has been placed and needle removed it is essential that you confirm the wire placement in both the longitudinal and cross-sectional view. Once the wire is confirmed to be in the correct target vessel, the cannula is advanced over the wire and using ultrasound you can once again confirm the cannula remains in the vessel.[8-12]

As shown in **Fig. 50.1**, three different types of probes can be used for vascular access guidance in central venous pressure (CVP) line insertion.

The Short-Axis Approach to IJV

The short-axis or out-of-plane approach means that the vein is visualized in cross-section as a black or anechoic circle. Now, the needle is inserted "out of plane"; that is to say, it is perpendicular to the beam axis. The needle enters the skin at an acute angle and nearly parallel to the probe. The complications of this is that the needle tip is invariably, not seen with this procedure; thus, the neighboring structures may suffer injury. If the probe is moved toward the needle, then it may be possible to visualize the needle tip by following the forward movement of the needle. The three main advantages of the short-axis approach are summarized in **Boxes 50.2** and **50.3**. It is easy to learn, when surrounding anatomy is seen.

The In-plane, Long-Axis Approach

In this technique, the probe is placed orthogonally, to the long-axis of the vessel, where the needle is seen as an echogenic white line and the vessel to be punctured is observed as a "Rectangle" in the center of the screen. Now the needle

Box 50.2 Advantages of a lung ultrasound at the end of an IJV USG-guided cannulation

- Accessible
- Shortens time to catheter when lung ultrasound is combined with point-of-care ultrasound (POCUS)
- Lung ultrasound to rule out or verify the presence of pneumothorax is superior to chest X-Ray
- It can be integrated into the end of the procedure[15]

Abbreviations: IJV, internal jugular vein; USG, ultrasonography.

Box 50.3 Advantages of "out-of-plane" approach

- It offers better visualization of the anatomy of the surrounding structures
- It is an easy-to-learn technique even for the novice
- It can be used for small caliber vessels as well
- Can be used easily in short-necked patients as it is feasible to perform this as two-operator techniques[16]
- The key to the success of the out-of-plane approach is to keep a sharp eye on exact position of the needle tip

Box 50.4 Advantages of in-plane long-axis approach

- Use of coaxial systems makes in-plane method of IJV cannulation easier.
- There is free movement of the needle in a larger surface area.[18]

is inserted into the vein, which in the long axis, is seen as an anechoic rectangle/cylinder. In this approach, the image plane is parallel to the course of the vessel and also to the needle, hence the terminology "in-plane." The advantages of this technique are outlined in **Box 50.4**, and chiefly include good visualization of the needle tip and its shaft, which thus prevents the structure of the posterior wall of the vessel and

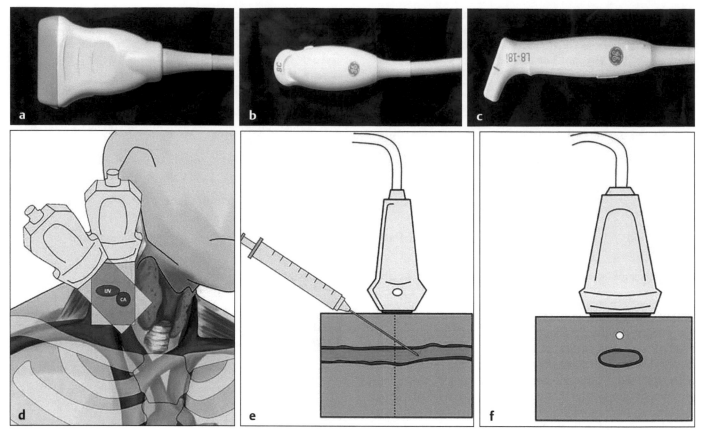

Fig. 50.1 Types of probes used for vascular access guidance in central venous pressure (CVP) line insertion. **(a)** A high-frequency, linear probe (5–11 MHz). **(b)** A microconvex ultrasound probe for subclavian vein visualization; it has a lower frequency. **(c)** It is an ultrasound probe shaped like a hockey stick. It has a smaller footprint which is ideal to interrogate obese patients and also the pediatric population. The lower panel of this figure shows probe positions on the patient's anatomy of internal jugular vein (IJV). **(d)** Probe is placed at an angle to align for the internal jugular vein (IJV) from arterial to medial axis, rather than the anteroposterior (AP) diameter. **(e)** In-plane, long-axis position, wherein posterior wall vein structures can be avoided and the needle trajectory from skin to IJV observed clearly on the ultrasound screen. **(f)** The short-axis position, which is out of plane.

also injury to adjoining structure.[17] It is a more challenging approach to perform in-plane approach as it is technically more difficult as the operator has to simultaneously image the thin needle and its trajectory and at same time align with the transducer the vein in the long axis, all throughout as shown in **Fig. 50.1** using a very narrow ultrasound beam.

Lung Ultrasound Integration to Rule Out Pneumothorax

The incidence of pneumothorax after cardiovascular catheterization using the landmarks techniques is 98%, following IJV cannulation is 0.3 to 1%, and following SCV cannulation is 1.6 to 2.5%. Ultrasound usage of vascular access not only reduces the incidence of pneumothorax, but also has a high sensitivity and specificity for detecting pneumothorax.

Alrajab et al showed in a meta-analysis that the sensitivity of ultrasound to detect pneumothorax is much higher than that of chest X-ray (**Box 50.4**).[19–22]

It can be integrated into the end of the procedure[23,24] and has several advantages: accessibility at the bedside, speed (no need to wait for the chest X-ray), and accuracy. Combining lung ultrasound with point of care ultrasound (POCUS) examination during the procedure can potentially shorten the time to catheter utilization.[25]

Other Uses

In addition to central venous cannulation, ultrasound has been used in both arterial cannulation and peripheral venous cannulation in adults and pediatric patients. As these are usually smaller vessels than central venous vessels a higher frequency probe such as a hockey stick or even a high-frequency micro ultrasound (50 MHz) may be useful. When using ultrasonography to access radial artery the probe should be a high-frequency setting and smallest probe should be used as the radial artery is very shallow. Since the radial artery is thin, a cross-sectional approach is preferred to ensure the needle is in the center of the artery to allow for proper wire placement. Brachial, axillary, and femoral arteries access also lend themselves to ultrasound-guided placement.

Training for Ultrasound-Guided CV Access

CVC cannulation, which is ultrasound guided, requires acquiring technical skills such as ultrasound scanning, identifying adjoining anatomical structures, learning tracking the ultrasound-guided needle insertion, and performing vascular cannulation. There should be a core curriculum, which should teach to the fellow, all above, along with its complications and limitations. A systematic, guided approach at each step is a must. In a study done on emergency medicine and anesthesiology-related fellowships with a competent core curriculum, it was concluded that it is only by the fourth session of a simulation-based curriculum that the performance of the novice candidate improved and reached a mean performance. Most studies today have shown that a smaller portion–based cubiculum is much better retained than a complete, whole training session. Not just the students, but also the experienced teachers and clinicians, today understand the value of ultrasound-based training. In a cohort of ICU-based physicians, Nguyen et al have demonstrated that 50% of the intensivists who were new to the ultrasound technique of CVP placement before the training said they benefitted immensely from the training. The parameters they learnt most were CVP line in placement with ultrasound-guided techniques. As more ultrasound-guided procedures are done and their practice increased, then the number of punctures in ICU for vessel line increase placement decrease and confidence level increase.[26] Other studies have shown the superiority of a portioned, session-based curriculum rather than teaching as whole.[27] The value of training pertains not only to trainees but also to experienced clinicians. Nguyen et al demonstrated this on a cohort of intensivists of whom 50% were novice to ultrasound-guided CVC placement. Furthermore, before implementation of the training, even for intensivists with prior CVC or ultrasound experience, the time between skin puncture and aspiration of venous blood was not significantly shorter than for intensivists who were novices to ultrasound. Yet, this time decreased rapidly with the number of procedures for all intensivists, suggesting that even senior intensivists have to master this technique.[28]

Conclusion

According to jolly et al, the use of ultrasonography for femoral access did not reduce bleeding or vascular complications. However, ultrasonography did reduce the risk of veni-puncture and number of attempts. Larger trials may be required to demonstrate additional potential benefits of ultrasonography-guided access.[29]

References

1. Ullman JI, Stoelting RK. Internal jugular vein location with the ultrasound Doppler blood flow detector. Anesth Analg 1978;57(1):118
2. Yonei A, Nonoue T, Sari A. Real-time ultrasonic guidance for percutaneous puncture of the internal jugular vein. Anesthesiology 1986;64(6):830–831
3. Troianos CA, Hartman GS, Glas KE, et al; Councils on Intraoperative Echocardiography and Vascular Ultrasound of the American Society of Echocardiography. Guidelines for performing ultrasound guided vascular cannulation: recommendations of the American Society of Echocardiography and the Society of Cardiovascular Anesthesiologists. J Am Soc Echocardiogr 2011;24(12):1291–1318
4. Hind D, Calvert N, McWilliams R, et al. Ultrasonic locating devices for central venous cannulation: meta-analysis. BMJ 2003;327(7411):361
5. Gualtieri E, Deppe SA, Sipperly ME, Thompson DR. Subclavian venous catheterization: greater success rate for less experienced operators using ultrasound guidance. Crit Care Med 1995;23(4):692–697
6. Terkawi AS, Karakitsos D, Elbarbary M, Blaivas M, Durieux ME. Ultrasound for the anesthesiologists: present and future. Sci World J 2013;2013:683–685
7. Gayle JA, Kaye AD. Ultrasound-guided central vein cannulation: current recommendations and guidelines. Anesthesiol News 2012:1–6
8. Kaye AD, Fox CJ, Hymel BJ, et al. The importance of training for ultrasound guidance in central vein catheterization. Middle East J Anaesthesiol 2011;21(1):61–66
9. Castillo D, McEwen DS, Young L, Kirkpatrick J. Micropuncture needles combined with ultrasound guidance for unusual central venous cannulation: desperate times call for desperate measures: a new trick for old anesthesiologists. Anesth Analg 2012;114(3):634–637
10. Sofi K, Arab S. Ultrasound-guided central venous catheterization in prone position. Saudi J Anaesth 2010;4(1):28–30
11. Rupp SM, Apfelbaum JL, Blitt C, et al; American Society of Anesthesiologists Task Force on Central Venous Access. Practice guidelines for central venous access: a report by the American Society of Anesthesiologists Task Force on Central Venous Access. Anesthesiology 2012;116(3):539–573
12. Schindler E, Schears GJ, Hall SR, Yamamoto T. Ultrasound for vascular access in pediatric patients. Paediatr Anaesth 2012; 22(10):1002–1007
13. Hartman GS. Ultrasound facilitated vascular cannulation improving performance and avoiding the disasters. Perioperative Echo Basic, 2010; 104–111
14. O'Grady NP, Alexander M, Burns LA, et al; Healthcare Infection Control Practices Advisory Committee. Guidelines for the

prevention of intravascular catheter-related infections. Am J Infect Control 2011;39(4, Suppl 1):S1–S34

15. Ueda K, Ahmed W, Ross AF. Intraoperative pneumothorax identified with transthoracic ultrasound. Anesthesiology 2011;115(3):653–655

16. Amir R, Knio ZO, Mahmood F, et al. Ultrasound as a screening tool for central venous catheter positioning and exclusion of pneumothorax. Crit Care Med 2017;45(7):1192–1198

17. Stone MB, Moon C, Sutijono D, Blaivas M. Needle tip visualization during ultrasound-guided vascular access: short-axis vs long-axis approach. Am J Emerg Med 2010;28(3):343–347

18. Schofer JM, Nomura JT, Bauman MJ, Hyde R, Schmier C. The "Ski Lift": a technique to maximize needle visualization with the long-axis approach for ultrasound-guided vascular access. Acad Emerg Med 2010;17(7):e83–e84

19. Ebrahimi A, Yousefifard M, Mohammad Kazemi H, et al. Diagnostic accuracy of chest ultrasonography versus chest radiography for identification of pneumothorax: a systematic review and meta-analysis. Tanaffos 2014;13(4):29–40

20. Ding W, Shen Y, Yang J, He X, Zhang M. Diagnosis of pneumothorax by radiography and ultrasonography: a meta-analysis. Chest 2011;140(4):859–866

21. Alrajab S, Youssef AM, Akkus NI, Caldito G. Pleural ultrasonography versus chest radiography for the diagnosis of pneumothorax: review of the literature and meta-analysis. Crit Care 2013;17(5):R208

22. Abdalla W, Elgendy M, Abdelaziz AA, Ammar MA. Lung ultrasound versus chest radiography for the diagnosis of pneumothorax in critically ill patients: a prospective, single-blind study. Saudi J Anaesth 2016;10(3):265–269

23. Lamperti M, Bodenham AR, Pittiruti M, et al. International evidence-based recommendations on ultrasound-guided vascular access. Intensive Care Med 2012;38(7):1105–1117

24. Bedel J, Vallée F, Mari A, et al. Guidewire localization by transthoracic echocardiography during central venous catheter insertion: a periprocedural method to evaluate catheter placement. Intensive Care Med 2013;39(11):1932–1937

25. Galante O, Slutsky T, Fuchs L, et al. Single-operator ultrasoundguided central venous catheter insertion verifies proper tip placement. Crit Care Med 2017;45(10):e994–e1000

26. McGraw R, Chaplin T, McKaigney C, et al. Development and evaluation of a simulation-based curriculum for ultrasoundguided central venous catheterization. CJEM 2016;18(6):405–413

27. Chan A, Singh S, Dubrowski A, et al. Part versus whole: a randomized trial of central venous catheterization education. Adv Health Sci Educ Theory Pract 2015;20(4):1061 1071

28. Nguyen BV, Prat G, Vincent JL, et al. Determination of the learning curve for ultrasound-guided jugular central venous catheter placement. Intensive Care Med 2014;40(1):66–73

29. Jolly SS, AlRashidi S, d'Entremont MA, et al. Routine Ultrasonography Guidance for Femoral Vascular Access for Cardiac Procedures: The UNIVERSAL Randomized Clinical Trial. JAMA Cardiol. 2022;7(11):1110–1118

51

POCUS-Based Protocols and Assessment of Fluid Responsiveness

Poonam Malhotra Kapoor and Sanchita Garg

Introduction

Over the past decade, there has been an increasing emphasis on patient safety and evidence-based medicine. Protocolized patient care has been shown to decrease errors, standardize patient care, and improve outcomes.[1] In recent years, the scope and usage of ultrasound (US) has expanded to the extent that point-of-care US (POCUS) has been considered by some as the modern stethoscope.[2] If used judiciously, US-based protocols that incorporate screening of multiple organ systems can impact the accuracy of the patient's diagnosis and also hasten the management of critically ill patients.[3] When applied in a stepwise manner, these protocols have the potential to assist the intensivists in rapidly "ruling in" or "ruling out" a plethora of diagnoses. In a busy, resource-constrained intensive care unit (ICU) or emergency room (ER), POCUS can allow triage of patients such that unnecessary costly and time-consuming investigations and interventions can be avoided. By allowing the intensivists to perform these assessments at the bedside, POCUS reduces the risks associated with transportation of critical patients. It also mitigates the risks inherent with exposure to ionizing radiation. An additional advantage is that these assessments can be repeated periodically and can thus be used to assess the patient's dynamic response to interventions and therapies and can lead to improved outcomes.[4]

Today, US-based protocols have been designed for aiding in the diagnosis and management of patients presenting to the ER and ICU with a multitude of medical situations, such as trauma,[5] hypotension and shock,[6,7] heart failure,[8] dyspnea,[9] and cardiac arrest.[10,11]

About every fifth patient coming into a cardiac critical care unit is suffering from shock.[12] Therefore, it is essential to have knowledge of protocols that elucidate the differential in such instances. The commonly used protocols are described in **Table 51.1**.

Rapid Ultrasound for Shock and Hypotension Protocol

In 2006, Weingart et al introduced an ultrasound-based assessment protocol for patients arriving to their ER with shock, known as rapid ultrasound for shock and hypotension (RUSH).[5] They later published this in 2009. The RUSH exam is designed to be a rapid screening tool rather than

Table 51.1   Pathological findings on a RUSH exam and their clinical relevance

Organ assessed	Possible pathologies	Interpretation
H (heart)	Reduced EF	Systolic heart failure
	Hyperdynamic ventricle	Distributive or hypovolemic shock
	Pericardial effusion	Tamponade
	RV strain RV > LV	Pulmonary embolism
	RWMA	Myocardial infarction
	Low CO	Cardiogenic shock Hypovolemic shock Obstructive shock
	High CO	Distributive shock
I (IVC)	Noncollapsible IVC	Obstructive shock Cardiogenic shock
	Collapsible IVC	Hypovolemic shock Distributive shock
M (Morison pouch/e-FAST)	Hemoperitoneum	Hemorrhagic shock
	Hemothorax	Hemorrhagic shock
A (aorta)	Dissecting flap	Aortic dissection
	Increased aortic diameter	Abdominal aortic aneurysm
Femoral vein	Noncompressible echogenic material	DVT
P (pulmonary)	Absent lung sliding	Pneumothorax
	Confluent B-lines	Fluid overload Heart failure

Abbreviations: CO, cardiac output; DVT, deep vein thrombosis; EF, ejection fraction; IVC, inferior vena cava; LV, left ventricle; RUSH, rapid ultrasound for shock and hypotension; RV, right ventricle; RWMA, regional wall motion abnormality.

a comprehensive assessment of every component listed. It helps to exclude the major pathologies that can cause hypotension (and shock) in a patient. Once practiced, this exam can be completed in as little as 2 to 5 minutes at the bedside or in the ER.

The components of the RUSH exam are given by the mnemonic HI-MAP, as explained below:

1. Heart (probe positioning, **Figs. 49.5–49.9**).
2. Inferior vena cava (IVC) (probe positioning, **Figs. 49.5, 49.10,** and **49.11**).
3. Morrison/e-FAST (focused assessment with sonography for trauma) abdominal views (probe positioning, **Figs. 49.12–49.14**).
4. Aorta.
5. Pneumothorax.

It describes both the sequence and the structures to be examined. A simpler method to recall and assess the components of the RUSH exam is as follows:

- PUMP (heart): Tamponade, LVEF (left ventricular ejection fraction), and RV (right ventricular) size.
- TANK (intravascular): IVC, thoracic and abdominal compartments.
- PIPES (large arteries/veins): Aorta and femoral/popliteal veins.

If we recall the popular mnemonic 5Hs and 5Ts for the reversible causes of cardiac arrest, the RUSH protocol examines one of the Hs (hypovolemia) and four out of five Ts (cardiac tamponade, tension pneumothorax, pulmonary thromboembolism, and cardiac thrombosis or myocardial infarction). The remaining ones are ruled by sending basic lab tests and air blood gas (ABGs) analysis and monitoring the vitals.

Bedside Lung Ultrasound in Emergency (BLUE) Protocol

Due to the inability of US waves to pass through air, the USG was assumed to have a limited role in imaging the lung. Lung ultrasound (LUS) is basically a study of the different patterns of artifacts produced by presence or absence of air and fluid in and around the lung. BLUE protocol[9] is made simple by its dichotomous nature and can rapidly be used in ICU and ER to delineate the likely cause of respiratory distress. The normal lung USG gives a "sandy beach sign" (**Fig. 49.18**). The two commonest causes of acute respiratory distress are pneumonia and acute pulmonary edema.[9]

It scans three standardized points, called BLUE points (**Fig. 51.1**), over each hemithorax in patients with acute respiratory failure. It looks for the presence or absence of ten standard signs (lung sliding, Batwing sign [**Fig. 49.17**], A-lines [**Fig. 51.1**], quad sign, sinusoid sign, shred sign, tissue-like sign, anterior lung rockets/multiple B-lines [**Fig. 49.20**], stratosphere sign [**Fig. 49.19**], lung point sign, fluid) and generates a pathophysiological profile (**Table 51.2**). At the

posterior chest wall, consolidations and pleural effusions (**Fig. 51.2a, b**) are assessed together. Both disorders can coexist and gravity and recumbent posture allow best screening at the PLAPS (posterolateral alveolar or pleural syndrome) point. Based on these profiles (**Table 51.2**) a rapid tentative diagnosis can be made with an accuracy just over 90% when compared with computed tomography (CT) scanning.[10]

The Sonography in Hypotension and Cardiac Arrest (SHoC) Protocols[11]

It consists of two protocols: one for hypotension and the other for cardiac arrest. The SHoC-hypotension protocol consists of basic views focused on distinguishing between cardiogenic and noncardiogenic causes of hypotension.

1. Cardiac views (the subxiphoid window and/or parasternal long-axis window to look for pericardial fluid, cardiac form, and ventricular function; **Figs. 49.6–49.9**).
2. Lung views to look for the presence of pleural fluid and presence/absence of B-lines as a surrogate for filling status.
3. IVC views for assessing the filling status (**Figs. 49.10** and **49.11**).

When appropriate or needed, supplementary/additional views are taken, for example, if patient is suspected of having abdominal aortic aneurysm (AAA) or deep vein thrombosis (DVT).

The SHoC-cardiac arrest protocol consists of assessing cardiac function using subxiphoid or parasternal long-axis (PLAX) views during the pause in chest compressions for rhythm check. It is to rule out pericardial fluid (**Fig. 51.3**) and RV strain. Also, this opportunity is used to differentiate between asystole and organized cardiac activity.

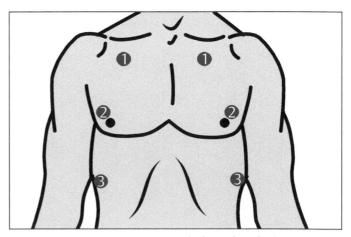

Fig. 51.1 BLUE points. 1. Just below clavicle (upper BLUE point). 2. Close to the nipple (lower BLUE point). 3. Junction of the horizontal line from the lower BLUE point and the posterior axillary line (**posterolateral alveolar and/or pleural syndrome** [PLAPS] point).

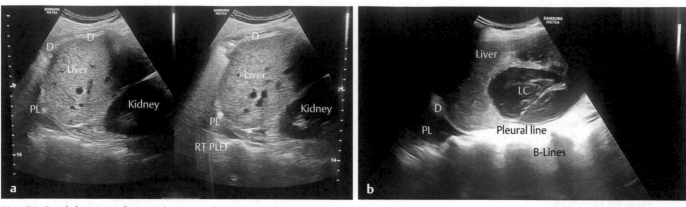

Fig. 51.2 **(a)** Point-of-care ultrasound (POCUS) showing the relations of right lung, liver, and right kidney. A small right-sided pleural effusion. **(b)** POCUS showing large hepatic collection and a right-sided pleural effusion. Abbreviations: D, diaphragm; LC, liver collection; PL, pleural effusion.

Table 51.2 Pathophysiological profiles seen in BLUE protocol and their clinical interpretation

Profile	Description	Possible diagnosis (with signs)
A-profile	Anterior A-lines present with lung sliding	Normal lung
A′-profile	Anterior A-lines present with absent lung sliding	Possible pneumothorax (stratosphere sign in M-mode and lung point)
B-profile	Lung sliding with lung rockets	Interstitial syndrome/pulmonary edema
B′-profile	Absent lung sliding with lung rockets	Pneumonia
A/B-profile	Unilateral lung rockets	Pneumonia
A-profile with PLAPS	Positive findings at PLAPS point	Pneumonia
C-profile	Anterior lung consolidation with thick irregular pleural line	Pneumonia
Nude profile	A-profile with no DVT and no PLAPS (compressible veins)	Asthma and COPD
A-profile with V	A-profile with noncompressible veins	Pulmonary embolism
A′-profile without lung point	Sliding sign absent but no lung point seen	Diagnosis unclear

Abbreviations: BLUE, Bedside Lung Ultrasound in Emergency; COPD, chronic obstructive pulmonary disorder; DVT, deep vein thrombosis; PLAPS, posterolateral alveolar and/or pleural syndrome.

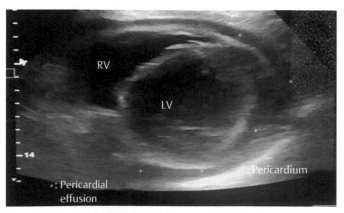

Fig. 51.3 Parasternal short-axis (PSAX) view showing anechoic (*black*) rim indicating the presence of fluid around the heart (i.e., pericardial effusion). Abbreviations: LV, left ventricle; RV, right ventricle.

The **C.A.U.S.E. protocol**[12] is also based on two US views to rule out the commonest causes of cardiac arrest. A four-chamber view of the heart is visualized to rule out severe hypovolemia, cardiac tamponade, and pulmonary embolism, and a two-probe position to quickly rule out pneumothorax.

The **SESAME protocol**[13] is an abbreviated version of SESAMOOSSIC. This mnemonic stands for "Sequential Echographic Scanning Assessing Mechanism Or Origin of Severe Shock of Indistinct Cause." There are several purported advantages and utilities of using this protocol. First, it advises using only one microconvex probe and thereby saves time in an emergency situation (cardiac arrest). The sequence of scanning is different from most other protocols, in that the first step is LUS, then lower femoral vein ultrasound, or abdominal ultrasound to detect DVT (**Fig. 51.4**) or free fluid in the abdomen (**Fig. 51.5**) and lastly pericardial and cardiac ultrasound is done.

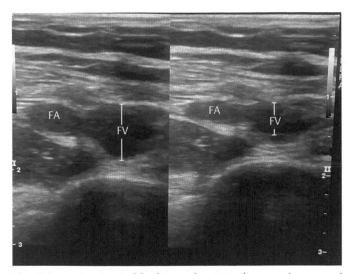

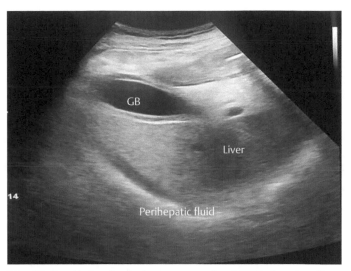

Fig. 51.4 Compressible femoral vein indicates absence of deep venous thrombosis (DVT). Abbreviations: FA, femoral artery; FV, femoral vein.

Fig. 51.5 Abdominal ultrasonography (USG) showing liver with perihepatic fluid. Abbreviation: GB, gall bladder.

Global ultrasound check for the critically Ill (GUCCI)[14] is another protocol, which integrates multiple US-based protocols and create a unified approach to the acutely ill patient. The target is to diagnose and differentiate between the most common ICU syndromes (acute respiratory failure, shock, cardiac arrest) and it also incorporates US-guided procedures such as thoracocentesis and pericardiocentesis. It is easier to follow as compared to other integrated protocols and is also directed toward making management decisions such as US-guided tapping and starting of inotropes when hypotension occurs.[16]

POCUS and Fluid Responsiveness

Shock is a potentially life-threatening condition and if not treated promptly, it can lead the patient into a rapid downward spiral ending in death.[17] Intravenous fluids (IVFs) are considered the first-line therapy for shock and are routinely used in ICUs and hospitals in order to restore effective blood volume and maintain organ perfusion.

Patients are transfused fluids with the premise that increasing stressed venous volume and consequently improving stroke volume and cardiac output (CO) will result in better tissue oxygenation and organ function. In the early 1970s, when the use of the pulmonary artery catheter was in vogue and fluid therapy was being titrated to fixed targets of central venous pressure (CVP) or pulmonary artery occlusion pressure (PAOP),[18] the landmark EGDT (early goal-directed therapy) study by Rivers et al[19] showed that massive fluid administration (30 mL/kg) during the first 6 hours of resuscitation of patients with severe sepsis and septic shock improved outcomes. This study heralded an era of large volume resuscitation and rigid targeted protocols.

However, there is a growing body of evidence[20–25] that has shown that indiscriminate use of fluids without giving due regard to the patient's hemodynamic status and response to the purported boluses can be detrimental to the patient's health. The harmful effects of a positive fluid balance can present in the form of pulmonary edema, hypoxemia, tissue edema, renal dysfunction, intra-abdominal hypertension, delirium, cerebral edema, intestinal dysfunction, impaired wound healing, prolonged ventilator days, and hospital stay, and increase in mortality as well.[22,23,24,25] Recent literature has in fact shown that maintaining a negative fluid balance can improve the chances of survival in patients with septic shock and acute kidney injury.[26] It is important, therefore, to determine whether giving more fluids will result in benefit or harm.

When tissue perfusion is threatened, it is prudent to ascertain which of the three is the appropriate choice: optimization of preload status (fluids), ionotropic support and vasopressors, modulation of afterload, or a combination of the above.

Studies have shown that only about half the hemodynamically unstable patients in a critical care unit will be fluid responsive.[27] To make matters worse, the FENICE investigators[28] found that majority of the clinicians used fluids in an empirical, liberal, and unstructured manner, without due consideration to response to fluid challenges. The time has come that IVFs are given the same respect as that afforded to any other pharmaceutical preparation, and should be given only after due assessment.

A patient whose stroke volume or CO rises by a fixed percentage (commonly 10–15%), in response to a predetermined volume of fluid challenge (commonly bolus 500 mL, 100 mL in minifluid challenge), over a predetermined period of time is defined to be "fluid responsive." Several validated tools and technologies exist today that allow assessment and continuous monitoring of fluid responsiveness (FR), such as those based on analysis of arterial pulse contour,[29] transpulmonary thermodilution, and bioreactance. Though quite a few show promise, most of these need invasive lines and expensive monitors that carry with them their own inherent risks such as pneumothorax and central line–associated blood stream infections. The need of the hour is a tool that is inexpensive, noninvasive, easily accessible, fairly accurate, with reproducible results. The European Society of Intensive Care Medicine has in fact issued a consensus statement on circulatory shock, wherein it was proposed that bedside echocardiography be used as a first-line modality in the evaluation of patients with shock.

Theoretically speaking, it appears simple to give fluids to patients that lie on the steep part of the Frank-Starling curve and to restrict fluids for patients on the flat part of the curve. However, it is not always possible to pinpoint the patient's position on the curve, especially when the steepness of the curves varies with changes in LV systolic function. A static parameter/marker is measured at a given LV function and presumed to reflect preload at a given point on the Frank-Starling curve. It also assumes that a lower value of preload implies FR. Evidence supports discontinuing the use of static markers of preload, such as CVP and PAOP, because one isolated value does not predict FR.[30] Dynamic indices, on the other hand, involve the delivery of a preload challenge and therefore assess the actual response of the cardiovascular system to the said challenge.[31] This preload challenge could be external (fluid bolus), internal provoked (end-expiratory occlusion or passive leg raising [PLR]) or provoked spontaneously by mechanical ventilation.

In addition, there is a physiological variability in the dynamic parameters secondary to variations in intrathoracic pressure occurring during both spontaneous and mechanical breaths. Positive pressure ventilation by increasing the intrathoracic pressure during inspiration decreases the RV preload and consequently decreases the RV stroke volume (as described by the Frank-Starling relationship). These phenomena are transmitted to the LV pressures after pulmonary transit time. This manifests during expiration as a decrease in LV preload and LV stroke volume.[32] These changes in stroke volume caused due to heart-lung interactions are monitored before and after a preload challenge. The change is more pronounced when the patient is preload dependent; greater the volume deficit, the larger is the change in the

dynamic parameters. The magnitude of the changes indicate the patient's position on the Frank-Starling curve. Heart-lung interactions form the basis of most tests for FR. This forms the basis of the multitude of stroke volume variation monitoring systems and can also be assessed by calculating the flow through valves, vessels, or outflow tracts by using Doppler echocardiography. There are certain prerequisites to be fulfilled for stroke volume variation and its derivatives to be good predictors of FR.[29] These limitations hold true for all continuous CO monitors as well. Few echocardiographic indices can overcome these limitations.

There are several POCUS-guided indices that help the clinician ascertain the state of FR. Some of these are explained below and others are described in **Box 51.1** and **Tables 51.3–51.6**.

A. LV Size (Left Ventricular End-Diastolic Area and Index): The ventricular size, best judged visually (eyeballing) in parasternal short-axis (PSAX) view, can give a rough estimate of patient's preload state. Fluid response is to be expected in small, chinked, or kissing ventricles (papillary muscles seem to meet each other at end systole) and is unlikely when dilated poorly contracting ventricles are observed. Left ventricular end-diastolic area (LVEDA) can also be measured but cut-off values are yet to be suggested (**Table 51.6**).[34]

B. Inferior Vena Cava Assessment: In a spontaneously breathing patient, inspiration causes the IVC to collapse and vice versa during exhalation. The reverse is true in a mechanically ventilated patient.[35] IVC diameter and its respiratory variation has been extensively studied and can be used to estimate CVP semiquantitatively (**Table 51.5**). Use of respiratory variations in IVC diameter to predict FR has been validated in both mechanically ventilated (distensibility index) and spontaneously breathing patients (collapsibility index). However, as with CVP measurements, recommendations are still unclear due to several confounding factors. It is most useful when the values at of FR (fluid responsiveness) are either too lower too high. The formula is $(D_{max} - D_{min}/D_{min}) \times 100$. Current literature casts doubts about validity of respiratory variation of IVC as an accurate index for FR.[36]

C. Superior Vena Cava Assessment (Using Transesophageal Echocardiography): Respiratory variability in the superior vena cava (SVC) diameter can be assessed using transesophageal echocardiography (TEE). The main disadvantage of this approach is that its use is restricted to

---

Box 51.1   Calculation for IVC variability

- **For spontaneously breathing patients**
  IVC Collapsibility Index = (maximum diameter on expiration – minimum diameter on inspiration)/maximum diameter on expiration
- **For mechanically ventilated patients**
  IVC Distensibility Index = (maximum diameter on inspiration – minimum diameter on expiration)/minimum diameter on expiration

Abbreviation: IVC, inferior vena cava.

Table 51.3 Various protocols for POCUS

Name of protocol	Purpose/Utility	Views involved	Abnormalities detected
• BLUE: Bedside Lung Ultrasound in Emergency[9]	• Diagnosis in acute respiratory failure	• LUS	• A-profile • B-profile
• FALLS: Fluid Administration Limited by Lung Sonography protocol[10]	• Management of unexplained shock	• CUS • BLUE protocol	• Sequentially rules out obstructive, cardiogenic, hypovolemic shock and finally excludes distributive shock
• Sonography in Hypotension and Cardiac Arrest (SHoC) protocols[11]	• Two protocols: one for hypotension and the other for cardiac arrest	• CUS • LUS • IVC	• Pericardial fluid, cardiac form, and ventricular function • AAA or DVT
• C.A.U.S.E.: Cardiac arrest ultrasound exam[12]	• Rule out causes of cardiac arrest (nonarrhythmogenic)	• LUS • CUS	• Pericardial tamponade • Tension pneumothorax • Pulmonary embolus • Hypovolemia
• SESAME protocol: Sequential echographic scanning assessing mechanism or origin of severe shock of indistinct cause[13]	**Utility of SESAME:** • Rule out pneumothorax • Rule out pulmonary embolism • Fluid therapy can be guided following the falls protocol **Falls protocols:** • Fluid administration limited by lung ultrasound	• CUS • LUS • IVC • AUS • DVT	• Pneumothorax • Pulmonary embolism • Guiding fluid therapy • DVT
• Global Ultrasound Check for the Critically Ill (GUCCI)[14]	• Diagnose and differentiate between the most common ICU syndromes (acute respiratory failure, shock, cardiac arrest)	• CUS • LUS • IVC • AUS • DVT	• Rules out common diagnoses and incorporates US-guided procedures such as thoracocentesis and pericardiocentesis
• PIEPEAR workflow[15]	• Seven-step protocol with decision and management tree for cardiorespiratory compromise	• LUS, AUS/DVT, CUS	• Includes a complex seven-step algorithm that deals with pathophysiology, etiology, and actions needed
• ACES: Abdominal and Cardiac Evaluation with Sonography in Shock	• Establish diagnosis and deliver goal-directed therapy for nontraumatic undifferentiated shock in ED	• Cardiac, peritoneal, pleural, inferior vena cava, and aortic views	• Common causes of shock
• VExUS: Venous Excess Ultrasound grading system of the severity of venous congestion	• Evaluates venous congestion in the IVC, liver, kidneys, gut, and correlates with risk of AKI	• IVC • Hepatic, portal, and renal vein Dopplers	• 0–3 VExUS grades

Abbreviations: AAA, abdominal aortic aneurysm; AKI, acute kidney injury; AUS, abdominal ultrasound; CUS, cardiac US; DVT, deep vein thrombosis; IVC, inferior vena cava; LUS, lung US; POCUS, point-of-care ultrasound.

Table 51.4 Interpretation of IVC diameter and variability and recommendation for fluids

IVC diameter	IVC variation	Estimated CVP	Recommendation for fluids
>2.5 cm	<50% collapse	15–20 mmHg	Not recommended
1.5–2.5 cm	<50% collapse	10–20 mmHg	Indeterminate
1.5–2.5 cm	>50% collapse	10–20 mmHg	Indeterminate
≤2.5 cm	>50% collapse	0–5 mmHg	Should be given

Abbreviations: CVP, central venous pressure; IVC, inferior vena cava.

Table 51.5 POCUS-based indices for assessment of fluid responsiveness (static)

Index	View	Interpretation
LVEDA	PSAX	≤10 cm²: significant hypovolemia ≥20 cm²: volume overload
E/A ratio	4C A	E/A >2, DT < 160 s: PCWP >18 mmHg
IVC Dia	SC	≤10 mm: CVP < 5–10 mmHg ≥20 mm: CVP > 15–20 mmHg

Abbreviations: 4C A, apical four-chamber view; CVP, central venous pressure; IVC, inferior vena cava; IVC Dia, IVC diameter; LVEDA, left ventricular end-diastolic area; LVEDI, left ventricular end-diastolic index; POCUS, point-of-care ultrasound; PCWP, pulmonary capillary wedge pressure; PSAX, parasternal short-axis view; SC, subcostal view.

Table 51.6 POCUS-based indices for assessment of fluid responsiveness (dynamic)

Index	View	Threshold value (Δ)[a]	Advantages	Limitations
ΔLV area	PSAX	>16%	Easy to perform	• Image acquisition
IVC D	SC		Easy to perform	• RV dysfunction: tamponade, RV infarct
IVC C	SC	>18%		• Obesity • Open chest cavity • ↑ IAP • Big swings in ITP • Image acquisition
ΔVmaxAo	5C A	>12%		• Spontaneously breathing patients
VTI		≥20%		• TV < 8 mL/kg • High RR (HR/RR <3.6) • Poor lung compliance, ARDS • Arrhythmias • Open chest cavity • ↑ IAP
PLR	5C A	>10±2%	Can be used in: spontaneously breathing patients patients with arrhythmias	• V ↑ IAP • V ↑ ICP • Pregnancy • Open chest cavity • Lower limb/pelvic fractures
ΔSVC	Longitudinal 90 to 100 degrees view	>36%	Can be used in: spontaneously breathing patients patients with arrhythmias patients with ↑ IAP	• Availability and access • Training • Invasive • Upper airway or esophageal disease • Image acquisition • Skill set
EEO		>5%	Easy to perform Can be used in ARDS	• Patients not intubated

Abbreviations: 5C A, apical five-chamber view; ARDS, acute respiratory distress syndrome; Δ, delta or change; EEO, end-expiratory occlusion test; HR, heart rate; ↑ IAP, increased intra-abdominal pressure; ↑ ICP, increased intracranial pressure; ITP, immune thrombocytopenic purpura; ΔIVC, variations of the diameter of the inferior vena cava; IVC C, IVC collapsibility; IVC D, IVC distensibility; ΔLV area, left ventricular area; PLAX, parasternal long-axis view; PLR, passive leg raising; POCUS, point-of-care ultrasound; PSAX, parasternal short-axis view; RR, respiratory rate; SC, subcostal view; ΔSVC, variations of the diameter of the superior vena cava; TV, tricuspid valve; ΔVmaxAo, variation in peak aortic flow velocity; VTI, velocity time integral.
[a] Threshold value is the value which differentiates between fluid responders and nonresponders.

sedated and mechanically ventilated patients because of assessment using TEE. It has the potential advantage to avoid all confounding elements associated with changes in intra-abdominal pressure (IAP), concerns regarding spontaneous respiratory efforts, and can even be used in patients with irregular cardiac rhythms. As compared to assessment of respiratory variability in IVC, the SVC (cut-off >36%) performs better as a marker for FR in terms of sensitivity and specificity.[37] The distensibility index used for respiratory variation in mechanically ventilated patients and its formula is $(D_{max} - D_{min}/D_{min}) \times 100$.

D. **Aortic Blood Flow Variations:** Stroke volume can be estimated by multiplying area of LV outflow tract (LVOT) with velocity-time integral (VTI), using a pulsed-wave (PW) Doppler signal. The LVOT area can be measured from the PLAX view and PW Doppler signal acquired in the apical five-chamber view.[38] The LVOT area is assumed to be constant; therefore, changes in velocity-time integral (VTI), averaged over three respiratory cycles, can be used as a surrogate of stroke volume variation (SVV). This index has been validated with as little as 100 mL of hydroxyethyl starch as a bolus given over 1 minute.

With the assumption that LVOT area is constant, changes in aortic blood flow would be proportional to changes in stroke volume. Peak aortic blood flow velocity can be estimated by using continuous wave or PW Doppler with the sweep speed set to include several respiratory cycles in a screen.

E. **Passive Leg Raising Test:** Another innovative test designed to detect FR is the passive leg raising[39] (PLR) test. The PLR examines the impact of an internal preload challenge to estimate changes in stroke volume and determine FR. The main advantages are that it can be employed reliably even in spontaneously breathing patients, patients with irregular rhythms, and has been used in patients receiving extracorporeal membrane oxygenation. An added benefit is that no external volume is added to the circulation. There are some technical challenges faced in maintaining correct probe angle with LVOT. It is not reliable in the presence of raised IAP, which precludes use in many surgical patients.[40] It is also not feasible in patients who are pregnant, have lower limb fractures, and is not recommended in patients with raised intracranial pressure (ICP).

F. **End-Expiratory Occlusion Test:** The changes in preload caused during regular respiration are normally transmitted from right-side to left-side circulation after one pulmonary transit time. By stopping mechanical ventilation for more 15 seconds, there is a transient increase in cardiac preload. If the end-expiratory occlusion test results in an increase in CO or SV, it indicates FR.[41]

G. **Corrected Carotid Flow Time Index:** Corrected carotid flow time index (CTI) is calculated as a ratio of the systolic flow time and square root of the cardiac cycle time

(to correct for impact of heart rate). A PW Doppler waveform of carotid blood flow is generated and the flow time between the onset of systole and dicrotic notch is recorded. A fluid bolus or PLR associated with an increase in the Corrected carotid flow time index (CFTI) value of 10 to 15% indicates FR.[42]

Clinical Pearls

- In some instances, such as an actively bleeding polytrauma patient or early untreated septic shock, FR is obvious. Don't waste time.
- FR is not to be tested when CO needs to be increased for reasons other than circulatory shock, for example, a case of tissue hypoxia.
- All patients who are deemed FR cannot be given fluids. Sometimes, the benefits of fluid administration are greatly outweighed by the risks. For instance, in a patient with acute respiratory distress syndrome (ARDS) and circulatory shock, or ischemic or dilated cardiomyopathy with poor LV function and septic shock. In such situations, repeated assessments with added emphasis on assessment of extravascular lung water are needed. Don't drown the patient.
- No test is 100% sensitive or specific. Always correlate clinically. Treat the patient not the test result.

Sample Cases

Case 1: A 79-year-old man, a known case of diabetes, hypertension, chronic kidney disease, was shifted to ICU after an abdominal surgery for colonic perforation with fecal peritonitis. He is tachycardiac and hypotensive. He has already received 5 L of IVFs in the OR. Preoperative labs showed an elevated creatinine and lactates. Patient is sedated and ventilated and has spontaneous inspiratory efforts. POCUS was used to ascertain the type of shock and guide further management. IVC was found to be small and collapsing >50%. Cardiac ultrasound showed kissing ventricle sign indicative of severe hypovolemia. LUS showed no B-lines. This case is a classic example of distributive shock where patient will need fluids. After the initial bolus, repeated examinations of IVC and the lung need to be done to find the end point.

Case 2: A 54-year-old patient with history of diabetes, cardiomyopathy, alcohol abuse, and a recent total knee replacement (TKR) was brought to ER. Patient was tachycardiac, hypotensive, breathless with low saturations. IVC was big and noncollapsing. Cardiac ultrasound showed large RV >> LV and McConnell sign on apical view, D-shaped LV on PSAX indicative of acute RV strain probably secondary to a pulmonary thromboembolism. LUS was clear. Femoral vein

Doppler scan showed noncompressible femoral vein with echogenic material suggestive of DVT. This case is a classic example of distributive shock where patient will need fluids. After the initial bolus, repeated examinations of IVC and the lung need to be done to find the end point.

Case 3: A 71-year-old woman, a known case of chronic renal failure with congestive heart failure presents the emergency. Patient was breathless and hypotensive having difficulty lying down in bed. IVC was dilated and noncollapsing. Echocardiogram showed biatrial dilation with poor LV ejection fraction. LUS showed multiple confluent B-lines. Patient treated for interstitial lung disease the B lines or "COMET TAILS" are vertical reverberations indicating decreased lung aeration. Three or more B lines if seen in a single image between two ribs are considered significant for pneumonitis interstitial ling disease pulmonary fibrosis.

Take-Home Points

- POCUS assessments can be useful for monitoring and obtaining rapid diagnosis in emergency situations. Its acceptance is growing.
- Clinical impact and benefit of several protocols remains to be documented.
- One formula fits all is no longer an acceptable standard of care.
- Assess FR and tailor fluid therapy to the unique needs of each individual patient.
- Some questions have to be answered: Does my patient need fluids? How much fluid should be given? When do I stop?
- Repeated assessments are more useful than isolated readings.
- Use dynamic indices versus static ones to assess for FR.
- Values at the extremes, either too low or too high, are most useful in determining the course of action.

Conclusion

Analogous to the National Board of Echocardiography training and certification standards for echocardiography, standardizing POCUS education and delineating competency levels also are central to ensuring appropriate quality assurance. This is even more critical as POCUS use increases and more physicians seek to attain POCUS expertise to incorporate this technology more widely into routine clinical practice. With the current available and growing evidence of clinical value of POCUS, its utility across the perioperative arena adds enormous benefit to clinical decision-making.[43]

References

1. Cox EGM, Koster G, Baron A, et al; SICS Study Group. Should the ultrasound probe replace your stethoscope? A SICS-I sub-study comparing lung ultrasound and pulmonary auscultation in the critically ill. Crit Care 2020;24(1):14
2. Graham ID, Harrison MB. Evaluation and adaptation of clinical practice guidelines. Evid Based Nurs 2005;8(3):68–72
3. Melniker LA, Leibner E, McKenney MG, Lopez P, Briggs WM, Mancuso CA. Randomized controlled clinical trial of point-of-care, limited ultrasonography for trauma in the emergency department: the first sonography outcomes assessment program trial. Ann Emerg Med 2006;48(3):227–235
4. Kanji HD, McCallum J, Sirounis D, MacRedmond R, Moss R, Boyd JH. Limited echocardiography-guided therapy in subacute shock is associated with change in management and improved outcomes. J Crit Care 2014;29(5):700–705
5. Scalea TM, Rodriguez A, Chiu WC, et al. Focused assessment with sonography for trauma (FAST): results from an international consensus conference. J Trauma 1999;46(3):466–472
6. Weingart SD, Duque D, Nelson B. The RUSH exam: rapid ultrasound for shock. 2008. https://emcrit.org/rush-exam/
7. Volpicelli G, Lamorte A, Tullio M, et al. Point-of-care multiorgan ultrasonography for the evaluation of undifferentiated hypotension in the emergency department. Intensive Care Med 2013;39(7):1290–1298
8. Anderson KL, Jenq KY, Fields JM, Panebianco NL, Dean AJ. Diagnosing heart failure among acutely dyspneic patients with cardiac, inferior vena cava, and lung ultrasonography. Am J Emerg Med 2013;31(8):1208–1214
9. Lichtenstein DA, Mezière GA. Relevance of lung ultrasound in the diagnosis of acute respiratory failure: the BLUE protocol. Chest 2008;134(1):117–125
10. Lichtenstein DA. BLUE-protocol and FALLS-protocol: two applications of lung ultrasound in the critically ill. Chest 2015; 147(6):1659–1670
11. Milne J, Atkinson P, Lewis D, et al. Sonography in hypotension and cardiac arrest (SHoC): rates of abnormal findings in undifferentiated hypotension and during cardiac arrest as a basis for consensus on a hierarchical point of care ultrasound protocol. Cureus 2016;8(4):e564
12. Hernandez C, Shuler K, Hannan H, Sonyika C, Likourezos A, Marshall J. C.A.U.S.E.: cardiac arrest ultra-sound exam—a better approach to managing patients in primary non-arrhythmogenic cardiac arrest. Resuscitation 2008;76(2):198–206
13. Pyo SY, Park GJ, Kim SC, Kim H, Lee SW, Lee JH. Impact of the modified SESAME ultrasound protocol implementation on patients with cardiac arrest in the emergency department. Am J Emerg Med 2021;43:62–68
14. Tavares J, Ivo R, Gonzalez F, Lamas T, Mendes JJ. Global ultrasound check for the critically Ill (GUCCI): a new systematized protocol unifying point-of-care ultrasound in critically ill patients based on clinical presentation. Open Access Emerg Med 2019;11:133–145
15. Yin W, Li Y, Wang S, et al. The PIEPEAR workflow: a critical care ultrasound based 7-step approach as a standard procedure to manage patients with acute cardiorespiratory compromise, with two example cases presented. BioMed Res Int 2018;2018:4687346

16. Atkinson PRT, McAuley DJ, Kendall RJ, et al. Abdominal and cardiac evaluation with sonography in shock (ACES): an approach by emergency physicians for the use of ultrasound in patients with undifferentiated hypotension. Emerg Med J 2009;26(2):87–91

17. Dellinger RP, Levy MM, Rhodes A, et al; Surviving Sepsis Campaign Guidelines Committee including The Pediatric Subgroup. Surviving sepsis campaign: international guidelines for management of severe sepsis and septic shock, 2012. Intensive Care Med 2013;39(2):165–228

18. Marik PE, Baram M, Vahid B. Does central venous pressure predict fluid responsiveness? A systematic review of the literature and the tale of seven mares. Chest 2008;134(1):172–178

19. Rivers E, Nguyen B, Havstad S, et al; Early Goal-Directed Therapy Collaborative Group. Early goal-directed therapy in the treatment of severe sepsis and septic shock. N Engl J Med 2001;345(19):1368–1377

20. Rosenberg AL, Dechert RE, Park PK, Bartlett RH; NIH NHLBI ARDS Network. Review of a large clinical series: association of cumulative fluid balance on outcome in acute lung injury: a retrospective review of the ARDSnet tidal volume study cohort. J Intensive Care Med 2009;24(1):35–46

21. Marjanovic G, Villain C, Juettner E, et al. Impact of different crystalloid volume regimes on intestinal anastomotic stability. Ann Surg 2009;249(2):181–185

22. Balogh Z, Moore FA, Moore EE, Biffl WL. Secondary abdominal compartment syndrome: a potential threat for all trauma clinicians. Injury 2007;38(3):272–279

23. Cordemans C, De Laet I, Van Regenmortel N, et al. Fluid management in critically ill patients: the role of extravascular lung water, abdominal hypertension, capillary leak, and fluid balance. Ann Intensive Care 2012;2(Suppl 1 Diagnosis and management of intra-abdominal hyperten):S1

24. Boyd JH, Forbes J, Nakada TA, Walley KR, Russell JA. Fluid resuscitation in septic shock: a positive fluid balance and elevated central venous pressure are associated with increased mortality. Crit Care Med 2011;39(2):259–265

25. Micek ST, McEvoy C, McKenzie M, Hampton N, Doherty JA, Kollef MH. Fluid balance and cardiac function in septic shock as predictors of hospital mortality. Crit Care 2013;17(5):R246

26. Alsous F, Khamiees M, DeGirolamo A, Amoateng-Adjepong Y, Manthous CA. Negative fluid balance predicts survival in patients with septic shock: a retrospective pilot study. Chest 2000;117(6):1749–1754

27. Michard F, Teboul JL. Predicting fluid responsiveness in ICU patients: a critical analysis of the evidence. Chest 2002;121(6): 2000–2008

28. Cecconi M, Hofer C, Teboul J-L, et al; FENICE Investigators; ESICM Trial Group. Fluid challenges in intensive care: the FENICE study: A global inception cohort study. Intensive Care Med 2015;41(9):1529–1537

29. Marik PE, Cavallazzi R, Vasu T, Hirani A. Dynamic changes in arterial waveform derived variables and fluid responsiveness in mechanically ventilated patients: a systematic review of the literature. Crit Care Med 2009;37(9):2642–2647

30. Marik PE, Cavallazzi R. Does the central venous pressure predict fluid responsiveness? An updated meta-analysis and a plea for some common sense. Crit Care Med 2013;41(7):1774–1781

31. Vincent JL, Pelosi P, Pearse R, et al. Perioperative cardiovascular monitoring of high-risk patients: a consensus of 12. Crit Care 2015;19:224

32. Mahmood SS, Pinsky MR. Heart-lung interactions during mechanical ventilation: the basics. Ann Transl Med 2018; 6(18):349

33. Argaiz ER, Koratala A, Reisinger N. Comprehensive Assessment of. Fluid Status by Point-of-Care Ultrasonography. Kidney360. 2021, 2(8):1326–1338

34. Franchi F, Vetrugno L, Scolletta S. Echocardiography to guide fluid therapy in critically ill patients: check the heart and take a quick look at the lungs. J Thorac Dis 2017;9(3):477–481

35. Feissel M, Michard F, Faller JP, Teboul JL. The respiratory variation in inferior vena cava diameter as a guide to fluid therapy. Intensive Care Med 2004;30(9):1834–1837

36. Orso D, Paoli I, Piani T, Cilenti FL, Cristiani L, Guglielmo N. Accuracy of ultrasonographic measurements of inferior Vena Cava to determine fluid responsiveness: a systematic review and meta-analysis. J Intensive Care Med 2020;35(4): 354–363

37. Vieillard-Baron A, Chergui K, Rabiller A, et al. Superior vena caval collapsibility as a gauge of volume status in ventilated septic patients. Intensive Care Med 2004;30(9):1734–1739

38. Feissel M, Michard F, Mangin I, Ruyer O, Faller JP, Teboul J-L. Respiratory changes in aortic blood velocity as an indicator of fluid responsiveness in ventilated patients with septic shock. Chest 2001;119(3):867–873

39. Cavallaro F, Sandroni C, Marano C, et al. Diagnostic accuracy of passive leg raising for prediction of fluid responsiveness in adults: systematic review and meta-analysis of clinical studies. Intensive Care Med 2010;36(9):1475–1483

40. Cherpanath TG, Hirsch A, Geerts BF, et al. Predicting fluid responsiveness by passive leg raising: a systematic review and meta-analysis of 23 clinical trials. Crit Care Med 2016;44(5): 981–991

41. Messina A, Dell'Anna A, Baggiani M, et al. Functional hemo-dynamic tests: a systematic review and a metanalysis on the reliability of the end-expiratory occlusion test and of the mini-fluid challenge in predicting fluid responsiveness. Crit Care 2019;23(1):264

42. Barjaktarevic I, Toppen WE, Hu S, et al. Ultrasound assess-ment of the change in carotid corrected flow time in fluid responsiveness in undifferentiated shock. Crit Care Med 2018; 46(11):e1040–e1046

43. Kalagara H, Coker B, Gerstein NS, et al. Point-of-Care Ultrasound (POCUS) for the Cardiothoracic Anesthesiologist. J Cardiothorac Vasc Anesth. 2022;36(4):1132–1147

Index